NLN
PRESS

NURSING RESEARCH

A Qualitative Perspective, Third Edition

Patricia L. Munhall, Ed.D., ARNP, PsyA, FAAN

Professor, University of South Carolina
President, International Institute
of Human Understanding
Columbia, South Carolina

JONES AND BARTLETT PUBLISHERS
Sudbury, Massachusetts
BOSTON   TORONTO   LONDON   SINGAPORE

National League for Nursing

World Headquarters
Jones and Bartlett Publishers
40 Tall Pine Drive
Sudbury, MA 01776
978-443-5000
www.jbpub.com
info@jbpub.com

Jones and Bartlett Publishers Canada
2406 Nikanna Road
Mississauga, ON L5C 2W6
CANADA

Jones and Bartlett Publishers International
Barb House, Barb Mews
London W6 7PA
UK

Library of Congress Cataloging-In-Publication Data

Nursing research : a qualitative perspective / [edited by] Patricia L. Munhall.—3rd ed.
   p.cm.
   Includes bibliographical references and index.
   ISBN 0-7637-1135-7 (alk. paper)
   1. Nursing—Research. I. Munhall, Patricia L.

   RT81.5 .N866 2001
   610.73'07'2—dc21

                                                                00-069418

Production Credits
Acquisitions Editor: Penny M. Glynn
Associate Editor: Christine Tridente
Production Editor: AnnMarie Lemoine
Editorial Assistant: Thomas Prindle
Manufacturing Buyer: Amy Duddridge
Cover Design: AnnMarie Lemoine
Design and Composition: Carlisle Communications, Ltd.
Printing and Binding: Malloy Lithographing

Printed in the United States of America
05 04 03 02 01   10 9 8 7 6 5 4 3 2 1

CONTENTS

This book represents a continuing conversation, which started before 1987, the year in which the first edition of this book was published. The many people who joined that conversation were apparent in the publication of the second edition in 1993, which was rereleased in the year 2000. The second edition was longer than the first edition by 216 pages. The interest, growth, and recognition of the value of qualitative methods for nursing research are again evident in the enlarging conversation, which has grown from the 288 pages of the first edition to the 671 pages of the third edition.

So, welcome to the third edition of *Nursing Research: A Qualitative Perspective*. Indeed, the book *is* larger, not only in the number of pages in the literal sense, but also in the representative sense as a semiotic signifier. What does such an enlarging conversation from 1987 to 2001 mean to nurse researchers? During these years (a relatively short period of time), nursing research has burgeoned. Doctoral programs in nursing have tripled. Research courses for nurses are required in undergraduate education, and many more research courses are required in graduate education.

Research and the concomitant dissemination of results are required of faculty and are essential for promotion and tenure. Graduate students are writing research proposals; some students are completing theses for master's degrees; and, of course, the dissertation must be completed for the doctoral degree. A profession that was once housed in 3-year diploma schools affiliated with hospitals is now, 40 years later, ensconced in the university setting and has responsibly taken on the values of an academic profession. One of the most important values is the search for truth. Broadly speaking, this search for truth is a search for new knowledge for the profession. One of the most remarkable changes since 1987 is what is sometimes called "the knowledge explosion," which is simultaneous with the "explosion of technology." Technology has enabled advances in the health sciences, changes in the health care system, and the rapid communication of knowledge in a moment-to-moment, if not nanosecond, development.

Today when we embark on a research project, we see a change more in "how" we believe something than in "what" we believe. Before the introduction of qualitative methods of research in nursing, the profession had embraced the scientific method as the paradigm for nursing research. The reasons are discussed in the Preface and in Chapters 1 and 2 of this text. Some nurse researchers had a bent, so to speak, to look for other ways of coming to know. Other disciplines, other than the natural sciences, had methods that interested nurse researchers and, for those pioneers of qualitative research in nursing, the rationale for their use was as strong and compelling as the use of a natural science method. As with most new ideas, and we need to remember that this pursuit of qualitative research was a new idea for nursing research, some conflict ensued.* Professional legitimacy was seen as affiliation with the "hard" sciences.

Linear progress, absolute truths, and rationality were all thought to be ideals for a science. Before nursing entered the academy, it was popular to say that nursing was an art and a science, but, once in the academy, the art piece was subsumed and the science component was elevated for reasons that were socially constructed within the context. This social construction also is explained in the beginning chapters of this book.

The sands of science itself are shifting, as more and more scientists, including nurse scientists, realize that science cannot be a field of absolute and final truth but is an endeavor focused on illuminating an ever-changing body of ideas. For many, though, this focus is still not accepted and is considered a grievous loss; others find the shifting sands exhilarating and liberating.

In 1987, few dissertations and publications indicated an acceptance of qualitative methods of inquiry in nursing. And, ironically and I might add unfortunately, in the year 2001, qualitative nurse researchers and quantitative nurse researchers, who often call themselves nurse scientists, do not garner the same prizes. In the year 2001, we have the National Institute for Nursing Research, a branch of the National Institutes of Health, mostly rewarding quantitative/scientific research proposals.

---

*An acknowledgement of nurse researchers who pursued doctorates in fields such as sociology or anthropology in the earlier years needs to be made, because they steadfastly stood their ground in the promotion of other ways of coming to know.

Colleges of nursing pride themselves on establishing Centers for Nursing Science, or the Science of Nursing. Of course, a Center for Nursing Research would be more embracing, at least in name, of various approaches to the pursuit of knowledge. As you will read in this text, the situated context in which we live influences what we want to be "like" and how we wish to appear—in this instance, in the academic or medical setting.

Here a reader might pause and wonder, "Is this the way a discipline or profession chooses ways of being in the world?" Qualitative researchers who are often interested in the "meaning" of being in the world understand this question and understand nursing's desire to affiliate with the natural sciences. I have yet to meet a qualitative nurse researcher who believes his or her method of doing research is the "only" and the legitimate way of coming to know and advancing knowledge. I suppose this belief itself is reflective of the philosophical underpinnings of qualitative research methods, so that it should not come as a surprise that here we see the difference about "how" we believe.

It would certainly be unfair to portray all of nursing scientists who are based in the natural science method as not being accepting of qualitative nurse researchers, but it would also be unfair to have a student of nursing research not be aware of the dichotomy, which persists within the field. Yet, I am very encouraged that, in spite of what some may view as the superiority of the scientific method, more and more nurse researchers change their whole view of research once they become acquainted with this alternative paradigm. Some have said that they have come home. They have found a home in this world of research.

Hence the conversation enlarges, the text is more substantive, new methods are added, new issues are addressed, and the need for this type of knowing is acknowledged. But more needs to be said to explain, in spite of some resistance in the field, why qualitative research methods not only are appropriate for nursing but actually propel us to a "new" science reflective of the contemporary world.

Let us begin with the personal and set aside the political (to the extent possible) for the moment. Nurse researchers, as in any field that involves human beings, have different propensities. First, when students begin studying nursing, most are not even aware that nurses do research. If they were entering a field such as physics or chemistry, they would know at the outset that they were going to become scientists and their propensity for the logic and rationality of the scientific method with its mathematical equations would have already been a choice.

How different, then, for students in nursing. They enter the profession not aware that nurses do research and, if they happen to hear that they have to take nursing research courses, cannot imagine what it is that nurses research. So the initial socialization of nurses, from the perception of others (guidance counselors, peers, parents), does not include research. When this idea is introduced to them at the undergraduate level, the standard research textbooks, which are larger than this one, include perhaps one chapter of 30 on qualitative research. I believe that readers of this text on qualitative research need to have an acute awareness of the disproportionate attention to quantitative methods in the early years of socialization of nurse researchers. So we have created a context in which entering students of nursing do not have an awareness that research is a part of the nursing role and then, when it is introduced, the scientific method, the method of the natural sciences, seems to be the method of choice.

Now another fluke that makes nursing students different in regard to research is that most will not make a career in research, unlike the aforementioned physics and chemistry students. Few will ever be solely nurse researchers, and those who do research will share their time with other responsibilities, such as being a faculty member. Because of all these differences, we do not have in our educational preparation of nurses the inherent faculty–student expectation of research mentorship, where research is the primary goal of education, as in the natural sciences. Yet, research *is* one of the many goals of nursing education.

Nurse educators expect students to read, critique, and utilize nursing research and that becomes a goal of nursing education. However, is it realistic to think that graduates of undergraduate schools can understand and critique research? In particular, if it is presented in an advanced mathematical format, which the student has little preparation to understand?

Readers need to be aware of the socialization of nursing students to research. The readers of this text are the future nurse researchers and are the ones who will make the changes necessary to address these critical problems. They will continue the conversation because that is what needs to be done to expand the dialogue.

Within the dialogue and within this text are many reasons to consider just how critical qualitative research methods are for a human science field, a profession dedicated to alleviating suffering and promoting well-being. The need for the scientific method is not in dispute here. In fact, it is celebrated for specific problems and questions. However, it is inappropriate for seeking answers and solutions to other problems and questions.

Consider the world that we human beings inhabit in the year 2001. We have the breakdown of the "enlightment project," where there was the belief that there were rational explanations for all phenomena. With that belief was the idea that there was only one possible answer to any question or problem. Yet, at the same time, we are acknowledging the real influence of the "local," the subjective, the meaning, the heterogeneity, the myriad perceptions, the polyvocality, and the fact that we are overwhelmingly pluralistic and living multiple realities of experience.

Science, with a capital "S," fascinated us and was and still is an interesting story, but it is only one story to describe you and me and the world that we inhabit. It is interesting to note that we discuss science in a somewhat dispassionate discourse—a statement of a discovery, a theory proved, a theory refuted, so to speak. And, though sometimes dispassionate, there are moments of passion when a cure for some terrible condition arrives and indeed the quality of life is improved. Ironically, many of these "scientific" discoveries are found by accident; while something else is being searched for, a serendipitous discovery is made.

As nurses, though, we have much to contribute to understanding the multistoried world—the diversity and the plurality of the people whom we serve—through other methods of science, through qualitative methods. I have seen the excitement of students when they come upon these methods. It seems as though our students are pluralistic as well.

Bear with me, I would like to emphasize—We are all blessedly pluralistic: students, faculty, patients, family, and the community. There is not one best answer and there is not one best way of doing research. In reference to the earlier example, because the incoming student is often not aware of the research component, when it is introduced we should be aware that our students might separate into groups in which some seem mathematically inclined and the others seem linguistically inclined, and it is imperative to sort that out, for ourselves and for our students. Toward that end, our research endeavors become enlarged as we help to develop the multitalented group of students in their specific propensities. Because we have both the mathematically minded and the linguistically/philosophically inclined student, our potential is magnified, as is our field of understanding.

Those who are linguistically and philosophically inclined need our encouragement to develop their talents and propensities in their research endeavors. No one way is superior to another. Students and faculty alike might have noticed that many students develop a dislike for research. Perhaps this dislike is because only one language is spoken and those students need to hear and learn the other languages of discovery.

Because in our practice we are exposed to the languages, semiotics, and beliefs of different cultures, we need to have the nurse and nurse researcher who hears the differences and who questions generalizations. We need to have researchers who will tell us the meaning of different realities—personal, subjective realities—so that we approach individual persons with an individual prescription and an individual protocol, once again remembering that there is no right answer to everything.

Today there is an emphasis on interventions and taxonomies. I ask, how can this be? Interventions need to be based on meaning because, without knowing the meaning of a patient's behavior, the intervention will undoubtedly be meaningless. The patient will be labeled noncompliant, a negative judgment against the patient. Measures will be taken against such noncompliance, and they also will be doomed until a qualitative research study into the meaning of events or behavior for the patient is carried out. And this qualitative study is done to acknowledge the plurality, the diversity, and the different ways of being that most nursing philosophies ascribe to in their descriptions of a human being.

The patient undoubtedly has different perceptions of reality from those of the "inventor" of the intervention. The inventor's intervention without the language of the person who is to be the recipient of the intervention is probably why so many health and social educational programs fail. The intervention—for example, to stop smoking in children or adults, reduce obesity or teenage pregnancy, or combat homelessness—all too often comes from the perception of reality of the professional, who is far removed from the interior of the experience and the interior meanings of the behavior. This is where the qualitative researcher is at home.

There is so much difference that goes unacknowledged, as we try so earnestly to create human laboratory systems, untainted by the outside world. Then the human being must eventually return to the outside world, to the entire context and all the contingencies of his or her life. These are the concerns of the qualitative researcher: the meanings within context, the interpretation of the individual person, how he or she narrates his or her own story, how a self is socially constructed, and how truth is an interpretation. Truth arrived at by numbers is even held suspect by qualitative researchers, because they worry about all the variables that were not in the equations. They also worry about how individual people interpret words differently and assign different values to numbers. Qualitative researchers have a different propensity and different worldview. Given the freedom to grow and develop in their methods, they can provide to the profession understanding, description, theory, interpretation, and direction concerned with the intricateness and interconnectedness of being in this world—a world that is not one but many in perception; a world that is not one but many in language. One language has many languages within that language, as does one culture. Qualitative researchers search for the differences not only between cultures but also within cultures. They challenge stereotypes, presuppositions, and assumptions.

Qualitative researchers break new ground by revealing what had been concealed, because they look beyond appearance. They provide the reconstruction that time demands of us, as the sands shift and the known is no longer valid. In their quest for discovery, qualitative researchers legitimate the existence of others in their differences. Conformity is not the object; we know that a universal concept of meaning is not possible and doubt that it is desirable.

By 2001, the narrative had enlarged, as manifested in this text, and I believe we need in nursing research a growing appreciation for what every method has to offer to our understanding. The dichotomy is old and refers to a dualistic way of perceiving reality. Let us encourage and reward those researchers who are more linguistically inclined, because there are those who believe that language constitutes reality, instead of languaging reflecting reality. How important it is then to ensure that these researchers are rewarded in their search to seek knowledge of others in their worlds and in their language and to understand how others negotiate their own meanings.

Although we may choose our friends because we value "compatibility," as nurses part of the challenge of our work is our incompatibility with many of our patients. Part of the intrigue of our work is understanding a "newness," a very different negotiation of meaning. What I personally value most about qualitative research is that, in that "incompatibility," I am awakened to new ways of being. What I think qualitative nurse researchers return through their research and practice, is legitimization, understanding, acceptance, and compassion. What qualitative nurse researchers want to provide to the knowledge base of nursing is discovery, description, explanation, interpretation, critique, understanding, and sensitization among other ways of knowing the meaning of being. Overall and critically, the work of the qualitative nurse researcher offers to us through the interpretation of meaning and experience, as well as the critique of his or her own methods, an expanding and wakeful consciousness to others and to self.

Contrary to some preconceptions, qualitative researchers do like numbers. Numbers are a part of our language, and they are imbued with meaning. So to return to the beginning of this preface, where the increase in page numbers of the three editions was mentioned, I would like to shape the differences a bit more for clarity.

The first edition was divided, like all three editions, into three sections. As in the first two editions, Part I of the third edition sets the context, which is compatible with and an example of the philosophical underpinnings of qualitative research. In Part I, three chapters undergird the text, in that language, epistemology, and philosophy are discussed. At the conclusion of Chapter 2 is a complete outline of the chapters with authors in a section called Reading the Following Chapters, which will guide you in a more specific manner.

The reader needs to know that a textbook is limited in its abilities to convey a specific amount of what can be known and so, if you are captured by the essence of qualitative research, I hope you will delve into the references as well.

Part II, as in the preceding editions, consists of chapters on "how to do" different qualitative methods, followed by exemplar chapters. In this edition, two new qualitative methods have been added: interpretive analysis (hermeneutics) and action research, both with exemplars. Another method—a phenomenology method—has been added in a different way. In the first and second editions, there were overviews of different approaches to phenomenology; in this edition, the overviews are maintained and an enlarged method is offered in a separate chapter. The methods of grounded theory, ethnography, case study, and historical research have all been updated.

All exemplars of the seven methods presented are current and new studies. With the exception of the two new methods, the reader can return to the first and second editions to read other exemplars representing different studies, using the same method to amplify understanding. Additionally, as the field has grown, so has sophistication in the use of these methods. I think, in this third edition, that the methods and exemplars demonstrate the very talented and gifted contributors' abilities to critique and narrate in a style that represents the growing acknowledgment of creativity and interpretation that has had a liberating effect on qualitative researchers.

Part III, which in the first edition had one chapter and in this edition has seven chapters, concerns issues and considerations that generally affect all qualitative methods. The effects of time are very evident when one considers that, in 1987, most of us were not using the Internet; now we wonder when it did not exist. Is it a coincidence that the year is 2001, the year of Staley Kubrick's film named for that year, with Hal the computer, and that our last chapter is about getting help on-line?

However, if you are spending more time with your computer and if you are looking for software to assist you in categorizing, Hal might be taking over. To paraphrase Husserl, remember to the people themselves, to the experiences themselves.

I often think of qualitative research with reverence and awe. As researchers, we are allowed to enter the experience of others as they openly convey their pain and joy. So it really is not the research that inspires this reverence and awe: it is the generosity and courage of human beings, who allow us to return to them. It is to these people to whom this book is dedicated.

Patricia L. Munhall

January, 2001

To consider the qualitative perspective in nursing research, we are well advised to come to terms about the meanings of *science, scientific, humanistic,* and *research.* The mere fact that a text such as this one can be distinguished from other nursing research texts as being *qualitative* testifies to the presence in our work of a massive dichotomy that finds expression in our practice experiences as well as our research endeavors.

Science, as it is customarily used, sometimes poses a threat to humanistic ideals because it is frequently promoted as the single true vision of reality and route to truth. Nursing's concern with developing a body of knowledge and assuming professional status in the health care arena has resulted in an identification with empirical science as the model for intellectual endeavor in the field. The isolation of parts suitable for scientific analysis in the empirical model discourages those who envision the acceptance of other ways of knowing, particularly ways of grasping wholes and complex meanings in nursing situations.

In commenting on positivistic assumptions and approaches in the sciences of man, Merleau-Ponty (1964) states: "All of us live in the natural attitude—that is, in the conviction that we are a part of the world and subject to its action on us, which we passively receive from the outside" (p. 56). The term *objective* refers in positivism to a reality independent of the observer, and the aim thus becomes one of eliminating as much observer bias as possible to arrive at the truth of objective reality. The scientific observer of the objective world is ideally a camera of the reality that he or she studies. In this way, a dichotomy between the objective and subjective worlds has been created.

The tension resulting from this splitting of the world into objective and subjective realities has been acknowledged and described by nurses striving to express and share what they know about nursing. This has been particularly apparent in nurses' writings during the 1960s about such skills as listening and touching. Travelbee, for example, developed an argument that sympathy and compassion are nursing assets in response to a growing effort to become more objective in nursing assessment (1964). Other nurse authors found support in existential philosophy for their development of subjective themes in nursing (see Arnold, 1970; Black, 1968; Clemence, 1966; Ferlic, 1968; Raymond, 1968). Either vestiges of our prescientific era or reactionaries to a rapidly growing observance of scientific mores in nursing practice, these nurses' ideas did gradually disappear from the nursing literature.

The significance of such subjective experience in nursing as nurses' attitudes, their empathetic awareness, and their emotional responses to clients continues to be recognized. What remains unresolved, however, is the tension that they constitute in a discipline striving to establish itself as a scientifically based profession. Science, as we have come to understand it, demands that these subjective experiences be operationalized in terms of those objective manifestations that attest to their reality. Apart from this, there is no basis for knowing whether they are real. The problem arising from this demand, of course, is that of locating such evidence in measurable terms.

This last realization serves to explain why nursing's pursuit of truth through empirical methodology warrants a critical examination for its fit with nursing reality. Davis (1973) argues that "the nature of the scientific method has not been and is not now a fixed, established datum" (p. 216). Further, Davis states that research in nursing and nursing itself are social acts and that social science is not qualitatively continuous with natural science. It is the social nature of nursing that lends credence to the ideas that the observer exists in the world and that reality is the observer's interpreted experience. In this sense, there is no objective reality, apart from the observer's experience in the world, to be captured by scientific methods.

Science is, by definition, both a process of coming to know and the product of knowledge. It is characterized by being systematic in nature. Strictly speaking, there is nothing in the term *science* that excludes, for example, philosophical inquiry as a process of knowing, and philosophical insight as knowledge. Yet, science has come to assume a narrow meaning that does exclude philosophy, intuition, and much of nursing. It is opposed in its usage to belief, art, and other subjectively based knowledge.

It is well known that science referred initially to the process and product of study of the natural or physical world. Over time, this process was refined and principles emerged to guide scientific inquiry and to serve as gatekeeper to the world of science. What are the assumptions and principles of natural science as they have come to such disciplines as philosophy, sociology, education, and nursing?

First, the universe is assumed to be orderly. For every effect, there is a cause. The social scientists recognize that the cause may be complex. There may be, and often are, multiple causative factors in complex interaction; nevertheless, human behavior is understandable in stimulus–response terms. For these patterns, the experimental design, which controls variables to isolate cause–effect relations, is sacrosanct.

Second, human reality is assumed to be two-dimensional—that there is no pure consciousness, void of the world. We are always conscious of something in one way or another. The complex modes of consciousness unique to human beings open up multiple realities, no one less true than the others. This, then, is an alternative assumption about the world and reality from which scientific study might proceed: objective reality is grounded in our subjective experience in the world.

> The whole universe of science is built upon the world as directly experienced, and if we want to subject science itself to rigorous scrutiny and arrive at a precise assessment of its meaning and scope, we must begin by reawakening the basic experience of the world of which science is the second-order expression. Science has not and never will have, by its nature, the same significance qua form of being as the world which we perceive, for the simple reason that it is a rationale or explanation of that world. (Merleau-Ponty, 1962, p. viii)

Adherents of the scientific method in nursing recognize, of course, the limitations of research findings vis-à-vis the complexities of nursing situations. Further, understanding is for all nurse researchers, regardless of their methods, the ultimate aim of study. Merleau-Ponty's statements, however, draw attention to several significant considerations.

First, the scientific attitude is but one view of the world, rather than the means to a grasp of a single reality. Further, that view is one of commenting on lived reality as it appears from the dictates and limitations of its methods. Second, this characteristic of science as a commentator on reality negates the idea that scientific knowledge is equivalent to reality itself. In the qualitative researcher's view, the human experience underlies conceptual understanding and needs to be reawakened in the researcher. The more sedimented this original experience is in the researcher's inquiry, the less meaning will be possessed by scientific expressions. Conversely, the observer's awareness of his or her position in the world, which grounds inquiries in subjective experience, enhances the significance of his or her scientific description as a presentation of reality. Scientific description in this view is recognized as a presentation of the observer's reality as it appears in the context of the position that he or she has taken in the world.

Qualitative researchers suggest that lived reality serve as the focus of inquiry, toward the end that subjective and objective realities merge or unify in a closer alliance between lived reality and our knowledge of it. Because the perceived world, or lived reality, underlies scientific explanation and because human experience is the focus of concern in nursing practice, some means of describing lived experience in nursing situations is a paramount need in nursing research. In the view of the qualitative researcher, subjective experience is not merely a private, inner world; rather it is inextricably bound with objective reality and the basis from which scientific knowledge is derived.

Subjective involvement in the objective world, then, is the origin of inquiry for researchers interested in contributing to a body of knowledge concerned with the variety of human experiences in nursing practice. Nurse researchers can profit from study of the methods and techniques developed by qualitative researchers in other disciplines—notably, philosophy, psychology, sociology, and anthropology. They may also be stimulated to discover new methods and techniques in this research perspective, which is characterized by an openness to the search for access to human experience. Nurse researchers will find a congruence between nursing's philosophical embrace of humanism and holism and qualitative methodologies.

Not every research interest can be accommodated by the qualitative perspective; nor should nursing, in our view, adopt a single method for developing knowledge about our wonderfully complex, multidimensional nursing world. To do so is to impose a conformity in nursing that is inconsistent with the variety of roles, settings, goals, and styles that constitute a societal service that is comprehensive, flexible, and dynamic.

Qualitative research is, like empirical method, a tool of science. Each qualitative approach is structured by principles and methods that endow it with the systematic, disciplined quality that is requisite to science, as opposed to superstition, propaganda, tradition, or prejudice. Like empirical method, each qualitative approach requires certain steps, in a certain order, and according to certain rules and is thus subject to certain measures of the value of the research findings.

Qualitative approaches are scientific; they are legitimate members of the realm of science; and they lead to knowledge about the world.

Readers are invited to consider them, first, in the context of how they compare with the more familiar quantitative approach on a philosophical level and, second, in a more detailed examination of selected qualitative approaches in nursing inquiries.

REFERENCES

Arnold, H. (1970). I-thou. *American Journal of Nursing*, 70, 2554–2556.

Black, K., Sr. (1968). An existential model for psychiatric nursing. *Perspectives in Psychiatric Care*, 6, 178–184.

Clemence, M., Sr. (1966). Existentialism: A philosophy of commitment. *American Journal of Nursing*, 66, 500–505.

Davis, A. (1973). The phenomenological approach in nursing research. In E. Garrison (Ed.), *Doctoral preparation for nurses*. San Francisco: University of California Press.

Ferlic, A. (1968). Existential approach in nursing. *Nursing Outlook*, 16, 30–33.

Merleau-Ponty, M. (1962). *Phenomenology of perception* (C. Smith, Trans.). New York: Humanities Press.

Merleau-Ponty, M. (1964). *The primacy of perception* (J. Edie, Trans.). Evanston, IL: Northwestern University Press.

Raymond, M., Sr. (1968) Existentialism and the psychiatric nurse. *Perspectives in Psychiatric Care*, 6, 185–187.

Travelbee, J. (1964). What do we mean by rapport? *American Journal of Nursing*, 63, 725–728.

ACKNOWLEDGEMENTS

Just last week I had the pleasure of reuniting with some of the contributors in this book and in that moment I had an overwhelming sense of my interconnectedness with them. A few of us had not seen each other for six or seven years but our common bond and search for understanding has resonated over long distances and time—perhaps as long as twenty years! During the conference that brought us all together, I had the opportunity to express my appreciation for their wonderful work in this volume to Sarah Steen Lauterbach, Carol P. Germain, Zane Robinson Wolf, and Mary Colvin. All of us were presenting at a research conference and moaned and complained about how overworked we all were. So I had to doubly thank them; however, my gratitude could not be more authentic.

When I arrived home, the awareness of our extended connections became apparent as I read E-mail or spoke to other contributors. Maureen Duffy, who just finished a marathon with a challenged knee, Carolyn Brown and Julie Evertz who sent abstracts for the upcoming IIHU conference, Jody Glittenberg who wrote to tell us all that funding for qualitative research is available outside of our usual agencies, and Sally Hutchinson, just back from Tibet, all have my admiration and gratitude for their contributions to this book. I know they, too, suffer from our generation's most common malady, "self over-extension," or "over-extension of self" (O.E.S.).*

Also afflicted with O.E.S. is Richard MacIntyre, who agreed just this week to do a book project with me and Janice Morse, who is always involved in our qualitative dialogues. Carolyn Oiler Boyd's chapters are classics and have always inspired qualitative researchers, and Carla Mariano's and M. Louise Fitzpatrick's updated chapters are exemplified by two new contributors to this book, the already mentioned Mary Colvin, and Lynne Dunphy. JoAnne Weiss brings a new exemplar chapter to this volume with Sally Hutchinson. Sally's chapter on grounded

---

*The overextended self (Munhall) is an upcoming title scheduled for publication by Jones and Bartlett Publishers.

theory is co-authored with her best friend and a former contributor Holly Skodal Wilson. Julie Maureen, Richard, Janice Lynne, Mary, JoAnne, and Jody are all new over-extended contributors.

I have such close feelings for the ongoing contributors, the ones who began in the first and second editions and then who so generously came through again for the third edition. I am thrilled with our new contributors and what they bring to the third edition. The reader should know this gratitude is based so much on their willingness to present new materials and brand new chapters. For example, Sally, Zane, Sarah, and Carolyn have all written entirely new chapters. Every study within this edition is a new study. An editor could not be more grateful for such dedicated scholarship. One characteristic of individuals with O.E.S. is their generosity to sacrifice energy, talent, and time toward a goal they believe will benefit the quality of life of other individuals.

I will always be grateful to Allan Graubard, former Director of the NLN Press, for all his assistance in the second edition and other books, but now have new individuals to whom to express my gratitude and appreciation. The individuals at Jones and Bartlett I graciously thank for their competence and encouragement in bringing this project to fruition. I am most grateful to Christine Tridente, Associate Editor, who I asked to pester me and she did not fail! (People with O.E.S. need to be reminded a lot!) I thank Christine for her persistence, talent, encouragement and clear headedness. I wish also to thank Dr. Penny M. Glynn, the visionary Nursing Acquisitions Editor, and Production Editor Ann-Marie Lemoine, both at Jones & Bartlett, and Janet Kiefer, the wonderful project editor at Carlise Communications. They represent a wonderfully professional group of individuals to whom I am most grateful.

How fortunate I am to have these wonderful professional and personal friends in my life. They have so much to offer me and to you the reader. The readers of this book, past and present, are part of this interconnectedness, as well. We have begun to weave a quilt, one still being woven into a multipatterned, vibrantly alive, in the present, representative of the polyperceptual world in which we inhabit. The quilt is our everchanging knowledge base for practice. I hope the knowledge quilt will continue to emerge and continue to replace worn out parts no longer useful, with the authentic intersubjective, multistoried experiences which create our ever changing body of knowledge.

Every contributor in this edition, including myself, is always grateful to those individuals who become our research participants and who allow us into the interior of their beings and cultures, and share with us the meaning of their experiences. It is our participants to whom the greatest acknowledgement of gratitude belongs.

Editor and Contributing Author

Patricia L. Munhall, Ed.D., ARNP, PsyA, FAAN
Professor
University of South Carolina
President
International Institute of Human Understanding
Columbia, South Carolina

Contributing Authors

Carolyn L. Brown, RN, Ph.D.
President
e-HealthEd.com
Boca Raton, Florida

Mary Colvin, RN, MSN
Doctoral Student
College of Nursing
University of South Florida
Assistant Professor
Barry University
Miami Shores, Florida

Maureen Duffy, Ph.D.
Professor and Chair
Department of Counseling
Barry University
Miami Shores, Florida

Lynne M. Dunphy, Ph.D., FNP, ARNP
Associate Professor
Graduate Program Coordinator
College of Nursing
Florida Atlantic University
Boca Raton, Florida

Julie Evertz, RN, MSN
Doctoral Student
College of Nursing
Barry University
Miami Shores, Florida

M. Louise Fitzpatrick, Ed.D, RN, FAAN
Dean and Professor
College of Nursing
Villanova University
Villanova, Pennsylvania

Carol P. Germain, RN, Ed.D, FAAN
Chairperson, Science and Role Development Division
Associate Professor
School of Nursing
University of Pennsylvania
Philadelphia, Pennsylvania

Jody Glittenberg RN, Ph.D. FAAN, HNC
Professor of Nursing and Anthropology
Research Professor of Psychiatry
The University of Arizona
Tucson, Arizona

Sally A. Hutchinson, Ph.D., RN, FAAN
Professor
College of Nursing
University of Florida
Gainesville, Florida

Sarah Steen Lauterbach, RN, MN, MSPH, Ed.D
Associate Professor
College of Nursing
The University of Southern Mississippi
Hattiesburg, Mississippi

Carla Mariano, Ed.D, RN
Associate Professor and Director
Advanced Education in Nursing Science
Division of Nursing
New York University
New York, New York

Richard C. MacIntyre, Ph.D., RN
Professor and Division Chair
Nursing and Health Sciences
Mercy College
Dobbs Ferry, New York

Janice M. Morse, Ph.D. (nurs), Ph.D. (anthro), D.Nurs (Hon.), FAAN
Director, International Institute of Qualitative Methodology
Professor
Faculty of Nursing
University of Alberta
Edmonton, Canada

Carolyn Oiler Boyd, RN, GNP, Ed.D
Researcher and Practitioner
West Virginia

JoAnne Weiss, RN, Ph.D., FNP, CS
Assistant Professor
College of Nursing
Florida Atlantic University
Treasure Coast Campus
Port St. Lucie, Florida

Holly Skodal Wilson, RN, Ph.D., FAAN
Professor Emerita
Department of Community Health Systems
School of Nursing
University of California at San Francisco
San Francisco, California

Zane Robinson Wolf, RN, Ph.D. FAAN
Dean and Professor
School of Nursing, LaSalle University, Philadelphia, Pennsylvania
Associate Director of Nursing for Research
Albert Einstein Medical Center
Philadelphia, Pennsylvania

Part I

Language, Epistemology, and the Qualitative Paradigm

In the first three chapters of this volume, a cumulative discussion supports the foundation of qualitative research. Readers are invited to contemplate the emergence of nursing research and the evolution of qualitative research in nursing. In the first two chapters there is a contextual discussion to provide the background necessary to understand the differences in language, the philosophical perspectives, and the contexts in which nursing research first developed and continues to grow and evolve. Additionally, an effort has been put forth to explicate patterns of knowing, the purpose of science, what it is we want to know about, how we go about knowing and what commitments are needed to engage in qualitative research.

Chapter 3, the final chapter of Part I, by Carolyn Oiler Boyd, continues the discussion of the philosophical foundations of qualitative research in more depth and breadth. The reader, upon completion of Part I, will be ready to read specifically how one goes about knowing and researching from a qualitative perspective and to study actual qualitative methods from a critical stance so essential to scholarship.

Language and Nursing Research

Patricia L. Munhall

> Discussing or talking is the way in which we articulate significantly the intelligibility of Being-in-the-world.
>
> The way in which discourse gets expressed is language.
> (Heidegger, 1962, p. 204)

> So the main function of a language symbol is not to stand for or represent an object to which it corresponds. Rather, it initiates a total movement of memory, imagery, ideas, feelings, and reflexes, which serves to order attention to and direct action in a new mode that is not possible without the use of such symbols.
> (Bohm, 1998, p. 68)

Being in the world, for those nurse researchers who embark on the path of discovery through qualitative research designs or methods, has many challenges. One of these challenges has to do with the limits and power of language. Our world is narrated and organized through language. The use of language is one way in which we communicate meaning. We also experience moments when we cannot find the language to express a feeling, an emotion, or a response. So our language at once allows expression and also constrains expression. In the very way that we narrate with language, the particulars of our context, personal, social, and cultural agendas are set. So too in our research language; values, beliefs, and aims are communicated from which varying meanings of being in the world will evolve.

For many years, nurse researchers and theorists have engaged in a lively and enlightening dialogue of various paradigms, the two most common being the logical positivist or empirical–analytic paradigm and the contrasting one, phenomenology. This dialogue was prompted by many nurse researchers who initiated what was to become an "interpretive turn" in nursing research (Munhall, 1989). These nurse theorists and researchers began to raise these questions:

- Was nursing a natural science, like that of chemistry and biology, and therefore based on similar linguistic assumptions?
- Was nursing a human science based on differing linguistic assumptions?
- Was nursing research ready for a poststructuralist perspective (Dzurec, 1989)?

The purpose of this chapter is to place in context the words and perspectives that gave rise to these discussions. Nursing language is both concealing and revealing of the stances and perspective that we pose to nursing as we interact with the phenomenon of concern. For some nurse researchers, this discussion will be historical because they have chosen one paradigm over another for various reasons. For other nurse researchers, it will also be historical because they see a postmodern perspective of multiple research paradigms as not only acceptable but essential. At this point in time, many nurse researchers are encouraging moving beyond what they see as an unruly dualism between what in the early 1980s was structured as a debate. The debate was centered on two different research paradigms, the quantitative and the qualitative. These two research paradigms were often compared and contrasted, elucidating their different philosophical underpinnings. However, it remains extremely important to students studying qualitative research at the outset to become familiar with some of the fundamental and basic assumptions, beliefs, and outcomes of these two paradigms. Using the concreteness of placing paradigms in stark relief to one another should be of assistance to our beginning understanding of various worldviews.

In this chapter, we will see, in the form of contrasting systems of language, competing articulations—in other fields as well as our own—that are characteristic of various philosophical orientations. This particular focus on philosophical analysis is further elucidated in Chapter 3 and again in Chapter 4.

Research in nursing will be at the center of this linguistic exploration. Methods of doing research are still divided into two purportedly ideological (and thus far considered conflicting) schools of thought with two distinct language systems. These schools of thought have been categorized as the qualitative and quantitative approaches to research. By quantitative methods of research we mean the traditional scientific methods as presented in most of the contemporary nursing research textbooks. These methods are characterized by deductive reasoning, objectivity, quasi-experiments, statistical techniques, and control. In contrast, the qualitative methods, many of which are described within this text, are characterized by inductive reasoning, subjectivity, discovery, description, and process orienting (Reichardt & Cook, 1979). The outcome, depending on the method, can be derived from description, interpretation, and analysis (Ashworth, 1997).

This chapter will explore this qualitative-quantitative dichotomy and perhaps will appear culpable of unnecessary polarization. This is done for the pedagogical advantage of clearly revealing the possible differences between these two research traditions. I hope to absolve myself of this polarization as the second chapter of this book begins. In that chapter a cyclical continuum is suggested that finds its origins in qualitative research and its validation in quantitative research. Others have also suggested moving to postpositivism and reconciliation (Clark, 1998).

The present chapter begins with a discussion of the living aspect of language and then progresses to a contextual analysis of nursing research so that we may ferret out the meanings of our linguistic expressions, their origins, and subsequent propulsions. This motion of transition from our earliest identification with medicine represents a broad worldview transition or paradigmatic shift. Nursing research and the quest for nursing theory development are discussed from the perspective of language development and language usage as we seek out the pattern and process of our articulation of meaning and experience. Before we begin our exploration, see if you can hear the words of encouragement from David Allen (1995).

> The emphasis on language, and particularly the insistence that individuals inherit and are constituted by their language, is a helpful corrective to the solipsistic and individualist models that continue to plague our theory and research about practice. (p. 181)

LANGUAGE AND LIVED EXPERIENCE

Long before children speak actual words, they have learned effectively to express their physical, mental, and emotional states of being. Very early in our childhood we learn that laughing, crying, pouting, and looking quizzical stimulate a response from those who are "significant others." We are indeed beginning to learn the power of expressive language.

Eventually, we begin to develop a vocabulary and, interestingly, by the time we are 2 years of age or so, we have learned to treasure the word "no." Individuation, assertiveness, posturing, and a continuing desire for power in our environment render this one of the most important words in any language. People have written entire books on how, when, and where to say "no" effectively.

Nursing as a profession, concomitantly with women as a social force, is still very much involved in those processes of individuation, assertiveness, posturing, and claiming power in our environment. Like the significance of the word "no," our language and the use of specific sets of words simultaneously reveal and conceal who we are, both to ourselves and to the world at large.

Thus, in our quest for individuation—and, we should mention, our autonomy (*auto-no-my*)—we are in the process of developing a language system that defines our particular role with our clients. This focus on autonomy correlates well with the point of the revelatory and concealing power of language and the exemplary word "no." Nursing has claimed the power to say "no" through the Greek word autonomous, meaning *self-ruling*. Thus, we see language alive in a word that says, "I have a right to be self-determined." The living of autonomy expresses the position of a profession and, in nursing, has called attention to our transition from the physician's handmaiden (just look at that word!) to an independent *self-ruling* practitioner. This posturing of ourselves is consistently illustrated in our transition from the primary usage of medical language to our concerted efforts to develop a nursing language, taxonomy, nomenclature, and nursing diagnostic system.[1]

The moment-to-moment language that we choose defines the posture or stance that we assume in the space that we believe is ours in the health care _____ (fill in the blank):

1. system
2. arena
3. delivery system
4. field

---

[1] There is considerable ambivalence within the profession about the usage of the term "nursing diagnosis" and developing taxonomies. Many view these systems as reductionistic, acontextual, and a continued imitation of medicine.

For example, in the preceding multiple-choice option, we find it most interesting to study such words in their starkness for their literal or metaphorical meaning. Is health care "delivered"? Is there a "system" of health care? The word "arena," which is frequently used with health care, is a word that is often associated with a circus or sports. (The temptation is too great to resist pointing out how that word, with its noted association, may be the most apt description of the present so-called health care system.) The word "sports" is also associated with the word "field," where many games are played, with winners and losers. So, of these words, which one or two or perhaps one not mentioned would characterize, for you the reader, the state of health care today?

As noted, nursing language, like that of other professions, is revelatory of the stance and perspective that we suppose as we interact with the phenomena of our experience. The symbols that we choose as expressions either implicitly or explicitly lay open our assertions, propositions, assumptions, beliefs, values, and priorities. The significance of such expressions is centered in our emergence: our expressions bring us into existence. The noumenal, or "thing in itself," depends on the phenomenal for its expression.

DeVries (1983) succinctly and humorously illustrated the noumenal emerging from felt obscurity into shared, understood experience in the following passage:

> In the beginning was the word. Once terms like identity doubts and midlife crisis become current, the reported cases of them increase by leaps and bounds, affecting people unaware there is anything wrong with them until they have got a load of the coinages. You too may have an acquaintance or even a relative with a block about paper hanging or dog grooming, a high flown form of stagnation trickled down from writers and artists. Once my poor dear mother confided to me in a hollow whisper, "I have an identity crisis." I says, "How do you mean?" and she says, "I no longer understand your father." Now we have burnout, and having heard tell of it on television or read about it in a magazine, your plumber doubts he can any longer hack it as a pipefitter, while a glossary adopted by his wife has turned him overnight into . . . a male chauvinist pig, something she would never have suspected before. (p. 4)

Though satirized, we can identify readily in the foregoing what is referred to as a concept development. The "thing itself" (the noumenal) existed, was felt; yet we needed the description and language of shared experience to connect us within the world and provide a way of perceiving the phenomenon. There are other recent contemporary phenomena that we have developed into abstractions of concrete events or, from some intuitive sense, into empirically expressed concepts and words that are commonly used to express our or others' positions/posture/stance in the world. Thus, we have codependency, women who love too much, deficit spending, premenstrual syndrome (PMS), and seven steps to obtain almost anything you would like—success, financial freedom, a good marriage, and more to come! The proliferation of support groups for various conditions of life as well as the many 12-step programs speak also to our need for shared language to connect us within the world with one another. The internet has provided many ways of using language ranging from informational purposes to once again allowing language to connect one human being to another.

The various forms of language that we use, as with all disciplines, bring us into emergence. We need to recognize and articulate our points of contact in this pluralistic world, and we need language with the referent of nursing phenomena to have a recognized place in that world. Qualitative research is poised with its emphasis on language and meaning to assist us in understanding the meaning of our various places in experience.

The word "undeveloped," describing Third World countries, was judged to be a pejorative adjective and was discontinued. The word "emerging" was used instead, to express optimism. Our emergence, like that of children and emerging countries, will depend on our ability to express ourselves clearly within the context of this pluralistic world. Let us look at the lived experience of nursing through a contextual analysis of our language development.

THE CONTEXT OF NURSING RESEARCH

Meshier (1979) argued that there is *no meaning* (italics added) without context dependence. Allen (1995) encourages us to recognize the social, political, and historical location in the role of nursing research. The historical context in which individuals live places them in a world specific to that time and place, of contingencies that must be recognized and acknowledged if research or discourse is to be meaningful (Rorty, 1991). So it appears appropriate, especially in a text on qualitative research that readily acknowledges and embodies its search within the context of "things," that we begin this exploration of language in nursing research by attending to the context in which it has occurred and is continuing to evolve.

Context is defined as "that which leads up to and follows and often specifies the meaning of a particular expression" and "the circumstances in which a particular event occurs" (*American Heritage Dictionary*, 1992). We believe that within this definition of context the following three antecedents and their evolutionary concurrent factors should be acknowledged with the contiguous expressions. They are:

1. Research in nursing evolved predominantly when nursing education became a part of higher education and was seeking its own body of knowledge, different from that of medicine.
2. Nursing's first researchers were being prepared in fields other than nursing and have brought to nursing the various paradigms from those fields.
3. Derivation and/or deduction for nursing research was (is) being drawn from disciplines other than nursing.

Each factor will be explored from the perspective of its contributions to our nursing research language.

Transition in Worldviews of Nursing

During the 1950s, as an outgrowth of the development and acceptance of new theoretical approaches to understanding physical and human phenomena emerging from other fields (approaches such as systems perspectives, quantum physics, adaptation, and ecological views), nurse scholars began questioning the prevalent acceptance and alignment of the medical model as the basis for nursing practice. Nursing was also entering the university setting at that time. These two historical events converged, and the need for our own distinct body of knowledge, a benchmark of a profession and the research imperative of the university, spurred a revolution in nursing.

These two factors, the acknowledgment of a major scientific revolution in other disciplines, as well as our own, and the desire to attain a level of professionalism where we would base practice on a distinct body of nursing knowledge, led to a perceptual shift in the way that we spoke about nursing phenomena and simultaneously led to the scientific investigation of nursing phenomena.[2] It seemed, though, that the way in which we *spoke* about nursing and the way in which we *investigated*

---

[2]For a more detailed explanation of the scientific revolution that eclipsed determinism and objectivism, the reader is referred to works on quantum physics, Heisenberg's principle of uncertainty, and Bohr's principle of complementarity. In Floyd Matson's *The Broken Image*, a most readable discourse can be found, and Larry Dossy's *Space, Time and Medicine* is wonderfully explicit and enjoyable reading on this topic.

nursing phenomena often reflected assumptions, propositions, beliefs, and priorities of two different worldviews, the first reflecting one worldview and the other reflecting a different worldview. We will see shortly that this is a characteristic of paradigmatic shift within a discipline.

The spoken language in nursing began to change, reflecting this perceptual shift from the medical, atomistic, causal model to a distinct nursing, holistic, interactive model. This represented a paradigmatic innovation for nursing. The way in which phenomena were viewed in nursing was changing in a way that was considered by some to be irrevocably conflictual in its basic premises and assumptions with the medical model.

This shift, which was well recognized in the discipline of physics, began to permeate the language of other fields as well as nursing. The change is representative of a transition from a mechanistic to an organismic perspective, from the reliance on objectivity to intersubjectivity, and from the received view to a nonreceived view (Watson, 1981). Today, Watson (1999) urges us farther "away from the reaction worldview, past the reciprocal and into the transformative-simultaneous" and urges nurses to create nursing's own postmodern paradigm. Many of the qualitative methods of research, before the language of postmodernism became more commonplace, had as underpinnings many of the values and beliefs of postmodernism.

Illumination of the differences between and among these worldviews and/or paradigms can be demonstrated in the scrutiny of the respective language systems. It seems appropriate, though, to be clear at this point as to what a worldview or paradigm is. Patton (1978), in terms consistent with those of Kuhn (1970), defined a paradigm as:

> A worldview, a general perspective, a way of breaking down the complexity of the real world. As such, paradigms are deeply embedded in the socialization of adherents and practitioners: paradigms tell them what is important, legitimate and reasonable. (p. 203)

If we accept the premise that things come into being through language, the language paradigm of a discipline will tell the practitioner what is important, legitimate, and reasonable. Kuhn (1970) suggested that a paradigm is a discipline's specific method of solving a puzzle, of viewing human experience, and of structuring reality. It is a worldview, a way of viewing phenomena in the world.

Laudan (1977), in a similar vein, used the phrase "research tradition" to communicate the same theme:

A research tradition . . . is a set of assumptions about the basic kinds of entities in the world, assumptions about how these entities interact, assumptions about the proper methods to use for constructing and testing theories about these entities. (p. 97)

Morgan (1983) called our attention to the significance of these assumptions. He stated: "Assumptions make messes researchable, often at the cost of great simplification, and in a way that is highly problematic" (p. 377).

This reference about assumptions becomes more powerful when, as Morgan suggested, researchers choose their own assumptions on which to base their studies. One could then say that this latitude or freedom gives the means for achieving what the researcher values. In the paradigms introduced in this chapter are assumptions about the world, believed in some way to be true, though they are actually the "taken for granted" views of human scientists. In a fundamental sense, then, researchers choose the values, "truths," and perspectives on which they base their research endeavors.

Another way of expressing this shift was the idea that nursing was a human science. Nursing seems to be philosophically expressed through language to be compatible with the ideas and concepts of a human science. German philosopher-historian Wilhelm Dilthey (1926; as translated in Atwood & Stolorow, 1984) held these assumptions about a human science:

The supreme category of the human sciences is meaning. (p. 2)

The natural sciences investigate objects from the outside whereas the human sciences rely on a perspective from the inside. (p. 2)

The central emphasis in the natural sciences is upon causal explanation: The task of inquiry in the human sciences is interpretation and understanding. (p. 2)

Our transition in worldviews then seems to have moved from a narrowly defined type of science to a much broader connection of what constitutes science. However, in that broader view, there remain two very distinct sciences: natural science and human science. Some would even question the idea of a human science, if using the strict parochial rules of *science*. However, as the human sciences have evolved, there is little doubt that they have legitimated their place as a science, one with a different philosophy from the philosophy of natural science.

THE LANGUAGE OF WORLDVIEWS

What follows now are expressions belonging to different ways of viewing phenomena (worldviews). The language reveals different assumptions, beliefs, and values concerning human and physical reality. In essence, the paradigm or research tradition is a philosophy: it conceptualizes fundamental beliefs. For this reason, the research paradigm as a puzzle-solving method should be congruent with the discipline's larger paradigm, that is, the paradigm of nursing or nursing's philosophy.

Although this idea of congruency is not held as essential by all researchers, the most sophisticated or reasonable response to any either-or discussion would be to choose a dialectic approach (Moccia, 1988; Morgan, 1983). This approach, as Morgan (1983) stated, "also accepts the diversity of assumption and knowledge claims as an inevitable future of research and attempts to use the competing perspectives as a means of constructing new modes of understanding" (p. 379). A postmodern perspective would transcend the either-or stalemate as an unnecessary obstacle to understanding and would beg the question with an emphasis on plurality of perspectives, which would be context dependent.

As was said at the start of this chapter, to assist students in understanding the different language systems of various fields, the tables present language in its stark relief. They are purposely presented to demonstrate the different meaning systems and are more for explicitness than for the subtleties that, of course, also can be discussed.

Each of the five tables (Tables 1–1 through 1–5) of paradigmatic-type language presents two contrasting belief systems. The language of the systems in the left-hand columns is often the same language or, if not literally the same, it is at least consistent in syntax and meaning, reflecting the underlying continuity of beliefs, values, and assumptions. The same continuity in language will be observed in the systems presented in the right-hand columns of the tables. The observations are important when we take into account that the paradigm preserves and perpetuates the disciplinary matrix of a field (Kuhn, 1970).

A major premise that this text suggests is that the language expressed within the left-hand columns and found within the paradigms of the mechanistic, the realists, the received view, the medical model, and behaviorism is consistent with the scientific method or quantitative research. In contrast, the language expressed in the right-hand columns reflects the paradigms of the organismic, the idealists, the nonreceived view, humanism, and many nursing models and is consistent with qualitative research methods.

We know well that there are more cultures than the two described by C. P. Snow in *The Two Cultures and the Scientific Revolution* (1959). Today, there are hundreds, and there are disciplines and subdisciplines of those disciplines. Often, the subdisciplines of a discipline speak in foreign tongues to one another. For this reason, it is important to understand the overall fundamental differences so that we may intelligently see what Kirby (1983) called "the points of contact in a plural world." Illustrating the plurality of worldviews, he optimistically stated that "there could be an underlying unity . . . and thus a single earth-centered perspective from which all problems may be viewed" (p. 25). Seventeen years later, which is just a blip on the time screen, we have yet to come to this perspective. The following tables and the language should illustrate the fundamental differences. Perhaps the reader can surmise possible points of contact and propose an alliance where all sorts of evidence will contribute to the richness of our comprehension and our ability to make sense of the world around us.

Paradigms in Psychology.   It has been said that all contemporary psychological systems are derivative of either the mechanistic or the organismic paradigms (Table 1–1) (Looft, 1973). Many philosophers and psychologists argue that the assumptions of each are unbridgeable. Either humans are reactive organisms, as Skinner (1953) would have them, or individuals are active and thinking organisms, as Piaget (1970) would predicate. One lays before us a thesis; the other, an antithesis.

TABLE 1–1   PARADIGMS IN PSYCHOLOGY

MECHANISTIC	ORGANISMIC
Human being reacts and responds to the environment	Human being acts on and creates the meaning of an experience
Predictable response sets from human beings can be determined	Understanding comes from individual human perspective—variable responses
Empirical reality	Social construction of reality
One reality—same rules	Dynamic reality—different responses
Human beings can be controlled	Human beings can be self-determined
Behavior—should be prescribed	Behavior—many possibilities acceptable and desirable

The reader is asked to contemplate the differences in meaning as expressed in the descriptive language of the mechanistic and the organismic paradigms of psychology (Table 1–1).

Are the perspectives unbridgeable? With these paradigms, as well as the ones that follow, discussion about the bridgeability of these perspectives should prove lively and fruitful.

Paradigms in Philosophy.   Filstead (1979, p. 34) stated that at the core of the distinction between the quantitative and qualitative methods of research lies the classical argument in philosophy between the schools of realism and idealism and their subsequent derivatives (Table 1–2). The Baconian reality of "seeing is believing" led to believing in the "real" as the only reality about which one could be positive. Hence, those who ascribed to that belief system were called "positivist." When reality could be held static, observations made, and experiments performed, science was done and the truth revealed. Those philosophers who questioned this positivist logic and method of science when it was applied to the understanding of human beings became known as "idealists" (Kneller, 1964). Today, the same questions asked by the "idealists" have been amplified by postmodernists. Science is no longer absolute or the final truth. Science is an ever-changing body of ideas, and we have daily shifts about beliefs. The whole concept of universality and generalizability are put into question. We have come to see that "being in the world" may be more aptly stated as "beings-in-the-worlds." There are multiple worlds, multiple realities, and multiple perspectives (Anderson, 1995).

Although the idealists acknowledged the existence of a physical reality, they argued that the mind was the creator and source of knowledge. In addition to the language expressed in Table 1–2 from the idealist school, the following short Zen parable is indicative of idealists' ideas and the place of human perception (*Zen Buddhism*, 1959):

TABLE 1–2   PARADIGMS IN PHILOSOPHY

REALISM	IDEALISM
Static conception of world	Evolving conception of world
Seeing is believing	There is more than what meets the eye
Logical positivism	Dynamic, chaotic
Social world as given	Social world as created
Independent physical reality	Reality is mentally perceived—sense perception

One windy day two monks were arguing about the flapping banner. The first said, "I say the banner is moving, not the wind." The second said, "I say the wind is moving, not the banner." A third monk passed by and said, "The wind is not moving. The banner is not moving. Your minds are moving." (p. 52)

Although briefly presented, inherent here is the great debate between the objective and subjective means of knowing. We are about to see now how research methods as worldviews are an inherent outgrowth of a philosophical worldview that precedes it and establishes its epistemological ways of coming to know about the world.

Subsequent Paradigms in Epistemology. Flowing from the paradigms of philosophy should be congruent paradigms or research traditions for the way in which each school of thought establishes how it comes to know about its particular account of the world. Epistemology is the branch of philosophy that concerns itself with the nature of knowledge. Each school of philosophy will have an epistemology. In other words, each belief system will have a congruent belief system about *coming to know* about the world and the nature of knowledge.

For our purposes, the realist philosophy is connected with the epistemological paradigm of the received view and the idealist is connected with the nonreceived view (Table 1–3). We must acknowledge at this point or perhaps call attention to this very simplified version of what is most complex to philosophers. We are examining the gist of language differences, yet we strongly recommend further study in this area for those who are interested in greater in-depth knowledge. (Chapter 2 provides a further base to this aspect of the discussion.)

TABLE 1–3 PARADIGMS IN EPISTEMOLOGY

RECEIVED VIEW	NONRECEIVED VIEW
Logical positivism	Uncertainty
Materialism	Mental Perception
Reductionism	Holism
Laws—quantification	Patterns—qualification
Predictions	Interpretations
Objectivity	Subjectivity
Neutrality	Human values
Operationalization	Context integration
Knowing something	Understanding meaning

The expressions of the received view are those of the positivists and/or realists (Suppe, 1977; Watson, 1981). They are consistent with the scientific method[3] and are representative of expressions found most often in our present nursing research texts. The nonreceived view of coming to know about nursing phenomena is emerging, and those expressions are found in the language of qualitative epistemology as well as most nursing philosophies.

Paradigms in Education.   The mechanistic and organismic paradigms are reflected in the field of education as behaviorism and humanism (Table 1–4). Learning theories emerging from these two paradigms are distinctively different, because they are reflective of differing beliefs, values, and assumptions about the world and the nature of human beings. The reader may find it interesting here to reflect on which paradigm is more prevalent in nursing education and discuss the relative merits of each and, again, the bridgeability or points of contact (Munhall, 1992a).

Paradigms in the Health Professions.   Table 1–5 seems to reflect nursing's congruity with the preceding paradigms of the organismic, the idealists, the nonreceived view, and humanism. In contrast, the language of medicine seems to have the same congruity with the mechanistic, the realists, the received view, and behaviorism. It seems important to note, then, that our language system is congruent with some paradigms and not logically consistent with other paradigms. This is particularly relevant when we acknowledge that each paradigm should have a compatible research paradigm or method. The rele-

TABLE 1–4   PARADIGMS IN EDUCATION

BEHAVIORISM	HUMANISM
Homogeneous group	Heterogeneous group
Human reactiveness	Human activeness
Human malleability	Self-determination
Human passiveness	Unique interpretation of reality
Human objectivity	Subjectivity
Shaping concrete behavior	Changes in consciousness
Measurable outcomes	Hoped-for outcomes—variable
Preparation for specific roles	Preparation for world at large

[3]As defined in the traditional sense. All the methods presented in this text are considered scientific methods of research.

TABLE 1–5   PARADIGMS IN HEALTH PROFESSIONS

MEDICINE	NURSING
Reductionism—treating the part; treating the symptom	Holism—coming to the whole care for the whole person, whether "sick" or well
Reactive human being—reacts as prescribed	Active human being—transformative
Physical symptomatology	Integrated human being
Linear causality—cause and effect	Multiple interaction—self, others, environment, cosmos
Closed system	Open system
Steady state	Dynamic
Objective	Subjective
Manipulation	Self-determination
Control	Choice
Paternalism	Advocacy

vance is demonstrated in the philosophical paradigms of the realistic and idealistic and in the concomitant epistemological paradigms of the received view and nonreceived view, respectively. The languages of the medical model and most nursing models are readily distinguishable as to their perspectives, worldviews, tradition, or paradigms.

We believe it is important to return here to our first consideration: "Research in nursing evolved predominantly when nursing was in transition between broad philosophic worldviews."

The language represented in Table 1–5 as the language of medicine was for a long time that of nursing. When the worldview for nursing began changing, as reflected in proposed nursing models, the activity of nursing research concomitantly was underway. Ironically, the research activities that occurred in a parallel fashion often were not congruent with the premises of the nursing model. However, this incongruity is quite understandable when we review the second consideration in our language development: "Researchers in nursing were being prepared in fields other than nursing."

Early Preparation of Nurse Researchers
It is so commonplace today that our nurse scholars and researchers have doctorate degrees in nursing that we need to reflect on the influence of the earlier doctoral preparation of nurses. Before the opening

of specific nursing doctoral programs in the United States, nurse faculty and others sought this degree in other disciplines that seemed to relate to nursing. On completing these degrees, many of those doctorally prepared nurses began to think of developing nursing's own degree, a doctoral degree in nursing. Because our doctoral education evolved in this way, we will proceed to examine its influence rather than discuss the merits and limitations of such evolution.

The outcome was the development of a community of nurse researchers who were educated in the better established disciplines and who subsequently developed a commitment to that discipline's research method (Chinn, 1983, Corbin, 1999). Although this development offered nursing a wide array of methods from which to choose, it soon appeared evident that the scientific method, with its own language, was adopted to such an extent that, according to Watson (1981), "The scientific method is considered the one and only process for scientific discovery, experimental quantitative research methodology and design" (p. 414). Swanson and Chenitz (1982) stated: "While nursing exists almost exclusively in the empirical social world, the profession uses the laboratory method of the basic sciences in its research design" (p. 241).

Norris (1982) attributed this supremacy of the scientific method in part to nursing's "desperate attempt" to become a legitimate science by embracing the experimental research model as the way to proceed. Indeed, "science" and "scientific" cannot be considered neutral words (if there are such words!). In today's world, they are extensively value laden as expressing truth, goodness, worthwhileness, and legitimacy. Kaplan (1964) emphasized this legitimacy point:

> There are behavioral scientists who in their desperate search for *scientific status*, give the impression that they don't much care what they do if only they do it right: substance gives way to form.
> (p. 406)

However, as Norris (1982) pointed out in a discussion of nursing's leap to experimental research, many nurse researchers are hampered by the lack of concept clarification, theory development, and descriptive methods of research, all of which are linked to qualitative research methods. Norris (1982) observed that, during the period from 1958 to 1975, nursing scholars made a concerted effort to develop a body of nursing knowledge without the necessary training in the methods of concept clarification, which are prerequisite to experimental research.

This "scientific" influence continues to exercise its exclusivity, as is evidenced in the following scenario (Tinkle & Beaton, 1983):

It was her first dissertation committee meeting. The topic of discussion was the proposed research methodology. Two of the committee members (well-known for their "hard" research) began to dialogue about the "softness" of the approach in the proposal before them—the lack of control, the lack of quantitative measurement, and the lack of manipulation of variables. Before long, the committee was in accord about the relatively low scientific merit of this type of research methodology as opposed to an experimental approach. The student found herself agreeing to shift her methodology to one involving experimental manipulation. (p. 27)

What makes this anecdote relevant 17 years later is that, in some colleges of nursing, this belief system has become even more prominent. The status and sometimes the requirement to attain NINR-NIH funding to advance, obtain a position, and even earn tenure demonstrates how fundamental to the research enterprise this commitment to "hard" science is.

Downs (1982), in response to a similar theme, observed: "This distorted value system rode in on the coattails of the idea that scientific method was equivalent to experimental research" (p. 4). Bronowski (1965), with a broader conception of science, surpassed this narrow view of the scientific method and enlarged the aperture. Science, he said, is:

Nothing else than the search to discover unity in the world variety of nature or . . . in the variety of our experiences. Poetry, painting, the arts are the same search. (p. vi)

In a cogent argument for a poststructural perspective, Dzurec (1989) commented on the tenacity of logical positivist methodology in nursing:

The period beginning in the 1960's and stretching to today is perhaps the first in which the power relations in nursing and in human sciences in general, have allowed the recognition of logical positivism as a single philosophy of science rather than as science itself. (p. 74)

We now know that our worldview has opened to allow for other methods of research. Coming to know and coming to discover rather than verify have become acknowledged as essential to the base of nursing knowledge.

Watson (1981) attributed this increased acknowledgment to the same processes of scientific development that have taken place in other sciences. She stated that our commonality with other fields lies in the process of first adopting the received-view idea and then undergoing processes of rejection of that particular paradigm. We would not advocate the abandonment of all the characteristics of the received view or the scientific method, but two important points need to be made about the early preparation of nurse researchers (and, to a large extent, the present preparation of nurse researchers). These points are still discussed today and will lead us into the next contextual consideration (Clark, 1998, Ashworth, 1997, Watson, 1999). They are:

1. Nurse researchers predominantly use the scientific method of inquiry and that language system.
2. The scientific method is used in nursing research prior to the description and understanding of the phenomenon within the nurse–patient context. In other words, we take leaps to a step without the necessary conditions for that step. Often we take those leaps within the context of deduction and derivation from theories from other disciplines and from nursing theories representing a totality paradigm (whose assumptions are congruent with those of natural-science research).

A third possible point here is that some of nursing research is research done by nurses but not research in nursing.

Deduction and Derivation from Theories: From Then to Now

Walker and Avant (1983, p. 163) defined theory derivation as "the process of using analogy to obtain explanations or predictions in another field." These authors make a good distinction between theory derivation and borrowing theory (p. 163), but, for our purpose here, we are speaking about a process in which the description and explanations of phenomena for the development of nursing theory evolved from a discipline or field of knowledge other than nursing. Therefore, the language originates from a world other than the nurse–patient world. Nursing researchers identifying similarities from other fields believe a specific theory to be appropriate to a nursing or a patient situation and proceed to generate deductions and/or hypotheses from that theory. This theory derivation is asserted to be useful when there are no available data or when the phenomenon is poorly understood (Walker & Avant, 1983). Thus, we had almost 25 years of nursing research based on theoretical frameworks that did not originate within a nursing or patient context.

One point that should be considered at this juncture is that many borrowed and derived theories in nursing are based first on the natural and behavioral sciences and, with that, a mechanistic paradigm. Subsequently, the hypothesis deduced from such theories originated from how physical matter behaves, how people respond to forced choice questions, and, probably all too often, how college students respond to questionnaires and various experiments.

It is amazing to realize with a simple perusal of psychology texts that one experiment after another, leading to the development of theory, has been performed on college students. In these many instances, theories evolved from a very specific age sample and then were generated to the population at large. The very specific sample has been for researchers of human behavior a real convenience sample, that is, their 19-year-old sophomore students.

Another potential problem with theory derivation and language development from other fields is the male bias inherent in many of our developmental theories (Belenky, Clinchy, Goldberg, & Taub, 1986; Chinn, 1985; Gilligan, 1978). Pinch (1981) proposed that we should critically examine theories of development generated by Freud, Piaget, Erickson, and Kohlberg to recognize how we have accepted worldviews as developed and evolved from a male perspective (this topic is further discussed in Chapter 2). When we apply a hypothesis derived from such theory to individuals who may be ill—whether the derivation is from a male perspective, a college student's perspective, a well person's perspective, and so on—we will always have problems of authenticity, validity, and, most important, contextual meaning.

In our history of knowledge development, Dickoff and James (1968) proposed a schema of four levels of theory (factor-isolating theories, factor-relating theories, situation-relating theories, and situation-producing theories), which dominated the development of nursing theory. We now need to evaluate how well we have proceeded with each of the four levels of theory. Often, when borrowing or deriving from theories from other fields, we proceed directly to situation-producing theories, sacrificing meaning and true significance to expedience. As far back as 1968, Dickoff and James cited this lack of attention to the beginning levels of theory development as being detrimental to the development of nursing theory. Wald and Leonard (1964) suggested that nurses develop their own concepts for nursing theory from inductive analysis of nursing experience rather than from deductive analysis from others' experiences. Perusal of many of the nursing research articles published today still indicates dependence on deducting hypotheses from unrelated contexts or unrelated populations.

Diers (1979), in a context correlative to the work of Dickoff and James, provided us with another classification of levels of theory (Table 1–6). Germain (see Chapter 9 of this book) demonstrates how the qualitative method of ethnography fits into the factor-searching level of inquiry proposed by Diers (1979, p. 54) and shown in Table 1–6.

Indeed, all the qualitative methods of research presented herein seem essential to the beginning steps of theory development. In the first and second levels of inquiry, the questions "What is this?" and "What's happening here?" are answered within our own nurse–patient context. With qualitative research methods, theory is not derived, borrowed, or modified from other fields but rather springs from observation of and participation in an actual phenomenon. Norris (1982) believed that the phenomena with which nurses have the social prerogative and mandate to manage concern human health, illness, and

TABLE 1–6   LEVELS OF INQUIRY AND STUDY DESIGN

LEVEL OF INQUIRY	KIND OF QUESTION	STUDY DESIGN	KIND OF ANSWER (THEORY)	STUDY DESIGN
1	What is this?	Factor-searching	Factor-isolating (naming)	Exploratory Formulative Descriptive Situational
2	What's happening here?	Relation-searching	Factor-relating (situation-depicting, situation-describing)	Exploratory Descriptive
3	What will happen if . . .?	Association-searching	Situation-relating (predictive)	Correlational Survey design Nonexperimental Natural experiment Experimental Explanatory Predictive
4	How can I make . . . happen?	Prescription-testing	Situation-producing (prescriptive)	

From *Research in Nursing Practice* (p. 54), by D. Diers, Philadelphia-Lippincott, 1979.

comfort. Newman (1983, 1986) identified additional patient-nursing phenomena, such as reciprocities, patterns, configurations, rhythms, and composition, and emphasized context dependency, recognizing the simultaneity of our human-environmental processes.

The Social Policy Statement of the American Nurses' Association (1995) specified that the phenomena of concern to nurses are human responses to actual or potential health problems. All are phenomena researchable through qualitative methods and in the end may well stimulate the development of knowledge grounded in the experience of the patient, in complex interactions and situated in an individual life-world. In the last edition, I had voiced hope that these discussions and debates of a socially constructed dichotomy would be a historical curiosity. Although some literature speaks to moving beyond this debate (Clark, 1998) and Watson (1999) offers a strikingly contemporary worldview for nursing, the old traditions largely dominate.

A TRANSITION: NURSING WORLDVIEWS, NURSING RESEARCHERS, AND THEORY DEVELOPMENT

One of the purposes of this chapter is to explore nursing's coinages (language), its situatedness in this world, and how we choose to express ourselves. The foregoing discussion is an attempt to place in context our present posture in nursing research and to suggest the origin and evolution of how we have come to express ourselves and the language that we use to bring nursing phenomena into being. We suggest that this text on qualitative research methods is a natural outgrowth of this context. It is contemporary, evolutionary, and congruent with changing worldviews. Expanding research horizons, acquiring new languages, and bringing phenomena into view constitute a reconstructing process.

Transitions in worldviews or paradigms are a gradual process wherein beliefs, values, and practices of the old and the new overlap (Kuhn, 1970). This is a time when there may be conflict, incongruity, and confusion. It is, though, a wonderful time for self-reflection, self-consciousness, and clarification. Thesis, antithesis, and paradigmatic shifting are all parts of scientific revolutions or, in Laudan's (1977) terminology, the evolution of research traditions. They are the history and essence of science.

Returning now to the three identified factors that seem to influence the context of nursing research most, let us consider them from the perspective of Kuhn's language in an application to nursing research. Kuhn (1970) observed:

> During the transition period [of worldviews] there will be a large but never complete overlap between the problems that can be solved by the old and by the new paradigm. But there will also be a decisive difference in the modes of solution. When the transition is complete, the profession will have changed its view of the field, its methods and goals. (p. 84)

Evidently, we have not reached this stage, with two paradigms ironically being taught in some cases simultaneously: the totality paradigm and the simultaneity paradigm. Each of these paradigms indicates a method of research. The former yields best to the scientific method and the latter to qualitative methods of research.

Chapter 2 discusses epistemology in nursing and the qualitative and quantitative methods of knowing, but let us see here the role of transition.

Nursing Worldviews

Nursing has attempted to abandon the language of the medical model and, concomitantly, to reject the mechanistic paradigm expressed by that language. To a lesser extent, medicine itself appears to be in transition from its own medical model to one that seems more aligned with some of the beliefs that we have most recently been espousing. There is within that field an emerging language that focuses on holism, psychosomatic phenomena, and the influence of environmental factors.

Even though nursing has attempted to develop nursing language, it often continues to retain the philosophical foundations of the medical model for research and to express its significance and importance in the symbols and practices that traditionally belong to medicine. Perhaps readers will consider some of these nonverbal symbolic forms of language that nursing continues to use and even seeks to acquire from the perspective of paradigmatic transition (Roberts, 1973).

In view of Kuhn's suggestion (1970, p. 84) that when "the transition is complete, the profession will have changed . . . its methods . . . ," we repeat a question raised in an article by Munhall (1982b):

> Could it be that when nursing abandoned the medical model and the language of that discipline, it retained the research paradigm that perpetuated what nursing was seeking to dissociate from? (p. 68)

Because transitions are gradual and because of the aforementioned contextual variables, I am inclined to view this question as characteristic of a trajectory of transition in worldviews. Things do not change at once; Kuhn's (1970) words were: "When the transition is *complete*, the profession will have changed . . . its *methods* . . ." (italics added). Our transition is far from complete. However, many nurse researchers and scholars are catalyzing the progress and process of this transition.

Nurse Researchers and Scholars

Many of our nurse researchers and scholars, many of whom were socialized into the scientific method, are emerging strongly from that orientation (often meaning experimental research) and are contributing now to the logical shift in research paradigms that would be congruent with the shift in the larger philosophical worldview and new perspective of viewing phenomena. What seems to have occurred is that questions and problems of the profession with its new and unique nursing perspective, that is, holism versus reductionism and/or simultaneity versus totality, cannot be answered or solved by the old methods, at least not at first.

Laudan (1977) reassured us with the following observation:

> But there are times when two or more research traditions, far from mutually undermining one another, can be amalgamated, producing a synthesis which is progressive with respect to both the former research traditions. (p. 103)

Although we have moved from what Norris (1982, p. 6) identified as "the occasional nurse who used the podium or the literature to support a descriptive route to knowledge [as] a 'voice crying in the wilderness'" to regular publication of the merits of qualitative research, the need for qualitative methods, research programs highlighting qualitative research, and, in general, the recognition of the advantages of a broadened repertoire of research methods, we seem now in the year 2001 to have divided ourselves into two different schools. When we first debated the various methods, it was as though we were seeking a place for each method for a specific purpose. Now we see conferences, journals, and particular programs specializing in either quantitative or qualitative methods. It is an interesting evolution, and we need to be cognizant of the need to hear one another's voices, regardless of the orientation. Hardly hidden in the agendas of various schools or organizations is a strong bias toward one orientation, and, unfortunately, there may even appear to be suspicion or disrespect of the other. Such suspicion or disrespect is so very counterproductive and, just as tolerance for individual differences is part of our nursing philosophy, it needs to extend to differences in research orientations; these differences need to enrich us and assist us in ultimately meeting the needs of our patients.

At this point it might be helpful to analyze not only the syntactical parallelism but also the contextual congruency of our larger philosophical paradigm with our most prevalent research method. The language that we use in the expression of the two demonstrates for us the emergence of the new worldview and the residual of the old worldview. .

The expressions in Table 1–7 are provided to demonstrate the transitional nature of our worldviews and research paradigms. Table 1–7 illustrates the expressions of competing paradigms and Kuhn's overlap as we examine the contextual parallelism for logical syntax. This overlap has stimulated for many nurse researchers the proliferation of competing views, debates about methods, and discontent over the effect of nursing research on practice. Kuhn (1970) believed such debates are symptomatic of a "transition from normal to extraordinary research," but, as just mentioned, we should beware of splintering. The wholeness and the interaction that we propose in nursing models should be reflected in our own community of nurse researchers.

For the sake of conceptual clarity, the various paradigms have been presented in a dichotomized way, however, the practice is used more for its illustrative purpose. The goal here is to build bridges rather than erect walls. The bridge may well represent a transcendence of the two competing worldviews with the emergence of a research paradigm that either utilizes the two views or goes beyond them.

Theory Development

The transition from one paradigm to another paradigm or to the inclusion of another paradigm will be reflected, as has been suggested, in our language and expressions. We previously mentioned the borrowed theoretical frameworks that are used so prevalently in nursing research. We borrow freely from physics, biology, physiology, psychology, and sociology. We seem, as was mentioned, to also have two different nursing paradigms: the totality and the simultaneity. These practices often lead to fuzzy language and, in this context, the discovery of unique knowledge for nursing. Although the benefits of interdisciplinary work must be acknowledged and recognized, it still remains

TABLE 1–7 EXPRESSIONS IN NURSING PHILOSPHY AND RESEARCH PARADIGMS, AND CONTEXTUAL PARALLELISM

EXPRESSIONS OF CONTEMPORARY NURSING PHILOSOPHY

Humanism	Uniqueness
Individualism	Relativism
Self-determination	Autonomy
Active organism	Advocacy
Open system	Organismic
Holism	Situated context
Life-worlds	Simultaneity
Multiple realities	Multiplicity
Self-interpretive	

EXPRESSIONS OF THE SCIENTIFIC METHOD

Reductionism	Theory for the average
Objectivity–positivism	Categorization
Delimited problems	Prediction
Reality reduced to the measurable	Control
Human and environmental passivity	Mechanistic
Manipulation	Totality

CONCEPTUAL PARALLISM

Nursing Philosophy	Nursing Research Based on the Scientific Method
Individualism	Commonalities
Uniqueness	Generalizations
Relativism	Categorization
Open system	Closed system
Holism	Reductionism
Individual interpretations	Statistical analysis
Active organism	Reactive organism
Organismic	Mechanistic
Self-determination	Control
Simultaneous interaction	Totality
Situated context	Acontextual
Multiple realities	Objective reality
Subjective perceptions	Objectivity

essential for each discipline to develop its own essence, its own substance, its own reason for being, and its own meaning.

Paterson (1978) compiled a list of nursing phenomena (Table 1–8) selected by practicing nurses as being essential to nursing. We would ask the reader to compare these expressions with the expressions found in many of our contemporary research titles. It bears repeating to recognize just how pioneering Paterson and then with Zderad were. To pay tribute to them, their jointly written book *Humanistic Nursing*, was reissued in 1988, as being contemporary and relevant for the present after its first publication date in 1976. Read, think about, and respond to these words as perhaps the quintessence of nursing. Could any of us argue that they do not constitute nursing phenomena?[4] Would we not want them to? Are these not the words that express caring in experience? To those who wonder why there is not adequate description of such experiences in nursing literature, we believe the answer lies in the arguments for qualitative research. We eagerly await the extraordinary research that Kuhn promises as the outcome of scientific revolutions.

TABLE 1–8   THE QUINTESSENCE OF NURSING

ACCEPTANCE	GIVE AND TAKE
Authenticity	Laughing–crying
Awareness	Loneliness
Becoming	Openness
Caring	Patience
Charge	Readiness
Choice	Response
Commitment	Responsibility
Confirmation	Self-recognition
Confrontation	Sustaining
Dedication	Touching
Dying and death	Trust
Fold—its meaning	Understanding
Freedom	Waiting
Frustration	

From "The Tortuous Way Toward Nursing Theory," in *Theory Development: What, Why and How?* (p. 65), by J. Paterson, New York: National League for Nursing, 1978.

---

[4]Additional phenomena are discussed in Chapter 2.

LANGUAGE AND COMPREHENSIBILITY

The existential-ontological foundation of languages is discourse or talk. (Heidegger, 1962, p. 203)

Discourse is existentially language, because that entity whose disclosedness it articulates according to significations, has, as its kind of being, being-the-world and being which has been thrown and submitted to the world. (Heidegger, 1962, p. 204)

For in conversation, as in research, we meet ourselves. Both are forms of social interaction in which our choice of words and actions return to confront us in terms of the kind of discourse or knowledge we help to generate. (Morgan, 1983, p. 406)

And where does a nurse researcher thrown and submitted to the world learn to speak? In the pedagogical world of research, a new language is learned. We noted earlier that this language is sometimes chosen freely, sometimes encouraged in one or another direction, and sometimes "raised" to such high levels of abstraction that it becomes incomprehensible. From a qualitative perspective, language and the ability to express oneself to others is the only way in which we can bring experience into a form that creates in discourse a conversational relation (Van Manen, 1990).

Before this chapter ends, it seems essential to mention an obvious inherent component of language: listening. Discourse and conversing include keeping silent and hearing. The openness that is required for new ideas to penetrate into a belief system requires silence and hearing. Additionally, when considering language, many people silence themselves, they do not give voice to their experience, and what may be meaningful in the "said" may even be more meaningful in the "unsaid."

The language of human science or phenomenology may at first sound strange to people who are steeped in a natural-science language (see Table 1–9). Paterson and Zderad's (1976) first attempts to introduce this language into nursing were often met with firm preconceptions and assumptions about being in the world that were dramatically different. In 1993, the second edition stated that the desire herein was to lay a possible groundwork in many curricula to assist students in the language of understanding the meaning of both being human in our different perspectives and understanding those differences in nursing and nursing research. This third edition will be published in the year 2001 and, like

TABLE 1–9 Expressions of Qualitative Research Methods

Subjective experience	Closeness to the data
Intuition	Process orientation
Variability	Dynamic reality
Communication	Open system
Individual perceptions	Time and space considerations
Shared language	Patterns
Interrelatedness	Configurations
Lived experience	Context dependence
Holism	Complementarily
Naturalism	Human development
Nonmanipulated observation	Life-worlds
Self-interpretation	Contingencies
Multiple perspectives	Multiple realities
Intersubjectivity	Narratives/stories
Existential meaning	

the theme from the film of that title, technology run amock and then rebirth, it seems fitting once again to call attention to learning new languages and ways of expressing ourselves in our worlds. The symbols, signs, and words that we use have inherent meaning. They are signifiers of who we are, what we are, and what is meaningful to us.

SUMMARY

The intent of this chapter can be summarized by borrowing Paterson's (1978) word:

> For responsible, effective existence the professional requires *language* (emphasis added) to relate authentically the purposes, beliefs, concerns, and events experienced continually to the nursing world. (p. 51)

A mystery exists in those phenomena listed by practicing nurses, but each seems to be a "thing in itself"—something waiting for description to bring it into our everyday awareness and to give it significance. It is as though we need to assert these events as belonging to nursing, to articulate our authentic experience with patients, and to claim what we and our patients believe to be essential to health and to our quality of existence. We then assign language to what is uniquely the abstract and the concrete, the enduring and the relevant meanings of shared human experience between patient and nurse. It is indeed a privilege and a calling to assist a patient in finding meaning in experience.

Qualitative research methods have much to offer as a research paradigm that is congruent with nursing's larger worldview, paradigm, or model. These methods offer ways to approach individuals in experiences, to encourage their giving voice to their experiencing, and to care enough to search for meaning within the experience. We refer again to Table 1–9 as an illustration of the language of the qualitative research methods, and leave our readers to draw their own conclusions. If this is your first time encountering the language of qualitative research, play the compact disc from the film 2001 to experience your new birth in language through music.

REFERENCES

Allen, D. (1995). Hermeneutics: Philosophy, traditions, and nursing practice research. *Nursing Science Quarterly,* 8(4), 175–181.

Anderson, W. *The Truth About Truth.* New York: Putnam, 1995.

American Heritage Dictionary. (1992). New York: American Heritage.

American Nurses' Association. (1995). *Nursing: A social policy statement.* Washington, DC: American Nurses' Association.

Ashworth, P. D. (1997). The variety of qualitative research (Part 2: Nonpositivist approaches. *Nurse Education Today* 17(3), 219–224.

Belenky, M., Clinchy, B., Goldberg, N., & Taub, J. (1986). *Women's ways of knowing: The development of self, voice and mind.* New York: Basic Books.

Benner, P. (Ed.). (1994). *Interpretive phenomenology: Embodiment, caring, and ethics in health and illness.* Thousand Oaks, CA: Sage.

Bronowski, J. (1965). *Science and human values* (rev. ed.). New York: Harper & Row.

Chinn, P. (1983). Editorial. *Advances in Nursing Science,* 5(2), ix.

Chinn, P. (1985). Debunking myths in nursing theory and research. *Image: The Journal of Nursing Scholarship,* 17(2), 45–49.

Clark, A. M. (1998). The qualitative-quantitative debate: Moving from positivism and confrontation to post-positivism and reconciliation. *Journal of Advanced Nursing,* 27, 1242–1249.

Corbin, V. (1999). Misusing phenomenology in nursing research: Identifying the basic issues. *Nurse Researcher* 6(3), 52–65.

DeVries, P. (1983). *Slouching towards Kalamazoo.* Boston: Little, Brown.

Dickoff, J., & James, P. (1968). A theory of theories: A position paper. *Nursing Research*, 17, 197–203.

Diers, D. (1979). *Research to nursing practice*. Philadelphia: Lippincott.

Dilthey, W. (1926). *Meaning in history*. London: Allen & Unwin. [Cited in G. Atwood & R. Stolorow. (1984). *Structures of subjectivity: Explorations in psychoanalytic phenomenology*. Hillsdale, NJ: Analytic Press.]

Downs, F. (1982). It's a great idea but it won't work. *Nursing Research*, 31(1), 4.

Dzurec, L. (1989). The necessity for and evolution of multiple paradigms for nursing research: A poststructuralist perspective. *Advances in Nursing Science*, 11 (4), 69–77.

Filstead, W. (1979). Qualitative methods: A needed perspective in evaluation research. In C. Reichardt & T. Cook (Eds.), *Qualitative and quantitative methods to evaluation research*. Beverly Hills, CA: Sage.

Gilligan, C. (1978). In a different voice: Women's conception of self and of morality. *Harvard Education Review*, 47, 481–517.

Heidegger, M. (1962). *Being and time* (J. Macprairie & E. Robinson, Trans.). New York: Harper & Row.

Kaplan, A. (1964). *The conduct of inquiry*. Scranton, PA: Chandler.

Kirby, D. (1983). Seeing the points of contact in a plural world. *The Chronicle of Higher Education*, 26(7), 25.

Kneller, G. (1964). *Introduction to the philosophy of education*. New York: Wiley.

Kuhn, T. S. (Ed.). (1970). *The structure of scientific revolutions*. Chicago: University of Chicago Press.

Laudan, L. (1977). *Progress and its problems: Toward a theory of scientific growth*. Berkeley: University of California Press.

Light, R., & Pillemer, D. (1982). Numbers and narrative: Combining their strengths in research reviews. *Harvard Education Review*, 51 (1), 1–23.

Looft, W. (1973). Socialization and personality throughout the life span: An examination of contemporary psychological approaches. In P. Baltes & K. Schaie (Eds.), *Life-span developmental psychology*. New York: Academic Press.

Meshier, E. (1979). Meaning in context: Is there any other kind? *Harvard Education Review*, 49(1), 1–19.

Moccia, P. (1988). A critique of compromise: Beyond the methods debate. *Advances in Nursing Science*, 10(4), 1–9.

Morgan, G. (1983). *Beyond method: Strategies for social research* (pp. 377–382). Newbury Park, CA: Sage.

Munhall, P. (1982a). Ethical juxtaposition in nursing research. *Topics in Clinical Nursing*, 4(1), 66–73.

Munhall, P. (1982b). Nursing philosophy and nursing research: In apposition or opposition? *Nursing Research*, 31(3), 176–177, 181.

Munhall, P. (1986). Methodological issues in nursing: Beyond a wax apple. *Advances in Nursing Science,* 8(3), 1–5.

Munhall, P. (1989). Philosophical pondering on qualitative research methods in nursing. *Nursing Science Quarterly,* 2, 20–28.

Munhall, P. (1992a). A new age ism: Beyond a toxic apple. *Nursing and Health Care,* 13 (7), 370–375.

Munhall, P. (1992b). Holding the Mississippi River in place and other implications for qualitative research. *Nursing Outlook,* 10(6), 257–262.

Munhall, P. (1993). Toward a fifth pattern of knowing: Unknowing. *Nursing Outlook,* 41, 125–128.

Munhall, P. (1994). *Qualitative research: Proposals and reports.* New York: National League for Nursing.

Munhall, P. (1997). *Déjà Vu,* Parroting, Buy-ins, and Opening. In J. Fawcett & I. King, *The language of nursing theory and metatheory.* Indianapolis, IN: Sigma Theta Tau International.

Newman, M. A. (1983). Editorial. *Advances in Nursing Science,* 5(2), x–xi.

Newman, M. A. (1999). The rhythm of relating in a paradigm of wholeness. *Image: Journal of Nursing Scholarship,* 31(3), 227–230.

Norris, C. (1982). *Concept clarification in nursing.* Rockville, MD: Aspen.

Paterson, J. (1978). The tortuous way toward nursing theory. In *Theory development: What, why and how?* New York: National League for Nursing.

Paterson, J. A., & Zderad, L. J. (1976, reissued 1988). *Humanistic nursing.* New York: National League for Nursing.

Patton, M. Q. (1978). *Utilization focused evaluation.* Beverly Hills, CA: Sage.

Piaget, J. (1970). *Structuralism.* New York: Basic Books.

Pinch, W. (1981). Feminine attributes in a masculine world. *Nursing Outlook,* 12, 29–36.

Reichardt, C., & Cook, T. (Eds.). (1979). *Qualitative and quantitative methods in evaluation research.* Beverly Hills, CA: Sage.

Roberts, S. (1973). Oppressed group behavior: Implications for nursing. *Advances in Nursing Science,* 5(4), 21–30.

Rorty, R. *Essays on Heidegger and others.* New York: Cambridge University Press, 1991.

Skinner, B. (1953). *Science and human behavior.* New York: Appleton-Century-Crofts.

Snow, C. P. (1959). *The two cultures and the scientific revolution.* Cambridge, England: Cambridge University Press.

Suppe, F. (Ed.). (1977). *The structure of scientific theories* (2nd ed.). Champaign: University of Illinois Press.

Swanson, J., & Chenitz, C. (1982). Why qualitative research in nursing? *Nursing Outlook,* 30(4), 241–245.

Tinkle, M., & Beaton, J. (1983). Toward a new view of science: Implications for nursing research. *Advances in Nursing Science*, 5(2), 27–36.

Van Manen, M. (1990). *Research lived experience: Human science for an action sensitive pedagogy.* New York: SUNY Press.

Wald, F., & Leonard, R. (1964). Towards development of nursing practice theory. *Nursing Research*, 13, 4–9.

Walker, L., & Avant, K. (1983). *Strategies for theory construction in nursing.* Norwalk, CT: Appleton-Century-Crofts.

Walters, A. J. (1996). Nursing research methodology: Transcending Cartesianism. *Nursing Inquiry*, 3(2), 91–100.

Watson, J. (1981). Nursing's scientific quest. *Nursing Outlook*, 29(7), 413–416.

Watson, J. (1999). *Post modern nursing and beyond.* New York: Churchill Livingston.

West, M. (1983). *The world is made of glass.* New York: Morrow.

Zen Buddhism. (1959). Mount Vernon, NY: Peter Pauper Press.

ADDITIONAL REFERENCES

Allen, D., Benner, P., & Diekelmann, N. (1985). Three paradigms for nursing research: Methodological implications. In P. Chinn (Ed.), *Nursing research methodology issues and implementation* (chap. 3). Rockville, MD: Aspen.

Baer, E. (1979). Philosophy provides the rationale for nursing's multiple research directions. *Image*, 2(3), 72–74.

Benoliel, J. (1984). Advancing nursing science: Qualitative approaches. *Western Journal of Nursing Research*, 6(3), 1–8.

Chenetz, W. C., & Swanson, J. M. (1986). *From practice to grounded theory: Qualitative research in nursing.* Menlo Park, CA: Addison Wesley.

Dossey, L. (1982). *Space, time and medicine.* Boulder, CO: Shambala.

Fawcett, J. (1983). Hallmarks of success in nursing theory development. In P. Chinn (Ed.), *Advances in nursing theory development* (chap. 1). Rockville, MD: Aspen.

Field, P., & Morse, J. (1985). *Nursing research: The application of qualitative approaches.* Rockville, MD: Aspen.

Gorenberg, B. (1983). The research tradition of nursing: An emerging issue. *Nursing Research*, 32, 347–349.

Harden, J. (2000). Language, discourse and the chronotope: Applying literary theory to the narratives in health care. *Journal of Advanced Nursing*, 31, 506–512.

Johnson, J. (1991). Nursing science: Basic applied or practical implications for the art of nursing. *Nursing Research*, 14, 7–15.

Leininger, M. (1985). *Qualitative research methods in nursing.* New York: Grune & Stratton.

Ludemann, R. (1979). The paradoxical nature of nursing research. *Image, 2,* 2–8.

MacPherson, K. I. (1983). Feminists methods: A new paradigm for nursing research. *Advances in Nursing Science, 5,* 17–25.

Matson, F. (1964). *The broken image.* New York: George Brazillier.

Meleis, A. (1985). *Theoretical nursing: Development and progress.* Philadelphia: Lippincott.

Moccia, P. (Ed.). (1986). *New approaches in theory development.* New York: National League for Nursing.

Morse, J. M. (1999). Qualitative methods: The state of the art. *Qualitative Health Research, 9,* 393–406.

Newman, M. A. (1979). *Theory development in nursing.* Philadelphia: Davis.

Newman, M. A. (1986). *Health as expanding consciousness.* St. Louis, MO: Mosby.

Oiler, C. (1982). The phenomenological approach in nursing research. *Nursing Research, 31*(3), 178–181.

Oiler, C. (1986). Qualitative methods: Phenomenology. In P. Moccia (Ed.), *New approaches to theory development.* New York: National League for Nursing.

Omery, A. (1983). Phenomenology: A method for nursing research. *Advances in Nursing Science, 5*(2), 49–64.

Reeder, J. (1987). The phenomenological movement. *Image, 19,* 150–152.

Sarter, B. (1988). Philosophical sources of nursing theory. *Nursing Science Quarterly, 1,* 52–59.

Silva, M. C. (1977). Philosophy, science, theory: Interrelationships and implications for nursing research. *Image, 9*(5), 59–63.

Watson, J. (1985). *Nursing: Human science and human care and theory of nursing.* Norwalk, CT: Appleton-Century-Crofts.

Epistemology in Nursing

Patricia L. Munhall

> . . . since we have come to the understanding that science is not a description of "reality" but a metaphorical ordering of experiences, the new science does not impugn the old. It is not a question of which view is "true" in some ultimate sense. Rather, it is a matter of which picture is more useful in guiding human affairs.—Willis Harman

I qualified in the preceding chapter that perhaps I might appear culpable of unnecessary polarization of worldviews; so I hope the reader understands that this indulgence is for ease in conceptual clarity and pedagogical purposes. Furthermore, I could not agree more with Gould (1984) when he observed that

> Dichotomy is the usual pathway to vulgarization. We take a complex web of arguments and divide it into two polarized positions—them against us. We then portray "them" as a foolish caricature of extremes in order to put "us" in a better light. (p. 7)

However, complex webs are starker when placed in contrasting systems; the differences between the systems become more focused. Our intention is not to see one system as the truth but to see each as different. As Harman (1977) stated, "It is not a question of which view is true [but which] is more useful in guiding human affairs." This is our connectedness with the subject. In this chapter, we propose an epistemology for nursing research that, as a whole, incorporates the qualitative and quantitative methods of research. This does not represent a conciliatory effort at compromise but rather a belief in a cyclical continuum that begins with discovery and moves toward verification. These activities represent, respectively, the first- and second-order activities of science. We believe there are appropriate research methods for different questions, and errors occur when a method is used prematurely or acontextually to answer a specific question or solve a problem. As was suggested in Chapter 1, there are times when many research traditions are amalgamated to produce a synthesis that is progressive to both traditions (Laudan, 1977). Perhaps at this time in our development we are witnessing a search for ontological and epistemological authenticity (Guba & Lincoln, 1989) in which we recognize the multiplicity of perspectives and perception of reality and in which postmodernism

> . . . is an intellectual movement (and as such) challenges the
> ideas of a single correct approach to knowledge development, of
> a single truth, and has a single meaning of reality, rejecting the
> ideal that there is one true story about reality (Uris, 1993, p. 95).

In this chapter, there will be an overview discussion of paths to knowledge, the purpose of science, research paradigms, and research traditions. I will attempt to answer the questions "Knowing about what?" and "How do we get to know?" as well as "Toward what end?" and will then propose a qualitative-quantitative cyclical continuum for knowing. Emphasis throughout is on qualitative research methods in response to a need identified by Johnson (1978), who stated: "We are beginning at the wrong end . . . engaging in experimental research before the variables significant to that research have been determined" (p. 9). In the year 2000, we saw, because of the situated context of the necessity of grant funding, this same process. We witnessed once again the dominance of the scientific method for funding purposes. As researchers and students of research, it is critical that we understand that, for any research enterprise to be authentic, we must begin with qualitative inquiry as a foundation from which we can identify variables, understand the context of experiences, and develop instrumentation. In this chapter, the theme as articulated by Morgan (1983), will guide us:

> To steer clear of the delusion that it is possible to know in an
> absolute sense of "being right" and devote our energies to the
> more constructive process of dealing with the implication of our
> different ways of knowing. (p. 18)

I also envision a postmodern perspective where the necessity for and evolution of multiple paradigms for nursing research will create new possibilities of coming to understand and develop the knowledge that is necessary to nursing practice par excellence.

This is the study of epistemology in nursing, that branch of philosophy that deals with knowledge and how we come to know about the world as we experience it.

PATHS TO KNOWLEDGE

Knowledge for nursing, about nursing, in nursing—where does this knowledge come from? In Chapter 1, we mentioned knowledge (theory) borrowed from related disciplines. Other disciplines are indeed one source of knowledge, perhaps more accurately stated from the perspective of Stevens's notion (1979, p. 85) of "shared knowledge": because disciplines have indistinct boundaries, there are areas "where the inquiries and answers of one field overlay those of another." At the turn of this century, we have almost abandoned the term "borrowed theory," recognizing the interconnectedness of various disciplines, and so today interdisciplinary research is encouraged by nurse researchers and often a requirement for funding.

However, caution must be used when identifying similarities to other disciplines and then utilizing those respective theoretical frameworks to derive hypotheses for nursing. We need to understand that, if the first- and second-order activities are not from the same world or discipline, there is a risk that the inquiry will not be logically consistent or experientially valid. In other words, the first-order activities of coming to know, discovering, and understanding are coming from another discipline and from that discipline's perspective. The second-order activities of validation and verification are then performed within the nursing discipline and applied to nursing's particular perspective. Before we go farther, however, let us in a foundational manner consider where knowledge generally comes from and some of the structures of knowing.

In a pedantic fashion, philosophers who study the way that we come to know (epistemologists) have identified specific sources of knowledge, generally acceptable as structures of knowing. Among them are (Kneller, 1971):

1. Revealed knowledge—knowledge that God has disclosed. Revelations of truth are found in the Bible, the Koran, and the Bhagavad-Gita. In the past decade, we have seen a growth of

research on spirituality—for example, religion as a source of comfort and inspiration; belief as having curative power; and so on. We do know that from revealed knowledge comes the imperative to care for and about one another.

2. Intuitive knowledge—knowledge within a person, in the form of insight that becomes present in consciousness; an idea or thought produced by a long process of unconscious work. This process of discovery is nurtured through experience with the world.

3. Rational knowledge—knowledge from the exercise of reason. This knowledge takes the form of abstract reasoning and is exemplified in the principles of formal logic and mathematics.

4. Empirical knowledge—knowledge formed in accordance with observed or sensed facts and associated with scientific hypotheses that are tested by observation or experiments.

5. Authoritative knowledge—knowledge accepted on faith because it is vouched for by authorities in the field.

In the foregoing brief description of the sources of knowledge, the one least attended to, but the one holding much potential for nursing, is intuitive knowledge, which for the purpose of this text will be experiential knowledge. The repudiation of intuition as a source of knowledge was one of the major themes when nursing moved toward establishing itself as a science. Intuition was unscientific; it was associated with women, who themselves were thought to be unscientific. More confident today, women of science—including nurses—recognize the vitalness of intuition and have come to trust and value this important source of knowledge.

Belenky, Clinchy, Goldberg, and Taub (1986), in describing the different ways in which women come to know, have legitimized to a great extent the place of intuition, personal meanings, and the connection to ideas as means of knowing. Rather than focusing on "proof," these women scientists seek understanding. The work of Gilligan (1982), Belenky et al. (1986), and Freiri (1971) challenges us all to rethink our concepts about epistemology—underlying assumptions and the critical consequences. Critical theory is one way to analyze the underlying structural and power relations inherent in the "sanctioned" ways of knowing (Allen, 1991). Allen (1995) expands the importance of critique in his discussion of critical hermeneutics with great emphasis on the subjective "reality" that research can socially construct.

Carper's (1978) framework of four fundamental patterns of knowing continues to be a way in which nursing identifies its epistemological interests. These patterns of knowing are described as follows:

1. Empirics—the science of nursing; emphasis is on the generation of theory and of research that is systematic and controllable by factual evidence. Within this pattern of knowing, there is a need for emphasis on knowledge about the empirical world, knowledge that will be organized into general laws and theories for the purpose of describing, explaining, and predicting phenomena of concern to nursing.

2. Esthetics—the art of nursing; emphasis is on expressiveness, subjective acquaintance, individual perceptions, and empathy. Rather than uniformity and general laws, there is recognition of alternative modes of perceiving reality, which then clearly asks for a "many different ways" approach to designing and participating in nursing care.

3. Personal knowledge—the focus is on the importance of the interpersonal process and the "therapeutic use of self"; on knowing the self, knowing the other as a subject, and striving toward authentic personal relations.

4. Ethics—the focus is on matters of obligation or what ought to be done. Knowledge within this domain requires an understanding of ethical theories, conditions of society, conflicts between different value systems, and ethical principles.

All of the foregoing patterns are rich and essential sources of nursing knowledge that can be studied from various perspectives of science.

I have suggested a fifth pattern of knowing, while at the same time questioning the categorizing of knowledge in this way (Munhall, 1993). The fifth pattern is one of "unknowing." "Knowing," in contrast with "unknowing," leads to a form of confidence that has the potential of a state of closure to alternatives and differences. "Unknowing," from an epistemological perspective, is a condition of openness and seems essential to the understanding of intersubjectivity and perspectivity. Kurtz (1989) stated:

[K]nowledge screens the sound the third ear hears, so we hear only what we know. (p. 6)

We can become limited by our own belief systems. Often, once we believe something or think we "know" something, we cease further exploration or explanation. Many practitioners in all fields will continue to hold the body of knowledge that they attained in their formal education. The impractibility and danger of continuing to do so in an unsurpassed age of knowledge explosion is apparent.

Only by unlearning comes wisdom.

—James Russel Lowell

Although the patterns of knowledge are presented for historical and pedantic reasons, they are organized as categories; I think we can see them as mutually interdependent, not mutually exclusive. Intuiting in the empirical world while using one's personal knowledge embedded in an ethical context or founded on a philosophical perspective is a holistic approach to theory development.

We move now from general structures of knowing to the purpose of exploring those structures. Because nursing has identified itself as a science, let us review the purpose of science or science in general. How does nursing conceptualize itself as a science?

PURPOSE OF SCIENCE

Laudan (1977), a philosopher, simply stated that the purpose of science is to solve problems, and theory tells us how to do so. He further proposed that the rationality and progressiveness of a theory are not linked with its confirmation or its falsification but instead with its problem-solving effectiveness. This conception of science opens the windows and doors in the hallowed halls of science to include important nonempirical and even nonscientific knowing in the traditional sense. This provides a broader perspective that Laudan suggested was necessary to the "rational development" of science. Insight, spontaneity, accidental findings, mutability, vicissitude, and fortune all play a role in science.

On the basis of this conception of science and theory, it seems to us that all sources of knowledge and patterns of knowing are essential sources for problem solving. Nursing research, in its earliest years, began its quest to become a legitimate science with an almost unilateral pattern of knowing that can be categorized as empirics, logical empiricism, logical positivism, or, as described in most nursing research textbooks, "the scientific method."

Laudan (1977) set forth—in contrast or in explanation—a philosophy of science of historicism that incorporates the human elements of science; the study of scientific knowledge is often fostered by illogical and nonrational decision making. The following two quotations may illuminate this point:

> That no major scientist ever has proceeded in his work along either Baconian or Catesian lines has not prevented the *consecration of method* by these two powerful minds from exacting a dismal toll [our italics]. (Nesbitt, 1976, p. 14)

> Insight announces itself in mental images. Newton's conception of gravity and Einstein's notion of the constant speed of light came to them as perceptions, as images, not a hypothesis or conclusions drawn from logical deduction. Formal logic is secondary to insight via images, and is never the source of new knowledge. (Bohm, 1981, p. 444)

Van Manen (1990), in contrast with Laudan's emphasis on problem solving, summarized what a phenomenological human science cannot do: "Phenomenology does not problem solve" (p. 23). Van Manen believed, from a research perspective, that phenomenological questions are "meaning" questions. However, one might wonder: If we did understand the meaning of specific phenomena, might we not have the basis for problem solving? Furthermore, might we also have understanding that could significantly contribute to the promotion of health and well-being? From his perspective, Van Manen stated:

> [N]atural science studies objects of nature, "things," "natural events" and the way that objects behave. Human science, in contrast, studies "persons" or beings that have "consciousness" and that act purposefully in and on the world by creating objects of "meaning" and that are expressions of how human beings exist in the world. (p. 4)

Allen (1995) argues further that meaning, understanding, and interpretation gleaned from acontextual research will lead us back to foundationalism. He describes foundationalism as referring "to the claim that there is a way to anchor knowledge by referring to ahistorical, nonsocial, non-contextual criteria" (p. 175). This adds to Lauden's science of historicism, of not only incorporating the vicissitudes of the scientist, and so forth, but also to enlarge; what is necessary to "knowing something" is the essential nature of also knowing what is going on in the contingencies of history and life-worlds when that knowing something occurs (see Chapter 5 for further discussion). We return to the postmodern idea that truth is not immutable and is indeed an ever-changing body of ideas and meaning contingent on multiple factors.

These ideas are not necessarily contradictory; rather, they seem to be woven together as a whole. In addition, discussions about sciences and methods of sciences often seem to lead us away from concrete, lived experiences unless "that" lived experience is the discussion of sciences. Researchers, I believe, need to be well grounded in the pedantic and philosophical underpinnings of the research enterprise but not for conformity, which can sacrifice creativity. We suggest to students that it is far more scientific to find a phenomenon that interests them, peaks their curiosity, and perhaps even fills them with passion than to become befuddled by method.[1] Substance should lead the way to form. Interest in some "thing" or "experience" should light many sparks of imagination and light the path to method.

However, it is essential to understand the influence and power of research paradigms and traditions in interweaving the ways of knowing and shaping them into a body of knowledge. They can be restricting or liberating, depending on their own ontology and supporting constituencies. Qualitative research methods seek to be of the liberating, illuminating, and emancipatory kind.

The critical nature embedded in research paradigms and traditions is found in the circumstance that they are rarely questioned in the study of a discipline. It is a rare undergraduate or graduate student in any field who questions the research methods prevalent in that field. If most of us find guidelines helpful and a research tradition provides us with those guidelines—and if success within the field will be determined by how well one follows those guidelines—the importance of those guidelines can hardly be overstated! The next section describes the nature of research paradigms and traditions connected with our discussion of paths to knowledge and the purpose of science. It is paradoxical to hear the purpose of education to be one of liberation and then to hear students cite the common wisdom of "just do what they tell you to do," subsuming to the unfair power structure that we often encounter in our educational settings.

---

[1]Van Manen's (1990) interpretation of why Gadamer's (1975) book *Truth and Method* became popular in North America is relevant and recommended to readers.

Paradigms and Research Traditions

Kuhn (1970) believed that a paradigm structures the questions to be asked within a discipline and systematically eliminates those kinds of questions that cannot be stated within the concepts and tools supplied by the paradigm. This function then is enormously powerful. A paradigm can actually prevent questions from being answered!

Laudan (1977), elaborating on his definition of a research tradition, wrote:

> A research tradition is a set of general assumptions about the entities and processes in a domain of study, and about the appropriate methods to be used for investigating the problems and constructing the theories in that domain. (p. 81)

In both these ways, as suggested by Kuhn and by Laudan, the research paradigm and tradition will specify the domain of study, the legitimate modes, and the methods of inquiry open to a researcher within a discipline. This directedness is seldom questioned; in fact, complicity is usually required as well as rewarded.

Why one proceeds in this fashion is explained by Laudan's idea that we need to explore the scientists' work and their reasoning processes. Laudan suggested that scientific knowledge is often developed by illogical and nonrational decision making. Let us now tie together that idea with nursing's historical acceptance of the logical empiricist's worldview or, as stated, the large reliance on logic and empirics as our primary paths to theory development.[2]

The preparation of many nurse researchers in fields in which the research tradition was one of logical empiricism was considered in Chapter 1. Let us look for evidence that supports the further use of this tradition and that may exemplify the nonrational or illogical side of science. This evidence is not always negative, but let us reflect on nursing research and on the subtle and not so subtle ways in which this paradigm or tradition has been perpetuated and still prevails today to a large extent.

The answers to the following questions, which were asked in the first edition of the book (1986), demonstrate how the values of scientists and their practices influence the general account of human nature. I believe it is quite significant that the same questions are relevant almost

---

[2]Silva and Rothbart (1984) have written a most readable and highly recommended work synthesizing this material. Dzurec (1989), presenting a poststructural perspective, should also be considered.

14 years later. I attempted to explain the reason for their relevance in a discussion of life-world fittingness (Munhall, 1992):

1. If you were to request a research grant from the Division of Nursing of the Department of Health and Human Services or the Center for Nursing Research, what research method do you believe would be viewed most favorably?
2. If you wanted guidelines for doing research and consulted the most prevalent nursing research textbooks, which research method would seemingly be the only one available? What is the research method most taught in our research classes?
3. If you wish to submit an abstract of research for a research conference, what research method is represented in the format for the abstract?
4. If you wanted to critique a research study, what method is most represented under criteria for evaluation?

Now in the third edition of this book, I might further ask us to consider additional questions:

1. If you are enrolled in a Ph.D. program, for what method does your required courses program you? (There are exceptions!)
2. If you are seeking a faculty position, how will you get the evidence of extramural funding that is required to be demonstrated?
3. Peruse the list of recent NINR (National Institute of Nursing Research) grants and ask, Which paradigm is most rewarded?

I believe that those nurse researchers who have been questioning the general acceptance of the answers to these questions begs the suggestion to enlarge our lens, to broaden our scope, to widen our perspective. Furthermore, the answers to these questions demonstrate the subjectivity of the entire research enterprise. Human beings determine which paths to explore. We need to explore all the paths to knowledge and all the patterns of knowing, because in some intuitive way we would then be celebrating the whole of the human condition.

Capra (1982) stated our need almost two decades ago:

> What we need, then, is a new vision of reality—a fundamental change in our thoughts, perceptions and values. The beginnings of this change, of the shift from the mechanistic to the holistic conception of reality, are already visible in all fields and are likely to dominate the entire decade. (p. ix)

My endeavor here, built upon the works of many nursing scholars, among them the contributors to this book, is to encourage this vision, to incorporate the qualitative and quantitative methods of research as representative of an epistemology of wholeness, and to respect and reward all patterns of knowing. Despite the answers to those questions, the processes and rewards of doing qualitative research certainly have continued to grow, and we have become more sophisticated and savvy. In fact, many NINR grants today require a qualitative section. That is progress!

It has been said that your research question should determine your research method. I am not sure that is the best way to think about choosing one's research method. Over many years, I have seen students have specific leanings toward one or another way of thinking. I believe these leanings reflect a natural attitude toward the world at large, and students, just as we acknowledge having different ways of learning material, also have different philosophical orientations toward questioning and how one answers those questions. I believe most of my colleagues respect these innate tendencies. Actually they should make the whole research enterprise holistic, more consistent with the times in which we live, and contribute to a much greater depth and breadth of knowing and understanding. Our differences enrich us and an inspire us to see the new.

Let us move now to a consideration of an epistemological question: "What is it that we want to know about?"; "What is it that we wish to understand?"

EPISTEMOLOGICAL INTERESTS OF NURSING

As stated earlier, one of the purposes of science is to solve problems, and the subsequent theory development involves the solution of problems (Laudan, 1977). Qualitative researchers would want to qualify that purpose with the caveat that, before you can solve a problem, you need to understand the many facets of "a" problem. In this section, we explore schemata that have been developed by nurses in an effort to focus nursing research on nursing phenomena.

Six nursing perspectives are summarized in an effort to identify our epistemological interests. They are presented chronologically and may demonstrate consistency, overlap, complementarity, and/or much variation. I begin with Paterson and Zderad, out of great respect for their major groundbreaking work of 1976, in which they were the first nurses to actually use the language and the method of phenomenology. It is important to understand these different perspectives so that one can debate the merits or lack of merit of the various perspectives. Each provides varying answers to the question, "What do nurses study?" We will also reexamine the ideas of Donaldson and Crowley (1978), The American Nurses' Association's Social Policy Statement (1995), Fawcett's (1984) metaparadigm for nursing, and the emphasis on care (Newman, Sime, & Corcoran-Perry, 1991; Watson, 1985), and we will conclude with Watson's (1999) ideas of what nurses should be studying as we move into this new century. I need to let the reader know that this summary does not do justice to the field of theory development, nor does it intend to, because the intent of this section is to consider exemplars and a historical perspective. Undoubtedly, if you are reading this book, you probably are very knowledgeable about theory and can ask, What does a particular theorist think we should "know" and "how" should we research their particular phenomena? These questions would provide a good seminar discussion.

Paterson and Zderad (1976), to the question "What do nurses study?" (or "What should nurses study?"), might reply in this manner. Because the act of nursing is "the intersubjective transactional relation, a dialogue experience, lived in concert between persons where comfort and nurturance produce mutual human unfolding," nurses would do well to study the following situations (Paterson, 1978, p. 51):

1. Comfort—persons being all that they can be in particular life situations.
2. Nurturance—promoting growth through relating.
3. Clinical—presence in the health situation, reflected and acted upon.
4. Empathy—imaginative moving toward oneness with another, sharing his or her being in a situation, resulting in an insightful knowledge of another's perspective.
5. All-at-once awareness of living many concepts, emotions, desires, and beliefs in a particular instance.

From these situations, the phenomenon of concern to nurses is one in need of quality nursing descriptions of those experiences inherent in the preceding situations and suggested in Table 1–7. Paterson and Zderad (1976) called our attention to existential, humanistic, phenomenological phenomena that should be our epistemological interests. This they did in 1976 and the reader can see how future oriented they were. I urge students of current theory to read through their pioneering book that prompted reissuing the same book in 1988.

Widely cited and more traditional, yet showing promises of a new worldview, were Donaldson and Crowley (1978), who identified three major themes of nursing:

1. Concern with the principles and laws that govern the life processes, well-being, and optimum functioning of human beings, sick or well.
2. Concern with the patterning of human behavior in interaction with the environment in critical life situations.
3. Concern with the processes by which positive changes in health status are affected.

Concepts within the nurse–client world that relate to the preceding themes need to be discovered, and the methods of the first order of scientific activity, the qualitative methods of science, are essential to this process. Within this book, an effort is made to demonstrate this basic activity of discovering what is there, naming it, understanding it, and explaining it. We can then give examples of what is *meant* and what is the potential within the scope of these themes.

Our own professional organization, The American Nurses' Association, has consistently revised its definition of nursing according to society's needs and has focused nurse researchers' perspective on human responses within the following context: "Nursing is the diagnosis and treatment of human responses to actual or potential health problems" (1995). Possible phenomena that bear investigation from this perspective of nursing are further suggested. They include:

1. Self-care limitations
2. Impaired functioning–physiological needs
3. Pain and discomfort
4. Emotional problems, such as anxiety, loss, loneliness, and grief
5. Distortion of symbolic functions
6. Deficiencies in decision making
7. Self-image changes
8. Dysfunctional perceptual orientations
9. Strains related to life processes
10. Problematic affiliative relations

Readers familiar with the works of Rogers (1970), Roy (1976), Johnson (1980), Orem (1980), King (1981), Watson (1985), and other nursing theorists can readily see the influence of these theorists on the various phenomena that would constitute human responses.

Fawcett (1984) identified in her earlier works a metaparadigm for nursing in pursuit of establishing boundaries within which the purview of nursing can be delineated. She proposed that the metaparadigm comprises the central concepts and themes that represent the phenomena of interest to the discipline. Paradigms, then, are the conceptual models that provide "distinctive contexts for the metaparadigm concepts and themes" (p. 2).

The metaparadigm of nursing that has evolved, according to Fawcett (1984, p. 2), consists of four major concepts: person, environment, health, and nursing. These central concepts are defined as:

1. Person—the recipient of care.
2. Environment—significant others and the surroundings of the recipient of care; the setting in which nursing care takes place.
3. Health—the wellness or illness state of the recipient at the time when nursing occurs.
4. Nursing—actions taken by nurses on behalf of or in conjunction with the recipient of care.

Fawcett (1984) added the themes explicated by Donaldson and Crowley, presented earlier, to the metaparadigm of nursing by indicating the central concepts and the themes that should represent the phenomena of interest to nurse investigators. She then suggested that the four patterns of knowledge, as discussed by Carper (1978) and in this chapter, link the concepts and themes.

With these varying perspectives had come articles that called for a focus of the discipline of nursing. Newman et al. (1991) pointed out that its domain of inquiry distinguishes a discipline. As is readily apparent in the foregoing paragraph, nursing has a rather large domain of inquiry. Newman et al. (1991) suggested that nursing should have a focus statement. They pointed out that, from the time of Florence Nightingale to the present era of Leininger (1984), Watson (1988), and Benner and Wrubel (1989), health and caring have been linked. Incorporating Pender's (1987) use of the term "health experience," Newman's focus statement at the time was:

Nursing is the study of caring in the human health experience. (p. 3)

Nursing's domain of inquiry was then stated as "caring in the human health experience" (p. 3).

Present-day perspectives in nursing research and theory seem to have evolved from this eclecticism of thought. This eclectism is philosophically congruent with the world at large. Today the prefixes "multi" and "poly" are frequently used to reflect the shift from foundationalism to hermeneutics, or interpretation of phenomena. Newman (1986) and Watson (1999) are among the many nursing scholars who have expanded the worldview of nursing and the domains for nursing inquiry. Postmodern in their perspectives, they recognize that whatever is studied must be viewed within the context and possibility of multiple realities. The idea that individuals, families, cultures, and societies construct their own realities is readily evident in a world that all of a sudden has found itself so interconnected—that what we hear is polyvocality, what we see is individually perspectival, and what we read is contextually interpreted. Multiple realities are recognized as being based on subjective experience; so multiplicity and multimind emerge. Qualitative researchers are most synchronous with these conditions of uncertainty, flux, discontinuity, and indeterminacy. Qualitative researchers have long recognized the social construction of reality, contingencies, and the situated context as critical parts of their research efforts. This topic will be further considered in the next section, but, for our purposes here, whatever domains or phenomena nurses want to research, it is most important to take into account the situatedness of a person in a multiworld of endless variations.

Perhaps we should enjoy the complexity of our profession because it affords us an opportunity to study and research an almost infinite variety of human and environmental phenomena. Some could say we are "all over the place"; and, in actuality, nurses themselves are all over the place, in every developmental phase of an individual's life, in health and in crisis, in private practice, in schools, in hospitals, in foreign countries, and in the homes of patients. They are practitioners, educators, administrators, writers, researchers, and politicians. With all this complexity, it is quite understandable why nurses would need a variety of research methods or approaches from which to choose.

EPISTEMOLOGICAL COMMITMENTS TO QUALITATIVE RESEARCH

In the foregoing discussion, we presented different perspectives or views of what nurses might investigate. Their broad scope reflects the expansiveness of the profession of nursing. Discussions among theorists and researchers often revolve around narrowing this scope, perhaps by adopting one model or accepting, for equally good reasons, a multiple-perspective approach. I, personally, do not think we have any choice but to be representative of the world and, being in the world, that demands a multiperspectival epistemological commitment. In Chapter 1, we defined quantitative methods of research as:

> The traditional scientific method as presented in most of the contemporary nursing research textbooks, characterized by deductive reasoning, objectivity, quasi-experiments, statistical techniques, and control.

In contrast, we defined the qualitative methods, many of which are described within this text, as "characterized by inductive reasoning, subjectivity, discovery, description, and process orienting" (Reichardt & Cook, 1979). Benoliel (1984) enhances that description in this observation:

> Qualitative approaches in science are distinct modes of inquiry oriented toward understanding the unique nature of human thoughts, behaviors, negotiations and institutions under different sets of historical and environmental circumstances. (p. 7)

We should view these two approaches from a historical perspective. During the seventeenth century, empiricism, as the scientific method, reigned supreme. That form of empiricism proceeds through sense knowledge, and that which connects with our senses is matter. This often is the origin of conceived objectivity, in which the physical world can be seen, touched, or measured. The hold that matter (materialism) has on us is connected with the simple fact that we think we can get hold of matter and control it. Thus, we have the controlled experiment with validation, significance, and the premise of confidence and prediction. As has been suggested, nursing research has, to a large extent, aligned itself with this positivistic and materialistic view of science.

In the 1993 edition of this book, we discussed the postpositivistic perspective articulated by Polkinghorne (1983), who cited recognition and acceptance of the following factors as enlarging the scope of science:

1. Different language systems reflect different perceptions of the same reality (as was illustrated in Chapter 1).
2. The essential study of complex wholes is through system theory, and human beings are complex wholes.
3. The ideas of purposive and intentional activity explain human action.
4. All knowledge, instead of being truth, is an expression of interpretation.

Such beliefs and assumptions have contributed to the acceptance of the worthiness and credibility of methods of knowing other than the positivistic worldview. Additionally, there has been growing acceptance and recognition of the differences between the material and the experiential nature of human behavior and relationships. Benoliel (1984) cited some of these differences as follows:

1. Social life is the shared creativity of individuals and their *perceptions* [emphasis added].

2. The character of the social world is *dynamic* and *changing* [emphasis added].

3. There are *multiple realities* and frameworks for viewing the world: the world is not independent of mankind and objectively identifiable [emphasis added].

4. Human beings are active agents who *construct* their *own* realities [emphasis added].

5. There are not any response sets that are highly predictable. (p. 4)

Since that edition, one can easily see how these ideas have come to expression in most contemporary philosophies of nursing. Because the emergent nursing philosophies reflect, whether stated or not, post-structualist or postmodern perspectives, the stated beliefs and values about the individual are congruent with the research methods presented in this text. We are involved in an emergent shift from the modern characteristics of science to a postmodern perspective on science. This shift is not a negation of science but recognition of a "more." Science expands its boundaries from strict materialism and recognizes the need for accommodating a dynamic reality and describing individual situatedness to be essential to good research.

The shifts that are most prevalent in the qualitative domain are: the focus on meaning of experience, understanding what it means to be in this world, or that world, listening to others to provide us with this material, and interpretation by both the research participant and the researcher.

Contrary to the traditional scientific method, where the problem is stated at the outset of the research project, the qualitative researcher usually begins with a phenomenon or an experience. Going to the people who are involved in the phenomenon or experience, the qualitative researcher engages with the participant and the environment and lets both speak to her or him. The narratives, semiotics, and interaction allow for the development of coming to understand some "thing." Problems may emerge as part of the wholeness of the experience, but the identification of the problem comes from the source, the individual in experience.

This involvement calls for the nurse researcher to have many characteristics of her or his own. I would say that it is important for qualitative researchers to have a grasp on the complexness of experience, of its wholeness. Rather than compartmentalizing experience into two or three different variables, which may be necessary in experimental research, experience needs to be met with "openness" by the researcher. In addition to steps that qualitative researchers take to be open and are described in the various method chapters, the researcher needs to be the one who is "unknowing." The participant is the expert who is imparting to us existential material that should be cointerpreted and then interpreted for its implications for nursing practice.

For many years, I have interacted with colleagues and students, and as much as I attempt not to categorize individuals, there does appear to be propensities among and between us. These propensities are grounded in each of own lived world and experiences; so we seem to find our own paths, our own journeys, and our own commitments, all of which assist us in forming our own ontology. Your beliefs and values about being and the meaning of being should be the guideposts to your choosing methods of inquiry. As stated elsewhere in this text, I do not believe that your research question in its specifics should be the determining factor in selecting a method.

I believe that, before specific questions for research are formulated, overarching questions and commitments should guide researchers in choosing a research method. What is it that interests you? Do you think of yourself as more concrete and more comfortable with structure? Do you like discovering relations, correlations, and possible solutions to problems? Do you find beauty in a perfect scientific design with complex statistical analysis? If you have these propensities, so to speak, then what we are calling quantitative designs are probably what you will enjoy doing and be successful at, as well as contributing to nursing's body of knowledge.

For those who are considering qualitative research methods, such researchers need to be more comfortable with uncertainty and not necessarily problem oriented. The primary focus is on meaning, and the aims of inquiry are found in understanding and interpretation. A critical commitment is to faithfully, without your own presuppositions or judgments, represent another's experience, meaning, and interpretation. There needs to be an authentic caring about how another person perceives his or her world, and there needs to be authentic respect for many differences.

These considerations do not in any way imply that a nurse researcher cannot combine these commitments. Indeed many hold all these commitments toward research. Yet, in the years of my own experience, students and researchers seem to "show" different ways of being in the world, and reflection and recognition of one's leanings should be clearly thought out before embarking on learning a specific method, because that is a commitment itself.

And that brings us to considering the last commitment in this section. This text on qualitative methods and considerations is an overview, as are most textbooks. If you are interested and even excited about a specific method, this is your first step: reading the chapter on method and the exemplar. The real commitment is to the further in-depth and breadth study of the particular method, its philosophical, ontological, theoretical, and conceptual underpinnings and the human requirements, abilities, and characteristics needed to implement the method well. With more and more reading and practice, you will evolve, change, understand, have your own insights, and truly understand what it is that you are doing in a way that becomes a part of you. So the first "meaning," "understanding," and "interpretation" are those of the experience itself, those of coming to grasp the wholeness and complexity of the method.

An Epistemological Circle

Questions are often asked about the relatedness of quantitative and qualitative methods or if there is a relation at all. Chapter 18 of this book addresses this question. Reading Chapter 18 might not yield the following epistemological circle, but here it is offered as one perspective. This conceptualization is one of process and demonstrates how theory evolves, is revised by a nuance, and is first discovered through qualitative inquiry and validated in some way by quantitative inquiry. Quantitative inquiry in a human science, I believe, should always have its origins in qualitative inquiry. Otherwise the researcher is the "knower" of the experience and the phenomenon, and therefore, whatever instrument is developed or intervention tested, it is grounded in the life-world of the researcher, rather than the life-world of those who are experiencing "knowers" and who can inform, through their sharing with us, the descriptions and interpretations necessary for congruency grounded in specific contexts.

My own dissertation was an example of "not" following this sequence (Munhall, 1982). Using an instrument, which was derived and tested on an only male population, Kohlberg (1976) derived a theory on moral development based solely on his male sample. Unknowingly, I used an instrument based on his theory on women, and they performed much "lower" in scores than the norms. The norms, I did not realize, were based only on males. After Carol Gilligan's (1982) groundbreaking work, *In A Different Voice*, I came to realize why my own sample of nurses did not fare so well.

The article that I wrote critiquing my own study and illustrating that the utilization of a theory and instrument derived from another population was a great epistemological error was rejected by a nursing research journal. The grounds for rejection were "that the last thing we need in nursing research is criticizing ourselves." The manuscript found a home (1983), and I do hope it called attention to the need for this epistemological circle and the thorough thinking through of any method, as well as the critical need for self-critique of one's research.

The purpose of this nonlinear schema, in which qualitative descriptions, interpretations, and understandings lead to quantitative analysis (when that is appropriate) and from that analysis, nuances or what Kuhn (1970) terms anomalies, become sources of further qualitative inquiry. For example, many studies statistically support the proposition that preoperative teaching reduces anxiety for the majority of preoperative patients. There are some patients, however, in whom such teaching increases anxiety. This is a nuance and calls us back to a qualitative study: "What about those patients?" We need now to discriminate further within our populations. Theories always need reevaluating, and the nuances or the exceptions often alert us to alternative or evolving ways of viewing phenomena. Thus, the qualitative–quantitative cyclical continuum represents the dynamic and changing life-worlds. The linkages of the qualitative and quantitative methods are circular, as shown in Figure 2–1. This circularity does not have to be the outcome of all qualitative research. The findings of qualitative research can stand on their own merit with implications for nursing practice found in the descriptions, interpretations, and narratives by the researcher. However, for congruency in arriving at hypothesis, a qualitative base line from the same situated context—that is, people, place, time, culture, sex, and other characteristics—should be the origin of good quantitative research. Perhaps Campbell (1975) summarizes this point best when he says:

> After all, man in his ordinary way is a very competent knower, and qualitative common sense is not replaced by quantitative knowing. Rather quantitative knowing has to trust and build on the qualitative, including ordinary perception. We methodologists must achieve an applied epistemology which integrates both. (p. 191)

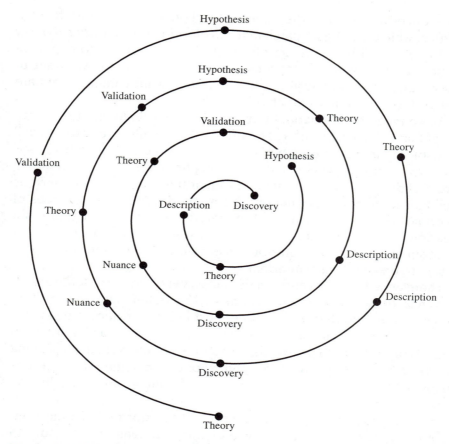

Figure 2–1 Qualitative–quantitative cyclical continuum. A nuance is defined here as a variation or a subtle aspect or quality.

READING SUBSEQUENT CHAPTERS

At this juncture I hope that you the reader hold with me the belief in the rich potential that qualitative methods of research have to offer to our practice, our understanding of ourselves, patients, the multi-worlds in which we live, and what it means to be human at this time in history. I think we have come to understand the importance of the subjective experience of the one who experiences to the development of nursing theory. In the first two chapters, there has been an attempt to provide the background necessary to understand the differences in language, the philosophical perspectives, and the contexts in which nursing research first developed and continues to grow and evolve. Additionally, an effort has been put forth to explicate patterns of knowing, the purpose of science, what it is we want to know about, how we go about knowing, and what commitments are needed to engage in qualitative research.

As we move on to Chapter 3, by Carolyn Oiler Boyd, the final chapter of Part I, the philosophical foundations of qualitative research will be explored in more depth and breadth. We will then be ready to read specifically how one goes about knowing from a qualitative perspective. Readers will become aware of similarities among the methods as well as variations in carrying out the methods. The term "degrees of freedom" is not associated with qualitative research, but there is a freedom about qualitative research, a flexibility, room to move about in, room to explore. Our contributors exemplify the courage often necessary to deal with such freedom.

There are similarities and congruencies, yet there are differences. As this chapter began, we quoted Harman in his belief that it matters less which view is true than what will be most helpful in guiding us in theory development. The studies reported here as examples of qualitative research seem to us excellent examples of the humanistic, caring perspective that embraces the philosophy of nursing. They are descriptive of experience at the very core of human caring and human understanding.

In Chapter 4, Carolyn Boyd describes the major philosophical underpinnings of phenomenology and some prevalent methods. In Chapter 5, I present a phenomenological method, which has evolved from my interactions with colleagues, students, and patients. Sarah Lauterbach in Chapter 6 presents new research, which is a longitudinal phenomenological study in which she returns to the mothers who experienced prenatal death of a wished-for baby 5 years ago. The first part of that study is in the second edition of this book and the reader is encouraged to study that phenomenological inquiry for an example of phenomenology inquiry when it is closer to the experience in a temporal sense. Reading about the experience of these mothers 5 years later is extremely moving and demonstrates the need for this kind of understanding for nursing practice, as did Sarah's first study.

Sally A. Hutchinson and Holly Skodal Wilson, in Chapter 7, introduce us to the potential and possibilities of the Grounded Theory Method, another qualitative research method. JoAnne Weiss and Sally Hutchinson provide us with an exemplar study titled "Understanding Clients

Health-Care Decisions." This study, Chapter 8, challenges our current beliefs about health care education and directs us to the perceptions and processes that patients use when given information.

Carol P. Germain clearly describes the method of ethnography in Chapter 9. Zane Robinson Wolf, in Chapter 10, demonstrates the richness derived from this method with findings critical for cardiac patients and their symptom management.

The Case Study method is presented by Carla Mariano in Chapter 11 and is poignantly illustrated by Mary Colvin in her compelling study: Drifting Without Consciousness.

The historical method of research is described by M. Louise Fitzpatrick in Chapter 13 and demonstrated in a fascinating historical study by Lynne Dunphy. This study, Chapter 14, is a history of nursing care of patients in iron lungs, from 1928 to 1955.

New to this edition is the method of Interpretive Analysis, written by Richard MacIntyre in Chapter 15. Richard then goes on in Chapter 16 to demonstrate the role of critical theory in his interpretive analysis of "Religion as Metaphor" in a study involving people with AIDS or HIV.

Another new method, called Action Research, and exemplar are added to this third edition. Carolyn Brown, in Chapter 17, provides us with a description of this method, and Jody Glittenburg, Chapter 18, provides us with a "snowball" exemplar!

These chapters conclude Part II of this text, and Part III consists of a general discussion about various considerations, techniques, and conditions for qualitative research that influence all of the foregoing methods.

Chapter 19 presents ethical considerations in qualitative research and, closely related to ensuring the ethical dimensions, a discussion on institutional review boards is the topic of Chapter 20.

Chapter 21 is a new chapter on interview strategies and analysis by Janice Morse. Carolyn Oiler Boyd describes the issues and the possibilities of combining qualitative and quantitative methods in Chapter 22.

Chapter 23, by Julie Evertz, describes the evaluation and critiquing of qualitative research. Chapter 24 helps the researcher with suggestions for qualitative research proposal and reports.

Chapter 25 is another new chapter in which Maureen Duffy presents the sources for qualitative researchers to be found on the Internet.

For students who would like to read further exemplars of the first five methods articulated in this book, those different exemplars or examples of the method can be found in the first and second editions of this book (Munhall & Oiler, 1986, 1993). Those studies are well worth returning to, not only for their richness, but to further explicate the particular method.

Returning to nursing's epistemological domains for inquiry, the reader can see in all these studies the humanistic, caring, and compassionate characteristics that envelop both researcher and participant. They are descriptive and interpretive of persons in experience, providing us with a "knowing" that cannot ever be known without listening to the best "knower" of all, the one who experiences and gives meaning to the phenomenon of inquiry.

REFERENCES

Allen, D. (1991). Applying critical social theory to nursing education. In N. Greenleaf (Ed.), *Curriculum revolution: Redefining the student-teacher relationship*. New York: National League for Nursing.

Allen, D. (1995). Hermeneutics: Philosophy, traditions, and nursing practice research. *Nursing Science Quarterly*, 8:4 (175–181).

American Nurses' Association. (1995). *Nursing: A social policy statement*. Kansas City: American Nurses' Association.

Anderson, W. (1995). *The truth about truth*. New York: Putnam.

Appleton, J. V., & King, L. (1997). Constructivism: A naturalistic methodology for nursing inquiry. *Advances in Nursing Science*, 20(2), 13–22.

Belenky, M., Clinchy, B., Goldberg, N., & Taub, J. (1986). *Women's ways of knowing*. New York: Basic Books.

Benner, P., & Wrubel, J. (1989). *The primacy of caring*. Menlo Park, CA: Addison-Wesley.

Benoliel, J. (1984, March). Advancing nursing science: Qualitative approaches. *Western Journal of Nursing Research in Nursing and Health*, 7, 1–8.

Bohm, D. (1981). Cited in H. Smith, Beyond the modern western mind set. *Teachers College Record* (Columbia University), 82(3), 444.

Bohm, D. (1998). *On creativity*. New York: Rutledge.

Bolster, A. (1983). Toward a more effective model of research on teaching. *Harvard Education Review*, 53(3), 294–308.

Brenner, P. (Ed.). (1994). *Interpretive phenomenology: Embodiment, caring, and ethics in health and illness*. Thousand Oaks, CA: Sage.

Campbell, D. J. (1975). Degrees of freedom and the case study. *Comparative Political Studies*, 8, 178–193.

Capra, Z. (1982). Foreword. In L. Dossey (Ed.), *Space, time and medicine* (p. ix). Boulder, CO: Shanibhala.

Carper, B. A. (1978, October). Fundamental patterns of knowing in nursing. *Advances in Nursing Science*, 1, 13–23.

Clark, A. M. (1998). The qualitative-quantitative debate: Moving from positivism and confrontation to post-positivism and reconciliation. *Journal of Advanced Nursing*, 27, 1242–1249.

Dahlberg, K., & Drew, N. (1997). A lifeworld paradigm for nursing research. *Journal of Holistic Nursing*, 15, 303–317.

Diers, D. (1979). *Research in nursing practice*. Philadelphia: Lippincott.

Donaldson, S. K., & Crowley, D. M. (1978). The discipline of nursing. *Nursing Outlook*, 26, 113–120.

Drew, N., & Dahlberg, K. (1995). Challenging a reductionistic paradigm as a foundation for nursing. *Journal of Holistic Nursing*, 13, 332–345.

Dzurec, L. (1989). The necessity for and evolution of multiple paradigms for nursing research: A poststructural perspective. *Advances in Nursing Science*, 11(4), 69–77.

Fawcett, J. (1984, October). Hallmarks of success in nursing research. *Advances in Nursing Science*, 7, 1.

Freiri, P. (1971). *Pedagogy of the oppressed*. New York: Seaver.

Gadamer, G. H., Sheed & Ward, Ltd. (1975). *Truth and Method*. New York: Crossroad.

Gilligan, C. (1982). *In a different voice: Psychological theory and women's development*. Cambridge, MA: Harvard University Press.

Gould, S. J. (1984, August 12). Science and gender. *The New York Times Book Review* (book review).

Hall, E. O. C. (1996). Husserlian phenomenology and nursing in a unitary-transformative paradigm. *Vard-I-Norden Nursing Science and Research in the Nordic Countries*, 16(3), 4–8.

Harman, W. (1977). *Symposium and consciousness*. New York: Penguin.

Johnson, D. E. (1978). State of the art of theory development. In *Theory development: What, why, how?* (p. 9). New York: National League for Nursing.

Johnson, D. E. (1980). The behavioral system model for nursing. In J. P. Riehl & C. Roy (Eds.), *Conceptual models for nursing practice* (2nd ed.). Norwalk, CT: Appleton-Century-Crofts.

King, I. M. (1981). *A theory for nursing: Systems, concepts, process*. New York: Wiley.

Kneller, G. (1971). *Introduction to the philosophy of education*. New York: Wiley.

Kohlberg, L. (1976). Moral stages and moralization. In T. Lickona (Ed.), *Moral development and behavior*. New York: Holt Rinehart & Winston.

Kuhn, T. S. (Ed.). (1970). *The structure of scientific revolutions*. Chicago: University of Chicago Press.

Kurtz, S. (1989). *The art of unknowing*. Northvale, NJ: Aronson, Inc.

Laudan, L. (1977). *Progress and its problems: Toward a theory of scientific growth*. Berkeley: University of California Press.

Leininger, M. (Ed.). (1984). *Care: The essence of nursing and health.* Thorofare, NJ: Slack.

Light, R., & Pillemer, D. (1982). Numbers and narrative: Combining their strengths in research reviews. *Harvard Education Review, 52,* 1–23.

Lincoln, Y., & Guba, E. (1985). *Naturalistic Inquiry.* Newbury Park, CA: Sage.

Lutz, K. F., Jones, K. D., & Kendall, J. (1997). Expanding the praxis debate: Contributions to clinical inquiry. *Advances in Nursing Science,* 20(2), 23–31.

Morgan, G. (1983). *Beyond method.* Newbury Park, CA: Sage.

Morse, J. M. (1999). Qualitative methods: The state of art. *Qualitative Health Research* 9, 393–406.

Munhall, P. (1982a). Methodic fallacies: A critical self appraisal. *Advances in Nursing Science,* 41–47.

Munhall, P. (1982b). Nursing philosophy and nursing research: In apposition or opposition? *Nursing Research,* 31(3), 176–177, 181.

Munhall, P. (1982, April). Ethical juxtapositions in nursing research. *Topics in Clinical Nursing,* 4, 66–73.

Munhall, P. (1986). Methodological issues in nursing: Beyond a wax apple. *Advances in Nursing Science,* 8(3), 1–5.

Munhall, P. (1989). Philosophical pondering on qualitative research methods in nursing. *Nursing Science Quarterly,* 2, 20–28.

Munhall, P. (1992). Holding the Mississippi River in place and other implications for qualitative research. *Nursing Outlook,* 10(6), 257–262.

Munhall, P. (1993a). Toward a fifth pattern of knowing: Unknowing. *Nursing Outlook,* 41, 125–128.

Munhall, P. (1993b). Unknowing: Toward another pattern of knowing. *Nursing Outlook,* 41, 125–128.

Munhall, P. (1994a). *Qualitative research: Proposals and reports.* New York: National League for Nursing.

Munhall, P. (1994b). *Revisioning phenomenology: Nursing and health science research.* Sudbury, MA: Jones and Barlett.

Munhall, P., (1997). Déjà Vu, Parroting, Buy-ins, and Opening. In J. Fawcett & I. King, *The language of nursing theory and metatheory.* Indianapolis, IN: Sigma Theta Tau International.

Munhall, P., & Oiler, C. (1986). *Nursing Research: A Qualitative Perspective.* Norwalk, CT: Appleton-Century-Crofts.

Munhall, P., & Oiler, C. (1993). 2nd ed. *Nursing Research: A Qualitative Perspective.* Sudbury, MA: Jones & Bartlett.

Nesbitt, R. (1976). *Sociology as an art form.* New York: Oxford University Press.

Newman, M. (1983, January). Editorial. *Advances in Nursing Science,* 5(2), x–xi.

Newman, M. (1986). *Health as expanding consciousness.* St. Louis, MO: Mosby.

Newman, M., Sime, A., & Cocoran-Perry, (1991). The focus of the discipline of nursing. *Advances in Nursing Science*, 14, 1–5.

Norris, C. (1982). *Concept clarification in nursing*. Rockville, MD: Aspen.

Orem, D. E. (1980). *Nursing: Concepts of practice* (2nd ed.). New York: McGraw-Hill.

Paterson, J. (1978). The tortuous way toward nursing theory. In *Theory development: What, why and how?* New York: National League for Nursing.

Paterson, J., & Zderad, L. (1976). *Humanistic nursing*. New York: Wiley.

Pender, N. J. (1987). *Health promotion in nursing practice*. Norwalk, CT: Appleton-Lange.

Polkinghorne, D. (1983). *Methodology for the human sciences*. Albany: SUNY Press.

Reichardt, C., & Cook, T. (Eds.). (1979). *Qualitative and quantitative methods in evaluation research* (pp. 33–48). Beverly Hills, CA: Sage.

Rogers, M. E. (1970). *An introduction to the theoretical basis of nursing*. Philadelphia: Davis.

Rorty, R. (1991). *Essays on Heidegger and others*. New York: Cambridge University Press.

Roy, C., Sr. (1976). *Introduction to nursing: An adaptation model*. Englewood Cliffs, NJ: Prentice-Hall.

Silva, M. C. (1997). Classic image. Philosophy, science, theory: Interrelationships and implications for nursing research. *Image: Journal of Nursing Scholarship*, 29(3), 210–215.

Silva, M., & Rothbart, D. (1984, January). An analysis of changing trends in philosophies of science on nursing theory development and testing. *Advances in Nursing Science*, 6(2), 1–12.

Stevens, B. J. (1979). *Nursing theory: Analysis, application, evaluation*. Boston: Little, Brown.

Thorne, S. E., Kirkham, S. R., & Henderson, A. (1999). Ideological implications of paradigm discourse. *Nursing Inquiry*, 6(2), 123–131.

Uris, P. (1993). Postmodern feminist emancipatory research. Unpublished doctoral dissertation, University of Colorado, Denver.

Van Manen, M. (1990). *Research on lived experience: Human science for action-sensitive pedagogy*. New York: SUNY Press.

Watson, J. (1985). *Nursing: The philosophy and science of caring*. Boulder: Colorado Associated University Press.

Watson, J. (1988). New dimensions of human caring theory. *Nursing Science*, 1(4), 175–181.

Watson, J. (1999). *Post modern nursing and beyond*. New York: Churchill Livingston.

Wainwright, S. P. (1997). A new paradigm for nursing: The potential realism. *Journal of Advanced Nursing*, 26, 1262–1271.

Wilson, L., & Fitzpatrick, J. (1984, January). Dialectic thinking as a means of understanding systems in development: Relevance to Rogers' principles. *Advances in Nursing Science,* 6(2), 41.

ADDITIONAL REFERENCES

Arslanian, C. (1998). Taking the mystery out of research: qualitative nursing research. *Orthopaedic Nursing,* 17, 31.

Ashworth, P. D. (1997). The variety of qualitative research (Part 2): Non-positivist approaches. *Nurse Education Today* 17, 219–224.

Bunkers, S. S., Petardi, L. A., Pilkington, F. B., & Walls, P. A. (1996). Challenging the myths surrounding qualitative research in nursing. *Nursing Science Quarterly,* 9, 33–37.

Coyle, J., & Williams, B. (2000). An exploration of the epistemological intricacies of using qualitative data to develop a quantitative measure of user views of health care. *Journal of Advanced Nursing,* 31, 1235–1243.

Farrel, G. A., & Gritching, W. L. (1997). Social science at the crossroads: What direction mental health nurses? *Australian New Zealand Journal of Mental Health Nursing,* 6, 19–29.

Forbes, D. A., King, K. M., Kushner, K. E., Letourneau, N. L., Myrick, A. F., & Profetto-McGrath, J. (1999). Warrantable evidence in nursing science. *Journal of Advanced Nursing,* 29, 373–379.

Letourneau, N., & Allen, M. (1999). Post-positivistic critical multiplism: A beginning dialogue. *Journal of Advanced Nursing,* 30, 623–630.

Marks, M. D. (1999). Network. Reconstructing nursing: Evidence, artistry and the curriculum . . . including commentary by L. Nyatanga, & M. Johnson. *Nurse Education Today,* 19, 3–11.

Monti, E. J. & Tingen, M. S. (1999). Multiple paradigms of nursing science. *Advances in Nursing Science,* 21(4), 64–80.

Munhall, P. (1992). A new age ism: Beyond a toxic apple. *Nursing and Health Care,* 13, 370–376.

Munhall, P. (1998). Qualitative designs. In P. Brink & M. Wood (Eds.), *Advanced designs in nursing research* (2nd ed.), Newbury Park, CA: Sage.

Munhall, P. (2000a). *Qualitative research reports and proposals: A guide.* Sudbury, MA: Jones and Bartlett.

Munhall, P. (2000b). Unknowing. In W. Kelly & V. Fitzsimons (Eds.), *Understanding cultural diversity.* Sudbury, MA: Jones and Barlett.

Watson, J. (1995). Postmodernism and knowledge development in nursing. *Nursing Science Quarterly,* 8(2), 60–64.

3

Philosophical Foundations of Qualitative Research

Carolyn Oiler Boyd

The tension between our science and our practice serves as the primary impetus for qualitative research in nursing. The growing interest among nurse researchers in qualitative research represents a reaction against the prevailing view of subjectivity and the nature of reality that is established as premise in the positivist tradition. It is a reaction against a focus on an external reality, an existence of things and others independent of a subject who experiences them. In the quantitative paradigm, the dichotomization of reality as objective and subjective has propagated rather than resolved tensions in nursing practice between the technological and the humanistic aspects of that practice. Doing research in the dominant paradigm, nurse researchers have been led to view subjectivity as a private and personal reading of reality, given to error. For the researcher who identifies with and has allegiance to nursing practice, such a view is often contrary to the lived reality of nursing practice.

The idea of *client* subjectivity, however, is valued in two ways within the quantitative paradigm: as a data source and as an outcome variable in nursing. In keeping with a split vision of reality, many nurse practitioners and researchers focus on external reality, directing their observations to the world as object, including the patient's subjectivity. For many of us, basic inconsistencies arise from the premises concerning the nature of reality in the quantitative paradigm. Conflict is generated for us in several ways:

- Recognition of the nurse–client relation as the medium of care conflicts with scientific devaluing of nurse subjectivity in the caring process.
- Nurses suffer the tension of a scientifically polarized reality, which drives subjective experience underground and deprives nurses of control over their realities.
- Awareness of nurses' realities is narrowly confined in the requirements of the professional role, and a gap emerges between their realities as lived and facts about these realities offered in scientific comment.
- A narrow vision of what happens in experience leaves nurses with unexplained dimensions of reality.
- To preserve objective detachment in nursing situations and some sense of integrity for themselves, nurses withdraw from and deny their awareness. This deflects us from values that center nursing as a humanizing influence in the health care system.
- The cumulative effect of these tensions in distancing nurses from their experiences renders them inarticulate, and the development of nursing knowledge is thus hindered in the gap between experiential and theoretical knowledge.
- A heightened sensitivity to some of the implications of a science that aims for prediction and control in view of a growing appreciation for the importance of the valuing of self-determination in health care has contributed to an unrest about our emerging science and to unsettling questions concerning our future development.

The prevailing views about subjectivity and reality in nursing establish a need to explore other ways of thinking about what is real so that more in nursing might be considered real and true in a scientific sense. In this chapter, the tensions and conflicts generated by incompatibilities between nursing philosophy and practice and nursing science are the background for a discussion of the philosophical foundations for qualitative research. The aim is to resolve these tensions and conflicts through a research paradigm that coincides with nursing beliefs, values, and aims. Although the interest is in the nexus of philosophy with research methods, there is also a need to focus on the nexus with nursing practice and nursing education. The larger context for the discussion will not be addressed here, but its relevance is critical. (See, for example, National League for Nursing, 1988.)

Traditional nursing beliefs and values that shape and give expression to nursing in our society may change (or may already have changed), and this change would certainly alter the arguments for qualitative research in this book. In a sense, the strivings of qualitative researchers are efforts not only to maintain nursing's humanistic current in its present form, but also to establish it more soundly as a grounding for our practice and our science (Paterson & Zderad, 1976, pp. 3–9). This goal is not shared by all in what seems at times to be a denial of the tensions between science and humanism and, at other times, a turn toward beliefs, values, and perspectives that are severed from nursing's traditional humanistic stance in health care. The intentions of qualitative researchers are thus important in distinguishing their work as part of the qualitative paradigm rather than an opportunistic use of some of the techniques and strategies associated with qualitative research.

This chapter limits its concern to the features of the qualitative paradigm, fully recognizing that some who do qualitative research may not attend to these features as grounding for their work. Nevertheless, the view presented here about philosophical foundations is essentially congruent with other presentations in the literature and has broad implications for nursing practice as well as for research. Each qualitative approach (ethnography, grounded theory, phenomenology, case study, historical research) discussed in this text carries its own orientation or perspective, draws on its own selection of theorists, methodologists, and philosophers, and reflects the parent discipline for that approach. Nevertheless, common premises link the various qualitative approaches in a tradition or a paradigm. The aim of this chapter is to relate some of these common premises to common characteristics of qualitative research and thereby to articulate the philosophical foundations or framework of the qualitative paradigm. Such a philosophical grounding provides both direction and rationale for research design and method.

WHAT IS QUALITATIVE RESEARCH?

Definition

The very general term "qualitative research" encompasses a variety of designs and methods. Nevertheless, the various designs generally have the following features in common:

- A *holistic approach to questions—a recognition that human realities are complex.* Research questions tend to be very broad. Some examples are: What are the birth experiences of women in foreign cultures

(Sharts-Engel, 1989)? What is comforting? What is it like to feel lonely when hospitalized (Copel, 1984)?

- *The focus is on human experience.* This is a turn toward subjectivities or people's realities.
- *The research strategies used generally feature sustained contact with people in settings where those people normally spend their time.* There is careful attention to the contexts of human behavior.
- *There is typically a high level of researcher involvement with subjects; strategies of participant observation and in-depth, unstructured interviews are often used.*
- *The data produced provide a description, usually narrative, of people living through events in situations.*

A definition of qualitative research may be stated, then, as involving broadly stated questions about human experiences and realities, studied through sustained contact with persons in their natural environments, and producing rich, descriptive data that help us to understand those persons' experiences. The emphasis is on achieving understanding that will, in turn, open up new options for action and new perspectives that can change people's worlds.

Purposes

Knafl and Howard (1986) viewed the purposes of qualitative research as fourfold: instrumentation, illustration, sensitization, and conceptualization. For example, to serve the purpose of instrumentation, a researcher might use in-depth, unstructured interviews of wheelchair-bound adults to learn what it's like to live with impaired mobility. The information that these adults provide the researcher could then be used to construct an instrument that includes categories based on their actual experiences rather than on what we imagine them to be.

The purpose of illustration was served in Kramer's classic study of young baccalaureate graduate nurses' reality shock (1968). In this study, Kramer used qualitative interview data and subjects' journal entries to illustrate her quantitative findings about their role orientations. The purpose of sensitization is served by all qualitative studies to the extent that they effectively communicate insights about experiences that we need to understand vicariously. Learning of these findings functions to sensitize research consumers to their patients and thereby to contribute to the quality of care. The researcher may also profit from the heightened awareness and meaning that emerge in the research process. Lastly, qualitative studies may be undertaken to serve the purpose of conceptualization or theory development. For example,

Hutchinson (1986) used the grounded-theory method to learn more about what it is like to be a nurse in a neonatal intensive care unit. After a protracted period of in-depth observation, participation, and interviews, Hutchinson constructed a theory descriptive of the coping strategies of these nurses.

This classification of qualitative research purposes reveals the very broad interpretation of the term "qualitative research" in contemporary usages. On the one hand, qualitative research is seen as a precursor to quantitative study. Researchers whose purpose is instrumentation use qualitative strategies without necessarily adopting the beliefs, values, and orientation of the philosophical foundations or the set of features (heretofore outlined) commonly associated with the qualitative paradigm. When the purpose is illustration, there may be a similar commitment to the positivist tradition rather than to the qualitative paradigm. The purposes of sensitization and conceptualization are more strictly in keeping with the qualitative paradigm.

Another way to think about the purpose of qualitative research is in regard to establishing a phenomenological baseline that would be a thorough description of the life-worlds of patients, families, and nurses as they are experienced by participants (Oiler, 1986, pp. 99–102). It would provide fully developed nursing concepts that are faithful to the real world of lived nursing/patient experience. The theory constructed on such descriptions would possess a greater relevance in their comments about nursing/patient phenomena because they would adhere more closely to participants' lived experiences. Establishing a phenomenological baseline, a coherent and accurate description of lived experience, will be accomplished through qualitative studies. The qualitative process is one of theory development; that of empirical studies is one of second-order comment.

Qualitative researchers strive to suspend foundations in our views that support second-order comment on experiences rather than insight into those experiences. Nursing management of dependency in the nursing situation, for example, may suffer from a lack of attention to the meanings of dependency in various nursing situations. We might consider how being bathed might facilitate recovery through a mechanism such as therapeutic touch. Or, how uncontrolled diabetes facilitates another goal by maintaining the noncompliant diabetic patient's relation with a visiting nurse. Or, how ministering to clients makes it possible for nurses to be emotionally available to them. In this example of dependency, the phenomenological baseline for practice and research would provide a thorough description of human dependency in nursing situations. We would ask such questions as: Dependent on whom, for what, with what consequences? What are the alternatives, and how does being dependent relate to health, to striving toward and achieving one's goals in one's world? The baseline would provide us with the understanding needed for a clarified concept of dependency. This would be a nursing concept—one that might vary from the perspective in psychology or in sociology. On the other hand, when thoroughly grounded in lived experience, a nursing concept of dependency might be instructive to other disciplines. Establishing a phenomenological baseline for nursing knowledge is, from this point of view, the single overriding purpose for qualitative research.

As reflected in the working definition of qualitative research, the position taken here is that the mere use of qualitative strategies such as unstructured interviewing does not place a study in the qualitative tradition. Research that does belong in the qualitative tradition is characterized by a commitment to a philosophical grounding that orients us to particular views on the nature of being human and the nature of reality; in nursing research, this grounding includes particular views on the nature of health and of nursing. This position directs the discussion in this chapter.

History of the Qualitative Tradition

Bogdan and Biklen (1982) provided a description of the historical context of qualitative research, noting that, although its recognition as a tool of science is relatively recent, its long and rich tradition in the United States began in the late 1800s. At that time, qualitative strategies were used to disclose the rapidly developing social problems in cities pursuant to industrialization, urbanization, and mass immigration. Qualitative descriptions encouraged social change by making urban problems visible to the public. The Pittsburgh survey, for example, not only provided statistics about the urban poor, but also gave us detailed accounts of urban life, conveyed through photographs, charcoal portraits, and interviews. The statistics were thus cast in human terms by the qualitative data (Bogdan & Biklen, 1982, pp. 3–8).

Concurrent with the productivity of social surveys at the turn of the past century, anthropological field research methods were being developed and taught in universities. The anthropological strategy of participant observation migrated to sociology, where it was used along with the case study method to study social problems in communities from a social interaction perspective. In the 1920s and 1930s, sociologists used qualitative strategies extensively to study such social phenomena as race relations, ethnicity, and delinquency. From the 1930s through the 1950s, qualitative research waned as worthy scientific endeavor came to be defined in accord with the growing expectation that quantitative methods were the most promising means to solutions. Taking the lead primarily from medicine, public health, and sociology, nursing subscribed to this view; our short history of research activity meshed with the dominant quantitative paradigm in the scientific world (Bogdan & Biklen, 1982, pp. 8–18).

The 1960s, however, disrupted the scientific world's unquestioning faith in the promise of quantitative methods. A variety of social minority groups clamored to be heard, and there was a renewed interest in the power of qualitative methods to provide us with better understanding of minorities' views and circumstances. In this period, the grounded-theory method was developed (Glaser & Strauss, 1967). In nursing, this method was used to study nurses' and patients' experiences with death and dying (Quint, 1967). However, this kind of early work did not flourish nationally. Nurse researchers tended to focus their talents and energies on mastering quantitative methods.

Nevertheless, the social unrest of the 1960s, including the feminist movement, stimulated methodological debates in other fields. Education, sociology, and psychology in particular turned toward qualitative methods with renewed interest in the 1970s. These debates surfaced in the literature, in university courses, and at national conferences, and they gradually engaged nurses in a serious consideration of the merit and prospects of qualitative research (Bogdan & Biklen, 1982, pp. 18–26). Paterson and Zderad (1976) introduced phenomenology to nursing in a work that intrigued some but puzzled others. Nursing debates concerning the merit of qualitative research approaches took off in the early 1980s. (See, for example, Munhall, 1982; Oiler, 1982; Tinkle & Beaton, 1983.) Today, we are in a period of exploring qualitative methods and developing our expertise in their use. Although we continue to rely heavily on direction from other disciplines that have created qualitative approaches for their concerns, we are on the move and can look forward to increasing experimentation with new qualitative methods for the investigation of nursing problems. (See, for example, Newman, 1990; Parse, 1990; Paterson & Zderad, 1976.)

Structure and Characteristics

When qualitative researchers speak of subjectivity, they are referring to the ways in which people make sense of their experiences and lives. In nursing, this concern with subjectivity is one with meanings or "sense making" in situations. To understand the sense that a given situation bears for a person is to grasp something of that person's reality—to see what is true from his or her point of view. We have accumulated many facts, for example, about menopause, osteoporosis, and pain. However, these facts do not add up to an understanding of what it's like to live through menopause or to have osteoporosis or to suffer. Qualitative researchers are most interested in subjective meanings rather than facts alone. If a patient's experience is one of suffering, it matters little whether the facts about the patient's condition coincide with his or her experience from some other person's point of view (reality). In nursing, we have always attended as best we can to patients' experiences. To refer to their experiences as subjective is quite superfluous and quite dismissive, as if patients' subjectivities were erroneous. All realities are subjective if one means that the person interprets, lends meaning to, and makes sense of the facts of the world. The objective view of health care providers is simply *one way* of interpreting, forming meaning, and making sense of things. We worry when patients take on this kind of perspective, in recognition of its limited usefulness for them.

To construct methods that disclose subjectivity, qualitative researchers recognize that people construct meanings in relation to the world in which they exist. This is the second leading characteristic of qualitative methods: the natural settings in which people under study live, work, learn, and play are sought for the conduct of the study. The researcher strives to collect data descriptive of the person–environment relation in the belief that human behavior is best understood in the context in which it occurs. If a researcher wants to learn about what it is like to ambulate in a wheelchair, for example, the natural setting would be subjects' everyday lives. The study design would include finding ways to be with subjects for a period of time in their lives. A questionnaire, in contrast, would lift subjects away from their natural setting and experiencing and would obscure such data as their struggles with stairs and doors, their solicitation or rejection of assistance, and their myriad ways of accommodating a world of forms designed for ambulating with the use of the lower extremities. Many qualitative studies rely heavily, if not exclusively, on interview data rather than on joining subjects in the course of their day-to-day lives. The distinguishing feature of a qualitative approach in interviewing, however, is the researcher's and the researched's turn toward the researched's day-to-day life. The interview is less structured and more intimate, akin to an initial therapeutic interview when the focus also is on understanding the patient's reality.

Because the aim is to disclose subjectivity, the qualitative researcher strives to locate and collect data that serve to describe the experience under study. Words, in the form of field observation notes and transcripts of interviews, are the most common form of qualitative data. However, photographs, videotapes, and the researcher's perceptions of sounds, tastes, and smells are sometimes included as data. Similarly, diaries, memos, letters, and art might be included if they contribute to presenting and understanding the human experience under study. The end product—the findings—represents the researcher's best effort to organize and present an accurate picture of what has been learned by going to people in their natural settings and being with them for a time in order to gain as much information as possible about their lives.

The pictures that qualitative research produces are distillations of large amounts of various kinds of data that are tracked down by maintaining a research focus on human processes. For example, a quantitative researcher might study whether nursing home residents are lonely, and to what extent, by using a scale that measures loneliness. Facts are thus produced: yes, they are lonely (in the main); furthermore, the loneliness is extreme. The qualitative researcher, on the other hand, would pursue the question of how nursing home residents experience loneliness. Understanding is thus produced: loneliness as it is lived through is brought into focus. Other process-oriented questions are: What is it like to work in an NICU? (Hutchinson, 1986); How are attitudes about women expressed in the physician–nurse relation? (Katzman & Roberts, 1988); What happens to families when there is sudden death of a member? Such process-oriented questions guide the qualitative researcher in a rigorous search for elusive data that help to disclose complex human experiences that often defy attempts simply to report them in interviews or on questionnaires.

The organization and distillation of data that the researcher performs in order to present a picture of the experience under study constitute an essentially inductive process. Many instances of an event, process, or perception are grouped together to generate a characteristic that is then represented in the picture that the researcher provides in the report of the findings. This inductive approach to building knowledge is sometimes referred to as theory development from the bottom up. For example, in Copel's study of loneliness (1984), she identified "problems with relationships" as a component of loneliness. A few of the instances that were grouped together to form this component were patients' statements of feeling unloved, isolated, and secluded and of having a sense of loss and lack of support.

A PHENOMENOLOGICAL PERSPECTIVE AS PHILOSOPHICAL FRAMEWORK

Leading themes of phenomenological philosophy offer a perspective on the nature of human reality that supports qualitative research efforts. Some qualitative methodologists draw directly from phenomenology to articulate a rationale and grounding for social science methods. Others make no reference to phenomenology as such. Yet, despite the fact that various qualitative methodologists have been inspired by thinkers who are not categorized as phenomenological thinkers, phenomenological themes can be discerned and are one of the leading influences. Patton (1980) noted that qualitative methods derive from a variety of philosophical, epistemological, and methodological traditions but that, generally, the qualitative paradigm is based on perspectives developed in phenomenology, symbolic interactionism, naturalistic behaviorism, ethnomethodology, and ecological psychology. The integrating theme of these perspectives is the idea of *verstehen*:

> The advocate of some version of the *verstehen* doctrine will claim that human beings can be understood in a manner that other objects cannot. Men have purposes and emotions, they make plans, construct cultures, and hold certain values, and their behavior is influenced by such values, plans, and purposes. . . . The *verstehen* tradition stresses understanding that focuses on the meaning of human behavior, the context of social interaction, an empathetic understanding based on subjective experience, and the connections between subjective states and behavior. (Patton, 1980, pp. 44–45)

Bogdan and Taylor (1975), writing about qualitative research in its general sense, credited phenomenology with the inspiration that the *verstehen* idea lends to the qualitative paradigm:

> The phenomenologist is concerned with understanding human behavior from the actor's own frame of reference. . . . The phenomenologist examines how the world is experienced. For him or her the important reality is what people imagine it to be. (Bogdan & Taylor, 1975, p. 2)

Bogdan and Biklen (1982) acknowledged that the word "phenomenology" is used in many ways, but, in its most general sense, "[A]ll qualitative researchers in some way reflect a phenomenological perspective" (p. 31). Not all qualitative researchers would classify themselves as phenomenologists, yet the idea of the *verstehen* would be readily recognized as a central tenet in their work.

The relevance of phenomenological philosophy to the qualitative paradigm is thus established in this discussion of philosophical foundations. The variety of qualitative designs that springs from the philosophy attests to the openness of the philosophy; it inspires and encourages extrapolations both to practice and to research methods and processes. What is important to keep in mind, however, is that (because of our youth as an emerging science) the qualitative designs of grounded theory, ethnography, and phenomenology-as-method were extrapolations within other disciplines. They bear the perspectives of those disciplines, which do not coincide perfectly with the perspectives of the nursing discipline. To do grounded theory in a way that is faithful to the ideas of the methodologists (Glaser & Strauss, 1988, for example), a nurse researcher cannot be knowledgeable about the phenomenological roots alone—there is also symbolic interactionism to take into account.

On the other hand, when we borrow theory from other disciplines, we should be adapting it in the context of the nursing discipline. Paterson and Zderad (1976) and Benner (1994) provided examples of this kind of adaptation for phenomenologic method in nursing, but, to date, there is still a great deal of work to do in creating nursing methodologies for research.[1] An embrace of a philosophical foundation for qualitative research will enable us to carry the qualitative tradition forward in nursing without risk of losing sight of the intentions of the turn away from the positivist paradigm. We clearly do not need to introduce new research methods that will divide and repress us further, and a sound grounding in the philosophical foundation will reduce this risk. For this reason, qualitative researchers need to be knowledgeable about and committed to the philosophy that grounds the designs, methods, and strategies of the qualitative tradition. It bears mentioning, however, that, for such well-established designs as grounded theory, ethnography, and historical research, the leading methodologists may be sufficient for rationale and direction, particularly when acceptance and recognition of the scientific merit of such studies constitute the issue at hand. The grounded theory method of Glaser and Strauss, for example, is suffused with a philosophical grounding. Adopting their

---

[1] In Chapter Five of this edition, Munhall offers a phenomenological method for human sciences, including nursing.

grounded-theory methodology may satisfy any challenge to using a qualitative approach that may be encountered, without necessarily articulating that grounding. However, in a concern for scholarship and for a commitment to foundational beliefs and valuing, a grasp of the approach in a simplistic, technical way is not satisfactory. One can usually recognize qualitative studies that are not well grounded in philosophy; they tend to take on a positivist flavor, to be plagued with incongruencies from design through discussion of findings, *and* to fall short of being compelling reading.

The Nature of Reality

In a simple turn of preference, qualitative researchers direct their attention to human realities rather than to the concrete realities of objects. The distinctive valuing of and respect for people in qualitative research do not allow for their objectification as featured in quantitative research. People are thus centered in qualitative research in recognition that reality is constituted in human perspectives. There are always multiple realities (perspectives) to consider when a full grasp of a situation is sought. A question such as What is treatment in an intensive care unit like? may be considered from a number of perspectives—that of the patient, that of the family, that of the nurse, and that of the physician—each of which is decidedly unique and in some ways contradictory to the others. Further, each research participant's experience may be understood variously by him or her from a number of perspectives. Yet, each is equally "true"; each is equally real. The concrete objective reality of the intensive care environment is experienced differently by each of these people, creating different realities.

Human involvement in the world, then, is of primary concern to the qualitative researcher who, by choice, focuses on human realities. Schutz (1973) wrote:

> The origin of all reality is subjective; whatever excites and stimulates our interest is real. To call a thing real means that this thing stands in a certain relation to ourselves. (p. 207)

A focus on human realities must therefore take into account not only the "thing" but also the relation that it bears to the experiencing person. The facts of the world—what we may customarily think of as objective reality—and the facts of human consciousness coincide in this focus. The very meaning of objectivity and subjectivity changes in this view of the nature of reality. Merleau-Ponty (1962) reasoned that subjectivity as inner existence is false on the grounds that existence (or consciousness) is possible because we are present within the world. The world is assumed; experience in it and knowledge of it, however, are always through the subjectivity of presence in the world. There are not two views of reality; the view is always the subjective one of this presence. Reality as it can be known to us is thus unidimensional in this sense. The appearance of phenomena expresses this welded relation of subject and object and is the first or fundamental reality on which our sciences and understandings are built. The body is one's natural access to the world. Sensation, sexuality, language, and speech are all expressions of our existence, and all are constituted concretely in a bodily reaching toward the world around us. Even in the experience of feeling alone and lonely, one's reference is paradoxically to others in the world. Merleau-Ponty (1962, p. 70) regarded the body as one's point of view of the world; the body as access to the world produces for the subject what he referred to as one's gaze. He explained that existence is expressed in a particular manner of approach to the world, and the approach, or gaze, is brought into being by one's bodily existence in the world:

> Even if I know nothing of rods and cones, I should realize that it is necessary to put the surroundings in abeyance the better to see the object and to lose in background what one gains in focal figure, because to look at the object is to plunge into it, and because objects form a system in which one cannot show itself without concealing others. . . . The object-horizon structure, or the perspective, is no obstacle to me when I want to see the object; for just as it is the means whereby objects are distinguished from each other, it is also the means whereby they are disclosed. (Merleau Ponty, 1962, p. 7)

Concretely, we are able to experience the world through our bodies: we assume a position in the world, which in turn determines object–horizon structure, both spatially and temporally, available to us. We are able to focus, to be conscious of one object over others in a figure–ground relation of our choosing.

The human gaze reveals just that aspect of the object accessible through one's bodily involvement in the world in space and in time. Human experience and human reality are always perspectival in this sense. It is important to recognize here, however, that the subject's biography, past experience, knowledge of the world, and whatever social and political facticities may hold true are all qualifications of gaze. Merleau-Ponty (1962) described these qualifications by using a common experience:

> When I look at the lamp on my table, I attribute to it not only the qualities visible from where I am, but also those which the chimney, the walls, the table can "see"; but back of my lamp is

nothing but the face which it "shows" to the chimney. I can therefore see an object insofar as objects form a system or a world, and insofar as each one treats the others round it as spectators of its hidden aspects and as guarantee of the permanence of those aspects. (p. 68)

In this way, a perspective on the world is formed. It is not pure experience but an interpreted experience that constitutes reality.

In what Schutz (1973) called the "natural attitude of daily life," consciousness is expressed within and on the world. The reality of experience is taken for granted and shifting perspectives are assumed as dictated by one's biography and by the practical need to achieve chosen purposes in the world. In the natural attitude, the world as experienced and interpreted by our predecessors is handed down to our own experience and interpretation. In the fashion of layers, a current experience is shaped by a stock of previous experiences and interpretations—one's own and those of one's parents and teachers. The natural attitude, a type of mode of consciousness, presents us with interpreted experience.

The natural attitude characterizes most of our existence. We assume that the meanings brought to the world coincide with an absolute, objective reality. Other realities (arising from other modes of consciousness) and different attentions to life (presenting other meanings) are incompatible. Merleau-Ponty explained that, in interpreted experience, positing an object makes us go beyond the limits of actual experience. He discussed the phenomenon of the phantom limb to demonstrate the inescapable relation of subject and object, which he referred to as being "situated":

What it is in us which refuses mutilation and disablement is an I committed to a certain physical and inter-human world, who continues to tend towards his world despite handicaps and amputations and who, to this extent, does not recognize them de jure. (1962, p. 81)

Rejecting physiological and psychological explanations as inadequate, Merleau-Ponty acknowledged that the phantom limb can be related to both. The difficulty in these explanations resides in the experience of the presence of a limb:

The man with one leg feels the missing limb in the same way as I feel keenly the existence of a friend who is, nevertheless, not before my eyes; he has not lost it because he continues to allow for it. . . . The phantom arm is not a representation of the arm, but the ambivalent presence of an arm. (p. 81)

The body as a power is assumed at a preobjective level, and the amputated limb is assumed as a customary part of this being. The person with a phantom limb is living his body in the way to which he is accustomed.

This phenomenological view of the phantom limb is not a denial of physiological facts or of psychological explanations of memory, belief, or acceptance. Rather, it introduces a common ground for these facts—a situation for an existence. In an active engagement in present experiences, the person is committed to carrying through his intentions in the world. The patient with a phantom limb might try, for example, to reach for something with his amputated arm. In his lived body and in his attention to action, the reach makes perfect sense and is not simply a matter of psychological denial or physiological nerve transmission extension. Only when this engagement with the world in action is suspended can the patient consider the truth of the amputated limb and compensate for a lived body that may continue to press toward the world for some time.

The phantom limb is a transient phenomenon. The patient's perception ultimately is replaced with another perception from the new perspective given through his or her body. The amputated limb gives rise to experiences that, through time, direct attention to life in new ways. This is not accomplished by thinking about it but, rather, by living it over a span of time. "The world is not what I think, but what I live through" (Merleau-Ponty, 1962, p. xvii). It is not created by the subject's involvement with it; it is discovered through perception. Perception does not depend on external stimuli as if they were clear, defined, and unambiguous. Rather, stimuli are perceived in the context of the experience to which they belong:

> [T]o see is to have colours or lights, to hear is to have sounds, to sense is to have qualities. . . . But red and green are not sensations, they are the sensed, and quality is not an element of consciousness, but a property of the object. Instead of providing a simple means delimiting sensations, if we consider it in the experience itself which evinces it the quality is as rich and mysterious as the object, or indeed the whole spectacle, perceived. (Merleau-Ponty, 1962, p. 4)

To clarify these statements, Merleau-Ponty explained that seeing a red patch on a carpet is contingent on shadows and lights, size, and the fabric of the carpet. This red would not be the same in the absence of the meanings that reside in it. It is not possible to perceive sensations, such as the color red, without the overlays that form experience.

Perception is awareness of the appearances of phenomena, and one must see the red patch on the carpet as it really is, with shadow, light, size, and fabric. From this totality, one is able to conceive of this particular red; that is, one lends an interpretation or gives meaning to one's experience—in this case, the experience of seeing a red patch on a carpet. Perception is open to an infinite variety of perspectives; they merge in a unique, individual style to define one's reality. Perception has the potential for access to meaning as it is discovered in living rather than as it is interpreted after the fact. Perception of an amputated limb as an ambivalent presence is not truth, but it is reality for the patient. It is this particular perspective that is taken up in qualitative research.

Modes of Awareness and Expression

On the bases of experience and perception, other human capacities for awareness enable us to bring meaning to our lives and world. Scientific awareness, for example, is one mode, one possible perspective, for interpreting experience. Like other modes of awareness, it posits what is figure and what is ground. In so doing, it provides a particular way of looking at things and yields a particular interpretation or reality while opening up future experiences as possibilities. Experience becomes known to us after the fact, when we reflect on it. To know an experience directly and immediately is not strictly possible. When we turn back to see it, we are then in a new experience: we are reflecting on an experience that has just passed. In other words, knowing what one is living through is interpreted experience, and the best that we can do is to be aware of our awarenesses and recognize that knowledge is interpreted reality. Such self-consciousness expands awareness, confronts us with our freedom, and points us toward the necessity of choice and action. Qualitative research is not value free, in other words. There is a reverence for life, for the individual, and for self-determination. Reflection and heightened awareness are accepted as instrumental in being free to choose among alternatives.

Values are brought into being through the meanings that people attach to objects, events, or circumstances. People establish what is figure and what is ground, thereby bringing order out of chaos in the world. There are gaps between what is given and what is to be gained through human perspective, choice, and action; these gaps represent opportunities to perceive anew, to orient oneself in the world through choices, and to construct one's own world.

The natural attitude described by Schutz (1970) is one possible perspective on experience. Reflection on experience, however, opens up other possible modes of awareness. As noted earlier, scientific aware-ness is one of them. Others include: esthetic awareness; empathic and intuitive awarenesses; and imaginative, spiritual, and historical aware-nesses. There are also the awarenesses of dreams and hallucinations and of belief and remembrance. Each mode of awareness presents us with a particular kind of evidence of the world. Expressions of these awarenesses are equally varied and are a rendering of awareness in behavior. Research, art, humor, worship, habit and ritual, acts of courage and of aggression—all are expressions of awareness of expe-rience. They may be called consequences of the ways in which we make sense of our existence; they are sensible outcomes of perspec-tives taken up in the world.

Summary of Philosophical Themes

- To exist is to be conscious of something in the world. Reality and truth hinge on this fundamental relation of human existence in a concrete world of others, objects, events, circumstances, and sit-uations. Human realities are thus interactive and transactional with the world.
- One is tied to the world in a perspective created by being bodily situated in the world in a particular way. Because human reali-ties are contingent on one's turn of attention to the world in a perspective that comes into being by that turn, they are always subjective in nature.
- Experience refers to living through a situation, event, or circum-stance in time. It can only be known reflectively.
- Perception refers to original awareness of the appearance of phenomena in experience and is constituted in one's perspective.
- Various modes of awareness characterize human capability and are superimposed on perception through reflection, providing various ways of interpreting/constituting meaning in experience. Awareness in a particular mode is a matter of taking up a per-spective on experience.
- The range of human expression, or the ways in which to present one's awareness, strengthens one's links to the world through the effects of those expressions on the world and the constitu-tion of perspective in awareness and expression. The scientific mode of awareness and its various expressions constitute a per-spective that, in turn, creates a particular way of involvement with things, others, and ourselves.

Lincoln and Guba (1985) provided an alternative summary or overview of what they referred to as axioms of the naturalistic paradigm. The axioms are as follows:

- There are multiple constructed realities that can be studied only holistically; inquiry into these multiple realities will inevitably diverge so that prediction and control are unlikely outcomes, although some level of understanding can be achieved.
- The inquirer and the object of inquiry are independent; the knower and the known constitute a discrete dualism—they are interactive and inseparable.
- The aim of inquiry is to develop an idiographic body of knowledge in the form of "working hypotheses" that describe the individual case. Only time- and context-bound hypotheses are possible.
- All entities are in a state of mutual, simultaneous shaping; so it is impossible to distinguish causes from effects.
- Inquiry is value bound in at least five ways:
  1. By inquirer values as expressed in the choice and framing of the phenomenon to be studied;
  2. By the choice of research paradigm;
  3. By the choice of theory used to guide data collection, analysis, and interpretation;
  4. By values that inhere in the context;
  5. By value resonancy among problem, paradigm, theory, and context. (pp. 36–38)

Benner (1985) described the essential tenets of the philosophy that guided her work as follows:

1. Human beings are self-interpreting and these interpretations are constitutive of the self.
2. Human beings take a position on the kinds of being they are.
3. The meanings available to an individual are constrained by the person's particular language, culture, and history. (p. 5)

THE NEXUS OF PHILOSOPHY WITH RESEARCH PROCESS

The use of phenomenological philosophy to guide research methodology unquestionably modifies the researcher's involvement with his or her subject matter. In the recognition that researching is an experience for participants, there is a profound regard for how that experience might be perceived and interpreted. Stimuli that the researcher introduces include his or her observing, questioning, reacting presence. When a person agrees to be a participant, he or she has taken up a perspective that is oriented to the research and the researcher. Each question posed directs the participant's attention in certain ways, establishing a figure–ground relation and opening up possibilities for new meanings to emerge. The self-conscious concern for the individual and for the effects of the research on participants is a matter of valuing people in a certain way, and this valuation provides direction for a wide variety of choices in selecting a research design and creating a method for the research.

The doctrine of naturalism in qualitative research is, in part, a methodological choice that defers to this understanding that realities are at the very least influenced by the research process. More to the point, the research process itself becomes part of the context of the phenomenon under study.

In a discussion of research as praxis, Newman (1990) stated:

> The nurse researcher cannot stand outside the person being researched in a subject–object fashion. The researcher is part of the interaction pattern which is the process of pattern recognition and choice. (p. 40)

Drawing on critical social theory (see, for example, Allen, 1985; Lather, 1986), Newman explained that, in the course of her research on expanding consciousness, both the researcher and the researched were transformed:

> [W]e discovered that sharing our perception of the person's pattern with the person was meaningful to the participants and stimulated new insights regarding their lives. We discovered that our participation in the process made a difference in our own lives. We suspected that what we were doing in the name of research was nursing practice. (p. 37)

Not all qualitative researchers would embrace the idea that the research process is clinical nursing intervention, but the central message holds true. The aim of qualitative research in nursing arises from nursing's purposes and its intentions to intervene. Attending to patients' responses with an understanding of how realities are constituted enables us to introduce health care to them in ways that open up new perspectives for them, thereby perhaps expanding their choices and altering their realities.

Much of what makes nursing unique resides in our presence in people's lives when they are in crisis, as during illness and hospitalization, and when the nurse is the most qualified health professional available, as in some community-based practices. Nursing's ready access to clients' experiences is clearly a unique and fortunate twist for our qualitative researchers in several ways. Nurse researchers have clinical interviewing skills, for example, that transfer nicely in research interviews, and they may find that gaining access to informants is relatively easy, based on the general public's perceptions of nurses. Further, the nurse who combines his or her research with practice has the resource of different kinds of data that nurses and patients generate and use in the course of nursing care. The idea of combined purposes of clinical nursing and clinical research in the same situation has been opened up for exploration and is well worth the effort needed to address the ethical and logistical questions associated with the idea. Gadow (1977) described the nurse's range of awarenesses in the clinical situation; they include empathic and sympathetic, esthetic and ethical, and scientific and objective awarenesses. Attending a patient through a night when he has pain and cannot sleep has the potential of yielding different and infinitely richer data than does the most carefully executed qualitative interview. Benner (1983, 1985) explicated the nurse's contextual knowledge of a number of patient care situations that illustrate how that knowledge is used in nursing practice. Her idea of "uncovering the knowledge embedded in clinical practice" refers to this understanding that meanings (1) inhere in situations and (2) both constitute and are constituted by those situations. Case studies in particular have been too infrequently used to aggrandize the nurse clinician's role in knowledge development.

The idea in qualitative research of researcher-as-instrument refers to several philosophical roots. Primarily, it refers to:

1. The tenet that humans are capable of exercising a variety of modes of awareness. Method is developed with this in mind, and strategies are used to maximize the researcher's range of modes of awareness.
2. The understanding that realities are constituted in a welded subject–object relation.

Qualitative researchers know that their findings are a function of the research context that they create as well as the broader context of the phenomenon under study for the participant and for the researcher. In addition to searching for participant expressions that will help to disclose the phenomenon, the researcher plans strategies to track his or her subjectivity throughout the project. This plan contributes to the control of possible researcher distortions, but its greater value resides in "treating it (researcher's subjectivity) as data to be analyzed for the information that it contains and contributes to the study" (Drew, 1989, p. 436).

When we request research subjects to tell us anything, we are requesting them to reflect on experience. Meanings are constituted in the particular perspective taken up in reflection. When we ask, What is it like for you when you become short of breath out-of-the-blue, as you say?, the respondent looks back on the experience by taking on a mode of awareness that establishes a particular perspective. The respondent may, for example, regard the experience from a spiritual mode of awareness. The meaning that is constituted will be a function of that awareness, and the response to the question will be an expression shaped by the meaning. The fact that people often shift about from one mode of awareness to another will limit what can be learned from a single, short interview. An informant who is reflective by nature may have one thing to say today and another thing (perhaps contradictory) tomorrow.

When interviewing is used in qualitative research, in view of the task of grasping the complexity of another's reality, it can readily be seen that the success of the interview as an interpersonal dialogue has everything to do with how successfully the researcher obtains the desired data. Thus, a grasp of the elusiveness and complexity of human realities constitutes the philosophical root of the two qualitative features of collecting data (1) in subjects' natural settings and (2) over a protracted period of time. Merely interviewing people does not place a study in the qualitative paradigm. The nature of the relation between researcher and researched and the process of the interview determine the data. As Newman stated, the process is the content (1990, p. 38).

SUMMARY

Although new and still emerging for us, qualitative research approaches have been receiving considerable attention for some time in other disciplines. Along with philosophical debates, there are debates about whether there needs to be a debate. On a philosophical level, there is irreconcilable conflict between the quantitative and the qualitative paradigms. It is important to recognize this conflict, avoiding illogical compromise. Yet, proponents of each paradigm need to applaud both the existence of the other and the hybrid paradigms that inevitably are born of conflict. An apt beginning would be broader definitions of what constitutes science and research in nursing, eliminating the sense-organ bias that is so contrary to our philosophy for practice. Such definitions alone would provide qualitative nurse researchers with the sanction that they need to progress in their exploration of various approaches to creating a science and a body of knowledge in, for, and about nursing practice.

In the chapters to follow, readers will be introduced to several qualitative research approaches. Each approach is an interpretation of the qualitative paradigm in nursing research, grounded in the general perspective of phenomenological philosophy. This perspective focuses on phenomena as they appear and recognizes that reality is subjective and a matter of appearances for us in our social world. Subjectivity means that the world becomes real through our contact with it and acquires meaning through our interpretations of that contact. Truth, then, is a composite of realities, and access to truth is a problem of access to human subjectivity. This perspective guides the qualitative researcher in nursing to the subject matter of lived experiences, which are the original contacts with a world, and of the processes and content of interpretation—the meaning attributions that constitute realities and perspectives for a future of possibilities in the world. Other consequences of a phenomenological perspective in research include deliberate attention to the researcher's involvement in the study, engagement of multiple modes of awareness, and creative expression of findings. The product of efforts to establish a phenomenological baseline, a thorough and accurate description of nursing phenomena (a task that remains forever incomplete), will be clarified nursing concepts. If we encourage our qualitative nurse researchers, we can look forward to enhanced relevance in theoretical and empirical comments about nursing from studies guided by a mature nursing identity.

REFERENCES

Allen, D. (1985). Nursing research and social control: Alternative models of science that emphasize understanding and emancipation. *Image: The Journal of Nursing Scholarship, 17*(2), 58–64.

Benner, P. (1983). Uncovering the knowledge embedded in clinical practice. *Image: The Journal of Nursing Scholarship, 19*, 21–34.

Benner, P. (1985). Quality of life: A phenomenological perspective on explanation, prediction, and understanding in nursing science. *Advances in Nursing Science, 8*, 1–14.

Benner, Patricia (1994). (Ed.). *Interpretive phenomenology: Embodiment, caring and ethics in health and illness.* Thousand Oaks, CA: Sage.

Bogdan, R., & Biklen, S. (1982). *Qualitative research for education: An introduction to theory and methods.* Boston: Allyn & Bacon.

Bogdan, R., & Taylor, S. (1975). *Introduction to qualitative methods.* New York: Wiley.

Copel, L. (1984). Loneliness: A clinical investigation. Unpublished doctoral dissertation, Texas Woman's University, Denton.

Drew, N. (1989). The interviewer's experience as data in phenomenological research. *Western Journal of Nursing Research, 11,* 431–439.

Gadow, S. (1977, November 11). Existential advocacy: Philosophical foundation of nursing. Phase I Conference, Four-State Consortium on Nursing and the Humanities, Farmington, CT.

Glaser, B., & Strauss, A. (1988). *The discovery of grounded theory.* Chicago: Aldine.

Hutchinson, S. (1986). Creating meaning: Grounded theory of NICU nurses. In W. Chenitz & J. Swanson, *From practice to grounded theory* (pp. 191–204). Menlo Park, CA: Addison-Wesley.

Katzman, E., & Roberts, J. (1988). Nurse-physician conflicts as barriers to the enactment of nursing roles. *Western Journal of Nursing Research, 10,* 576–590.

Knafl, K., & Howard, M. (1986). Interpreting, reporting and evaluating qualitative research. In P. Munhall & C. Oiler (Eds.), *Nursing research: A qualitative perspective.* Norwalk, CT: Appleton-Century-Crofts.

Kramer, M. (1968). Role models, role conception, and role deprivation. *Nursing Research, 17,* 115–120.

Lather, P. (1986). Research as praxis. *Harvard Educational Review, 560,* 257–277.

Lincoln, Y., & Guba, E. (1985). *Naturalistic inquiry.* Newbury, CA: Sage.

Merleau-Ponty, M. (1962). *Phenomenology of perception* (C. Smith, Trans.). New York: Humanities Press.

Munhall, P. (1982). Nursing philosophy and nursing research: In apposition or opposition? *Nursing Research, 31,* 176–181.

Munhall, P. (1986). Methodological issues in nursing: Beyond a wax apple. *Advances in Nursing Science, 8* (3), 1–5.

Munhall, P. (1989). Philosophical pondering on qualitative research methods in nursing. *Nursing Science Quarterly, 2,* 20–28.

National League for Nursing. (1988). *Curriculum revolution: Mandate for change.* New York: National League for Nursing.

Newman, M. (1990). Newman's theory of health as praxis. *Nursing Science Quarterly, 3,* 37–41.

Oiler, C. (1982). The phenomenological approach in nursing research. *Nursing Research, 31,* 178–181.

Oiler, C. (1986). Qualitative methods: Phenomenology. In P. Moccia (Ed.), *New approaches to theory development* (pp. 75–103). New York: National League for Nursing.

Parse, R. (1990). Parse's research methodology with an illustration of the lived experience of hope. *Nursing Science Quarterly, 3,* 9–17.

Paterson, J., & Zderad, L. (1976). *Humanistic nursing.* New York: Wiley.

Patton, M. (1980). *Qualitative evaluation methods.* Newbury, CA: Sage.

Quint, J. (1967). *The nurse and the dying patient.* New York: Macmillan.

Schutz, A. (1970). *On phenomenology and social relations* (H. Wagner, Ed.). Chicago: University of Chicago Press.

Schutz, A. (1973). *Collected papers 1. The problem of social reality* (M. Natanson, Ed.). The Hague: Martinus Nijhoff.

Sharts-Engel, N. (1989). An American experience of pregnancy and childbirth in Japan. *Birth, 16*(2), 81–86.

Tinkle, M., & Beaton, J. (1983). Toward a new view of science: Implications for nursing research. *Advances in Nursing Science, 5,* 27–36.

ADDITIONAL REFERENCES

Appleton, J. V., & King, L. (1997). Constructivism: A naturalistic methodology for nursing inquiry. *Advances in Nursing Science, 20*(2), 13–22.

Avis, M. (1997). Letting sleeping dogmas lie: An examination of positivism in the nursing research literature. *Social Sciences in Health: International Journal of Research and Practice, 3,* 52–63.

Clark, A. M. (1998). The qualitative-quantitative debate: Moving from positivism and confrontation to post-positivism and reconciliation. *Journal of Advanced Nursing, 27,* 1242–1249.

Corben, V. (1999). Phenomenology revisited. Misusing phenomenology in nursing research: Identifying the issues. *Nurse Researcher, 6*(3), 52–66.

Dahlberg, K., & Drew, N. (1997). A lifeworld paradigm for nursing research. *Journal of Holistic Nursing, 15,* 303–317.

Farrel, G. A., & Gritching, W. L. (1997). Social science at the crossroads: What direction mental health nurses? *Australian New Zealand Journal of Mental Health Nursing, 6,* 19–29.

Geanellos, R. (1997). Nursing knowledge development: Where to from here? *Collegian: Journal of the Royal College of Nursing Australia, 4,* 13–21.

Heslop, L. (1997). The impossibilities of poststructuralist and critical social nursing inquiry. *Nursing Inquiry, 4,* 48–56.

Johnson, M. (1999). Observations on positivism and pseudoscience in qualitative nursing research. *Journal of Advanced Nursing, 30,* 67–73.

Letourneau, N., & Allen, M. (1999). Post-positivistic critical multiplism: A beginning dialogue. *Journal of Advanced Nursing, 30,* 623–630.

Lutz, K. F., Jones, K. D., & Kendall, J. (1997). Expanding the praxis debate: Contributions to clinical inquiry. *Advances in Nursing Science,* 20(2), 23–31.

Marks, M. D. (1999). Network. Reconstructing nursing: Evidence, artistry and the curriculum . . . including commentary by L. Nyatanga and M. Johnson. *Nurse Education Today,* 19, 3–11.

Monti, E. J., & Tingen, M. S. (1999). Multiple paradigms of nursing science. *Advances in Nursing Science,* 21(4), 64–80.

Newman, M. A. (1999). The rhythm of relating in a paradigm of wholeness. *Image: Journal of Nursing Scholarship,* 31(3), 227–230.

Oiler, C. (1983). Nursing reality as reflected in nurses' poetry. *Perspectives in Psychiatric Care* 21(3), 81–89.

Picard, C. (1997). Embodied soul: The focus of nursing praxis. *Journal of Holistic Nursing,* 15(10), 41–53.

Quint, J. (1966). Awareness of death and the nurse's composure. *Nursing Research,* 15, 49–55.

Silva, M. C. (1997). Classic image. Philosophy, science, theory: Interrelationships and implications for nursing research. *Image: Journal of Nursing Scholarship,* 29(3), 210–215.

Thorne, S. E., Kirkham, S. R., & Henderson, A. (1999). Ideological implications of paradigm discourse. *Nursing Inquiry,* 6(2), 123–131.

Wainwright, S. P. (1997). A new paradigm for nursing: The potential realism. *Journal of Advanced Nursing,* 26, 1262–1271.

Watson, J. (1995). Postmodernism and knowledge development in nursing. *Nursing Science Quarterly,* 8(2), 60–64.

Part II

Qualitative Methods and Exemplars

In Part II of this text the reader is invited to contemplate the range of qualitative methods, the "how to do" chapter followed by the "here is an example" chapter. Readers will become aware of similarities among the methods as well as variations in carrying out the methods and the different aims of the methods. The term "degrees of freedom" is not associated with qualitative research, but there is a freedom about qualitative research, a flexibility, room to move about in, room to explore. Our contributors exemplify the courage often necessary to deal with such freedom.

There are similarities and congruencies, yet there are differences. The studies reported here, as examples of qualitative research, seem to be excellent examples of the humanistic, caring perspective that embraces the philosophy of nursing. They are descriptive of experience at the very core of human caring and human understanding.

In Chapter 4, Carolyn Oiler Boyd describes the major philosophical underpinnings of phenomenology and some prevalent methods. In Chapter 5, I present a "new" phenomenological method, which has evolved from my interactions with colleagues, students and patients. Sarah Lauterbach, in Chapter 6, presents new research, which is a longitudinal phenomenological study where she returns to the mothers who experienced prenatal death of a wished-for baby five years ago. Reading about these mothers' experiences five years later is extremely moving and demonstrates the need for this kind of understanding for nursing practice, as did Selen's first study (1993).

Sally A. Hutchinson and Holly Skodal Wilson, in Chapter 7, introduce us to the potential and possibilities of the Grounded Theory Method, another qualitative research method. JoAnne Weiss and Sally provide us with an exemplar study entitled, "Understanding Clients' Health-Care Decisions." This study, discussed in Chapter 8, challenges our current beliefs about health care education, and directs us to the perceptions and processes that patients use when given information. Carol P. Germain clearly describes the method of ethnography in Chapter 9. Zane Robinson Wolf, in Chapter 10, demonstrates the richness derived from this method with findings critical for cardiac patients and their symptom management. The case study method is presented by Carla Mariano in Chapter 11 and so poignantly illustrated by Mary Colvin in her compelling study: Drifting Without Consciousness. The historical method of research is described by M. Louise Fitzpatrick in Chapter 13 and demonstrated in a fascinating historical study by Lynne Dunphy. This study, described in Chapter 14, is a history of nursing care of patients in iron lungs, from 1928-1955.

New to this edition is the method of Interpretive Analysis, written by Richard MacIntyre in Chapter 15. Richard then goes on in Chapter 16 to demonstrate the role of critical theory in his interpretive analysis of "Religion as Metaphor" in a study involving individuals with AIDS or HIV. Another new method and exemplar are added to this edition: Action Research. Carolyn Brown in Chapter 17 provides us with a description of this method and in Chapter 18 Jody Glittenberg provides us with a "snowball" exemplar!

For students who would like to read additional exemplars of the first five methods articulated in this book, those different exemplars or examples of the method can be found in the two preceding editions of this book (Munhall & Oiler, 1987, 1993). Those studies are well worth returning to, not only for their richness, but to further explicate the particular method.

These Chapters will conclude Part II of this text, and we will move on to Part III for a general discussion about various considerations, techniques and conditions for qualitative research which influences all of the above methods.

4

Phenomenology
The Method

Carolyn Oiler Boyd

In this chapter, overviews of the various interpretations of phenomenological method in nursing will be presented with the expectation
that readers who wish to make the method their own will follow through
on leads to other writings and other thinkers, to acquire a thorough understanding of any one or more of these interpretations. Despite the
many meanings of phenomenological method, an effort will be made
to distinguish it as a method, in contrast with other qualitative approaches. These distinctions are the author's interpretations and are
very much guided by the common longer-range goal of making phenomenology work well for us in nursing research—that is, of extrapolating nursing research methodology from phenomenology. Phenomenology invites this kind of effort and insists on an openness that can
protect such ideas about method from being reduced to dogma.

The discussion picks up where the presentation of phenomenological themes left off in the preceding chapter. Phenomenology will be
defined first as a philosophical method with an emphasis on its defining characteristics. Overviews of selected modifications of phenomenology in social science will then be presented to acquaint the reader
with the cluster of research approaches that may be properly referred
to as phenomenologies in nursing.

WHAT IS PHENOMENOLOGY?

As noted in the preceding chapter, phenomenology is a word that is used in a wide variety of ways, obfuscating efforts to locate a clear response to the question, What is phenomenology? Merleau-Ponty, in a 1956 publication, acknowledged that phenomenology had not managed to define itself, and began his defining comments by noting:

> [P]henomenology was practiced and recognized as a manner or style . . . it existed as a movement before arriving at a complete philosophical consciousness. It has been on the way for along time, and its disciples find it everywhere: in Hegel and Kierkegaard certainly, but also in Marx, Nietzsche and Freud. . . . It is to ourselves that we will find the unity and true meaning of phenomenology. . . . Phenomenology is accessible only to a phenomenological method. . . . [Through a deliberate synthesis of phenomenological themes], [p]erhaps then we will understand why phenomenology has remained so long in a state of beginning, a task yet to be accomplished. (pp. 59–60)

Phenomenology has a long history as a general way of thinking among a number of theorists who greatly affected Western culture. We can identify many ideas and ways of thinking about things that are phenomenological in spirit, almost as a kind of attitude or a set of predilections that produce a certain style. It is first, then, a continuing intellectual movement, an attitude, a style of regarding the world that in itself has been pervasively influential in the social sciences. For overviews of phenomenology as a movement, Cohen (1987) and Reeder (1987) are excellent sources in the nursing literature. For a fuller account, Spiegelberg (1976, 1981, 1982), a phenomenologist and historian of phenomenology, is the most widely used reference.

Phenomenology is more than a general movement; it has arrived at a "complete philosophical consciousness." Merleau-Ponty directed readers who seek definition to the task of comprehending the themes of phenomenological philosophy. Simply, to know what phenomenology is, one must know the themes that constitute the philosophy. Some of these themes were identified in the preceding chapter as the philosophical foundations of the qualitative paradigm generally. Others, notably phenomenological description and bracketing and phenomenological reduction, will be discussed in this chapter. These themes speak directly to phenomenological method, and, as Merleau-Ponty stated, phenomenology is accessible only through its method. The grounding in phenomenology is, in other words, in its philosophy and its method. Readers are advised to take advantage of the various presentations of phenomenology in the nursing literature (Anderson, 1989; Benner, 1983, 1985; Davis, 1973; Oiler, 1982, 1986, 1988; Omery, 1983; Parse, 1990; Parse, Coyne, & Smith, 1985; Paterson & Zderad, 1976; Ray, 1985). It is important to recognize, however, that these nurse authors' efforts to present and explain are not substitutes for the readers' efforts to get inside the phenomenological framework and to see from there what becomes visible concerning those phenomena of interest in nursing. The process of struggling to see is, in other words, phenomenological method.

Social science modifications of phenomenological method aside, it is reasonable to question how relevant phenomenological method, in its strict philosophical sense, is to nursing research. This judgment does not hold for qualitative research in general; we need to turn heartily toward the qualitative paradigm not only in nursing research but also in nursing education and nursing practice. To the extent that the qualitative paradigm is assumed by the nursing profession, there will be phenomenological study in nursing, in accord with phenomenological method as philosophical method. However, these methods will be intimately related to other kinds of research (particularly those inspired by phenomenological philosophy) that are pursued in the interest of a variety of nursing practice aims. In other words, this optimistic view of a perfect world rewards us with a vision of coherence within the nursing discipline.

METHODOLOGICAL THEMES

In addition to the phenomenological themes presented in the preceding chapter as foundational to qualitative research, others will be described here to disclose common features across the variety of phenomenologies that collectively indicate something of the scope of phenomenology. Progress toward clarity in the definition will be made by narrowing the sense of the word if not by achieving precision for its use. Recurring ideas among authors delineate an area of consensus that will help us to establish some kind of boundary for what is to be considered phenomenological research in nursing in contrast with other qualitative research approaches. A particular boundary will be proposed, but in the spirit of continuing consideration of criteria for phenomenologies in nursing.

Aim: Phenomenological Description

Merleau-Ponty (1956, p. 59) stated that the whole effort of phenomenology is to describe experience as it is and to describe it directly, without considering the various causal explanations that social scientists may give. This statement seems simple enough, but the difficulty resides in the meaning of experience as consciousness or existence itself. Husserl (in a 1965 translation) argued for phenomenology as rigorous science and explained that the focus on experience in phenomenology does not coincide with a natural science about consciousness:

> [P]sychology is concerned with "empirical consciousness," with consciousness from the empirical point of view, as an empirical being in the ensemble of nature, whereas phenomenology is concerned with "pure" consciousness, i.e., consciousness from the phenomenological point of view. (p. 91)

Experience is "something psychical, a phenomenon comes and so it retains no enduring, identical being that can be objectively determinable as such in the sense of natural science, e.g., as objectively divisible into components, 'analysable' in the proper sense." Experience "appears as itself through itself, in an absolute flow, as and already 'fading away,' clearly recognizable as constantly sinking back into a 'having been'" (p. 107). Experience can be recalled, having been perceived at some point in time.

For Merleau-Ponty (1962), the world is not perceived through a combination of sensations and perspectives. Reality is not constituted by perceiving representations of reality. Coherence in the world is lived. Relation to the world is a living and nonirreducible impulse that is understandable only as a unified experience. It is not knowledge of the world such as posed by an analysis of sensation. Perception is original awareness of the appearances of phenomena in experience. It is defined as access to truth, the foundation of all knowledge. Perception gives one access to experience of the world as it is given prior to any analysis of it. "To perceive is to render oneself present to something through the body; all the while the thing keeps its place within the horizon of the world" (p. 42). The focus on experience in phenomenology is, then, a focus on human involvement in a world; the oft used expression "lived experience" emphasizes this focus. Phenomenology recognizes that meanings are given in perception and modified in analysis. "By these words, primacy of perception, we mean that the experience of perception is our presence at the moment when things, truths, values are constituted for us" (p. 25). Perception presents us with evidence of the world, not as it is thought but as it is lived. Perception of an amputated limb as an ambivalent presence is not truth, but it is reality. It is this evidence that is considered to be the foundation of science and knowledge. Beyond this, there is nothing to understand (p. 365).

In essence, phenomenologists hold that human existence is meaningful and of interest only in the sense that we are always conscious of something. Existence as being-in-the-world is a phenomenological phrase that acknowledges that people are tied to their worlds and are comprehensible only in their contexts. Human behavior occurs in the context of relations to things, people, events, and situations, in what Merleau-Ponty refers to embodiment. People, in all their subjectivity, are inseparably caught up in the physical world in such a way that the truth searched for in nursing research efforts will be grasped only by attending to the realities constituted in individual experiencing. Lived experience is, however, layered with meanings brought to the relation of being-in-the-world.

> Man finds himself at any moment of his daily life in a biographically determined situation, that is, in a physical and sociocultural environment as defined by him, within which he has his position, not merely his position in terms of physical space and outer time or of his status and role within the social system but also his moral and ideological positions. (Schutz, 1970, p. 73)

Seeing experience directly is thus not strictly possible, on two grounds: first, experiencing is living forward and, to be self-conscious, it must be suspended to yield to the experience of reflecting back on it; and, second, to suspend one's biography is to lose one's tie to the world. We can, however, become more self-conscious in reflection and resist the ready-made interpretations offered up by our biography in order to see more clearly the ties that we have to the world.

Farber (1966) noted that a purely descriptive method is an ideal with numerous obstacles:

> It is the aim of description to give an account of all the pertinent facts; it cannot be an account of *all* the facts, because the facts are infinite in number. . . . There are not only the difficulties resulting from the individual or the group which conditions him, but also the problems caused by the facts themselves; and there is the necessity of weighing the evidence of events which continue to recede into the past. (pp. 45–46)

We are limited by our "blinkers" and "spectacles"; that is, we see world as an already interpreted phenomenon, the result of past scientific inquiry and fixed traditional conceptions. For Farber, the nature of perception and of other modes of experience is the proper theme of phenomenological inquiry (pp. 48–49). In contrast with the interpretations of phenomenology in the social sciences, this delineation of the aim of phenomenology limits it to philosophical inquiry into acts of consciousness themselves. Merleau-Ponty's (1962) phenomenology of perception is such an inquiry. Zderad's (1968) philosophical dissertation on empathy is another example. Other acts of consciousness that would be included in the realm of phenomenology from Farber's point of view are remembering, judging, intuiting, and valuing. The phenomenological questions concern how these ways of attending to the world are possible.

Merleau-Ponty (1956) stated that perception:

[I]s the basis from which every act issues and it is presupposed by them. The world is not an object the law of whose constitution I possess. It is the natural milieu and the field of all my thoughts and of all my explicit perceptions. Truth does not "dwell" only in the "interior man" for there is no interior man. Man is before himself in the world and it is in the world that he knows himself. When I turn upon myself from the dogmatism of common sense or the dogmatism of science, I find, not the dwelling place of intrinsic truth, but a subject committed to the world. (p. 62)

The evidence of perception is condemned to meaning. (p. 69)

All description of experience is thus inescapably interpretive. The various techniques that can be used in phenomenological method serve, in the unity of knower and known, to forward the project of seeing a phenomenon and the project of describing what has been seen. Phenomenological description is the final "step" of phenomenological method; in it, the other steps taken (and the degree of success with which they were accomplished are reflected such that the process is the content. The nature of the task of description in phenomenology can thus be understood only through a grasp of antecedent steps of phenomenological method.

Bracketing and the Phenomenological Reduction

The process of recovering original awareness (perception) is called "reduction" in phenomenology. Phenomenological reduction is a particular manner of rigorous reflection, and bracketing is the leading methodological technique used in phenomenology to aid in this process. To describe lived experience, it must first be disclosed. Bracketing and phenomenological reduction are the means to this disclosure. Merleau-Ponty (1956) described the scope of this task:

> Our relation to the world is so profound and so intimate that the only way for us to notice it is to suspend its movements, to refuse it our complicity . . . or to render it inoperative. (p. 64)

He instructed us to make our presuppositions and common sense appear by deliberately abstaining from them. He advised us to be astonished before the world; in other words, to describe lived experience, we must set aside the natural attitude toward the world that our biography has given us. In astonishment, the layers of meaning given by interpretation, knowledge, and explanation are carefully preserved but laid aside. Our ties to the world in roles, knowledge, belief, habit, common sense, and the like, are disrupted so as to make them apparent. Bracketing our presuppositions about the world is performed "not to deny them and even less to deny the link which binds us to the physical, social and cultural world" (Merleau-Ponty, 1964, p. 49). The reduction is performed so as to expose the link.

What is revealed in phenomenological reduction, then, is not "pure" experience; rather, it is experience constituted in one's ties to the world. Complete reduction is impossible, because consciousness is engaged in a world. Phenomenological description is contingent on the perspective given in experience and presented in perception. People are "always situated and always individuated" (Merleau-Ponty, 1964, p. 51). In the reflection of reduction, which strives to freeze time and suspend acts of consciousness, time nevertheless continues. There is always, in phenomenological description, then, the layer of this experience in time, the study of the experience that has just passed. "Our existence is too strictly caught up in the world to know itself as such at the moment when it is thrown forth upon the world" (Merleau-Ponty, 1956, p. 65). For this reason, phenomenological reduction and description will yield incomplete profiles of reality because one never goes beyond time" (Merleau-Ponty, 1964, p. 49).

Schutz (1973) illuminated the complex idea of reduction by acknowledging that, although the technique of bracketing in reduction is extremely difficult, it is yet within human capability. In performing the reduction, one assumes an attitude of doubt toward the world:

> What we have to put in brackets is not only the existence of an outer world, along with all the things in it, inanimate and

animate, including fellow-men, cultural objects, society, and its institutions. Also our belief in the validity of our statements about this world and its content, as conceived within the mundane sphere, has to be suspended. Consequently, not only our practical knowledge of the world but also the propositions of all the sciences dealing with the existence of the world, all natural and social sciences, psychology, logic and even geometry—all have to be brought within the brackets. (p. 105)

As the layers of meaning that give us interpreted experience are bracketed, the perceived world emerges. In the reduced sphere, objects appear in a figure–ground relation, with each object having a horizon that implicates other objects in a meaningful system of relations. This is the meaning of holism, and perception is the level at which holism occurs. Intuition figures prominently, grasping this meaningful system of relations as a mode of awareness that adheres closely to the perceived world.

Phenomenological reduction is a matter of refraining from judgments. Schutz's (1973) description of the natural attitude as layers of meaning helps us to understand that reduction as a process can be used in degrees. Layers can be peeled away one at a time. Perception can be revealed relative to a painstaking effort to peel away some of our ready-made interpretations of experience:

Our knowledge of an object, at a certain given moment, is nothing else than the sediment of previous mental processes by which it has been constituted. It has its own history, and this history of its constitution can be found by questioning it. This is done by turning back from the seemingly ready-made object of our thought to the different activities of our mind in which and by which it has been constituted step by step. (p. 111)

In its most important sense, phenomenological method is a call to reflective thoughtfulness of the most rigorous kind, at the most rigorous level. The point of the effort is to return to the natural attitude where insights gained within the reduced sphere can be put to use (Schutz, 1970, p. 59).

Essential Elements

In a description of the characteristic core in the various phenomenologies, Spiegelberg (1976) identified seven steps of phenomenological method. He noted that the first of these steps, investigating particular phenomena, is easily the most adoptable and has a completeness of its own. There are three operations in this step: intuiting, analyzing, and describing. Of the first operation, he wrote:

> [Intuiting] is one of the most demanding operations, which requires utter concentration on the object intuited without becoming absorbed in it to the point of no longer looking critically. Nevertheless there is little that the beginning phenomenologist can be given by way of precise instructions beyond such metaphoric phrases as "opening his eyes," "keeping them open," "not getting blinded," "looking and listening, " etc. (pp. 659–660)

Comparing and contrasting the phenomenon under investigation with related phenomena and studying phenomenologists' approaches to and accounts of phenomena are also offered as aids in learning to perform the operation of intuiting a phenomenon.

The second operation of investigating particular phenomena, phenomenological analyzing, requires identifying the structure of a phenomenon under study. Anderson (1989) drew our attention to the problem of knowing what is meant by the term "structure." She argued that the problem is not so much knowing what the nature of structure is as it is identifying whose structures are being described:

> It is not as if the researcher is describing structures that are out there and are independent of the researcher and informant. . . . [W]hat needs to be made explicit is that the structures described are those that one creates and imposes on the world— these structures are embedded in the system of relevances of the researcher; what gets produced as knowledge results from the dialectical process between researcher and informant. (pp. 22–23)

In her discussion, Anderson alluded to the difficulty introduced in phenomenology when experience is studied vicariously, as is the case in the social sciences. [Readers may wish to see Spiegelberg's discussion of phenomenology through vicarious experience for another treatment of this difficulty (1975, pp. 35–53).] Anderson stressed that knowledge is created ideally in a joint project in which the researcher and the researched are mutually committed to describing the phenomenon under study. The structure that is identified through phenomenological analyzing is, in the end, the researcher's structure. It is an identification of the phenomenon's elements and of the relations and connections of those elements' adjacent phenomena.

The third operation of investigating particular phenomena, phenomenological describing, is undertaken after phenomenological seeing has been accomplished through intuiting and analyzing the phenomenon.

> Phenomenology begins in silence. Only he who has experienced genuine perplexity and frustration in the face of the phenomena when trying to find the proper description for them knows what phenomenological seeing really means. (Spiegelberg, 1976, p. 672)

Spiegelberg cautioned that premature description is, in fact, one of the main pitfalls of phenomenology. The aim of this describing operation is to communicate; to guide the listener by giving distinctive guideposts to the phenomenon. The description serves to direct the listener to his own experience of the phenomenon, whether actual or potential:

> Describing is based on a classification of the phenomena. A description, therefore, presupposes a framework of class names, and all it can do is to determine the location of the phenomenon with regard to an already developed system of classes. (p. 673)

In regard to new phenomena or new aspects of familiar phenomena, there will not be any such existent framework to house the description. Spiegelberg advised that description by negation, metaphor, and analogy can then be used cautiously to indicate the phenomena in a suggestive manner. Phenomenological description is always necessarily selective and, as such, always represents a particular perspective or interpretation of the phenomenon under study.

To perform the reduction is to choose to perceive from another vantage point; one seizes experience and lives it through for oneself in phenomenological analyzing. Insight is communicated in the description. In performing the reduction, one suspends his or her preconceptions in order to explore the phenomenon not from what is known about it but from what might be so. Merleau-Ponty (1964) referred to this process as the imaginary free variation of facts:

> In order to grasp an essence, we consider a concrete experience, and then we make it change in our thought, trying to imagine it as effectively modified in all respects. That which remains invariable through these changes is the essence of the phenomena in question. (p. 70)

The task of phenomenological analyzing is a matter of identifying those elements of a phenomenon that entail a relation which, if omitted, would annihilate the phenomenon; that is, that which is essential for the phenomenon to be is isolated. This is a process akin to induction. Merleau-Ponty pointed out that the difference between induction and phenomenological reduction and description is a matter of degree. However incomplete phenomenological descriptions may be, to the extent that they succeed in disclosing experiences from some points of view, they bring us closer to understanding lived experiences.

Spiegelberg (1976) asserted that intuiting, analyzing, and describing particulars may be considered a common program for those who identify themselves as phenomenologists. The scope of phenomenology, however, goes beyond the study of particulars to include investigating general essences, essential relations among essences, modes of appearing, and the constitution of phenomena in consciousness; suspending belief in the existence of phenomena; and interpreting the meaning of phenomena. Investigation of general essences and relations among essences refers to looking at particulars as examples or instances to apprehend their natural affinity in a pattern common to particular phenomena that belong together in a natural grouping. Based on antecedent or simultaneous intuiting of particulars, this extension of phenomenology to a concern with essences draws on seeing particulars in their structural affinities. Their pattern or essence is the ground of those structural affinities (Spiegelberg, 1976, p. 678). When an essence is apprehended, the next step can be attempted: a search for relations within an essence or among several essences. Throughout, the operations of intuiting, analyzing, and describing must be performed. In the phenomenological steps of watching modes of appearing and exploring the constitution of phenomena in consciousness, phenomenology directs its attention not only to the sense of what appears, but also to the way in which things appear, establish themselves, and take shape in consciousness. The step of suspending belief is phenomenological reduction and was discussed earlier. Lastly, the step of interpreting concealed meanings refers to the attempt to interpret the sense of certain phenomena. Spiegelberg (1976) noted that this effort was focused and developed in hermeneutic phenomenology, a particular type of phenomenology. In a sense, all of phenomenology is concerned with meaning and interpretation:

> For not only our purposive behavior but our whole cognitive and emotional life, as phenomenology sees it, is shot through with meaning and meaningful intentions. No description can leave them out, even though it may refrain from accepting them at face value. Thus hermeneutic phenomenology must aim at

something different and more ambitious: its goal is the discovery of meanings which are not immediately manifest to our intuiting, analyzing, and describing. Hence the interpreter has to go beyond what is directly given. (p. 695)

The appearance of references to hermeneutic phenomenology in the nursing literature needs to be understood as one way in which to practice phenomenology (Allen & Jensen, 1990; Benner, 1985; Leonard, 1989; Parse et al., 1985). The common theme among the various phenomenologies is the concern for describing lived experience, which is understood to be a concern for human meanings and ultimately for interpreting those meanings so that they inform our practice and our science. The variations in accounts of phenomenology among nurse authors is best understood by recognizing the many ways to phenomenology and the exercise of choice among these paths in the design and conduct of a phenomenological study.

CRITERIA FOR PHENOMENOLOGIES

The divergencies of the various phenomenologists in their interrelations and prescriptions for phenomenological method are further embellished in the various translations and modifications of phenomenology in social science; they have made phenomenology an increasingly broad approach with multiple paths. For both the observer and the learner of qualitative approaches, acquaintance with the common ground of phenomenology assists with consideration of interpretations of method. Spiegelberg (1975) proposed a set of seven criteria for distinguishing phenomenological inquiry from other approaches (pp. 10–12). These criteria will be discussed briefly as a point of reference for consideration of selected interpretations of phenomenological method in nursing and for a closer look at some of the particulars associated with those interpretations. Although the criteria are not sacrosanct, they do at least establish a framework for considering phenomenological method in its many variations. Over time, as phenomenological methods are used in nursing, other criteria may emerge to designate more aptly what phenomenological method is for nursing.

Spiegelberg emphasized the aim of phenomenology as the premise for his comments on characteristics of phenomenologies; to give access to layers of our experience unprobed in our everyday living, thus providing deeper foundations for both science and life. The first characteristic of phenomenologies, then, is the focus on concretely experienced phenomena, as free as possible from conceptual presupposi- tions. The performance of phenomenological reduction to achieve a fresh approach to the study of experience distinguishes phenomenol- ogy clearly from the positivist tradition but is less powerful in distin- guishing it from other qualitative approaches. This is due, in part, to the influence of phenomenological method on aspects of other ap- proaches to qualitative research. The notion of bracketing, for exam- ple, is featured in all qualitative research designs.

The second characteristic is the inclusion of nonsensuous data as well as sense experience. Nonsensuous data include relations, ab- stract entities, and values, for example, as long as they present them- selves intuitively. An intuitive foundation and verification for all formal concepts is the third characteristic, and resistance transforming the given in interpretation is the fourth. The central role of intuition in phe- nomenology presents a quandary for us. Little understood and thus suspect, intuition is associated with a lack of rigor. Nevertheless, it in- troduces to research a unique relation between researcher and re- searched. Figure 4–1 represents this relation by contrasting researcher (R) and subject (S) relations among quantitative, qualitative, and phe- nomenological approaches to inquiry. In phenomenology, researcher and subject join in reflection on the experience under study, creating the circumstances for the researcher's inclusion in the study. Two nurs- ing studies come to mind as illustrations: Lynch-Sauer (1985) de- scribed the introduction of her diary entries as data in a study of post- poned childbearing; Drew (1989) described the use of her personal

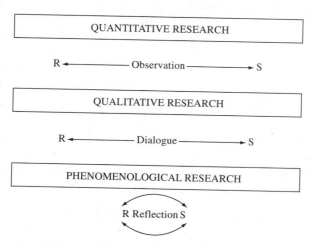

Figure 4–1 Comparison of researcher–subject relation.

responses in the interviewing process as data in a study of patients' experiences with caregivers.

The fifth characteristic is attention to the distinctions of the phenomena reflected in shades of ordinary language without sole reliance on language as a basis for study. The sixth and seventh characteristics concern producing as faithful a description as possible with cautious objectification of experience and responsible generalization based on insight into the relations between concrete experiences and abstractions.

PHENOMENOLOGICAL METHODS FOR SOCIAL SCIENCE

An overview of selected interpretations of phenomenological method will be presented to extend its description and to indicate its openness to interpretation as well as, indirectly, to point out some of the difficulties with this research approach. All these interpretations have been influenced by hermeneutic phenomenology to varying extents; all bear unique modifications to accommodate the aims of social science.

The Search for Structure and Essence in Experience

Phenomenological psychology introduces several interpretations for method taken up by a number of qualitative nurse researchers. Van Kaam's (1959) study of "really feeling understood" focuses on a psychological phenomenon and seeks to disclose the core of this experience. The research process in van Kaam's phenomenology requires posing the research question to a large number of subjects who are asked to respond by writing descriptions of their experiences with regard to a select phenomenon. It is presumed that people can express lived experience in such a way and that analysis of their descriptions will reveal an essential structure (core) of the human experience under study. Once the researcher obtains the descriptions from willing subjects, the analysis proceeds as follows:

1. Each expression (word or phrase) that describes some aspect of the experience is listed separately from the others.
2. Similar expressions are grouped together and labeled.

3. Irrelevant expressions are eliminated.
4. Groups of expressions that bear close relation to one another are clustered together and labeled.
5. The identified core of common elements is checked against a random sample of original descriptions by subjects. Discrepancies at this point direct the researcher to start again with the analysis.
6. The steps of analysis (1–5) are performed independently by judges to check the reliability of the results.

The essential structure of really feeling understood was reported in the following statement:

> The experience of really feeling understood is a perceptual-emotional gestalt. A subject, perceiving that a person co-experiences what things mean to the subject and accepts him, feels, initially, relief from experiential loneliness, and gradually, safe experiential communion with that person and with that which the subject perceives this person to represent. (van Kaam, 1959, p. 69)

The full report of findings includes justification and explanation of each phrase of the description of the essential structure.

A number of published nursing studies have used van Kaam's approach to phenomenology, often with some modifications of the process. These modifications usually are reduced sample size and/or the substitution or addition of interview for the written description. Sandelowski and Pollock (1986), for example, interviewed 48 women to identify recurring themes in their experiences of infertility treatment. Those themes were ambiguity, temporality, and otherness. The description of the experience of infertility pivots on these three themes (elements) and includes elaboration on varying expressions of them by participants in the study (p. 142). In Colaizzi's (1978) interpretation of the method, interview is the selected strategy for generating data. Often, lengthy and repeated interviews are necessary to facilitate subjects' descriptions of their experiences, thus accounting for there typically being fewer subjects in studies that use Colaizzi's approach. Haase (1987) used the Colaizzi method in her study of chronically ill adolescents' experiences of courage. She interviewed nine chronically ill, hospitalized adolescents and analyzed transcripts of these interviews in a process similar to van Kaam's (heretofore described). To illustrate this process of searching for themes in interview data, Haase

(1987) reported the following example of abstractions from subjects' words:

> Subject: "My mom just held my hand and talked to me. That made it better."
> Researcher's abstractions:
> 1. Mother holding hand and talking improved situation.
> 2. Touch and verbal expressions of caring by mother decreased feelings of despair to a tolerable level. (p. 67)

It can be seen from this example that the process of analysis is one of abstracting from subjects' words to formulate essential meanings in the experiences. Such meanings are grouped to constitute themes; themes are grouped into clusters; and clusters are grouped into categories. In Haase's study, 9 categories, 30 clusters, and an even larger number of descriptive themes within those clusters were identified. Figure 4–2 illustrates this inductive ordering of the data from the more concrete themes to the more abstract clusters and categories (Haase, 1987, pp. 77–78). This kind of inductive approach is a primary feature of both van Kaam's and Colaizzi's phenomenologies.

Perhaps because so much attention is given to analytic steps and because the data are formally limited to what people say in writing or in interview, both these phenomenologies appear to fall short of the aforedescribed criteria for phenomenologies. In Parse's (1990) phe-

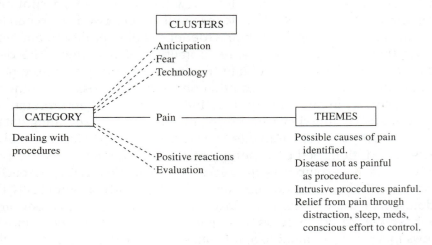

Figure 4–2 Illustration of inductive ordering in Haase's study of adolescent courage.

nomenology, some of these shortcomings were addressed. Parse identified lived experiences of health such as feeling lonely and feeling joyful as the entities for study, and stated, as the aim of phenomenology, understanding the structure of lived experience. Four processes are used to accomplish this aim:

1. Participant selection to achieve redundancy in or saturation of the data. From two to ten participants are usually sufficient.
2. Dialogical engagement of researcher and participant in an unstructured discussion. The quality of this engagement is one of intersubjective "being with" the other.
3. Extraction-synthesis of the data so that descriptions given in participants' language are moved up to the level of abstraction of the language of science. This process entails attentive study of the transcribed discussions and creative conceptualization. Creative conceptualization in turn requires various operations of abstraction and synthesis of abstractions to generate a structure that identifies core concepts and their relations to one another.
4. Heuristic interpretation of the finding of the study by relating it to Parse's man-living-health theory (pp. 10–12).

In a study of hope, Parse illustrated the use of her phenomenology. Ten patients were interviewed for 30 minutes or more while receiving hemodialysis. The process of extraction-synthesis is illustrated here:

Extracted essence: While waiting for a 2nd kidney transplant, looks forward to his situation getting better as he remembers and wishes for a life without the machine.

Synthesized essence: Anticipating is fostered by envisioning the was and will be as it is now.

Proposition: The lived experience of hope is anticipating through envisioning the was and will be as it is now while engaging in activities that create harmony and unfold in a different perspective. (p. 13) Ten propositions were created; one for each participant. (p. 14)

Extracted core concepts:

• Anticipating possibilities through envisioning the not yet.
• Harmoniously living the comfort-discomfort of everydayness.
• Unfolding a different perspective of an expanding view. (p. 15)

The structure of the lived experience of hope, then, is: "Hope is anticipating possibilities through envisioning the not yet in harmoniously living the comfort-discomfort of everydayness while unfolding a different perspective of an expanding view" (p. 15). Each core concept is then interpreted in terms of Parse's principles: "Hope is the persistent picturing of possibles (imaging) while incarnating opportunities-limitations all at once (enabling-limiting) which unfolds in viewing the familiar in a new light (transforming)" (p. 16). Last came the conceptual interpretation: "Hope is imaging the enabling-limiting of transforming" (p. 16). Parse's man-living-health theory provides the overriding framework in her phenomenological method, a feature that is viewed by some as contributing to the grounding of phenomenological inquiry in a nursing perspective. For others, this feature bleeds the work of phenomenological reduction and, from this point of view, transgresses what is regarded as the hallmark of phenomenology.

The Search for Expanded Consciousness

In another style of the phenomenologies, the work of Paterson and Zderad (1976) and Benner (1983, 1985), and Van Manen's interpretation in education (1990), may be grouped loosely together in contrast with the phenomenologies described in the preceding section. In the author's view, these approaches are more closely aligned with phenomenological philosophy and with Spiegelberg's criteria for phenomenologies.

Phenomenology was first introduced to a wide nursing audience in Paterson and Zderad's *Humanistic Nursing* (1976), which by their own account was a collection of metatheoretical essays about the nature of nursing. The phases of their phenomenological method are (pp. 76–81):

1. *Preparation of the researcher*: The researcher needs to be an open, self-aware person. These qualities can be nurtured especially well by ongoing studies in the humanities.
2. *Primary data collection*: Observations are made from *within* the situation under study. The researcher must therefore be a practicing nurse rather than an outside observer of nursing. Data will include *firsthand observations* inclusive of intuitive insights and empathic awarenesses.
3. *Scientific analysis*: The researcher conceptualizes and expresses understandings in a reflective turn toward the data collected from clinical experience.
4. *Scientific synthesis*: The researcher locates other related or similar situations (from past experience and in the literature) to compare and contrast the data with other known realities. This is

an interpretive activity performed to sort and classify the data thematically.

5. *Abstraction*: The experience is finally conceptualized to account for its relatedness to other knowledge and its variations. Nursing knowledge is thus expanded, and the researcher as clinician is transformed in perspective.

Paterson and Zderad's report of a study of comfort serves as an illustration of the use of their method for nursing research. Primary data were collected and recorded for several months from weekly interactions with 15 hospitalized psychiatric patients. Through reflective analysis and synthesis of these data, 12 nurse behaviors aimed toward patient comfort were identified, together with 4 criteria for estimating the degree of a patient's comfort and 52 items of knowledge needed by a nurse whose aim is to comfort (pp. 107–111, 123–129). The following theoretical construct of comfort emerged from this study:

> Comfort is (a universal nursing) aim toward which persons' conditions of being move through relationships with others by internalizing freedom from painful controlling effects of the past. These effects have inhibited their self-control, realistic planning, and prevented them from being all that they could be in accordance with their potential at any particular time in any particular situation. (p. 111)

An outline of Paterson and Zderad's approach for conceptualtion of nursing phenomena is presented in Figure 4–3. An intuitive grasp of a phenomenon is contingent on the researcher's openness to the phenomenon and encompasses the first two phases of the heretofore listed phenomenological method (preparation of the researcher and primary data collection). The techniques listed as aids to an intuitive grasp reflect bracketing and the phenomenological reduction and use of the researcher's access to an array of modes of awareness. Analytic examination coincides with the third phase (scientific analysis) and directs the researcher to what have been noted in Spiegelberg's discussion of phenomenological analysis. Description and synthesis coincide with the fourth and fifth phases (scientific synthesis and abstraction). Again, the operation of phenomenological analysis is apparent in the techniques suggested to define, describe, and construct a conceptualization of the phenomenon under study. The overriding context for this phenomenology is the nursing situation; products of the inquiry speak directly to that context.

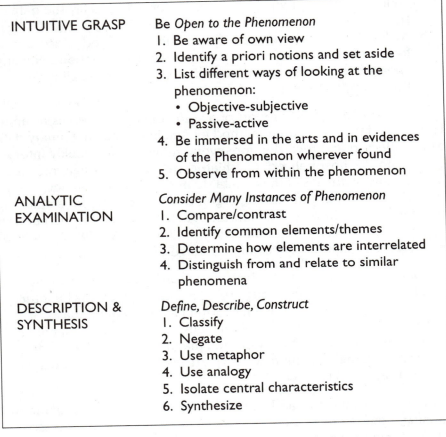

INTUITIVE GRASP   Be *Open to the Phenomenon*
                        1. Be aware of own view
                        2. Identify a priori notions and set aside
                        3. List different ways of looking at the
                           phenomenon:
                           • Objective-subjective
                           • Passive-active
                        4. Be immersed in the arts and in evidences
                           of the Phenomenon wherever found
                        5. Observe from within the phenomenon

ANALYTIC   *Consider Many Instances of Phenomenon*
EXAMINATION   1. Compare/contrast
                        2. Identify common elements/themes
                        3. Determine how elements are interrelated
                        4. Distinguish from and relate to similar
                           phenomena

DESCRIPTION &   *Define, Describe, Construct*
SYNTHESIS   1. Classify
                        2. Negate
                        3. Use metaphor
                        4. Use analogy
                        5. Isolate central characteristics
                        6. Synthesize

Figure 4–3 An approach for conceptualization of nursing phenomena.
Source: Adapted from *Humanistic Nursing* (pp. 71–91) by J. Paterson and
L. Zderad, 1976. New York: Wiley.

Benner (1985), Leonard (1989), and Allen and Jensen (1990) all provided presentations of hermeneutic phenomenology, one of the many
possible groundings in phenomenology. The particular is on human
nature as constituted by interpretive understanding (Leonard, 1989,
p. 47), and the aim is understanding through interpretation of the phenomenon under study (Allen & Jensen, 1990, p. 242). Benner (1985)
gave this overview:

The goal is to find exemplars or paradigm cases that embody
the meanings of everyday practices. The data are participant ob-

servations, field notes, interviews, and unobtrusive samples of behavior and interaction in natural settings. Human behavior is treated as a text analogue and the tack is to uncover the meanings in everyday practice in such a way that they are not destroyed, distorted, decontextualized, trivialized, or sentimentalized. (pp. 5–6)

Familiar phenomenological themes ground the method. Lived human meanings are understood to constitute and to be constituted by one's experiences. Understanding human experience, then, requires attending to what Benner refers to as the transaction between the individual and the situation (p. 7). Three phases of the research strategies of hermeneutic phenomenology were listed by Leonard (1989, pp. 53–55):

1. *Thematic analysis*: Interview material and observations are converted into text through transcription. A global analysis is performed to accomplish four tasks:
   a. Identify lines of inquiry from emerging themes and theoretical background of the study.
   b. Develop interpretive plan and coding protocol.
   c. Code the interviews.
   d. Identify general categories that form bases of study's findings.
2. *Analysis of exemplars*: An exemplar, by definition, is a "vignette or story of the particular transaction that captures the meaning in the situation" (Benner, 1985, p. 10) so that it is recognizable in other situations. It provides a presentation of the person in the context of his or her situation inclusive of "intentions of actors and meanings in the situation" (Benner, 1985, p. 10). In this phase, all aspects of a particular situation and the participant's responses to it are coded to capture the lived meanings of the participant's experiences.
3. *Identify paradigm cases*: A paradigm case, by definition, is a "strong instance of a particular pattern of meanings" (Benner, 1985, p. 10). In this phase of hermeneutics, analysis is carried forward to articulate both what the case depicts and why it stands out as an instance of a particular meaning. Paradigm cases are what Benner refers to as markers "so that once a paradigm case is recognized . . . other more subtle cases with similar global characteristics can be recognized" (p. 10). Presentation of a paradigm case provides the description necessary to understand how a person's actions and interpretations emerge from his or her situational context—that is, his or her concerns, practices, and

background meanings. Beyond this, such a presentation provides what Leonard (1989, p. 54) referred to as a family resemblance between the paradigm case and a particular situation that one is attempting to understand and explain.

Allen and Jensen (1990) illustrated the use of hermeneutics in a study of what it means to be visually impaired (pp. 246–249). In the context of interviews, these questions were addressed: What does it mean to have a visual impairment? How does the impairment affect day-to-day living? What changes have been made or will have to be made because of your visual impairment? What do you believe will happen in the future? Five major categories were identified to classify the data. These categories and the text as a whole were "used in a circular fashion to understand the meaning of visual impairment" (p. 247) so as to obtain a deeper awareness of participants' experiences. The identified categories served in this study to provide an organizational scheme for the narrative discussion of meanings associated with each category. The interpretive strategies of paradigm cases, exemplars, and thematic analysis served, as Benner noted, in the process of discovery of meaning as well as in the presentation of that meaning. They are distinct from grounded theory in that "the goal is not to extract theoretical terms or concepts at a higher level of abstraction" (Benner, 1985, p. 10); rather, the goal is to discover meaning and to achieve a deeper understanding of experience in the context of that meaning and the situation in which it occurs.

The last phenomenology to be considered here is Van Manen's human science (1990). Van Manen identified his phenomenology as hermeneutic, but the processes of inquiry were sufficiently different from those heretofore described to warrant their separate presentation. The human science that Van Marten proposed:

> [A]ims at explicating the meaning of human phenomena (such as in literary or historical studies of texts) and at understanding the lived structures of meanings (such as in phenomenological studies of the lifeworld). . . . The fundamental model of this approach is textual reflection on the lived experiences and practical actions of everyday life with the intent to increase one's thoughtfulness and practical resourcefulness or tact. Phenomenology describes how one orients to lived experience, hermeneutics describes how one interprets the "texts" of life, and semiotics is used here to develop a practical writing or linguistic approach to the method of phenomenology and hermeneutics. (p. 4)

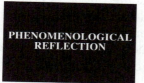
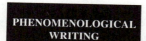

TURNING TO THE NATURE OF LIVED EXPERIENCE	1. Orienting to the phenomenon 2. Formulating the phenomenological question 3. Explicating assumptions and preunderstandings

THE EXISTENTIAL INVESTIGATION	4. Exploring the phenomenon:generating "data"
	   4.1 Using personal experience
	   4.2 Tracing etymological sources
	   4.3 Searching idiomatic phrases
	   4.4 Obtaining experiential descriptions from subjects
	   4.5 Locating experiential descriptions in literature, arts, etc.
	5. Consulting phenomenological literature

PHENOMENOLOGICAL REFLECTION	6. Conducting thematic analysis
	   6.1 Uncovering thematic aspects
	   6.2 Isolating thematic statements
	   6.3 Composing linguistic transformations
	   6.4 Gleaning thematic description from artistic sources
	7. Determining essential themes

PHENOMENOLOGICAL WRITING	8. Attending to the speaking of language 9. Varying the examples 10. Writing 11. Rewriting, etc.

Figure 4–4 Van Manen's method of phenomenology.
Source: Adapted from Practicing Phenomenological Writing by M. Van Manen, 1984, *Phenomenology and Pedagogy*, 2,5.

Doing phenomenology is a matter of questioning ways that we experience the world, bound through the research project to the world in a particular perspective. Researcher involvement thus has a particularly prominent place in his phenomenology, accounting for its growing appeal to qualitative nurse researchers. Figure 4–4 presents Lauterbach's outline (personal communication) of Van Manen's phenomenology and is adapted from Van Manen's presentations (1984, 1990). Van Manen (1990, pp. 8–13) oriented us to his phenomenology through the eight summative statements that follow.

1. *Phenomenological research is the study of lived experience.*
   Phenomenological inquiry is concerned with questions of what this or that experience is like and aims at understanding the meaning of the experience. The product of such inquiry is what Van Manen referred to as plausible insight that brings us in more direct contact with the world rather than theoretical

explanations which, by superimposing abstractions, distance us from the world as lived.

2. *Phenomenological research is the explication of phenomena as they present themselves to consciousness.* The phenomenological theme of consciousness as existence through a bodily involvement in the world is affirmed in this statement. Van Manen noted that one cannot reflect on experience while living through it, and stressed that phenomenological reflection is retrospective in nature.

3. *Phenomenological research is the study of essences.* By definition, an essence is a universal that is grasped intuitively through study of the internal structure of instances of the phenomenon under study. Phenomenological method is designed to disclose and describe the internal-meaning structures of lived experience. "The essence or nature of an experience has been adequately described in language if the description reawakens or shows us the lived quality and significance of the experience in a fuller or deeper manner" (p. 10).

4. *Phenomenological research is the description of the experiential meanings we live as we live them.* In a focus on meanings, description is interpretive by nature. The product of phenomenological inquiry articulates meaning embedded in experience—meaning as it is lived through.

5. *Phenomenological research is the human scientific study of phenomena.* Phenomenology is, Van Manen stated, systematic, explicit, self-critical, and intersubjective—all characteristics of scientific ways of knowing. It is always characterized by its concern for the subject matter of the structures of meaning of the lived human world.

6. *Phenomenological research is the attentive practice of thoughtfulness.* The impetus for doing research is the researcher's everyday practical concerns in his or her orientation as nurse, for sample. Doing phenomenology, then, is "in the service of the mundane practice of [nursing]: it is a ministering of thoughtfulness" (p. 12). The use of phenomenological research for nurses is "knowing how to act tactfully in [nursing] situations on the basis of a carefully edified thoughtfulness" (p. 8).

7. *Phenomenological research is a search for what it means to be human.* Ultimately, the aim of phenomenological research is to fulfill human nature, to actualize more fully who we are.

For example, to understand what it means to be a woman in our present age is also to understand the pressures of the meaning structures that have come to restrict, widen, or question the nature and ground of womanhood. Hermeneutic phenomenological research is a search for the fullness of living, for the ways a woman possibly can experience the world as a woman, for what it is to be a woman. (p. 12)

8. *Phenomenological research is a poetizing activity.* The presentation of phenomenological findings is characterized by the passion and aim that inspire the research process. The words that describe the experience are what Van Manen referred to as a primal telling, an original singing of the world. The language speaks the world rather than speaking of it.

And that is why, when you listen to a presentation of a phenomenological nature, you will listen in vain for the punchline, the latest information, or the big news. As in poetry, it is inappropriate to ask for a conclusion or a summary of a phenomenological study. To summarize a poem in order to present the result would destroy the result because the poem itself is the result. The poem is the thing. (p. 13)

Phenomenological description is, then, characterized by inspirational insight won through reflective writing. Research and writing are thus closely related. The task is to bring to speech one's understanding of a phenomenon achieved through rigorous reflection. Such description differs from poetry and literature in a concern for explicating universal meanings.

Chapter 5 presents aspects of Lauterbach's phenomenological research, guided by Van Manen's phenomenological method.

SUMMARY

Anderson (1989) argued that the proper focus for phenomenological nurse researchers is working out the problems and dilemmas of doing phenomenology well, rather than pondering the possibilities of triangulated research. Among those problems are questions concerning how and when one "brackets," how the researcher's self is featured, and the issue of rigor in analysis of phenomenological data. In accord with this position, the overview of phenomenological method in this chapter reveals a need to continue development of a phenomenology that produces nursing knowledge to guide nursing practices. It has been proposed that the qualities and characteristics of the researcher–researched relation are particularly important to reconsider.

The commonalities of the various phenomenologies that are engaging nurse researchers have been emphasized; their variations serve to raise methodological questions, redirecting us to yet another look at philosophical foundations for our science. The very subject matter of phenomenology is described variously. Some phenomenologies specify that the subject matter is such experiences as being in pain, doubting treatment, hoping to be well again, recovering from illness, or preparing for discharge. However, it may also be the mode of doubting or hoping or it may be a focus on ways that it is possible to be in the world, such as what it is like to parent a child with a chronic illness, for example. The product of phenomenological inquiry, the description of experience, is inescapably interpretive, but the extent of the interpretation is another variability among the phenomenologies. However, to the extent that the description is an effective communication of insights into an experience, its relevance is immediate and direct. As a particular qualitative approach in nursing research, phenomenology has the distinction of turning the researcher on the *self*, that is, on his or her own reflective and intuitive grasp of experience. The researcher's direct experience constitutes the data, whether immediate or vicarious. It also has the distinction of deliberate modification by nurses for its use in nursing. This development is fortuitous and well worth our attention as the qualitative paradigm in nursing continues to gain momentum in revolutionizing our science and our practice.

REFERENCES

Allen, M., & Jensen, L. (1990). Hermeneutical inquiry: Meaning and scope. *Western Journal of Nursing Research, 12*(2), 241–253.

Anderson, J. (1989). The phenomenological perspective. In J. Morse (Ed.), *Qualitative nursing research: A contemporary dialogue* (pp. 15–26). Rockville, MD: Aspen.

Benner, P. (1983). Uncovering the knowledge embedded in clinical practice. *Image: The Journal of Nursing Scholarship, 19,* 21–34.

Benner, P. (1985). Quality of life: A phenomenological perspective on explanation, prediction, and understanding in nursing science. *Advances in Nursing Science, 8,* 1–14.

Cohen, M. (1987). A historical overview of the phenomenological movement. *Image: The Journal of Nursing Scholarship, 19,* 31–34.

Colaizzi, P. (1978). Psychological research as the phenomenologist views it. In Valle and King (Eds.), *Existential phenomenological alternatives for psychology*. New York: Oxford University Press.

Davis, A. (1973). The phenomenological approach in nursing research. In E. Garrison (Ed.), *Doctoral preparation for nurses* (pp. 212–228). San Francisco: University of California.

Drew, N. (1989). The interviewer's experience as data in phenomenological research. *Western Journal of Nursing Research*, 11, 431–439.

Farber, M. (1966). *The aims of phenomenology*. New York: Harper & Row.

Haase, J. (1987). Components of courage in chronically ill adolescents: A phenomenological study. *Advances in Nursing Science*, 9, 64–80.

Husserl, E. (1965). *Phenomenology and the crisis of philosophy* (Q. Lauer, Trans.). New York: Harper & Row.

Leonard, V. (1989). A Heideggerian phenomenologic perspective on the concept of the person. *Advances in Nursing Science*, 11(4), 40–55.

Lynch-Sauer, J. (1985). Using a phenomenological research method to study nursing phenomena. In M. Leininger (Ed.), *Qualitative research methods in nursing* (pp. 93–107). Orlando, FL: Grune & Stratton.

Merleau-Ponty, M. (1956). What is phenomenology? *Cross Currents*, 6, 59–70.

Merleau-Ponty, M. (1962). *Phenomenology of perception* (C. Smith, Trans.). New York: Humanities Press.

Merleau-Ponty, M. (1964). *The primacy of perception* (J. Edie, Trans.). Evanston, IL: Northwestern University Press.

Oiler, C. (1982). A phenomenological approach in nursing research. *Nursing Research*, 31, 178–181.

Oiler, C. (1986). Qualitative methods: Phenomenology. In P. Moccia (Ed.), *New approaches to theory development*. New York: National League for Nursing.

Oiler Boyd, C. (1988). Phenomenology: A foundation for nursing curriculum. In National League for Nursing, *Curriculum revolution: Mandate for change*. New York: National League for Nursing.

Omery, A. (1983). Phenomenology: A method for nursing research. *Advances in Nursing Science*, 5(2), 49–63.

Parse, R. (1990). Parse's research methodology with an illustration of the lived experience of hope. *Nursing Science Quarterly*, 3, 9–17.

Parse, R., Coyne, A., & Smith, M. (1985). *Nursing research: Qualitative methods*. Bowie, MD: Brady Communications.

Paterson, J., & Zderad, L. (1976). *Humanistic nursing*. New York: Wiley.

Ray, M. (1985). A philosophical method to study nursing phenomena. In M. Leininger, *Qualitative research methods in nursing*. Orlando, FL: Grune & Stratton.

Reeder, F. (1987). The phenomenological movement. *Image: The Journal of Nursing Scholarship, 19*, 150–152.

Sandelowski, M., & Pollock, C. (1986). Women's experiences of infertility. *Image: The Journal of Nursing Scholarship, 18*, 140–144.

Schutz, A. (1970). *On phenomenology and social relations.* Chicago: University of Chicago Press.

Schutz, A. (1973). *Collected papers 1: The problem of social reality* (M. Natanson, Ed.). The Hague: Martinus Nijhoff.

Spiegelberg, H. (1975). *Doing phenomenology.* The Hague: Martinus Nijhoff.

Spiegelberg, H. (1976). *The phenomenological movement* (Vols. 1 and 11, 2nd ed.). The Hague: Martinus Nijhoff.

Spiegelberg, H. (1981). *The context of the phenomenological movement.* The Hague: Martinus Nijhoff.

Spiegelberg, H. (1982). *The phenomenological movement* (3rd ed.). The Hague: Martinus Nijhoff.

van Kaam, A. (1959). Phenomenal analysis: Exemplified by a study of the experience of "really feeling understood." *Journal of Individual Psychology, 15*, 66–72.

Van Manen, M. (1984). Practicing phenomenological writing. *Phenomenology and Pedagogy, 2*, 36–69.

Van Manen, M. (1990). *Researching lived experience: Human science for an action sensitive pedagogy.* Albany, NY: SUNY Press.

Zderad, L. (1968). A concept of empathy. Unpublished doctoral dissertation, Georgetown University, Washington, DC.

ADDITIONAL REFERENCES

Annels, M. (1999). Phenomenology revisited. Evaluating phenomenology: Usefulness, quality and philosophical foundations. *Nurse Researcher, 6*(3), 5–19.

Appleton, J. V., & King, L. (1997). Constructivism: A naturalistic methodology for nursing inquiry. *Advances in Nursing Science, 20*(2), 13–22.

Avis, M. (1997). Letting sleeping dogmas lie: An examination of positivism in the nursing research literature. *Social Sciences in Health: International Journal of Research and Practice, 3*, 52–63.

Beech, I. (1999). Bracketing in phenomenological research. *Nurse Researcher, 6*(3), 35–51.

Bergum, V. (1988). *Women to mother: A transformation.* South Hadley, MA: Bergin & Garvey.

Bergum, V. (1989). Being a phenomenological researcher. In J. Morse (Ed.), *Qualitative nursing research: A contemporary dialogue* (pp. 43–57). Rockville, MD: Aspen.

Bishop, A., & Scudder, J. (1990). *The practical, moral, and personal sense of nursing: A phenomenological philosophy of practice*. Albany: SUNY Press.

Corben, V. (1999). Phenomenology revisited. Misusing phenomenology in nursing research: Identifying the issues. *Nurse Researcher*, 6(3), 52–66.

Dahlberg, K., & Drew, N. (1997). A lifeworld paradigm for nursing research. *Journal of Holistic Nursing*, 15, 303–317.

Drew, N. (1986). Exclusion and confirmation: A phenomenology of patients' experiences with caregivers. *Image*, 18, 39–43.

Farrel, G. A., & Gritching, W. L. (1997). Social science at the crossroads: What direction mental health nurses? *Australian New Zealand Journal of Mental Health Nursing*, 6, 19–29.

Forbes, D. A., King, K. M., Kushner, K. E., Letourneau, N. L., Myrick, A. F., & Profetto-McGrath, J. (1999). Warrantable evidence in nursing science. *Journal of Advanced Nursing*, 29, 373–379.

Giorgi, A. (1970). *Psychology as a human science: A phenomenotogically based approach*. New York: Harper & Row.

Heslop, L. (1997). The impossibilities of poststructuralist and critical social nursing inquiry. *Nursing Inquiry*, 4, 48–56.

Johnson, M. (1999). Observations on positivism and pseudoscience in qualitative nursing research. *Journal of Advanced Nursing*, 30, 67–73.

Knaack, P. (1984). Phenomenological research. *Western Journal of Nursing Research*, 6, 107–114.

Lutz, K. F., Jones, K. D., & Kendall, J. (1997). Expanding the praxis debate: Contributions to clinical inquiry. *Advances in Nursing Science*, 20(2), 23–31.

Marks, M. D. (1999). Network. Reconstructing nursing: Evidence, artistry and the curriculum . . . including commentary by L. Nyatanga and M. Johnson. *Nurse Education Today*, 19, 3–11.

Monti, E. J., & Tingen, M. S. (1999). Multiple paradigms of nursing science. *Advances in Nursing Science*, 21(4), 64–80.

Oiler, C. (1980). A phenomenological perspective in nursing. Unpublished doctoral dissertation, Teachers College, Columbia University, New York.

Oiler, C. (1983). Nursing reality as reflected in nurses' poetry. *Perspectives in Psychiatric Care*, 21, 81–89.

Paige, S. (1980). Alone into the alone: A phenomenological study of the experience of dying. Unpublished doctoral dissertation, Boston University.

Paterson, J. (1971). From a philosophy of clinical nursing to a method of nursology. *Nursing Research*, 20, 143–146.

Picard, C. (1997). Embodied soul: The focus of nursing praxis. *Journal of Holistic Nursing*, 15(10), 41–53.

Proctor, S. (1998). Linking philosophy and method in the research process: The case of realism. *Nurse Researcher*, 5(4), 73–90.

Psathas, G. (1973). *Phenomenological sociology: Issues and applications*. New York: Wiley.

Riethen, D. (1986). The essential structure of a caring interaction: Doing phenomenology. In P. Munhall & C. Oiler (Eds.), *Nursing research: A qualitative perspective* (1st ed.), Norwalk, CT: Appleton-Century-Crofts.

Rose, J. (1990). Psychologic health of women: A phenomenologic study of women's inner strength. *Advances in Nursing Science*, 12(2), 56–70.

Schutz, S. E. (1994). Exploring the benefits of a subjective approach in qualitative nursing research. *Journal of Advanced Nursing*, 20, 412–417.

Silva, M. C. (1997). Classic image. Philosophy, science, theory: Interrelationships and implications for nursing research. *Image: Journal of Nursing Scholarship*, 29(3), 210–215.

Simons, S. (1995). From paradigm to method in interpretive action research. *Journal of Advanced Nursing*, 21, 837–844.

Stanley, T. (1978). The lived experience of hope: The isolation of discrete descriptive elements common to the experience of hope in healthy young adults. Unpublished doctoral dissertation, Catholic University of America, Washington, DC.

Strasser, S. (1963). *Phenomenology and the human sciences*. Pittsburg: Duquesne University Press.

Swanson-Kaufmann, K. (1988). Phenomenology. In B. Sarter (Ed.), *Paths to knowledge: Innovative research methods for nursing*. New York: National League for Nursing.

Thorne, S. E., Kirkham, S. R., & Henderson, A. (1999). Ideological implications of paradigm discourse. *Nursing Inquiry*, 6(2), 123–131.

van Kaam, A. (1969). *Existential foundations of psychology*. New York: Doubleday.

Van Amburg, R. (1997). A Copernican revolution in clinical ethics: Engagement versus disengagement. *American Journal of Occupational Therapy*, 51(3), 186–190.

Wainwright, S. P. (1997). A new paradigm for nursing: The potential realism. *Journal of Advanced Nursing*, 26, 1262–1271.

Zaner, R. (1970). *The way of phenomenology*. Indianapolis: Pegasus.

Phenomenology
A Method

Patricia L. Munhall

BEGINNING

This chapter, following Chapter 4 with a similar title, becomes at once one of continuation and, yet, one of departure. Since the last edition of this book, I have been encouraged to present to readers a more definitive "method"—one that would acknowledge phenomenology in interaction with patients, families, and communities in health care experiences.

The preceding chapter has guided readers with excellent overviews of the various interpretations of phenomenological methods that have been used in nursing. Readers have come to understand the philosophical underpinnings and the various perspectives reflecting the complexities of these various methods and their differences, which has advanced phenomenological research.

Quite often, the contrasting perspectives of Husserl, Merleau-Ponty, Schutz, Spiegelberg, and Heidegger can frustrate readers. They seem to have some similarities but more differences in beliefs, aims, and purposes; so, when reading Chapter 4, the reader could presumably choose among these philosophers and, coming to understand a particular belief system, arrive at a method consistent with one of them and proceed with an inquiry. However, it should always be kept in mind that the chosen approach represents one kind of phenomenology, one interpretation of the philosophy.

For example, Merleau-Ponty is considered more an existential phenomenologist, whose focus is on the individual's situatedness in the world through experience. Husserl is thought of as a transcendental phenomenologist, for whom consciousness in not empirical but "pure" consciousness. Then there is hermeneutical phenomenology, associated most often with Heidegger, where the focus is on understanding "being." Within Heidegger's phenomenology, one views all phenomenological description as interpretation. Then we could ask, What about analytical phenomenology? Is that the same? The answer to that question would be different, depending on whom you asked.

The different answers to the same questions are, in my experience, part of phenomenology. Yet, one could continue to categorize these different schools and arrive at one answer to the preceding questions and say that analytical phenomenology has more to do with the semiotic meaning structures of cultural practices or that gender phenomenology is most concerned with context sensitivity and is truth tentative (M. van Manen, workshop, 1998). So, the state of the art of phenomenology reflects the postmodern world that we inhabit in that there are multiple interpretations and multiple realities. It is like a mirror in that phenomenology celebrates reflection, where differences and the "particular" are unveiled.

OBSERVING

My own observations of phenomenological inquiry by nurses include reference to one of the French or German phenomenologists—say, the first generation—and then these nurse researchers move to a phenomenologist who has proposed a "method" for inquiry. Among them (for the sake of simplicity, I shall refer to them as second-generation phenomenologists) are Georggi, Colaizzi, van Kaam, and van Manen. The first three are, from the United States; they became the most influential methodolists for nurse researchers in the 1970s and 1980s. Faced with the requirement of finding a method to conduct a phenomenological study and lacking formal training themselves in this area, these nurse researchers understandably chose one of these three phenomenological methods. Many problems seemed to have arisen from this attempt at articulation.

Although the researchers became well versed in phenomenological thought by reading the first generation of phenomenologists, the transition to these other methods was often limiting and incongruent with the philosophy. Historically, this outcome is understandable if we remember the pedestal that "method" occupied; the closer a method could look like "the scientific method," the more acceptable it was in the academy.

The last phenomenologist, Max van Manen (1984,1990), changed this situation dramatically with a human science approach, about which, in Chapter 4, one reads how consistent his phenomenology is with many of the first-generation philosophers. The reason that he has been a particularly good phenomenolgist for those in the human sciences to follow is that he views phenomenology not only as a philosophy of being but as a practice as well. From this perspective, any methodic location can give a view of experiential understanding by questioning lived experience through reflective writing. Here and in this way, meaning can be understood and we can become practitioners of the "ever-fragile exercise of phenomenological wisdom" (M. van Manen, 1998 workshop).

Nurse researchers have elaborated on these various methods, including fine works by Benner (1994), and Parse (1987). In 1994, I wrote *Revisioning Phenomenology: Nursing and Health Science Research* and, as with previous editions of this work, I did not articulate "a method" in a formalized structured manner. The reader is referred to that work to supplement this chapter, and my aim here is to present "a method." This method has evolved from the work of countless doctoral students who used van Manen's method and often utilized work from the "revisioning" book but still raised questions and asked for clarification.

In "revisioning," I purposely was attempting to guide students through the process of inquiry from a phenomenological perspective. I referred the reader to van Manen's approach on the basis of a subjective appraisal that his method was the most consistent with phenomenology as philosophy. Still, I received requests to articulate "a method," because in my teaching I was apparently guiding students with what they perceived as "a method not yet written."

MOVING FORWARD

What has prompted me to move forward in print, are some criticisms being leveled at many studies. I am hoping that, perhaps by integrating those criticisms into the development of this method, they will be replaced by a more congruent philosophical approach. I want to do this now, because I do not want phenomenology to be misperceived or have its potential go unrecognized and respected. After 15 years of assisting students with either masters theses or doctoral dissertations, I have become acquainted with their questions and frustrations and with their sincere attempts to combine "a philosophy" with "a method."

If we were to accept the proposition that phenomenology as inquiry is aimed at understanding lived experience, as is sometimes written, or that the central purpose of phenomenology is to understand the meaning of being human, then the guiding word, I think, would be "approach." We would approach the project, the study, and be guided by the emergent material. The "experiences themselves" would show the way to understanding meaning. However "approach" does not do well in dissertation proposals or grant applications. The section is not labeled "approach" but "method." Because of the vast potential of phenomenology to our understanding, if I can contribute in some small way to its vitality, then I will stop quibbling about these two words!

"What is the meaning of being human?" is a phenomenal question. I believe the question is asked in order to come to a phenomenological answer: understanding the meaning of being human. For the most part, this question goes unanswered and the answer remains a mystery. All the phenomenology in the world is not going to solve the mystery altogether, and I am not sure that we would want all mystery removed. Yet, in many human experiences, the cry for human understanding cannot and should not be ignored.

What individuals have done with the foregoing question and its purpose has varied in responses and very different methods, even with the same philosophy of phenomenology. This chapter, though, is not to critique the various ways in which different schools of thought have developed methods to answer this question, but to give as example how phenomenology has been done by the wide use of humanistic psychological phenomenological methods. Studies following these methods, I believe, unfortunately have done little to enhance our understanding of meaning found in different experiences and have left us open to a well-founded critique that these methods reflect a form of reductionism and steplike studies that appear much like those based on logical positivism. Of course, using the same outlines for proposals and criteria for evaluation as those of the scientific method has not helped at all. Chapters 23 and 24 in this book offer alternatives.

Many of these methods, with all due respect to their origins, came about in order to gain acceptance within the academy. Many nurse researchers, when reviewing "phenomenological" research come away wondering what does all this "mean": lists of themes, lists of essences, structural definitions, categories of abstractions, meaning units, and other reductionistic descriptions of experience. Somehow, these methods eased qualitative and, in this instance, phenomenology, into the academy with rules to give these methods as much credence and respectability as the icon of "the scientific method."

RESISTING

So I have resisted and have argued for phenomenology as a process or phenomenology as an approach. Follow the "thing itself" wherever and whenever it appears, while being attentive, conscious, and alert to its appearance. Know that with appearance there is concealment as well. Explore that possibility. "Liberate yourself from prescribed steps" was my mantra. Methods will place you in a formula, where you cannot wander outside and that critical limitation, while a safeguard in the laboratory, is what will handcuff you from the spontaneous recognition of the appearance and the crucial exploration of the unforeseen.

For years, I would urge my wonderful colleagues to liberate students and let them follow the phenomenological process so that they can be free to journey where "being" reveals itself. My main argument to support this freedom was that where "being" reveals itself is largely unbeknownst at the outset of a phenomenological inquiry. The reader can see, in Sarah Lauterbach's phenomenological study (Chapter 6), that she did indeed wander into places, literally in her city backyard, which she had never known existed. One can see in her first study (second edition, 1993) a highly structured approach and in this edition a more phenomenological narrative of the meaning of losing a newborn child.

One could ask, Which one is more interesting to read? That really is not the point here, the point being that, in the academy, the first structured step-by-step presentation is the only one acceptable in nursing today, and the second is considered a luxury! Sarah states in both pieces that she combined van Manen's method and my approach in her study. This is the hybrid of which I spoke before. I believe that Sarah had all the freedom that she needed to find the "unbeknownst," but Sarah was also extremely well grounded in phenomenological philosophy. In her second piece, she even speaks to the life-world of temporality affecting her own self-knowledge of phenomenology and indeed influencing her study and interpretation.

This self-awareness is essential to conducting phenomenological inquiry. It actually "shows itself" and I am aware: I have shared Sarah's self-reflecting experience as well. So, before embarking on writing "a method" to phenomenological study, I reveal to the reader that it is the temporal nature of my life experience that brings me to this point. I have come to understand in the past 15 years that my own subjectivity, which is often the same as the interpretive belief about phenomenological inquiry as process and not as "method," can be substantiated philosophically. I have, though, also come to understand that nurse researchers and other human science researchers do not have the freedom to go about any inquiry without a "method."

CHOOSING

I have a choice here to be recalcitrant or, because of my experiential phenomenological understanding of students' experiences, act on the meaning of their experiences. Will that mean that I am capitulating my beliefs? The answer is negative; I still believe the phenomenological inquiry is a process of the unbeknownst that gives direction to the study and cannot be possibly known at the outset. How could we possibly come to understand the meaning of being human in experience if we were to follow linear prescribed steps? Each step taken would close that door and close it prematurely; or worse, if it opened another door, we could not go there, because it would not be part of the "steps" of the "method."

I also believe, at the same time, that such a liberated perspective will not be accepted in the academy, unless perhaps (and this is debatable) one is in a philosophy program. I have also taken note of the phenomenological "methods" and, with the exception of van Manen's, have become sufficiently alarmed about the problems inherent in them, such as naming "reactions" to an experience instead of meaning or even an understanding of the reactions; background of the experience is often a history of something other than "human experience" and always the appearance of ten transcribed interviews. Proceeding in this linear way, one then "extracts" essences or themes and provides a list or, worse, a definition of the lived experience! It is here that we are being critiqued as not understanding phenomenology (Crotty, 1996).

I am providing this background as an example of how I have come to use phenomenological understanding to justify presenting this pliable method. I am so troubled by so many studies that present themselves as phenomenological studies, when the researchers have followed a linear method and ironically can come out with, despite the experience under study, often the same list of what I have come to understand as "reactions" to experiences. For example, without naming the experience, studies often have the same essences or themes as findings: fear of the unknown, loneliness, anxiety, anger, depression, helplessness, and isolation. Listing themes or essences leaves us open to the accusation that we are categorizing human experience, much like a reductionism, found in quantitative studies.

If we recall that the major focus of phenomenological inquiry is understanding meaning of some "thing," some experience, something that is human so that we can better understand the meaning of being human, perhaps the fact that the responses to experiences are often similar may not be surprising. I would venture further and say that we have a fairly good sense of what kind of reactions (themes) people are going to have in a specific experience.

However, studies such as Sarah's demonstrate that we can be very wrong in our preconceived notions of reality. Where many studies leave off, and I would suggest because there is no "step," is not to inquire into the meaning of these essences/responses for the particular individual. Sarah demonstrates, with her participants, what the meaning of isolation is in the particular experience. So she demonstrates the going back and forth, seeking further explanation, pondering the responses, bringing them to bear on the experience in a unique manner, unique in that experience. Isolation has a different meaning in different experiences, and the researcher has to be able to narrate for the reader the understanding gleaned that enlightens us to the meaning of isolation in the experience of losing a newborn. There are reasons uncovered in the narrative of the participants that surprise us and give new direction to practice and most important to an understanding of human beings in experience.

MOVING BECAUSE OF PRAGMATISM

All this needs to be said because it provides the "situated context" that inspires me to move toward pragmatism. Students/researchers are required to present a proposal, which must include a method that is clearly spelled out and will lead to some kind of findings and must also pass the institutional review board. I have come to a place, as mentioned earlier, that I can draw upon the past 15 years, put aside for the sake of students that phenomenology is not a "method" but a process, a way of being toward meaning and experience, and present the "suggestions"

TABLE 5-1   METHOD FOR PHENOMENOLOGICAL INQUIRY

I. Immersion

II. Coming to the
    phenomenologial aim of inquiry

III. Existential inquiry, expressions,   IV. Phenomenological contextual
     and processing*   processing*

V. Analysis of interpretive
   interaction

VI. Writing the phenomenological
    narrative

VII. Writing a narrative on the
     meaning of your study

*Concurrent processes

with which I have guided students and now call a "method." As with phenomenology, these students, now researchers, have participated in a "going back and forth" with me and have been part of this work. Because of their work, they have demonstrated the "method." So I have come to understand this experience, mostly from them and unbeknown to them and me, we were all participants! Table 5–1, which represents the broad outline of this method and Table 5–2, which presents the method in greater detail, reflects this shared collaboration among former students, colleagues and myself.

DOING PHENOMENOLOGICAL INQUIRY: IMMERSION

Immersion is an essential and critical beginning of a phenomenological study. Phenomenological inquiry just cannot be done well or have any meaning if the researcher has not learned the language and come to understand the philosophical underpinnings of phenomenology. All philosophies are based on assumptions about the world and contain abstractions and concepts to explain, describe, conceptualize, and analyze the nature of being, the universe, truth, meanings, knowledge, ethics, and the many pursuits of philosophy.

Criticisms have been directed toward some researchers for simplifying the complexity and text of phenomenology. It is absolutely critical that, if one uses a method, the philosophical interpretation of phenomenology is consistent with the particular phenomenology of the inquiry. This does not mean reading one book on phenomenology. In this chapter, I will

TABLE 5–2   METHOD FOR PHENOMENOLOGICAL INQUIRY

I. Immersion	A. Describe and interpret the philosophical assumptions and underpinnings of a particular phenomenological perspective.
	B. Exemplify the meaning of phenomenological concepts.
	C. Elucidate the worldview of phenomenology as an approach to answering questions. (If you know the experience in which you are interested, use that one.)
II. Coming to the phenomenological aim of inquiry	A. Articulate aim of your study.
	B. Distinguish the experience that is part of your study.
	1. Describe if circumscribed experience or delimit context if broad experience.
	2. Articulate the situated context that is available to you in the moment.
	C. Decenter self and come to "unknow."
	1. Reflect on own beliefs, preconceptions, intuitions, motives, and biases so as to decenter.
	2. Adopt perspective of "unknowing."
	D. Articulate aim of study in the form of a phenomenological question.

	III. Existential inquiry, expressions, and processing*	IV. Phenomenological contextual processing*
III. Existential inquiry, expressions, and processing* IV. Phenomenological contextual processing*	A. Listen to self and others; develop heightened attentiveness to self and others. B. Personal experiences and expressions C. Experiential descriptive expressions: "the experiencer"	A. Analyze emergent situated contexts. B. Analyze day-to-day contingencies. C. Assess life-worlds.

*Concurrent processes

TABLE 5–2   METHOD FOR PHENOMENOLOGICAL INQUIRY (CONTINUED)

	D. Experiential descriptive expressions: "others engaged in the experience"
	E. Experiential descriptive expressions: "the arts and literature review"
	F. Anecdotal descriptive expressions: as experience appears
	G. Ongoing reflection in personal journal.
V. Analysis of interpretive interaction	A. Integrate existential investigation with phenomenological contextual processing.
	B. Describe expressions of meaning (thoughts, emotions, feelings, statements, motives, metaphors, examples, behaviors, appearances and concealments, voiced and nonvoiced language).
	C. Interpret expressions of meaning as appearing from integration.
VI. Writing the phenomenological narrative	A. Choose a style of writing that will communicate an understanding of the meaning of this particular experience.
	B. Write inclusively of all meanings, not just the "general" but the "particular."
	C. Write inclusively of language and expressions of meaning with the interpretive interaction of the situated context.
	D. Interpret with participant the meaning of the interaction of the experience.
	E. Narrate a story that at once gives voice to actual language as it simultaneously interprets meaning from expressions used to describe the experience.

TABLE 5–2 METHOD FOR PHENOMENOLOGICAL INQUIRY (CONTINUED)

VII. Writing a narrative on the meaning of your study	A. Summarize the answer to your phenomenological question with breadth and depth.
	B. Indicate how this understanding obtained from those who have lived the experience call for self-reflection and/or system reflection.
	C. Interpret meanings of these reflections to small and large systems within specific context.
	D. Critique this interpretation with implications and recommendations for political, social, cultural, health care, family, and other social systems.

reference some material presented in my own text titled *Revisioning Phenomenology* (Munhall, 1994b) and be very open with the reader that reading that book does not in any way suffice the process step of immersion. Nor does reading van Manen (1990) or Benner (1994).

Recall at the start of this chapter the reference to first-generation phenomenologists. They need to be read as well as those philosophers who followed and are referred to in Chapter 4. Certainly, the present chapter does not prepare a person to do a phenomenological study. It is an overview and the text itself is an introduction to many different qualitative methods.

Immersion also requires taking philosophy and method courses. If our colleagues are preparing to do quantitative studies with method and statistic courses, we cannot expect less from what we call qualitative research. One does oneself a disservice from the beginning if this formal study is not part of immersion. Reading unfamiliar language leaves the interpretation up to the reader, and it is in this particular activity where caution, in particular in the beginning of learning, needs to be heeded. Speaking and hearing others speak of the philosophical ideas, concepts, and assumptions must be part of the immersion.

This is the area where I have found the most breakdown in phenomenological studies. Although the lack of immersion or understanding may seem obvious, there are many students who move directly from reading about a method and how to carry the method out to doing the study. They often, to their own frustration, do not even understand what their aim is beyond some short definition of phenomenology that does not do it justice; that is, phenomenology is the study of lived experience. Certainly, as we read, we come to a much greater in-depth understanding of what a phenomenological inquiry is about, and it is certainly more than that phrase. Actually, "the study of lived experience" could equally apply to any kind of study that deals with experience.

As I write this, I think of my own recitation of that definition. For a long time, I would say it without comprehending the real sense of understanding. The goal of immersion, then, is not unlike the goal of phenomenology and that goal is understanding. If you are going to embark on phenomenological inquiry, I urge you to find courses specific to phenomenology. They are becoming more widespread and you may find them on-line. In addition, participating in workshops provides an interaction that enlarges the processes in phenomenological research.

Immersion also requires reading phenomenological studies, which can be a curious sort of immersion. Some of these studies can teach you from the perspective that the studies are not good ones, when you walk away and wonder what was the point. Other studies resonate with you and, after having read such a study, you come to realize that you understand the meaning of being in some experience or another much better than you ever had before or that you understand a human experience in a way that conflicts with what you once thought, as many people find when they read Sarah's study; this is good phenomenology.

Immersion also means learning what comprises what may be critiqued as good phenomenology. That means also reading articles from journals that discuss this topic and provide constructive criticism and remind the researcher of what must be of importance. The references from Chapter 3, 4, and 5 contain important readings and the Internet sites in Chapter 25 are also good sources, as well as doing a general search on the web.

This process of immersion is ongoing and I have found in my own life and my colleagues that the interest in the literature and the pursuit of greater understanding becomes a part of who you are as person. It is as though phenomenology takes part of you, becomes part of you, and you become phenomenolgically present to the world.

Becoming Phenomenological

Immersion allows one to understand what "becoming phenomenologically present to the world" means. Now, this is a process and cannot be reduced to a method, but over time one who comes from this perspective will begin to interact differently with others, whether in research or practice. One begins to become less assuming, often abandoning assumptions about another or another's experience, and adopts a stance of "unknowing" (Munhall, 1993b, 1994b). In this place, a person can be phenomenologically present to another person. Toward what end? To understand the other. To be open, nonjudgmental, and compassionate. How can one act toward another in a caring, compassionate way, if one has not suspended assumptions or judgments? How can one understand what kind of meaning an experience has for a person unless one suspends one's own preconceptions? In our giving of ourselves in nursing and in our personal lives, how do we know what to do, what to say, and when it is better not to say anything if we do not understand the meaning for the other. This is why immersion is so critical. Becoming phenomenologically oriented requires for many people a new and different way of perceiving reality.

So, part of immersion is to practice being phenomenological, which is a challenge but is essential to the interviewing step in most phenomenological methods. To interview in phenomenological inquiry is to be able to "decenter" and to be fully present to another (this topic will be discussed further).

I cannot overemphasize immersion as a step in this method. A researcher new to this method will be rewarded and less frustrated if she or he has studied. This step is challenging, but it is also one of the most intriguing and enlightening. If you are philosophically inclined toward understanding, this step will be one of the most intellectually stimulating and affectively moving experiences of your educational experience.

Without this step, phenomenological inquiry from my perspective is not possible. Without this step, you will be doing story telling, journalism, and impressionistic writing. Worse, you will be doing logical positivistic quasiqualitative research! None of those activities, with the exception of the last one, are negative; they are just not phenomenology. Phenomenology requires the philosophical underpinnings that those other activities do not require. And you can answer the question quite knowledgeably, when someone asks, "What is the difference?" or, as a colleague said so kindly to me after a phenomenological study, "That is not research, it's journalism!" After immersion, you can respond in such a way that the person will forever regret making the comment!

How Does One Fulfill the Step of Immersion in an Actual Study?

Remember, this method is for new researchers and primarily for those who might be doing a study for a dissertation or a part of a study for a masters thesis. Once this step is in process and has become a part of one's ongoing research program, then the step itself does not have to be on every proposal or study. However, it has been my experience that I am continually enlarging my understanding with new literature, as well as by returning to the classical literature.

This step is for those embarking for the first time or embarking for the second time, not having done this step the first time. Immersion is your research preparation for phenomenology (and is also preparation for any other method of inquiry; it is just spelled out more clearly for quantitative studies). Immersion as a step, then, is almost pedantic; yet, with practice, it can be concretely reported in ways such as the following:

I. Immersion
A. Describe and interpret the philosophical assumptions and underpinnings of a particular phenomenological perspective.

This section should include the evolution of phenomenology, the philosophers, and the different schools of phenomenology and how they differ from one another. The assurance that section A is done well is that you, your colleagues, and your professor come away from reading this section and agree that you do have a good understanding of phenomenology. If this is not the case, more immersion will be needed, but, again, I emphasize how much difficulty you are avoiding by learning this philosophy prior to any other activity concerning your research. Have I convinced you by now? I hope so because you will have an in-depth understanding of what it is you are doing.

B. Exemplify the meaning of phenomenological concepts.

In the process of writing part A, you most likely did not discuss the meaning of the various concepts. In this section, you explain what they mean. For instance, you give the meaning of:

- Situated context
- Intersubjectivity
- Perception
- Decentering
- Unknowing
- Appearance–Concealment
- Being
- Consciousness
- Life-worlds: temporality, spatiality, corporeality, relationality
- Contingency

- Preconceptions
- Shared perceptual fields

These and other phenomenological concepts are described in Chapters 3 and 4 of this text, as well as in *Revisioning Phenomenology*, so this chapter is enlarged for you (Munhall, 1994b).

The assurance that section B is done well is that, with each concept, the researcher demonstrates the meaning of the concept with a real-world example. Again, if colleagues and your professor understand you, you can be assured that you are understanding the meaning of concepts.

C. Elucidate the worldview of phenomenology as an approach to answering questions. (If you know the experience in which you are interested, use that one.)

This process prepares the researcher for phenomenological dialogue/interviews/conversations. The researcher, after studying decentering as an unknowing process and also understanding intersubjectivity, practices conversations with others. The best person to practice with is someone who can critique your listening skills. That notwithstanding, after a conversation in which you practiced decentered dialogue, write a description of the dialogue with an interpretation. Give this description to the person with whom you conversed to ascertain how and what you heard and if you overlaid the description or interpretation of the dialogue with your own assumptions or preconceptions. This excellent exercise should be repeated. The assurance that part C is done well is when your description and interpretation of what the "other" was saying is validated by that person as to your understanding of what she or he was saying and meaning.

This first step is so critical, that I do keep emphasizing its importance to doing inquiry from a phenomenological perspective. In my own experience with students and in my first attempts with phenomenology, a lack of this immersion is comparable to doing quantitative research without research courses in the scientific method, statistics, and measurement. This step enables you to be the "instrument" for your study. Your role in the study requires high-level skills and learned sophistication in communication.

Existential Interaction

Remember, in phenomenological inquiry, that you are going to be in constant interaction in the existential processing of phenomenological material. You will also be in transaction with persons in interviews or conversations and need to develop the consciousness of one who does not know. The researcher is in search of the meaning of a phenomenon, the meaning of being human in experience (phenomenon). Whether the researcher has or has not experienced the phenomenon, she or he needs to come to the phenomenological question as free as possible from assumptions, preconceptions, and forethought about the phenomenon or experience.

When you first begin phenomenological inquiry, it is important to be cognizant that you do not and should not have a hypothesis. To this, one may say, "Of course!" However, often we are not aware of some hidden belief that we may have and then try to find ways to document that belief. That is why decentering yourself from your own world of knowledge and hunches is so important.

As we go on with these steps, it is important to understand that, as was said, they are not linear. There is a going back and forth, and examining and reexamining, a thought and then a change in thought, and there are many middle-of-the-night ahas!

A major, if not the major, difference in doing phenomenological inquiry is a phenomenon that I call, for lack of a better description, "becoming your study." You become a repository for appearances of the experience or an example of the experience, and your attentiveness almost becomes unconscious. You are not actually looking for existential material for your study and, without notice, you will awaken to its presence. Some of us have marveled at the experience "of seeing it everywhere" or of realizing that "it was always there and I did not see it, hear it, understand it."

Another way of saying this is that the subject of your study, the phenomenon, the experience, takes up residence within you. Now, this will not occur if your inquiry is an academic exercise (although I have heard that, even then, it happens!). The taking up residence, to me, requires an intense longing to understand meaning—the meaning of something. So it becomes a passion, and then the process is so much easier because you have become engaged with the philosophy of phenomenology. Philosophers are thinkers and questioners of a different sort from scientists. One very important distinction is this very lack of linearity. Heideggar wrote that language generates and constrains the human life-world. When capitulating to this exercise of writing down a process as a method, I thought what a wonderful example. I am constrained by language because it expresses itself on paper in a linear way—line by line, when this method is, as was said, back and forth and circular and probably sometimes linear. So with that said on to the next "step."

II. Coming to the Phenomenological Aim of the Inquiry

Altogether the following four activities will assist you in focusing on the aim of your study. On completing this set of processes, what your aim is should be understandable to others who are taking part and are interested in your work.

A. Articulate aim of your study.

Here you want to be very clear about what you want to accomplish in conducting this inquiry. So often, the aim of the study is just listed as studying the "lived experience" of some experience, but that is not an aim. It is a means toward an end. So the researcher needs to think about what he or she is attempting to accomplish and for what purpose. I have discussed Crotty's (1996) main concern about the way in which North American nurse researchers were conducting phenomenological studies. His main contention, and perhaps not everyone agrees, is that phenomenology should be critical and offer philosophical criticism. Crotty asks for significance from phenomenological studies—that they go beyond describing and interpreting and suggest possibilities that may enhance or correct some experiences. Others who disagree say that their work is just to describe and interpret and that it is the work of other researchers to point out the problems inherent in the descriptions and to suggest implications leading to change.

My own response is that, because we do not add the critique or the suggestions to alleviate what we may have come to find in experiences or to actually suggest changing some prevailing theory, the needed change or needed research may never take place. The critique then of the experience may offer direction for infinite possibilities. At first I was defensive about Crotty's criticism and leaned toward a purist perspective, but, after much reflection, I came to believe that the addition of critique would certainly have the benefit of increasing the significance of phenomenological work and, in a pragmatic way, provide direction to practice or to theory. Additionally, I was beginning to find it difficult to argue with a suggestion that would ultimately enlarge our purpose and assist individuals toward attaining meaning and improved sensitivity, understanding, and change in conditions and approaches that were not enhancing the quality of their lives.

So, as a researcher, you need to enlarge your aim and you need to be clear about what the experience is that you are about to name, understand, and find the meaning of, as well as in the end critique your findings for larger implications.

You can be assured that this section is complete when you can persuade others of the significance of your aim and they agree that the way that you have stated the aim lends itself to phenomenological inquiry.

B. Distinguish the experience that is part of your study.
1. Describe if circumscribed experience or delimit context if broad experience.

Describing the experience: it is here where researchers seem to go two different ways, and some methodologists may have rules here. From my perspective, either direction is fine. So, one might choose an actual experience in the form of an activity or procedure or, as in Sarah's study, a life event. Or one might choose an emotion, or feeling state, such as restlessness, comfort, pain, anxiety, and so on. With emotions, or feelings, the researcher needs to be clear in distinguishing the range of the study. For example: studying pain is an extremely broad experience. I would suggest that the researcher think about what this inquiry is for and for what purpose. The researcher needs to distinguish in some way the kind of pain or the pain associated with a specific kind of experience.

There is experience within experience, and this is not a problem. Actually, it is part of any experience. No experience occurs in isolation. With this in mind, you might decide to study the meaning of pain experienced with a specific condition. If you felt confident and grounded in phenomenology, you could study the meaning of pain to persons who have experienced pain and actually not have a category or condition. That kind of study would be a grand study. A grand study of pain would be an attempt to understand the meaning of pain. All variations of experiences might be associated with pain and, in this type of study, one would distinguish the experience associated with the pain, but it would fall into the background and the meaning of pain would always be in the foreground. One advantage of doing a grand study is that this type of study could become one's research program, an area where one continuously explores the experience of pain in ongoing studies. Certainly, this study requires more time, is a subject for a larger study, and would find its major understandings narrated in at least one volume.

The assurance that distinguishing your phenomenon has been accomplished is when you have presented this phenomenon clearly, in a way that listeners will know that it is "this" that you are studying, not "that" along with it or any other fringe phenomenon. You are able to answer questions, clearly delineating what it is and what it is not that you are searching to find meaning in: the experience, the phenomenon.

2. Articulate the situated context that is available to you in the moment.

Experience is embedded in life-worlds and various contingencies. In this part of the study, you need to describe the context in which you and the study will be taking place. Life-worlds are described on pages 168–172 of this chapter.

C. Decenter self and come to "unknow."
1. Reflect on own beliefs, preconceptions, intuitions, motives, and biases so as to decenter.

Phenomenology has been said to liberate one from preconceptions. However, what may be ironical is that, often without their knowing, researchers design their studies or "hear" in a way that substantiates their preconceptions. That is why this process is so critical. The researcher in a phenomenological study is to use a metaphor, the "research tool" or the research "instrument." To be truly authentic and effective, the researcher is asked to do something that is impossible to do, but to do it to the extent that is possible.

Researchers are asked to clear their vision and thinking from assumptions, from prior knowledge, from their belief systems. In this step, in order for that to happen, one needs to adopt a perspective of "unknowing," where one listens with "the third ear" free, to the extent possible, of any prejudice or bias. In your journal, record your beliefs, assumptions, preconceptions, what you expect your findings to be, and any other noise that might prevent you from hearing about the meaning of the experience when you are listening to others. This is also an important step in seeing the experience in whatever forms it shows itself. Often, we see something and automatically overlay the sight with our own interpretation. We assumed we knew something about what we were seeing, only to find out that we had misperceived. Two films come to mind to assist the reader in this step. The film *As Good as It Gets* is a wonderful portrayal of preconceptions, biases, and prejudices, and *The Tail Wagging the Dog* demonstrates to us that we are on thin ice, believing what we see!

The assurance that you have accomplished decentering is obtained in practice listenening/interview/conversation sessions. As in Step C of Immersion, you practice decentering with any experience with a colleague or friend. Write in your journal what you are decentering from, listen to your friend tell of an experience, write a description of what you heard and what meaning your friend ascribed to the experience. Let your friend evaluate how accurate you were in grasping the essence of what he or she was saying.

During this practice, do not use a tape recorder and try not to listen in a way that you want to repeat ver batim what was said. Listen in order to grasp the meaning. Listen to get inside the person's perceptions. This often takes practice and with many different people and their experiences. It is quite a revelation to realize how different our perceptions are of the same event and how we take for granted that we both "saw" the same thing.

The following passage written by Jane Smiley (1989), describes the same phenomenon, the memory of a child at 2 years of age.

> As I sit on this hard bench I suddenly yearn for one last long look and not only of the phenomenon of little Joe and little Michael, but of the others too; Ellen, four, and Annie, seven months, sharing a peach. . . . As I watch them now as adults the fact that I will never see their toddler selves again is tormenting. (p. 120)

Ann Beattie (1989) wrote in a similar vein:

> When you are thirty, the child is two. At forty, you realize that the child in the house, the child you live with, is still, when you close your eyes, or the moment he has walked from the room, two years old. When you are sixty and the child is gone, the child will also be two, but then you will be more certain. Wet sheets, wet kisses. A flood of tears. As you remember him the child is always two. (p. 53)

2. Adopt perspective of "unknowing."

Decentering attempts to achieve the essential state of mind of unknowing as a condition of openness. In contrast, knowing leads to a form of confidence that has inherent in it a state of closure. The "art" of unknowing is discussed as a decentering process from the individual's own organizing principles of the world (Atwood & Stolorow, 1984). Unknowing in not simple but is essential to the understanding of subjectivity and perspectivity.

Unknowing paradoxically is another form of knowing. Knowing that you do not know something, that you do not understand someone who stands before you, and who perhaps does not fit into some preexisting paradigm or theory is critical to the evolution of understanding meaning for others.

To engage in an authentic encounter means standing in your own socially constructed world and, to unearth the other's world, saying:

I do not know you. I do not know your subjective world.

A person who engages another human being to form impressions, formulate a perception, and theorize from a place called knowing has confidence in prior knowledge. Such confidence, however, has inherent in it a state of closure. To be authentically present to a person is to situate knowingly in your own life and interact with full unknowingness about the other's life. In this way, unknowing equals openness (Figure 5–1).

Unknowing

The state of being decentered and unknowing is a challenging quest. Unknowing is an art and calls for a great amount of introspection. "Unknowing," as was said, remains essential to the understanding of intersubjectivity and perspectivity. In other words, it is essential to understand ourselves and the participants in our study as two distinctive beings, one of whom the researcher does not know. Each of us has a unique perspective of our situated context and a unique perspective of who we are as individuals in the world. This is our perspectivity, our worldview, and our reality. When the researcher and the participant meet, two perspectives of a situation need to be recognized. Thus the process of intersubjectivity begins to create a perceptual space (Figure 5–2).

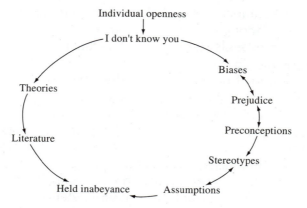

Figure 5–1 Unknowing openness.

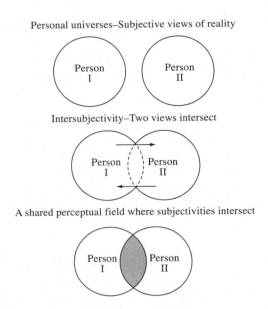

Personal universes–Subjective views of reality

Intersubjectivity–Two views intersect

A shared perceptual field where subjectivities intersect

Figure 5–2 Shared perceptual space of intersubjectivity.

Intersubjectivity

Intersubjectivity is not difficult to understand, though many writings seem intent on making the concept seem complex. What is complex is practicing it in a wide-awake manner. Intersubjectivity is the verbal and nonverbal interplay between the organized subjective worlds of two people in which one person's subjectivity intersects with another's subjectivity. The subjective world of any person represents the organization of feeling, thoughts, ideas, principles, theories, illusions, distortions, and whatever else helps or hinders that person. The real point here is that people do not know about anyone else's subjective world unless they are told about it. And even then, they cannot be sure. Figure 5–2 illustrates the concepts of intersubjectivity.

A film that I would suggest here to illustrate how two subjectivities that are extremely different because of the situated context of various life contingencies for individuals is *Whose Life Is It Anyway?* In the perceptual space in which the characters engage in dialogue, there are good examples of how decentering and unknowing by the health care providers would have contributed to an understanding of the patient. The patient is misunderstood, to the point of despair. I will not tell you the end, but watch and listen to a person being heard in a phenomenological manner as the film comes to its conclusion.

D. Articulate aim of the study in the form of a phenomenological question.

Coming to the point where you know the aim of your study, which is to understand the meaning of an experience, which you have clearly distinguished from other experiences, you are now able to begin to articulate questions. You have decentered yourself so as to be open and receptive to phenomenological material wherever and whenever it appears. So these processes of phenomenological inquiry allow you to proceed to the question.

Before Sarah began to articulate questions, she had an overarching interest and aim. Sarah said one day, "I am interested in how the mothers who were mourning for a lost infant and who were part of my first study are doing five years later." Thus what Sarah was interested in was, "I wonder if the passage of time has affected the meaning of their experience to them?" So the aim of her longitudinal study was to understand the meaning of the experience of losing a child when 5 years has passed. In her aim, we can see the question of what does it mean to be human in such an experience. This brings us to the critical aim of phenomenology, that of understanding the meaning of being human (Heidegger, 1927) and, as van Manen (1990) says, becoming more human. We can only become more human through understanding self and other. Self and other in individual life-worlds, situated context, and contingency. Internalizing the philosophy of phenomenology, distinguishing the phenomenon, and decentering from our own worldviews, we come now to the process of phenomenological questioning about the meaning of experience for individuals.

We can have many questions and will have more as material evolves. However, it is often helpful to have one overarching question. This question can then guide other questions. We must use caution here and not plan more than a few questions. When the existential material "speaks" to us and begs our attention, it will be the material from the study itself that will guide the researcher with questions and provide direction to the study as a whole. The overarching question, "the" question, should then reflect the underlying aim, that of understanding the meaning of being human and focusing on the experience that you have chosen to study.

There are different ways to articulate the question, which will often have to do with a philosopher or school of phenomenology in which you may be most interested in having your question reflect. My own experience has led me to find personal meaning in Heidegger's, Merleau-Ponty's, and van Manen's thinkings and writings. This does not mean that I am not influenced by many other philosophers and, indeed, in the next edition of *Revisioning Phenomenolgy*, the writing of the postmodernists will be accentuated. However, in regard to Heidegger, I find his curiosity about the question on "being" very compelling. "What does it mean, this idea we call being? What is the nature of being? What is the meaning of being?"

To wander down this path, one accepts that "beings" are always in experience. Therefore we go to the experience that the human being is in to attempt to answer the question of meaning for human beings. The experience may not necessarily be one that is concrete; it may be abstract, such as spirituality or even philosophizing. Beings are always being, even "being" asleep. So it is in what beings are being that enables us to find meaning in being!

The being is in experience. That is where the standard answer to "what is phenomenology?" evolved from: it is the study of lived experience. That definition, I believe, has led many astray, as they focus more on the experience than on human meaning in experience.

Like "being," "experience" should never be simplified. Merlau-Ponty believes that these experiences are layered with meanings, and he contributes to our understanding by emphasizing how these meanings create the way in which we perceive experience. This is where the life-worlds, contingency, and the situated context need to be addressed. This assists us in understanding the many layered and the multiplicity of considerations that there are in any one person's perception of experience.

Articulating the question calls on us to be very clear in what we are studying. The overall question, from a Heidegerian perspective would be: What is the meaning of being human in this experience (entity)? Many studies begin with the question, What is it like to be in this experience or to have had this experience? After many years of reading studies with the latter question, I have come to believe that if we keep "meaning" in the forefront of our study, we will have a richer study, one in which meaning is usually found in the participants' own words, as they form expressions of meaning. Keep in mind that you will have many questions that can be asked of participants in your study and "What's it like?" could actually be the first question. Often this will lead to a description of the experience. I think we need to go further. How were you feeling? thinking? and other variations can lead to the meaning of the experience, which will then bring into play the life-worlds, the situated context, and contingency.

Now, all this having been said, it is usually in the academic world when "the" question needs to be clearly articulated. Too-strict guidelines might prevent you from following where the participant wants to go. This needs to be avoided. Use common sense when trying to keep yourself, the researcher, and the participant focused. If the participant wanders from the experience, the researcher must make a decision about the relatedness or, better yet, ask the participant how he or she sees what he or she is saying to be connected.

A participant's wandering to areas whose relevance is not obvious to you can be extremely important to the participant. Refocusing participants needs to be done minimally. This wandering is part of the phenomenological study and, as such, has meaning. Because Sarah's study, which is presented in Chapter 6, was not prescribed by dissertation requirements, she was able to let the reader know what she was doing without specifically asking a question, as was heretofore noted. However, how would it be stated if she had to state it? She would simply take her aim and ask the question of it. Her overarching question then might be a version of the following one: What is the meaning of having lost a wished-for baby, with the passage of 5 years? Sarah's aim is to understand the meaning that the passage of time may have had on these women's lives who had this experience.

In one of my own studies, the question that was probably overarching was: What is the meaning of anger as it is experienced by women who are in therapy? The aim of that study was to begin to understand the meaning of anger of women who happened to be in therapy at the time (Munhall, 1994a).

The reader can see the difference in asking questions and stating aims, which are different from what we have become accustomed to reading. Remember the most frequent definition of phenomenology: the study of lived experience. Those studies would ask, What is the lived experience of anger of women who are in therapy? This is a matter of choice for the researcher and the "meaning as it is experienced" is a personal preference, for want of more meaning! I also believe that keeping "meaning" in the forefront of your study will produce a more phenomenological study. You will not be led astray to structures and categories.

I do not want to know just "what is it like," which was part of my own schooling, but "what is the meaning of." I am seeking an understanding of the meaning of "things" to individuals. Within this method presented here, that would be the ultimate aim and be reflected in the question.

III. Existential Inquiry, Expressions, and Processing
IV. Phenomenological Contextual Processing
Steps III and IV are two process steps that are conducted concurrently.

The existential inquiry by nature requires our "being-in-the-world" and takes place in the life-worlds of the researcher and the participant. That means, then, that, when we are engaging in dialogue with our participants, in addition to hearing the linguistic expressions they use to describe and interpret their experience, we need also to be hearing the situated context of their being-in-the-world. This has been called the horizon or the background of the experience.

Expressions of meaning cannot be acontextual. The thoughts, feelings, emotions, and questions are deeply embedded in the context of the participant's life, or life-world. So, while we are doing the existential inquiry, we are also doing contextual processing. They are separated out for pedantic purposes here and for ease in understanding, first as separate, then as concurrent. This concurrent process can be imagined by overlaying Figure 5–3 with Figure 5–4.

We will begin with Step III, The Existential Inquiry, Expressions, and Processing.

Existential inquiry, expressions, and processing constitute the step in which you gather the existential material; it requires specific processes, such as attentiveness, intuitiveness, constant reflection on decentering, active listening, clarifying, synthesizing, writing, taking photographs or creating verse, and almost anything that will reflect yours and your participant's consciousness and awareness to the experience.

Most phenomenological studies at present use some technique to collapse the material into groupings. This is part of the confounding nature of phenomenological research. Originally, phenomenology was a method used to interpret texts. What is the meaning of this book? However, since social and health care scientists started using the method with individuals to attempt to learn more about the experiences that their clients or patients were having, the problem of what to do with all the material has been approached in different ways. As was mentioned

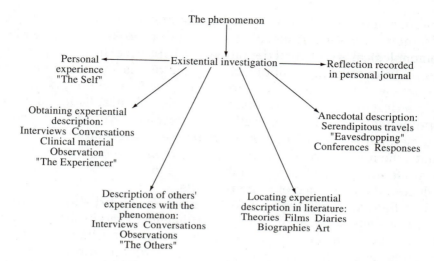

Figure 5–3 The Phenomenon—Existential Investigation.

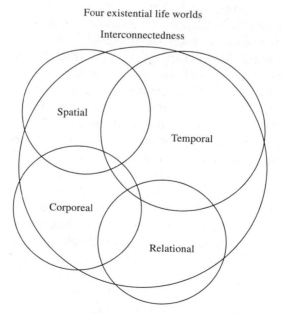

Figure 5–4 Four Existential Life Worlds.

before, some methods call for collapsing or condensing the material into themes, essences, meaning units, and, probably the least phenomenological, a structural definition. In Chapter 4 of this book, we see the prevalence of these approaches in the discussion of themes, essential elements, labeling, clusters, categories—all attempts to provide a description of an experience in a clear, logical listing of some type. Sometimes whatever method the researcher used to organize the material is then placed into a narrative. If there were 10 participants, the researcher searched for similar themes with perhaps a note or two for differences, but often then wrote the narrative in a way that reflected the mergence of 10 participants.

In a field such as nursing, where we are socialized strongly into a world of signs and symptoms, lists of diagnoses, and other kinds of classification, we tend to value this "shorthand" for its efficiency in communication. However, a major problem with this approach and in particular in using it in a phenomenological study is that words and signs do not have the same meaning for everyone. Both the health care provider and the patient interpret them differently. And, as with phenomenology, these words and signs lose further meaning if they are acontextual.

The signs and symptoms manifested by a patient have meaning only when placed in context—a historical, social, cultural and individual context. So we are in a dilemma. We cannot deliver a study of entire transcribed interviews. So what are some alternatives? Well, "dwelling with the data" used to be a popular phrase, which is heard or read less today. It is here where I think we need to return.

The researcher has either a transcribed interview of one person or notes that the researcher has taken over a series of interviews/dialogues. Within these texts are expressions of meaning. The expressions convey in words, as in art, a manifestation of meaning. Throughout the material, the researcher can highlight such expressions. They come as participants express themselves with emotions, thoughts, desires, questions, wishes, hopes, and complaints. It is to this that we need to turn our attention. People do not talk in themes; we do that to their "language." It seems more authentic to stay close to the participant's language and search through the material for the expressions of meaning.

Dwelling

Then, I believe, it is time to dwell. There are no shortcuts here and, for those who will invest the time and commitment to authenticity, they and their participants will be well served. Once again the researcher is called on to be the "instrument." Each individual participant needs our reverence for their individuality and their way of expressing meaning. You read the text of one participant, highlighting in your head the expressions of meaning, and then you actually do "dwell."

Contemplation is another word that could be used to describe this part of the study. The researcher needs to be alone to contemplate over a period of time the meaning that this participant was attempting to convey. After a certain amount of time has passed, time not measured in hours, insights, intuitions, and understanding emerge. The researcher begins to write. The researcher returns to the material and uses the language of the participant to illustrate the particular meaning. The researcher also returns to the participant and, depending on the participant's evaluation, will either have successfully captured that individual's meaning or will return after clarification to writing once again.

This is a departure from the collapsing or categorizing from interview materials in that there is no deliberate step of searching for similarities or differences. Each participant stands alone. The ending narrative does not homogenize 10 interviews but tells many different stories of meaning. Of course, the researcher will become aware of similarities and differences and write about them as well, while still holding the individual as the focus for meaning.

When I review some of my own work, I certainly see how I organized some material into categories, and I suppose for others and myself that there are times when this may be the most efficient way of organizing material. However, there is a chapter (Munhall, 1995) where I found Beverly's story, Lynn's story, Lisa's story, Victoria's story, and Carol's story. Each of these stories is different and has different meanings, and they challenged different normative commitments and unquestioned myths. Perhaps the experience that I was studying, (women's secrets) allowed for the individualistic interpretations, but there is something about the heterogeneity that, for me, has a feeling of "the experiences themselves" and of phenomenology.

So in this part of the study, where the researcher is gathering material that is spoken before it is read, dwelling and contemplation of "the said" needs to take place. This is a thinking through and at the same time a freeing of the mind so that insights spontaneously arise. Every phenomenologist must carry a small notebook for those moments. It is like taking a picture. There is the moment and, if you don't capture it, you might lose it. This process will happen to you, I promise you.

This is also the step in which you may, in a proposal, use specific areas to indicate where there will be "human subjects"; so in essence this is somewhat analogous to data collection. The difference in phenomenological inquiry is one of perception of the wholeness of the study. Once again, because the process is not linear, you are free to do the various processes of the existential process and phenomenological contemplation in a circular way. In actuality, all the steps should represent a circle. Toward the end of your study, you return to Immersion, Coming to the Phenomenological Aim, and so on. From a language perspective, because phenomenological inquiry has at once a subjective, objective, and intersubjective quality to it, we call the individuals who participate in our study "participants" and we call data "material."

Researcher as Participant and Instrument

Not only is the researcher the most important "instrument," he or she is a participant as well, as all come together to attempt to understand meaning in experience through this existential investigation. So in this part of the study you need to attend to the experience through amassing material and through processes.

Again, because this is not a textbook on phenomenology, I cannot possibly do justice to all that needs to be known and hope that the reader understands the general framework of the inquiry and the processes, which are critical to phenomenology. Now we proceed with the process steps of the existential inquiry.

(III) A. Listen to self and others; develop heightened attentiveness to self and others.

Listening and seeing in a phenomenological way bear further description. Part of what is required was discussed in the decentering process. Often times in phenomenological studies what we have seen consists of 10 or so transcribed interviews, with themes extracted, and then perhaps a discussion of those themes. As is said in *Revisioning Phenomenology*, if you feel you need to transcribe interviews in the beginning, then you should go ahead and do that. As you progress with this method, taping interviews and transcriptions become less necessary as you are able to grasp meaning in what might become a conversation rather than an interview.

When you choose your participants, you do not need to follow the sampling rules of quantitative research. Instead, you need to find individuals who are willing to speak to you about the experience that you are interested in understanding. Another qualification needs to be that they want to tell "their stories." Although there are many other sources to assist in attaining understanding, it is the language with all its intonation and inflection that will be the most revealing. Facial expressions and body language are also forms of languaging meaning. Needless to say, then, you want a willing and if possible enthusiastic participant.

Additionally, when you are listening, you must be cognizant that your participants are most likely telling you some things and not all things. As in any self-report, participants may think there is a "correct" way to respond to you. At the outset, this needs to be clarified and the participants must be reassured that these stories are their own, that you are interested in their own meaning and their own personal experience. The participant is the repository of meaning through narrative. Reminding your participants of their generosity in sharing often painful experiences demonstrates your sincerity. Clarify that there are no "right" answers or better answers and that what you value most is "their" exploring with you, in their own language, the meaning of the experience for them. If a participant asks you, "Is this what you want?" (which is often the case), you need to reassure the participant that it is "what" they want to share with you that you are interested in hearing.

At a dissertation hearing this past year, I heard a student say, "I had to keep bringing her back to the experience, she wanted to talk about. . . ." This outcome is frequent; it merits a response and is somewhat like the participant looking for the right answer. Instead, here the researcher apparently had in mind the range of focus that she wanted her participant to stay within.

Given that this is not psychotherapy but phenomenology, we do not have the luxury of free association. However, as was mentioned before, we need to hear what the participant is moving away from and where the participant is going. This can be in itself material from which meaning may be gleaned, and sometimes that meaning is the participant's wish to avoid further discussion. If you ascertain that the participant's comfort level is being disrupted for any reason at all, you need to attend to it and respect the participant's wishes at the time.

Significant Wandering

However, the participants may be communicating something other than avoidance; the wandering may in the end make significant sense. This will be discussed in greater detail under interpretation, but, for now, note that often there is great meaning in what is concealed. So, we are not only listening to what is said, but what is not said and also to where the participant goes to seek meaning, to another narrative.

Moving into a more conversational mode allows the researcher to gently probe as to the meaning of what is said. "Please go on, what are you thinking," if the participant falls silent, is good for the conversation. Once again, remember how important you are as well to this process. A good phenomenological researcher knows heightened consciousness, focusing intently, and continuous attentiveness to self and to the participant. If you, the researcher, find yourself wandering in thought, you must be always vigilant and bring your attention back to the dialogue. Make a quick mental note about where you wandered when you might have thought yourself to be distracted. This, too, may have significance in regard to its association.

(III) B. Personal experiences and expressions

Phenomenology begins with the personal, the subjective world in which you are present, a part of, and connected to in your own situated context, life-worlds, and different contingencies, which contribute to you as person. You begin your phenomenological study with self-reflection. You keep this self-reflection recorded in a journal. Because this kind of inquiry reflects a coming and going, a back and forth between and among parts of the study and the whole, your own personal experiential journey will change you.

Your self-reflection includes analyzing your life-world, situated context, and the contingencies, which bring you into relation to this human experience. Why do you, as person, want to study this experience? How did you become interested in this experience, in meaning, in understanding? This part of the study is ongoing, and the recording in your journal should reflect a deepening of "thinking," a "giving over" to the study, as well, as your frustrations, surprises, and questions, upon questions as your study evolves. Sarah, in the first study (1993) and in this study shares with us her own experience with what she is studying. She is intricately involved and at once "knows for herself" but puts that in abeyance to see the meaning for others.

This often raises the question of the researcher having had the experience that she or he is studying. Such questions are addressed in *Revisioning Phenomenology*, so in the interest of space I am referring the reader to that book because this component is an important one to think about.

The assurance that this personal expression section is being done well is that others who read your study understand in an authentic manner who you are in this study, your experiential perspective, and how and why you are engaged in studying the experience.

(III) C. **Experiential descriptive expressions: "the experiencer"**

This step pertains to experiences that may have a clinical component. Clinical, meaning the experience was in some way related to health care and in our particular domain, nursing care of individuals living through specific experiences. This is very broad and not limited to individuals who are actually in a clinical setting at the moment, but who have had an experience that has a clinical aspect. Examples could be experiences of physical, psychological, or psychosomatic illnesses, diagnoses, and the emotional and physical responses: worry, fear, hope, disorientation, loneliness. I would like to use loneliness as an example to delineate clinical from the next step, which has to do with either loneliness as experienced by an individual who is not necessarily lonely because of a clinical experience but who is experiencing loneliness as a generalized lived experience. There is no apparent clinical dimension to the loneliness. However, in the next step, those who are close to the individual who might be experiencing loneliness that is in some way related to a clinical situation can provide you with perceptions of their living with the phenomenon of loneliness. This enriches your study and gives additional material for interpretation.

Here is a concrete example: in a study related to Sarah's, a doctoral student also studied the same experience with mothers. She also asked the meaning or the experiences of the nurses caring for the mothers and found, as did Sarah, that many nurses had not had an awareness of the grief of the mother. A pragmatic defense seemed to be part of the nurses' and others' reactions to the experience. The belief that the mother has one healthy child and should be grateful for that overrode in almost all descriptions the belief that the mother had a need to mourn. Some "others" were even intolerant of such an idea. Now we find through Sarah's study that this mourning continues and is part of the dailiness of having the surviving twin. The surviving twin is a reminder of the one who died. These kinds of studies also remind us of the importance of phenomenology as a critical philosophy and that we need to go beyond interpretation to critique.

One can also see that an orthodox, 10 transcribed interviews as data collection could not provide the depth and breadth of all the varied materials of existential material.

Sarah, I believe, has a real interest in studying the experiential descriptions found in art, literature, music, photography, and other esthetic works. This interest has increased her focus on that dimension and someday could become a study of its own. One should note how a program of research could be had for those doing phenomenology and a very meaningful one as the study branches out and continues to shed light on the many facets of an experience.

When doing phenomenology, we need to be vigilant when we find ourselves looking to the rules for research from the scientific method. We do not have the limitations of operational definitions; nor do we have the limitations of linear steps.

We are searching for a full-of-meaning-and-detail narrative of experience, which will contain whatever adds to meaning. This is a simple and liberating criterion. If something contributes to the meaning of our understanding of an experience, one need not argue whether it belongs or not—of course, it belongs. The material enriches our understanding.

So, it is in this step that you begin to collect material from individuals who have experienced the phenomenon of interest in your study. *Revisioning Phenomenology* presents structural ways in which one can select themes and essences from transcribed interviews. I refer the reader to that book for more detail if you believe you need, at least at first, more structure to enable you to elucidate themes.

If you feel as though you can listen with "the third ear," asking individuals if they would be willing to share with you their experience in more than one sitting, then you might not need to tape the dialogue, but it is good practice, immediately afterward, to write as much as you can remember was said. Laptops make that a bit easier today.

Some Information About Interviews

In hermeneutic phenomenological human science the interview serves very specific purposes: (1) it may be used as a means of exploring and gathering experiential narrative material that may serve as a resource for developing a richer and deeper understanding of a human phenomenon and (2) it may be used as a vehicle to develop a conversational relation with a partner (interviewee) about the meaning of an experience (van Manen, 1990, p. 66).

In our evolution of the past 10 years or so, our studies using the phenomenological method often relied primarily on interviews. Researchers often asked the following questions or made observations:

1. What question should I ask?
2. How many people do I need to interview?
3. I can't seem to keep people focused.
4. What do I do with all this material (transcripts)?

As discussed earlier in this chapter, we must be careful in framing our question. The "what is it like" approach is fine, understandable, and concrete. Asking people to tell you about their lived experience of being cared for might prompt different responses from those in reply to asking what it is like to feel cared for: the first is asking for examples, and the second is asking for descriptions. There is no need here for either/or; both are fine.

Because of individuals' infinite differences, I find interactive dialogue, like conversation, to be very important. Additionally, stories, anecdotes, pictures, and any writing that the individual may be willing to share with you will enrich your study. I find the idea of being in dialogue to be one of a relation between two human beings. In this type of conversation, the unknower is seeking understanding of something from the speaker and not vice versa. It certainly is not a demographic interview and, though often tempting, it does not seek affirmation of your beliefs. Researchers sometimes find themselves saying:

- Don't you think . . .?
- Did you find that . . .?
- Do you think it was because they were . . .?

Such questions may appear to be harmless, but they have the potential to structure a person's story. They are the kind of questions through which you might be seeking to substantiate some of your own beliefs. The following lead-ins help explicate the person's unfolding of the experience.

- Could you give me an example of that?
- Do you remember how that made you feel (assuming there's a reason for a feeling question)?
- What did that do for you?
- (Or after a sentence) Go on. . . . Could you elaborate more on that?
- After a period of silence, ask, "Can you tell me what you are thinking about?"
- And never underestimate the "umm."

One student, after conducting some of her first interviews, told me that her mouth was sore from smiling. Although you might smile, it is certainly not a requisite and would sometimes be inappropriate. Try to follow the mood of the person whom you are interviewing. Also be aware of the body, the posture, the intonation in words, and the being of the other. Because the interview has sometimes assumed preeminence in the phenomenological approach, other considerations need to be taken:

- If you have never interviewed people before in the form of a dialogic conversation, then you need to practice. Practice with someone who has a background in psychiatric nursing, psychology, or psychoanalysis. In their disciplines, listening is elevated to an art. In phenomenology, listening also becomes an art.
- Listening is an art. Try to hear just what is being said. Try not to be anticipating what comes next—let there be pauses and silence.
- Silence is important. An individual said something. You listen. There is a pause. You are both reflecting. The pause will often yield additional reflection. Becoming comfortable with a silent or pregnant pause enables the storyteller to probe deeper within. Let the silence remain until you intuit that a prompt might be helpful.
- Many studies are a result of one-time interviews. As I have suggested elsewhere, two to three interviews with the same person may be more helpful. More "reflected upon" material is usually forthcoming, as is interpretation of what was said in previous interviews. A practitioner or researcher who ends a single interview with, " Is there anything else you might like to add?" is asking the question for that moment. Often, in the week that follows, more reflection occurs and the person desires to tell more about the experience.
- Imagine yourself in the interviewee's place for the first time. What might he or she be thinking about? Another reason that I strongly recommend additional interviews is that there is so much to process in the first encounter. You may need to use the first interview to establish trust and rapport, depending on what you are discussing. That effort will ensure the integrity of the material forthcoming.
- I believe it is critical to conduct these interviews/conversations where the participant is most comfortable. Just the choice of where the participant wants to be is material. Sometimes to find participants, you first need to go to where the experience is located; for example, school, office, clinic, or church.
- Be aware of your participant's holistic condition. You do not need to stop an interview because of crying or anger (as long as the interviewer knows very well whether it is therapeutic). How-

ever, you need good judgment. Even though informed consent ensures that the interviewee can stop the interview at any time, sometimes the interviewer needs to recognize that it is time to relax and change direction. Relief time, perhaps a little casual talk, may be comforting. Our intention here is not psychotherapy or nursing intervention. Our role must be clearly known, and we must act accordingly. So we need to be cognizant and attuned to our participant's psychological condition. Again, follow-up interviews help protect the psychological comfort of interviewees and demonstrate our genuine interest in them as persons.

Also include in your notes other observations that you or your participant have made. Phenomenology is not only the language of words but also the language of semiotics—the symbols and the signs in our environment that "speak" to us and tell us what is going on in this environment. They speak to your participants and are other sources of meaning as they attempt to make "meaning sense" out of their experience.

Your participant will most likely tell you in language his or her own description of various examples or observations, but you as a health care provider can also incorporate your own for comment and feedback. Again, this is an example of the "coming and going," the varying of examples, the varying of perspectives, and the looking upon a reflection with another reflection. This is what makes doing phenomenology so rewarding and worthwhile. The descriptions and interpretations attempt to be as inclusive as is feasible in the study, so as not to present a shallow description but a deeply embroidered tapestry of meaning.

The way in which you can be assured that this step is met is to bring your descriptions and reflections to your participants. If your descriptions and interpretations of the meaning of the experience resonate with the participants, then you will have assurance that you did indeed tell the meaning of their story.

Now does everyone share the same meaning? Of course not. So, first you go to the person with whom you have had several conversations to see if you captured his or her meaning. At the conclusion of your study, you will have reflected on all the material and will have begun to write a description and interpretation of your study. When that is completed, you once again return to your participants with the material woven into one narrative. Listen to the responses of your participants. Many will read an interpretation and remark that they did not have that experience or share that meaning. This returns us to the reason for separate stories and why it is critical to have in your narrative the similarities and differences found in the meaning of the same experience.

Some studies are written in which it seems that everyone in a particular study experienced the phenomenon in a similar manner. And that may be the case, as with Sarah's mothers. However, there may be other mothers in that experience who do not have this mourning phenomenon. This we do not know until we widen the scope of the study to include, perhaps, women from different cultures or backgrounds. Or perhaps most mothers do mourn a lost child when there was to be a multiple birth. We do not know and we cannot assume. We cannot generalize, because it is not our intent. However, because of Sarah's study, our consciousness has been raised to new possibilities and certainly a different way of being with these mothers.

However, I need to stress once again that, when one comes to writing a phenomenological narrative, one needs to heed the differences in meaning as well as the similarities. Phenomenology is not interested in generalizabilty. It is interested in how various individuals interpret the meaning of experience in their own individual ways.

(IV) D. Experiential descriptive expressions: "others" engaged in the experience

In this section your interviews/conversations are with other individuals who have lived through an experience in which you are interested but from another perspective. They have not experienced the phenomenon itself but have relationally interacted with the experience. This is like the example where the doctoral student also interviewed the nurses who cared for mothers who had lost one of their twin babies.

This becomes an additional source of material; the material gathered here will help vary the examples, provide different perspectives, and actually provide a source for another study or a furthering of one's study. In Sarah's study, she describes the reactions of others to her mothers and to herself. If you have the desire to broaden the depth of your study, you can talk to those individuals, as in a "going back and forth," to see if you can capture the various meanings from different individuals who may not be "directly" having the experience but are "directly" involved in the experience. Observing, once again, the language and semiotics of the "others" around the experience at hand is another source of material. The recognition that "others" play in phenomenological study is the belief that being in experience does not occur in isolation.

Imagine yourself painting a picture that is rich in detail and different colors and hues. The picture tries to capture, in the expression of individuals, their feelings and thoughts, which is an attempt to let the viewer know the meaning for those in the picture of an experience. Often times, in a museum or elsewhere, individuals gaze at a painting. This is like the phenomenological gaze. Searching for something in the picture that will speak to us, to tell us the meaning of this work of art. That is actually what you are doing when you lay out all the pieces of your study, always remembering that it is the pieces that have provided the meaning already, the individuals themselves. In the end it will be your phenomenological writing that will try to make sense of the experience in the many ways in which it has appeared or been concealed; and varying the material will enrich the text and fuse it with meaning.

Perhaps the lack of looking beyond interviews with the participants has led to findings that consist of lists of themes described in one or two sentences. We have moved beyond that phase of doing phenomenology, and I believe we should be allowing ourselves to "do" phenomenology in various ways, using various guiding philosophers, and experiencing the freedom to do what makes sense, sense making phenomenology.

Rather than being restricted by method, we are guided. We are not closed off from the appearance or concealment of some "thing," because the method does not allow us to look there. The method is different in intent from the one of scientism in that those delimiting steps must be respected or we will have distorted the experiment. Here, with phenomenology, if we do not go where participants lead us or where the experience leads us, then we will distort our findings. We will be sharing only some of the meaning, a limited part, grounded in rules about what to include and what to exclude.

In this existential investigation, if you the researcher have found some material that is not covered in the diagram (figure 5–3), you need to include it, if it helps you to understand the meaning of the experience. Husserl's famous direction, "to the things themselves" I take at face meaning. Although Husserl was often speaking of the world of objects, which has its place, the world of experience is more congruent with a human science. Can we take such a leap? If we are strict structuralists, perhaps not. Crotty (1996) has accused North American phenomenologists of overlaying continental phenomenology with pragmatism. Although this is an interesting observation and one, I might add, of which he is critical, for our purposes dwelling on objects probably will not add much to our understanding of human beings. If this is violating the purest sense of phenomenology, Crotty may be right in saying that we have a "new" phenomenology and that we should come forward and say so.

I am not so sure of his argument, in that Heidegger led the way to our interrogation of being. What he calls an entity, I believe we have translated logically to mean experience.

Although pragmatism has its share of proponents (and why not?), since in the health field we are most interested in results that will directly assist us in our work with individuals. Sometimes pragmatism becomes confused with doing something in an economical way, shortening time spent with patients, reducing costs and services. So it suffers from those connotations, but, nonetheless, pragmatism offers a way of thinking that acknowledges, with limited resources, here is the best way.

So, when nurses do phenomenology, it is not with the same aim, say, of a philosopher. We can say very directly that we are conducting a study with the aim of understanding the meaning of experience for our clients. We can acknowledge our values; that is, that we want to improve the quality of life for those we serve. So it is different. Nurses are interacting with "beings," and they are "being-in-the-world" in a service profession.

Perhaps another reason should be mentioned. Understanding meaning is the best way of designing interventions, so to speak. I must add, if interventions are called for, better they be from the patient's perspective of the experience than from the caregiver's assumptions.

One could argue that it is here where theory development must begin. Before all else, one needs a phenomenological baseline in order to describe, explain, predict, and control if that is what is needed in specific circumstances. The argument could be furthered with the observation of how poorly individuals "comply" with directions or education. If directions, interventions, and education are not derived from understanding what individuals experience and the meaning that they attach to their experiences, we have missed opportunities to be more effective. Individuals in experience are the ones to inform us of what it is they need, how we could be more helpful, and how we could assist in improving the quality of their health. Only from an understanding of the "other" in experience and the differences as well can we develop theory from "the individuals themselves." Theory needs to be grounded in the authentic experience of what is to be theorized, not from what an authority believes it should be. "Should be" theories usually lead to all sorts of "deficits"; the ideals are not grounded in the every day lives of individuals.

So perhaps it is a leap, and who gives us the authority to change continental phenomenology, as Crotty has suggested we have done? I would suggest that what is before us and what often cries out for our attention and seeks understanding at the deepest levels gives us permission. I would even go further and say that we have an ethical and moral imperative to use phenomenology to foster the highest and most humanistic standards of care. Wherever, then, you as researcher are able to hear, see, or touch material that has relevance to your study, remember that you are not bounded by rules. Your search is for as much experiential material as is available to you, so that your original aim is full of "life." And "real life" is what nurses are engaged in with others, and our lives are all intertwined.

You can then be assured that this is a process in work by observing, listening, and engaging in conversations with "others" who have had related experiences with the phenomenon.

(III) E. Experiential descriptive expressions: the arts and literature review

This step embodies the experience that you are studying, in coming into contact with others who have explored it either purposely or tangentially in esthetic work. The arts are poised to offer us a wealth of understanding if we engage in the search. Leaving yourself open to the experiential appearance, whether by accident or deliberate action, will often capture your imagination in ways that will literally excite you. I say this because I have watched countless students, colleagues, and myself act as though we have found gold when we come upon a film, a novel, biography, paintings, photographs, diaries, or other esthetic works that announce themselves to us through the experience that we are studying.

We are open to appearance. We are also aware of what may be concealed. So we come to these works and keep narratives of them—quotations, verse, a copy of a painting or photograph, lines from films and plays—to illustrate the meaning of the experience. We begin to understand more and more and sometimes stand in awe in regard to where our study has taken us.

We stand with the work or we view the film for the third time, we reread the play or the novel, and we are searching for the layers of meaning. This is just what we do when we return to an individual for the third time or maybe more. The researcher collects this material or records meaning and understanding gathered from these sources in his or her journal. The process becomes a way of being.

The reader can read how Sarah has found such deep meaning and understanding in esthetic engagement. However, it is critical to note that she is still engaged in the everydayness of her participants lives as their own form of art.

You can be assured that you have engaged in this process when you have found representations of the experience under study in the form of the various arts. If you find a paucity of material in this realm, begin to write verse, photograph, or paint to represent what you have heard from your participants or your own soul and spirit.

Reading the Literature

About experiential material in theoretical literature, one might think of the familiar literature review but, in phenomenology, it is used for a different purpose from that of the scientific method. Rather than reading all that is known about an experience thus far in the literature or in theories so as to support your hypothesis, you must find experiential descriptions of the experience or the meaning of the experience that have been written about from different perspectives. The intent is also different in that this step is considered part of your existential investigation, your gathering of material to deepen your understanding from these other perspectives.

Although it has been suggested not to do this step until you have had interviews/conversations with your participants, so as not to overlay the literature on your already "decentered self," literature about the experience may appear when you least expect it. In that case, it is a good idea to read it; just as with other existential descriptions, the content may lead you to pursue other avenues. In phenomenological research, material directs you to areas that you would never have thought of at the beginning of your study. As with all existential material, it shows itself to the researcher to be seen, to be read, to be touched, "as it is" within the life-worlds of the participants.

"As it is" for the participants and what is described in the literature may be at times very similar and also different. What is not in the literature is as important as what is in the literature and in many instances more important. The question of the literature reflecting, contrasting, and/or refuting what you have come to find in your analysis and interpretation is of critical importance to the advancement of understanding and our knowledge base.

Often our literature or theories are grounded in the knowledge base of the expert. If that knowledge base is deduced from other literature, from scientific observation of the scientific method mode, and from the perspective of the expert of "knowing," we may find an entirely different account of experience when we "go to the persons themselves."

Who can better tell us the nature, the meaning, and the "whatness" of an experience than the person who has had the experience? The question enlarges as previously described when we allow others engaged in different ways with the experience to give voice about what is going on, what it means, and how it is being perceived.

Actually, it would be preferable to postpone the experiential description in the literature until you have completed your interview/dialogues with your participants. I suppose that would assist you in staying as close to the participant's narratives as possible, without the influence of a literature review. However, as you progress in sophistication with the processes and the interview/dialogue becomes more conversational, you could introduce to the participant something that you have read and ask what the participant thinks about the material. This once again enriches the study, broadens its scope, and provides another perspective.

Whatever happens with this step, it should not appear under "literature review" in a research proposal. If you "must" have a literature review, the review should be of the philosophy of phenomenology and how you are planning to follow its underpinnings and suppositions.

More About Decentering

Here is an important point to clarify. Phenomenological inquiry does have suppositions. The suppositions are clearly articulated in the foundation of the phenomenological approach to being-in-the-world. We do not decenter ourselves from phenomenology; in fact, it guides us through the entire study.

What we do decenter from are presuppositions, beliefs, values, knowledge, thoughts, and ideas about the experience that we are studying and attempting to understand without the overlay of prior knowledge. Doing a literature review at the outset only serves the purpose of obtaining additional knowledge from which to separate ourselves.

You can be assured that you have done this section when you have gone to the literature on the experience that interests you and have obtained a good description of what is currently in the literature or in theories. This review will be another narrative to describe and interpret as it relates to your own findings and understanding of the experience.

(III) F. Anecdotal descriptive expressions: as experience appears

This process step is one that requires a consciousness of the experience or meaning of the experience when you are not necessarily expecting its appearance or concealment. The material appears in a serendipitous manner. You might be engaged in a conversation with a friend or neighbor who begins to talk about the experience without your prompting. You may hear about this experience at a conference in a formal presentation or in questions that people bring up in various formats. The more commonplace your experience is, the more often this will occur.

This type of serendipitous appearance can be a very important source of material, because sometimes people, without knowing it, become participants. They begin to converse with you about how "it is" with them to either be in this experience or to know of someone who is in it and how they are responding to that situation. This is anecdotal and not within the formal frame of your study. You did not expect it; nor did you ask for it. If you wish to pursue this with any one person and engage him or her in the study as a participant, then the rules that you agreed to regarding human subjects would need to be followed.

Other interesting sources of material for your study are people's responses to the subject. Just their reactions can be fascinating. I recall once discussing with a colleague the study of anger, and she angrily replied to me, "I don't ever get angry," apparently concealing to herself how she does experience anger. Your colleagues can provide not only feedback on how you are doing with your study, but also material from the perspective of their own initial responses to the experience. They may also be potential participants.

Again, as you become more familiar with this kind of inquiry, you will find yourself more awake to all experiences and engaging in the world in a different manner. Sometimes it seems to me, that "everything" said or seen has potential for a study of something and I collect material and write about "things" that I am not studying at the moment. I feel sometimes as though phenomenology has made me an "always" student of our everyday world.

Establishing a phenomenological perspective toward the world at hand stimulates attentiveness to the "every-day-ness" of life, its experiences, and objects, and you begin to see and articulate the taken-for-grantedness of much of experience. This attentativeness will further enrich your study with the addition of unforeseen appearances of material reflective of your experience.

You can be assured that this process step has been attended to by evaluating the material that you came upon in a serendipitous way and that you had not planned on. The serendipitous material comes about because of the aforementioned attentiveness by which a phenomeno-logical study takes up residence within you.

(III) G. Ongoing reflection in personal journal

This process step is ongoing from the very first day of your study or even thinking about your study. I cannot overemphasize the impor-tance of almost daily entries in your journal. After a conversational in-terview, the material in the journal should be either taped or recorded in another format; your responses, thoughts, associations, what you were feeling, what you thought the other person was feeling—all should be ongoing.

Your observations and your own reflective responses to them should be recorded. The responses of others to you should be recorded. This is your phenomenological journal and situates you in the life-world of your study. What happens to you during this time also should be included. Without recording as often as possible, you will lose this material; it will be naturally forgotten in the rush of your everyday life.

When you embark on description and interpretation, the material in this journal will most likely reflect a greatly enlarged view of the expe-rience and a greatly changed "you," as far as perspective and under-standing are concerned. That is why you would never want to lose a record of your own personal growth. Most likely you will see that you have enlarged your perspective in depth and breadth and have be-come much more sensitive and alert to the "taken for grantedness" of individual people and experiences.

In your phenomenological journal, beyond description try to incor-porate the meaning to you of "what is going on" and the meaning of the various experiences that you may be having in the course of this study. All phenomena within this study—the interactions, the responses, the good and the woeful times—will reflect in a back-and-forth way on your study. My journals during studies reflect this back and forth, both in tearful entries and in spontaneous "aha" entries. If you are a student doing a phenomenological study for a dissertation, you may have many tearful entries. Stay with it. Another promise: you will have traveled a journey that will make you more humanistic and sensitive than you thought possible. And your world will be so much more enlarged be-cause of it.

Your journal will read like a book when you are completed, and I think you will marvel at the richness of your own text as well as your own growth in awareness of meaning and of being human. You will be assured this process step is successful if the preceding sentence rings true!

IV. Phenomenological Contextual Processing

This process step is parallel to the process step of existential inquiry and processing. So what is presented here are your thoughts about the material gathered in that step. It is here where the researcher writes for the reader, the situated context of all who take part in the study, where his or her participants are located in the various life-worlds, and the contingencies of those in the study including the researcher. The experience is not separated from the participant so that context needs to be articulated as well.

A. Analyze emergent situated contexts.

This concept is actually quite literal. It refers to the situation that you and others are currently in, with all the contingencies that exist at the moment and as you progress in the study. Heidegger uses the term "thrownness" to express the perspective that the person is always "situated." The person is in context in his or her "being-in-the-world." From what we know thus far, we are without prior consultation, born into a historical time period, a culture, a family with a specific worldview and language. Other parts of the situated context are the experiences that we sometimes choose and sometimes do not choose. Because of our situated context, some choices are not available to us and others are not choices but required within the situated context.

B. Analyze day-to-day contingencies.

Contingencies are most often the reason for our action or inaction, decisions or avoidance of decisions, and voluntary change or involuntary change. Whatever the contingencies of one's life, they are within one's situated context and, in actuality, make a unity with the life-worlds. This unity will exert tremendous influence on the meaning of experience and a person's understanding of that meaning. A person's situated context allows certain actions and simultaneously limits other actions.

To truly understand another person, the researcher must engage in hearing and seeing that person by processing the material gleaned through the lens of that person's situated context.

C. Assess life-worlds.

The four existential life worlds are other dimensions from which we need to process phenomenological material to give meaning a perspective that tells us more about it. It is critical to understand that the life-worlds shown in Figure 5–4 on page 149 are a unity and reflect the interconnectedness of all four life-worlds. Contemplating on the spatiality, corporeality, temporality, and relationality furthers our understanding of the person in the world. As demonstrated in Sarah's study, a life world may also "stand out" as something very meaningful to an experience. Both temporality and relationality entered into her understanding of the experience of the mothers.

Spatiality refers to the space in which we are, our environment, which can assume different meanings for different experiences. So the phenomenological material needs to be processed once again through the lens of the environment. In regard to the study on women's anger, this was a very important world to discuss in many instances. The home for many of these women, especially those living in domestic-violence situations, needs to be part of the interpretation of her anger. An experience does not exist alone. It is always embedded and connected.

Corporeality refers to the body that we inhabit and is also referred to as embodiment. Rather than the idea that we *have* bodies, we think now that we *are* our bodies. Because we often speak as though our bodies and minds are separate, we know that the mind is embodied in this wonderful access to experience, the body. Then there are times that it is not such a wonderful experience. For this reason, the researcher must contemplate the connectedness of embodiment to the experience. The body intelligence is what experiences phenomena. We negotiate through experience through the unity of mind and body as one. Perceptions are what enter the body and therefore become the starting point of meaning. In the example of anger and domestic violence, not only is a woman's physical body shattered or damaged, but her whole perception of self can be shattered and damaged. The woman's embodiment is severely threatened, and readers familiar with the effects of this life-world understand the many different meanings of this experience for a woman. This is how all these ideas are interconnected. I write "as if this, then this" and need to occasionally focus on the interconnectedness of all these phenomena. Meaning and experience cannot exist in isolation.

Temporality is the time in which we are living always. We are always living through this concept called time. Our embodied bodies occupy a space and that space is located in time. Our participants often bring up the life-world of time, as is illustrated in Sarah's study. The passage of time, the temporal life-world, did little to ease the mourning process. Many readers of her study may express surprise, which is a sign of an excellent study. Sarah succeeds here in "liberating" some from their preconceptions.

The perception of time is another important concept to contemplate when listening to our participants and interpreting phenomenological material. The perception of time passing varies often in incredible ways with experience and is very meaningful. "Losing track of time" and "the time seemed endless" are phrases that the researcher needs to process with the participant. Actual interventions can be suggested from understanding the meaning of life-worlds in experience. Many readers will recall ICU patients who were diagnosed as being disoriented, because they did not know the time and day. They were in rooms without windows, so the orienting dark and light cycles were not present, not to mention that their space lacked clocks that could be seen. This is what might be called "everyday" experience for these patients. I believe the outcome of being in the world in a phenomenological way can lead a nurse to explore the space and time dimensions and arrive at a very practical solution: place large clocks showing time of day and the day of the week where patients can view them. Make sure that they indicate AM or PM. Some would say that it is obvious. Yes, and understanding of experience can come to the most obvious of solutions. Yet, for years, those patients were being labeled "disoriented."

Critical to temporality is history. We not only occupy a place in time, per se, but we are located in a historical period. That period is extremely influential in regard to our behavior, attitudes, beliefs, and where we are located (spatiality). The country and city or town is a critical influence, as is the family.

Relationality refers to the world where we find ourselves in relations with others. When studying phenomenological material, the researcher needs to contemplate the relationships within the experience being studied and as articulated by participants or found in other existential material. The importance of ourselves in relation to others is not just the phenomenologist's interest. This life-world seems to dominate popular culture in all of its manifestations. What is critical to phenomenologists is the recognition that the self is self-interpreting. We now can add to "to the persons themselves," "to the persons themselves for interpretation!"

Returning to women subjected to domestic violence, we as researchers or health care professionals could interpret their situations from all the literature there is available on this tragedy. Yet there are numerous interpretations, and to make the wrong one could be very harmful. To understand a particular woman in this situation, we must ask her for her interpretation. Otherwise we further violate her own unique life world of relationality.

In this process, the researcher begins to contemplate and look for meaning in all the materials gathered in the existential inquiry. Individuals provide meaning in their experiences through the expression of their feeling, thoughts, intentions, reflections, motives, desires, and emotions. These same expressions can be described by using many other existential modes of inquiry that researchers or participants have found illustrative of their own experiences. This concurrent contextual processing allows for integration of experience within context. The researcher is beginning to think in a narrative style, that there is a wholeness to it, a story with many different expressions of meaning.

What is critical here and in all sections of this method is to transcend the natural tendency to generate common emotions, themes, essences, categories, or meaning units. The narratives need to reflect one person's description of the experience with his or her own interpretation of his or her situated context.

Where researchers in phenomenology can divert from the philosophy of phenomenology is in the normal inclination to look for similarities, clusters, or themes. This is what has led critics to say that many of our studies are reductionistic. Of course, this reflects the dilemma, discussed earlier in this chapter, of how to understand individuals. Do we study the parts—in this case, the themes—and then put them back together as a "whole." We have long rejected the premise that man is the "sum total of his parts" and have adopted the maxim that "man is greater than the sum of his parts." Of all places, then, it is in phenomenology that we need to remember that "man is greater than the sum of his themes." This is particularly true when we put them in aggregates or categories.

This demonstrates itself in studies that have as findings for a group of people (an aggregate) a list of themes, which seem to describe the nature of an experience and how it is lived, through the perceptions of our sample of individuals, now being reported as a group. This is the principle used in quantitative research and, as challenging as it is to the phenomenologies, we need to use our imaginations to report meanings that acknowledge the individual in experience, not a synthesis of meanings. I would venture to say that, in Western culture, that remains the most challenging task of doing phenomenological research.

So, in this step, because it does not have the full richness of depth and breadth until it is combined with the next process step, we need to describe in narrative each individual's description and interpretation of the meaning of the experience. The researcher's main task is to very carefully choose from the participant's very long narrative the centrality of meaning that has been communicated and then to integrate the narrative with the life-worlds. One cannot exist without the other, if an authentic meaning is to be the outcome.

This is a subjective process, one, again, where our own assumptions, prejudices, and predilections can confuse an authentic delineation of what is most significant in one person's story. And we know that we cannot do this alone, without our participant's agreeing with our much shorter version of the meaning of the experience that was communicated.

People do not think or feel in terms of themes and essences for the most part. That is what researchers have been doing with phenomenological descriptions. This method varies from the practice of categorization, and asks the researcher to search through the material and begin writing narratives reflective of each participant's experience.

The interviews/conversations that you have had with individuals are in a verbal form, which by nature is much longer than descriptive summarizes in a narrative form. Recall that such narrative summation cannot take place until you have dwelled with the narrative, the memories of the interviews/conversations and contemplated the meanings that were communicated to you. However, narrative summation takes considerable practice, so as not to be writing through your own assumptions and frameworks, and, as was said, needs to be returned to the participant, as a written narrative, with the question, Does this reflect our interviews?

In the next process step, we will further answer the question, Why did we ever think we could find out "the" meaning of experience as though there was "one" meaning? While there are indeed common perceptions of experiences, they are quite different from common meanings. These differences depend on each individual's interpretive interaction.

V. Analysis of Interpretive Interaction

A. Integrate existential investigation with phenomenological contextual processing.

This step returns us to IV, "Contextual Processing." This is another step that needs to take place simultaneously with existential experiential expressions, or those descriptions will lack authentic meanings. Contextual processing, as described, called on the researcher and the participant to be historical, political, cultural, and social—in other words, being-in-the-world as it is in a specific time and place. Meaning cannot be found in an acontextual place or in an ahistorical time, if such notions even exist. However, in some descriptions, they have been completely ignored, and meanings gleaned from those studies are without the essentials that create and contribute to meaning.

In this interpretation of the interaction of the situated context in which individuals find themselves while in experience, we can arrive at a meaningful, holistic, simultaneous interpretation of an experience. Each participant in our study brings a personal biography and has already formed an interpretive system from which they will give voice to their experience. Each already has his or her own way of interacting with the larger world. Each has different situations in the life-worlds. Particular contingencies will influence his or her description, interpretation, and formulated meaning of experience.

B. Describe expressions of meaning (thoughts, emotions, feelings, statements, motives, metaphors, examples, behaviors, appearances and concealments, voiced and non-voiced language).

This analysis of the situated context, gives the thoughts, feelings, and emotions a "horizon," a context, knowledge, and a biography—in other words, a thick web of relational interactional processes that contribute to who the individual "is" among others and enable the researcher to capture meaning encapsulated in context.

In this process of interpretive interactionism, it is critical once again not to move into thinking in aggregates, categories, themes, or essences. Because two people were born in the same year or in the same family, town, or society does not mean sameness. We would be guilty of reductionism if we were to think in that manner. In quantitative terms, they are just variables, devoid of meaning. Only in interaction with all the other contingencies of individual life-worlds can we approximate phenomenological meaning. This is so complex that it is always an appoximation of meaning. I have viewed groups agreeing on a meaning of some "thing," only later to realize how divergent the agreed-upon meaning actually is.

C. Interpret expressions of meaning as appearing from integration.

To reemphasize, it is critical to understand the meaning of being human within context. From these understandings, we can give others the things that will assist them in generating further meaning, the "interventions" that they may need to increase the quality of life or minimize suffering. Such understanding allows us to individualize our approaches to individuals and enlarges our consciousness to a phenomenological way of being with others. We no longer have only one approach to an experience. We recognize that meaning for the individual is how we individualize care. Meaning should be at the core of our care, of what we do and plan with others.

One might ask, Then how can we have procedures, policies, treatments, and prescriptive theory? Well, we can have them, but we need to know why they often fail or meet up with "complications," or why we have a high rate of "noncompliance."

There are many reasons why such acontextual, homogenous approaches do not work. One of them is that large groups of people were reduced to "one" person, whether in a qualitative or quantitative study. The "one" person is a synthesis of many people and, in actuality, the "one" person does not even exist. This is critical to keep in front of you as you do phenomenological inquiry—that is, you are not homogenizing differences. What you are attempting to do is to have your participants and yourself interpret the interactions of their context with the experience at hand and to write a rich description of their experiences. Both these process steps combined lead to existential, experiential expressions.

Proceeding in this manner, you will have fulfilled some of the philosophical underpinnings of phenomenological inquiry. You will undoubtedly have varied examples, varied interpretations, and varied meanings.

I would like to interject here that, in nursing, we espouse phenomenological beliefs and values in our nursing philosophies—individuals are unique organisms in interaction with their environment—and then paradoxically have a nursing care model that fits all. Because why this does not work has already been discussed, let us proceed to the next step and see if it affords us better opportunities to generate knowledge that is more particular than general.

VI. Writing the Phenomenological Narrative
A. Choose a style of writing that will communicate an understanding of the meaning of this particular experience.

In this activity, an analysis of each individual's experiential expressions and interpretive interaction is narrated as one life-world vivid in description and detail. The narrative is reflective of the complexity of the interconnectedness of all the expressions spoken or "showing themselves" of the deeper contexualized meaning of experience.

There are many different ways to present your findings. For exemplars, I refer to two books: one by James Hillman, which he calls a phenomenology of emotion, and another by Robert Cole, a phenomenolgy in a series of stories about childhood spirituality. I do so to show the variation of presentations, for which there is no formula. Writing is a creative activity, and your subject and content should inspire your own presentation, sparked with your imagination.

James Hillman's (1997) book is titled *Emotion: A Comprehensive Phenomenology of Theories and Their Meanings for Therapy*. The introduction in this book is quite good: it presents phenomenology as method and describes how Hillman used this method for this book on human emotions. Not only is it an example then, but it also provides an interpretation of phenomenology as a method.

The other book, *The Spiritual Life of Children*, by Robert Cole (1991), states in the introduction that it is a phenomenological text. The book contains one narrative after another about an individual child talking about his or her spiritual life. Each chapter is one child's story. Cole finishes his book with a critique of spiritual life for children and its implications for our society. The book is a good example of presenting narratives for individuals and then doing a critique of the meaning of the study, which is the seventh step of this method.

Volumes 1 and 2 of *In Womens' Experience* (Munhall, 1995, 1996) contain 21 different phenomenological writings by different authors. As you read them, you will see a wide variation in style and creativity.

For further examples, use the many resources that are discussed in Chapter 25 of this book.

B. Write inclusively of all meanings, not just the "general" but the "particular."

In this method, there is a moving away from the idea of synthesizing experience into one narrative fits all. Surely there may be similar meanings voiced by individuals but, when they are contextualized, the interpretations may be different. Perception of experience is always grounded in the historical, political, social, and personal background. One might ask, then, Is this not several one-case studies placed together?

There are fundamental differences and they are articulated in phenomenological philosophy, the aim of phenomenology, and the method. The knowledge base of a person conducting phenomenological studies must be sophisticated, and the researcher herself needs to develop many different practices. The outcome of existential experiential expressions, within a deeply contextual world, produces a narrative that describes and interprets the heterogeneity of responses, which case studies do not do, the heterogeneity of meanings, which case studies do not do, and, yes, some similarities, which case studies do not do. However, because this method is phenomenological, we do not want to be reductionistic in "listing" those differences and similarities in the narrative. Once we do that, we have removed the deeply embedded contextual interpretations. In the narrative, similarities and differences will "show" themselves.

C. Write inclusively of language and expressions of meaning with the interpretive interaction of the experience of the situated context.

What we produce in these vivid life-world descriptions of our participants' meanings in experience are the possibilities of being-in-the-world for us to consider when we attempt to understand another individual. In casual conversations, "We are more alike than different" can be heard. Even if we were to base our theories on such an observation, the differences are probably the most important characteristics to consider when approaching patients, planning patient care, and developing nursing research ideas and projects. The similarities are easy, if indeed there are such entities. The differences are what challenge us and make all the difference in meeting the needs of patients. And the differences are paramount in our endeavor to understand individuals in their multiple realities, subjective worlds, life-worlds, and individual contingencies.

D. Interpret with participants the meaning of the interaction of the experience with the contextual processing (steps 3 and 4)

This is a process that has been ongoing in your research endeavor and can be referred to as co-interpretation of all the phenomenological material. The best sources the phenomenological researcher has are the participants and the other existential material that she or he has amassed. The researcher goes, as before, back to the participant and asks, "In this narrative am I interpreting the meaning of this experience for you?" This is the "mirror," the capturing of the whole: the participant's experiential descriptive expressions of the meaning of the experience *and* the same participant's situated context.

One cannot overemphasize the influence of the situated context on the meaning of an experience for an individual. This contributes to the complexity of understanding experience but without this complexity, a contextual meaning emerges, which essentially is meaninglessness. Every life world contingency will have influence on the interpretation of meanings of an experience. We do an injustice to individuals by minimalizing their life-worlds in our interpretations of experience or the meaning of being human.

From this interpretation will emerge the material for your own interpretive critique, which can be used for direction for theory, practice and change. This critique will be enriched if you ask your participant about ways the experience can become more meaningful, tolerable, understood and how health care professionals can demonstrate understanding of their meaning. Again referring to Sarah's study, the participants tell us how to understand their experience in ways we might not have thought about because of our own preconceptions.

> **E. Narrate a story that at once gives voice to actual language as it simultaneously interprets meaning from expressions used to describe the experience.**

How one captures this complexity in writing about meaning and understanding, I believe is about narrating the experiences in the language as told to us, in the material that appeared to us, and in the things that were concealed from us. The researcher's task is to accurately reflect, as if in a mirror, in words the interpretive analysis of interactions that have given meaning to experience. The integration is essential to the wholeness of experience. The researcher reconstructs from the existential inquiry and contextual analysis a narrative that captures the contingencies and meaning in which individuals have socially constructed this experience. The researcher narrates findings that were discovered and uncovered in the course of the study. New and unexpected meanings of experience are significant findings and lead to new possibilities of "being."

Discovering

Discovering the meaning in experience fosters the emergence of authentic encounters with one another. We come to understand the role of perception. We come to question our assumptions. And often we take phenomenology as not only a way to do research but also a way of being-in-the-world, in our every day lives. We often have developed an entirely new worldview, an entirely new understanding of how to encounter our existence.

VII. Writing a Narrative on the Meaning of Your Study

In this final descriptive and interpretive piece, as nurses, we have a moral and or ethical imperative to fill. We are ultimately in a profession that has aims and goals to assist others in attaining a better quality of life, by enhancing awareness of how life might be lived in a way that has meaning for the individual, in finding meaning in their situated context, and, among other goals, by enabling individuals to understand who they are as persons.

Our final research narratives of description and interpretation need to have implications for the profession. What does this meaning have for nursing practice? What does this meaning have for nursing theory? Does the final narrative contain implications that critique current practice? Does the interpretation introduce us to new ways of understanding experience? Does it free us from preexisting suppositions? In this way, does it liberate us from a way of thinking about an experience or its meaning that is no longer evident in our inquiry?

I do not believe that we can do phenomenology without answering these questions about its relevance. That relevance must extend beyond listing essences and themes, especially when they are acontextual.

We have come a long way in our phenomenological thinking and savvy, and we are more critical of our efforts, which is a sign of confidence and growth in our own understanding. In the final analysis, if we are studying meaning, then the ultimate paradox would be if our study itself did not have meaning!

A. Summarize the answer to your phenomenological question with breadth and depth.

For the purposes of this section, the researcher takes the narrative from the previous phenomenological writing and condenses it into a summary of major interpretations. Here, it would be good to return to the participants and ask for their reading of the summary. Explain that the summary is not the narrative of their experience, in that kind of detail, but will be used to look for meanings or direction for change in thought or practice.

B. Indicate how this understanding obtained from those who have lived the experience call for self-reflection and/or system reflection.

In the evaluation of your study, ask the meaning question of the study itself. Ask the interpretive interaction questions. Make sure your study is embedded in the situated context in which individuals and experiences are located. Be able to clearly articulate the meaning for nursing that your study has explicated and interpreted. Unveiling the meaning of experience contributes to human understanding.

We need to remember that this does not lend itself to predictive theory.

If we were to entertain that it may lead to descriptive theory, we would have to include many qualifications. The theory would have to be explicit to specific cultures, context, and contingencies. Recall that we want to avoid reductionistic formulations; we want to call our attention to differences in interpreting realities, yet, at the same time, usefulness becomes apparent in the realization of similarities. These similarities, as in Sarah's study, enlightened our understanding and, for many individuals, liberated mothers and then nurses from their presuppositions concerning this experience. These mothers can find comfort in the understanding that the meaning of their experience within this group is shared.

C. Interpret meanings of these reflections to small and large systems with specific content.

The outcome of phenomenological description and interpretation can have different purposes, as heretofore mentioned. However, there is a balancing act to this. As with balancing, we cannot lose concentration or reflection on what we are doing. Even as I write, I reflect and can see another possibility. If you have the tolerance for this uncertainty, are able to feel a bit unbalanced, and have a philosophical leaning to understanding the meaning of experience, phenomenology will enrich not only your professional life but your personal life as well. It becomes a way of being-in-the-world. And being-in-the-world, from a phenomenological perspective, calls for wide-awakeness and attentiveness. From our phenomenological narrative, we must ask, Are there implications for change in our situated context? Do our narratives contradict prevailing norms, or beliefs, and/or theories? If we are in agreement that critique should be an intricate part of phenomenology, we must interpret the narratives for their implications for social, cultural, political, health care, and educational change.

D. Critique this interpretation with implications and recommendations for political, social, cultural, health care, family, and other social systems.

The actual meaning question that is asked in the end about any study is, "So what?" We must be prepared to answer this question from a critical perspective. We have considered research about domestic violence. If we ended a phenomenological study on the experience of domestic violence as it is experienced by women or men who have been victimized, and provided an understanding of the meaning of that experience, I believe that the study is not completed from a moral-ethical perspective. Leaving the narrative for others to come up with solutions or interventions is part of what happens with phenomenological narratives and, if a researcher was working with a team of researchers, perhaps the researcher could be assured that his or her research had the requisite meaning to be followed up.

Without that assurance, I think we are on better ground if we critique the implications that are derived from the descriptions and interpretations and state them as direction for change. A "call to action" is sometimes the only response when one has done a phenomenological study. All too often, because this part was not highlighted or even narrated, the "very good" study did not fulfill all its potential and was left as a narrative without consequence.

In a field dedicated to improving the quality of life for members of all societies, we have a mandate to listen, beyond the participant's descriptions and interpretations, to how can we make this a better experience. We do this because in the meaning of our study lies an authentic caring about individuals in experience. We do this kind of research ultimately to bring to light what might otherwise be hidden and then to act on narratives with direction and implications for change toward quality experiences characterized by caring.

Coming to an End for Now

Phenomenology questions the consciousness of us, as we are in the world, how we experience the world, and how we give meaning to experiences. Meanings and interpretations emerge from our situated context and provide for heterogeneous perspectives of life's events. So, this chapter presents some interpretations of how one might go about doing a phenomenological study. I expect it to be flawed in many ways. There are always questions to ask about a claim, and so I must let the reader know that all claims are tentative. In the outlines and advisement of students conducting a study with this method and in my own journey, I am hoping that this method reflects the questions that students most frequently ask and clarifies the process of conducting this kind of inquiry.

Research guided by this philosophy seeks to unveil the meanings and will teach us about one another. So, this chapter will teach me and the critique will result in a clearer version, done by another or me. This is how we will advance our knowledge of phenomenology and its purposes.

Our Hope for Understanding

As a philosophy, phenomenology is our hope for understanding in this world. If we were to understand the meaning of events and experiences to people, we would approach them in a way that would reflect understanding of them specifically, not of theory reflecting aggregates of individuals. Our theories would acknowledge the many ways of being and that one way is not the best or the only way to be-in-the-world.

The health care provider would not be the author or the authority for patient care. Until the meaning of experience for a patient is known, the intervention is acontextual. "Noncompliance," I believe, results from not understanding the patient and the meaning of a behavior to the patient. Because nurses are often concerned in a caring way about behavior that may be detrimental to a patient, family, or community, they need to understand meaning. At the meaning level, we can offer to patients our understanding, and perhaps this generalization is well grounded; we all wish to be understood.

Phenomenology resists homogenizing responses to experiences, categorizing individuals, and placing them in stages. Unfortunately, individuals are viewed as atypical or, worse, abnormal if they deviate from the "mean" of a statistical equation or the goals of a theory.

In contrast, researchers following the path of phenomenology are interested in the "particular" of experience, while recognizing that there are similarities. However, they see the horizon of the experience, the context in which the experience occurs, and the contingencies affecting the individual as being integrated and critically influential. With this, there is no attempt at generalizing. The phenomenologist bears witness to individual consciousness and the consciousness of the same event perceived quite differently.

In the end, phenomenological studies raise and expand our consciousness and enable our understanding that, at the central core from which all things grow, lies meaning. The interpretation of the meaning allows for congruency in communication and in nurse-patient interaction. There is optimism in phenomenology, in its wide-awakeness to experience, in its reverence for differences and the subsequent possibilities, and in its ability to liberate us from our preconceptions and emancipate us from presuppositions that no longer work.

In coming to the end of this chapter I would like Sadler to have the last paragraph:

> Our experience is not less than an existential encounter with a world which has a potentially infinite horizon. This human world is not predetermined, as common sense or physicalist language would indicate; it is a world that is open for discovery and creation of ever-new direction for encounter, and hence open to the emergence of as yet undiscovered significance. Because our experience is a creative and thoroughly historical encounter in a lived world, one that is alive with our encounter of it, it is potentially open to new possibilities of significant existence (1969, p. 20).

REFERENCES

Anderson, W. (1995). *The truth about truth*. New York: Putnam.

Atwood, D., & Stolorow, R. (1984). *Structures of subjectivity*. Hillsdale NJ: Erlbaum.

Beattie, A. (1989). *Picturing Will*. New York: Random House.

Benner, P. (Ed.). (1994). *Interpretive phenomenology: Embodiment, caring, and ethics in health and illness*. Thousand Oaks, CA: Sage.

Coles, R. (1991). *Spiritual Life of Children*. Houghton Mifflin Co.

Crotty, M. (1996). *Phenomenology and nursing research*. South Melbourne, Australia: Churchill Livingstone.

Davis, S. F., & Finlay, L. (1999). Applying phenomenology in research: Problems, principles and practice. *British Journal of Occupational Therapy, 62*(9), 424.

Hammond, M., Howarth, J., & Keat, R. (1991). *Understanding phenomenology*. Cambridge, MA: Basil Blackwell.

Heidegger, M. (1927/1962). *Being and time*. San Francisco. Harper & Row.

Heidegger, M. (1949). *Existence and being*. Chicago: Regnery.

Hillman, J. (1997). *Emotion: A comprehensive phenomenology of theories and their meanings for therapy*. Evanston, IL: Northwestern University Press.

Koch, T. (1999). Phenomenology revisited. An interpretive research process: Revisiting phenomenological and hermeneutical approaches. *Nurse Researcher, 6*(3), 20–34

Lauterbach, S. (1993). In another world: A phenomenological perspective and discovery of meaning in mothers' experience with death of a wished for baby: Doing phenomenology. Chapter V in P. Munhall and C. Oiler-Boyd (Eds.), Nursing research: A qualtitative perspective (2nd ed.). Sudbury, MA: Jones and Bartlett.

Munhall, P., & Oiler-Boyd, C. (1993a). *Nursing research*: A qualitative perspective (2nd ed.) Sudbury, MA: Jones and Bartlett.

Munhall, P. (1993b). Unknowing: Toward another pattern of knowing. *Nursing Outlook*, 41, 125–128.

Munhall, P. (1994a). *In women's experience* (Vol. 1). Sudbury, MA: Jones and Bartlett.

Munhall, P. (1994b). *Revisioning phenomenology*: Nursing and health science research. Sudbury, MA: Jones and Bartlett.

Munhall, P. (1995a). *In women's experience* (Vol. 2). Sudbury, MA: Jones and Bartlett.

Munhall, P., & Fitzsimons, V. (1995b). *The emergence of women into the 21st century*. Sudbury, MA: Jones and Bartlett.

Munhall, P., & Fitzsimons, V. (2000). *The emergence of family into the 21st century*. Sudbury, MA: Jones and Bartlett.

Parse, R. (1990). Parse's research methodology with an illustration of the lived experience of hope. *Nursing Science Quarterly*, 3(1), 9–17.

Rorty, R. (1991). *Essays on Heidegger and others*. New York: Cambridge University Press.

Sadler, W. A. (1969). *Existence and love*: A new approach in existential phenomenology. New York: Scribner's.

Smiley, J. (1989). *Ordinary love and good will*. New York: Random House.

van Manen, M. (1984). *"Doing" phenomenological research and writing*. Alberta, CN: The University of Alberta Press.

van Manen, M. (1990). *Researching the lived experience*. Albany, New York: SUNY Press.

ADDITIONAL REFERENCES

Allen, D. G. (1995). Hermeneutics: Philosophical traditions and nursing practice research. *Nursing Science Quarterly*, 8(4), 174–182.

Allgood, M. R., & Fawcett, J. (1999). Acceptance of the invitation to dialogue: Examination of an interpretive approach for the science of unitary human beings. *Visions: The Journal of Rogerian Nursing Science*, 7, 5–13.

Annells, M. (1999). Phenomenology revisited. Evaluating phenomenology: Usefulness quality and philosophical foundations. *Nurse Researcher*, 6(3), 5–19.

Ashworth, P. D. (1997). The variety of qualitative research (Part 2): Non-positivist approaches. *Nurse Education Today*, 17(3), 219–224.

Astedt-Kurki, P. (1994). Phenomenological approach in nursing research: Experiences of health, well-being and nursing are studied from the point of view of clients and nurses. *Hoitotiede*, 6, 2–7.

Baker, C., Norton, S., Young, P., & Ward, S. (1998). An exploration of methodological pluralism in nursing research. *Research in Nursing and Health*, 21, 545–555.

Barnard, A., McCosker, H., & Gerber, R. (1999). Phenomenology: A qualitative research approach for exploring understanding in health care. *Qualitative Health Research*, 9(2), 212–216.

Forbes, D. A., King, K. M., Kushner, K. E., Letourneau, N. L., Myrick, A. F., & Profetto-McGrath, J. (1999). Warrantable evidence in nursing science. *Journal of Advanced Nursing*, 29, 373–379.

Finlay, L. (1999). Applying phenomenology in research: Problems, principles and practice. *British Journal of Occupational Therapy*, 62(7), 299–306.

Koch, T. (1999). Phenomenology revisited. An interpretive research process: Revisiting phenomenological and hermeneutical approaches. *Nurse Researcher*, 6(3), 20–34.

Proctor, S. (1998). Linking philosophy and method in the research process: The case of realism. *Nurse Researcher*, 5(4), 73–90.

Seymour, J., & Clark, D. (1998). Issues in research. Phenomenological approaches to palliative care research. *Palliative Medicine*, 12(2), 127–131.

Longitudinal Phenomenology: An Example of "Doing" Phenomenology Over Time
Phenomenology of Maternal Mourning: Being-A-Mother "In Another World (1992) and Five Years Later (1997)"

Sarah Steen Lauterbach

Time present and time past
Are both perhaps present in time future
And time future contained in time past. If
All time is eternally present
All time is unredeemable.
What might have been is an abstraction
Remaining a perpetual possibility
Only in a world of speculation.
What might have been and what has been
Point to one end, which is always present

—T. S. *Eliot*

This poem was included in my doctoral dissertation, "In Another World" (Lauterbach, 1992), as exemplifying the overarching dimension of *temporality*, a theme that was discovered to be running throughout mothers' experiences with death of a wished-for baby.

"Temporal" (lived time) was described by Munhall (1995) as one of four intersecting life worlds of human experience. In the 1997 (Lauterbach, 1998, 1999), 5-year follow-up research with participant mothers from the original study, the dimension of *temporality* became an increasingly important theme. It has led to an articulation of the need for a longitudinal perspective in some human science research. Further, in discussion with other researchers and practitioners, it has become apparent that *temporality*, or *lived time*, is of importance in other human experiences. It is thought to be particularly applicable to experiences that fall into the category of universal, common experiences.

"Using" Phenomenology over Time in Investigations of Lived Experience: Taking a Longitudinal Perspective

A longitudinal perspective is useful in investigations of highly sensitive human experience often requiring significant changes in life plans. Many human phenomena and experiences need to be investigated over time to gain full apprehension and understanding. Experiences that evolve and are developmental or have meanings and consequences that evolve and change over time perhaps should be investigated longitudinally. Living and dealing with some experiences takes time, especially those accompanied by unexpected or sudden losses. Meanings surrounding complex experience evolve and become more explicit over time.

The longitudinal perspective was found to be particularly important in research focused on investigating the death of a wished-for baby. This phenomenon called for an investigation and continuing phenomenology of mourning. At a qualitative research conference in 1999, where the follow-up research was presented, in an informal discussion with fellow qualitative researchers, Dr. Patricia Munhall, who was the dissertation chair, first suggested the term *longitudinal phenomenology* for phenomenological investigations over time.

Since completion of the follow-up investigation (Lauterbach, 1998, 1999), the researcher's continued human science and existential investigation surrounding the phenomenon has also illuminated methodological issues important to the particular investigation of maternal mourning. It warranted a continuing exploration and focus in thinking about human science research, particularly of sensitive phenomena. Meanings in this research, discovered and uncovered in the original research, continued to evolve and were also created through the research endeavor. Mothers' mourning is understood more fully and is potentially seen more clearly over time. The mothers described mourning as needing regular and thoughtful attention to become integrated into their and their families' continuing life.

BEING-A-MOTHER IN ANOTHER WORLD

Briefly, the findings from the investigation of mothers' experience with death of a wished-for baby will be presented. The title of the dissertation, "In Another World," was given to the original research at the completion of data analysis. The title is the overarching theme discovered, and serves as a metatheme, which is an interpretation of mothers' experience of having a wished-for baby die. Mothers' descriptions of their experience, which were embedded within their stories of loss, were interpreted to be an existential experience of *Being-a-mother* in another world. Heidegger's (1962) description was useful in providing this interpretation.

> In Being-with the dead [dem Toten] the deceased himself is no longer factically "there." However, when we speak of "Being-with," we always have in view Being with one another in the same world. The deceased has abandoned our "world" and left it behind. (p. 282)

This theme emerged as data from the first interview were analyzed with the first participant mother and was present in descriptions with each subsequent participant mother. It was a consistent, repetitive theme running throughout the data. Mothers stated that, with their babies' deaths, they experienced a dilemma of *Being*. They found themselves, existentially, in the world of *Being-a-mother* and **not** *Being-a-mother*. In reality, they were mothers **without** a baby to mother.

Three central dimensions in mothers' experience were identified as *context*, *connection*, and *temporality*. Mothers found that the particular life context, including work, family, and intimate relations, was important. In addition, the connections and relational contexts surrounding the death of the baby were critical. Finally, temporality, or lived time, influenced the meanings in experience. Mothers were shocked that many of their intimate relations and social contexts invalidated and contributed to a conspiracy of silence surrounding the significance of the loss. Mothers described how, having not chosen this particular outcome of pregnancy, each was then empowered to experience grief, in the words of one mother, "any damn way I chose."

Nine essential themes were identified as running throughout the three central dimensions of temporality, context, and connection: essence of perinatal loss; reflective pulling back, recovering, and reentering; embodiment of mourning loss; narcissistic injury; finality of death of the baby; living through and "with" death; death overlaid with life; changes in world views; and failing and trying again.

Themes Revisited Five Years Later

In the follow-up research (Lauterbach, 1998, 1999), *temporality* became an increasingly important dimension to mothers' mourning experience. All five mothers from the original research described 5 years later that meanings are continuing to evolve and exert their presence in continuing life experience. The essential theme of *integration of mourning into continuing life experience* was identified, and earlier original themes were revisited. Mothers said that meanings in the experience of having a wished-for baby die and that the reality and degree of loss experienced continued to emerge and change over time. One mother stated that she experienced a tremendous loss of being a mother to her baby at the moment she knew something was wrong. As time passed, she realized a much greater, more encompassing loss—the loss of a future relationship. This farsighted loss became evident over time and had been the most difficult. The passing of time was needed for the loss to emerge fully. Another mother stated that it was a loss not only for her, but for the world.

A year after the completion of the follow-up research, Princess Diana's death brought the theme of future loss home. Had Princess Diana's mother experienced a perinatal death, the world would have been deprived of her presence. In the original research, it was discovered that Shakespeare's mother had experienced two perinatal losses before he was born. What about those babies, and him? One of the children born to a participant mother, following the stillbirth of his sister, kept saying to his mother, "If she were here, I would not be here." The death of this sister and his life seem to be intimately connected.

In the follow-up research, the special relationship and status of children who follow a perinatal loss also constituted a theme. Making sense of the significance of death involved not only mothers, but their families, particularly the children who follow. There are many individuals, some famous or public figures, and very many "just ordinary folk" whose gifts and contributions have been missed because of dying too young, or "before their time." This theme was present in the experience of C. S. Lewis (1963), who, in A *Grief Observed*, stated, "And then one or other dies. And we think of this as love cut short; like a dance stopped in mid-career or a flower with its head unluckily snapped off—something truncated, and therefore, lacking its due shape" (p. 58).

The death of a human baby is considered by many "the ultimate loss" or "the grief that knows no words." The death of an infant person requires particular attention and mourning and is often invalidated by the social world. Denial of death seems to be a twentieth-century human phenomenon and has been greatly influenced by both time and technology. Technology has changed the definition of death and has provided us with opportunities for extending and preserving life that did not exist at the beginning of the century.

MORTALITY STATISTICS, TEMPORALITY, AND DENIAL OF DEATH

At the beginning of the twentieth century, the death rate in America was 17 per 1000, in contrast with approximately 8.6 (De Spelder & Strickland, 1995) in 1995. Life expectancy has increased from 47 to 76 years. In 1900, more than half of the deaths were of children under 14 years; now less than 3% occur in this group. It is now expected that a baby born will live into old age. The perinatal death rate at the beginning of the original research was 9.8 (U.S. Department of Health and Human Services, 1989). The infant mortality rate in 1900 was 140 (deaths on an annual basis per 100,000 live births) dropping to 17 in 1975 (Klaus & Kennell, 1980).

Because death has become a phenomenon that is often prevented by science and technology, there has been an accompanying denial and invalidation of death (Becker, 1973). Perhaps, denial and invalidation are more common with death experiences that are particularly painful human tragedies. Perinatal infant death is perhaps such a phenomenon. Even in the 1800s, when infant death was relatively common, postmortem photographs of infants were rare. The researcher found no infant funeral scenes with the family gathered around. However, in the mid 1800s, funeral postmortem photographs, with family around the coffin of an adult, are common. Even when death was a relatively public phenomenon, infant death was not a public affair.

In the anthology *The Oxford Book of Death*, Enright (1987) chose poetry and passages from literature that demonstrate varied and surprising reactions to dying as a final act and the bereavement that follows. He quotes a survivor of a concentration camp: "When in death we are in the midst of life." The following poem seems particularly related to social contexts surrounding death. It is from "Graveyard in Norfolk," by Sylvania Townsend Warner.

> Still in the countryside among the lowly
> Death is not out of fashion,
> Still is the churchyard park and promenade
> And a new-made grave a glory.
> Still on Sunday afternoons, contentedly and slowly,
> Come widows eased of their passion,
> Whose children flitting from stone to headstone facade
> Spell out accustomed names and the same story (p. 124)

Mothers' experience with perinatal death in this investigation show that the *conspiracy of silence* surrounding infant death takes its toll in the course of grief and mourning, often leaving mothers to grieve in isolation and privately. The particular wished-for baby and the joys and trials associated with mothering, of growing a person into a fully functioning adult person who is still a child to a mother, are forever lost, except in mothers' memories and memorials, when death occurs at birth. The acknowledgment of the particular baby who died and the subsequent existential "missing" the child are common themes with mothers and their families and have emerged over and over in discussions and conversations with other mothers in presentations of this research.

The temporality of infant death is further validated by the researcher's own experience. It is perhaps the temporality of the phenomenon that continues to engage the researcher. The personal experience with having a baby die is validated by the findings of the research. The longitudinal nature of the personal phenomenology of infant death, along with research, has led to a commitment to continuing research. When the researcher began the doctoral investigation in 1989, it had been 8 years since the personal experience with infant death. At the time of the writing of this chapter, the researcher experienced the death of her second twin baby girl, Amy Liv, 19 years earlier. Alexandra, the first twin baby girl, is now 19 and still experiences a bittersweet joy at family reunions and celebrations, such as her high-school graduation. She struggles with the experience of the death of her twin, experiences an existential missing *Being-a-twin*, and at times feels as if a piece of herself is missing. This is reflective of the *embodiment* theme described by mothers. Marlow, the researcher's first daughter and oldest child, who was 4 years old when Amy died, is now 25. Jared, who was just a 2-year-old toddler is 22. Jared and Marlow threw pink flowers into Amy's grave at the burial in the Hendry family cemetery, located near the childhood home and farm of the researcher's grandfather, the farm to which the researcher will eventually retire. Jared cried out unconsolably, for "my pinkest flower" as dirt was thrown into the grave and covered the urn of Amy's ashes.

Emergence of Life Worlds: Shifting Themes in Mothers' Experience over Time

Munhall (1992), in her article describing the four life-worlds through which human experience is lived, identifies them as: temporal (lived time); spatial (lived space); corporeal (lived body); and relational (lived relationships). In the dissertation (Lauterbach, 1992), three central dimensions were identified from which nine themes of meaning were identified. *Temporality*, *context*, and *connection* were the three central dimensions identified in mothers' experiences. Embodiment was identified as an essential theme in that research, and it is exemplified in Munhall's corporeality. However, in the 5-year follow-up, *embodiment* was articulated as one of the now four overarching dimensions in mothers' lived experience with mourning infant death over time.

Over time, seemingly small changes in themes are reflected in changing language, but they reflect fairly significant shifts in meanings. Thematic changes were reflected in mothers' use of language describing experiences. For example, the theme of *embodiment of perinatal loss* has been changed to *embodiment of loss*. Most importantly, over time the dimension of *temporality* has become a central, organizing dimension in mothers' experience. As time passed, with years of subsequent life experience and separation of mothers from the original experience of having a baby die, with continued reflection not only has there been the discovery of meaning in the experience, but, more importantly, research has made a contribution to the development of meanings. Thus, research has served not only to validate and uncover meanings, but to contribute to mothers' developing lived ongoing and unfolding meanings of the experience. *In this longitudinal phenomenology of maternal mourning, it appears that temporality of mourning is "almost" the thing itself.*

Longitudinal Methodological Perspectives: Using van Manen's (1990) Method

The Emergence and Importance of Temporality

Munhall's (1992) work and articulation of life-worlds in human phenomena validates the findings in the original (Lauterbach, 1992) and continuing investigation. The understandings related to life-worlds surrounding infant death, as abstractions, developed through time in the analysis, processing, and interpretation of meanings in mother's experiences. The researcher, in doctoral study as a beginning researcher and novice user of phenomenology, was not immediately aware of the significance of the abstraction and conceptualization. It was from the conversational and interview data that the three central dimensions were articulated, not from the abstraction. In retrospect, the analysis process and immersion in the phenomenology literature, plus the continued reflection on the phenomenon, have greatly contributed to the interpretation of the findings. The continuing investigation of death and bereavement literature and the continuing examination of human science material provided by the arts, continue to provide existential validation to meanings that were identified. In the original doctoral inquiry, *temporality* was identified as a central dimension in mothers' experience of losing a baby. Five years later, temporality continued to be articulated as a particularly important overarching dimension in mothers' experience of mourning the death of a baby.

Further, in the original study, the dimension of temporality was present and emerged as a central important theme in the first interview/conversation with the first participant mother. It was also in that first conversation that it became apparent that more than one session would be necessary to get a full description of the original experience of having a baby die. The dimension of temporality became a central focus in the unfolding existential investigation, particularly as examples of the phenomenon were sought in the creative arts and literature.

Temporality as Seen Through the Historical Perspective

The historical context surrounding the phenomenon of perinatal infant death, bereavement, and mourning rituals discovered in the existential investigation of human arts and literature began to appear *with increasing relief* against the landscape of mothers' descriptions of their experiences. The focus on mourning and bereavement within an historical context, along with the depiction of the phenomenon in the creative arts and literature, further lent validation to the temporal nature of mourning. Further, the fittingness of the phenomenon and van Manen's methodology is interpreted to have necessitated a continuing investigation and, as such, dictated the use of phenomenology longitudinally. The phenomenon "called out" for a continuing focus on meanings of mourning as seen in the enthusiastic participation of all five mothers in the original inquiry and in the follow-up. The phenomenon has directed the investigation from the beginning, once van Manen's method was used, which directed the researcher to *turning to lived experience of the phenomenon*, especially the arts, cemeteries, and creative literature.

Mothers' experiences with the phenomenon of perinatal infant death did not reflect the postmodern view of death and mourning— that the living separate from the dead and that death is followed by a rather brief mourning period during which the living select activities that are reflective of *"moving on."* Rather, mothers experienced not a separation but a need to "be with" the child. The mothers in this research described how they were often compelled, even in the midst of social pressure from loved ones, to engage in a very personal and private period, perhaps longer than is acknowledged or thought to be healthy, of intense grief and suffering, where mourning was the closest relation to "mothering" and *"being-with"* the very much missed and wished-for baby.

Originally, the doctoral research addressed a discrepancy between nursing practice and mothers' experiences. Phenomenology was the chosen methodology because its ultimate aim is to understand human phenomena. Even though the professional interdisciplinary literature investigated revealed much in the way of understanding death, there was a paucity of nursing literature that demonstrated understanding of this human phenomenon. Additionally, nursing care and nurses were perceived as providing perhaps well-meaning but uninformed care. Mothers described nurses who were very often helpful at the delivery time, but they related that they did not receive continuing care. Mothers also described how meanings surrounding the loss of the particular baby was invalidated by both the health care system and their friends. Focusing on loss was only a passing matter in care.

It is interesting that nurses in the early 1980s discovered that, by having postmortem photographs of their infants, mothers were aided in their journey through acute grief. Some of the earliest photographs taken in the middle 1800s were postmortem photographs. Interestingly, these prints are not often seen in public collections, but in the collectors' world or in private family albums. Since the 1980s, nursing protocols for delivery suites and hospitals have included the use of photography, taking a picture of each baby at risk at the time of delivery. The picture is usually added to the chart and discarded after a time if the parents have not requested it.

As the public has acknowledged the importance of memorials, taking pictures at funerals is becoming more common. In the mid-1800s, a postmortem photograph was often the only photograph taken of the deceased. The wealthy often commissioned paintings of their loved ones to be done from postmortem photographs. Death was thought of as part of everyday life, and planning for it was as common as planning for other ritual and nodal celebrations of life. Modern technology has obscured and prevented death, and the phenomenon is more removed from rituals and celebrations of everyday public human experience, even though it is still a universal human phenomenon.

Infant death is often seen as the ultimate tragedy and, as such, is even more removed from public life. However, the death experience has been embedded existentially through the creative arts and literature. The use of metaphor is particularly helpful when drawing attention to sensitive, and more common than usually thought of, painful lived experiences, such as perinatal death. Thus, illuminating objects and phenomena, such as mothers' lived experiences, along with full description of multiple backgrounds and contexts surrounding these experiences, is a necessary central feature in "seeing" and interpreting meanings in experience. Specifically, explicating the experience of one mother to that of another, and of one mother to the population of mothers who experience perinatal infant death, is important.

The artist, like the researcher, is concerned with images, especially the use of perspective and figure-to-ground images. Viewing an individual mother's experience as a unique experience, alongside viewing common experiences among mothers, gives depth and breadth to the experience. Individual and common meanings are used in the interpretation of the human experience. Perhaps more universal aspects of mothers' experiences are understood when considered along with contextual matters surrounding the phenomenon.

Temporality as Seen Through the Arts

"Art cleans life up," stated poet Robert Frost. " Art, in my view, depicts human experience with lived phenomena. Just as the artist is free to create, the viewer is free to experience art. Art allows a freedom for understanding and interpretation, depending on the artist's and/or viewer's personal intention, knowing, understanding experience.

Art has the potential for especially painful, sensitive human phenomena to be portrayed through various mediums and creative works. An example of art in creative literature and poetry can be seen in Robert Frost's poem titled "Home Burial." ". . . God, what a woman! A man can't speak of his own child that's dead. You can't because you don't know how to speak."(Untermeyer, 1964, p. 28) The gendered differences between a father's and a mother's experience with infant death and burial is described in this poem, which highlights differences in meanings in the separate, but shared experience of burying their child. Gendered differences existing in mourning were not the focus of this investigation, but there were common references to them in conversations with mothers.

A topographical map used as metaphor of maternal mourning depicts meanings of mourning as a growing relief over time with exacerbations of experience appearing at critical life events, anniversaries of the rituals of life and death. The topographical map of maternal mourning depicts the human phenomenon as a *Becoming*, living, human phenomenon with changes in the relief and landscape of grief, with mourning evolving along with human development over time. The temporality of mothers' experience of mourning is seen in the topographical relief that accompanied the appearance and creation of meanings as they evolved and became more explicit. Over time, especially over the 5 years between the original research and the follow-up, mothers experienced *participation in research as validation of mourning*. Mothers processed experience as they continued to both journey and "journal" and reflect with and separately from the researcher. Finally, in follow-up interviews/conversations, mothers began to interpret, using the original research process of fully describing their lived experiences, their own experience of mourning. It was important that, as mourning was validated, mothers continued to write and contemplate strategies to lead their families in developing meaningful memories and anniversary celebrations.

In the original research, mothers talked a good deal about the social world invalidating and thus silencing the private and public expressions of mourning. The participation in research originally served as key in mothers and others finding validity in their own view that mourning required attention, worthy of reflection and remembering. The existential validation of the experience of grief and mourning facilitated a full recognition of the significance and meaning in the experience.

Research, like art, has the potential to address sensitive, difficult phenomena. The qualitative researcher uses *self as an instrument of research*, thus facilitating discussion and attention to the phenomenon. This is very similar to the creations of the artist who uses various mediums of expression. The work of Edvard Munch, a symbolist artist, has themes of death running throughout his art (Prelinger & Parke-Taylor, 1996). He experienced the death of his mother as a young child, and at 14 his sister died. With the use of various mediums in his art, some of his work is closer to the "real life" experience of death than others. The lithographs of *The Sick Child* (p. 119), and *Head of Sick Child* (pp. 125–126) are explored through the use of different mediums and colors. The artist's sensitivity and portrayal of imminent death is evident.

In this research, loss was explicated through the use of phenomenology, which investigated human experience with the phenomenon in the creative arts as well as in mothers' experience over time. Phenomenological research began with focusing attention on the experience, eliciting remembrances and full descriptions of it. It provided the framework for mothers and others to reminisce, remember, process, reflect on, ascribe to, discover, and uncover meanings in experience over time. The potentials for meanings, embedded in the experience, were the originary, seminal perceptions, which, when reflected on, became partially or fully acknowledged meanings. Further, the *art of the research process* used enabled a continuing development of meanings. It also acknowledged that meanings evolve and, by attending to the experience, are more easily integrated into mothers' continuing life experience.

Further, as stated earlier, the process of research and inquiry was dictated by the phenomenon under investigation. The particular existential investigation into the arts, literature, and cemetery and memorial art was directed by the phenomenological method used. Once begun, the methodology used emphasized an attentive *listening* to the phenomenon and turned and focused attention on examples of the human lived experience with infant death in the humanities, the creative arts, literature, and poetry. The fittingness of the particular methodology used and developed in the continuing investigation, which continued to be provided by the phenomenon of perinatal loss, further validated findings.

Lived experience is the "originary" way in which we perceive reality. As living persons we have an awareness of things and ourselves which is immediate, direct, and nonabstractive. We "live through" life with an intimate sense of its concrete, qualitative features and myriad patterns, meanings, values, and relations. (Morse, 1989, p. 44, quoting Ermarth)

Temporality as Seen Through the Creative Literature and Poetry

The phenomenon of human grief and mortality is subject matter for poets, artists, and musicians, as well as scientists. John Milton, a reknowned English poet whose sister's infant daughter died when he was 19, had already lost two sisters in infancy. The infant, Anne Phillips, was buried on or around January 22, 1628. Milton wrote "On the Death of a Fair Infant Dying of a Cough" as a memorial (Hughes, 1957). Critics have debated what the death of this infant meant to Milton, but, in the continuing verses, the idea that grief is temporary is revealed, because it leads to a new pregnancy and a child to come.

Milton's poem reflects a common theme in the public responses to infant death, that a new pregnancy takes away the loss or that the infant is replaced by another child. However, mothers in this research described how they immediately looked to a new pregnancy the moment something was wrong but fully understood that the "particular" baby could not be replaced, and that was what was missed in the months that followed death.

T. S. Eliot's poem, quoted at the beginning of this chapter, was written in the early 1940s, at the same time of great interest in phenomenology in postwar France. In the analysis of textual data in this research, with the use of a process of phenomenological reflection and reduction, death as a phenomenon demonstrates temporality as a focus of concern. Universal human experiences exist and are lived over time. Interestingly, the poet Eliot, like other artists discovered by the researcher in the existential investigation of the creative and expressive arts, had themes of life and death running throughout his work. Themes of life and death were found in many examples in the creative arts of music, literature, and mourning and memorial art and jewelry. These themes represent, in addition, ultimate universal human experience and can be interpreted to be embedded with perhaps universal themes of meanings. Artists, creative writers, and poets often provide their interpretations, which are resonating themes in mothers' experience.

Recently, a colleague returned from a conference with a copy of *The Patient's Voice* (Young-Mason, 1997). The first chapter is by Herbert Mason, and is titled "The Memory of Death." Interestingly, Mason's (1970) *Gilgamesh, A Verse Narrative* was discovered and used in the dissertation. In the aforementioned chapter, Herbert Mason's experience when his father died suddenly and unexpectedly when Mason was 7 years old was the subject of discussion. He stated, "Grief, which is a spiritual illness derived from a loved one's death, has physical effects that cannot be diagnosed and treated simply. The impact is sudden. One's healing responses are unprepared and thwarted, and the expectation of recovery in indeterminate" (p. 6). Mason goes on to state,

> We learn from a loved one's death, most of all, that our deepest yearning for ourselves and all humanity is for that transcendent that compassion that can only come from the source that also gives life. And from that yearning and that compassion working in and through us can come a wisdom that enables us to resume living. (p. 6)

When the life that she has given, a newborn baby, dies before its time, a mother needs to articulate meanings and come to understand meanings surrounding the particular loss. This has been revealed in the continuation research as mothers, through understanding, are enabled to continue their own personal and family development and living, integrating the death and loss experience, with reflection and continuation of meanings. Dr. Mason's life and work, which are sources of insight into grief, are relevant to mothers' experiences and reflect, in this author's view, the temporality of death and mourning, as well as the endless effects of the experience of having a baby die, not only on the mother, but on the family and society. In the search for literature reflective of the lived experience with death, a poem was discovered that provided a good example of the human experience of living through the death of a child. Shakespeare's poem, written in 1596, described his lived experience with his son's death. In a search for the context within which the poem was written, it was discovered that Shakespeare's mother had experienced two perinatal deaths shortly before her pregnancy with him. Had his mother experienced a third perinatal infant death, the world would have been denied the literary contribution of probably the world's greatest playwright. The poem's description of embodiment of mourning the loss of Shakespeare's 11-year-old twin son is evident. The temporal experience of mourning this loss was very like that in the Mother's Day poem, which follows this one by Shakespeare:

> *Grief fills up the room of my absent child*
> *Lies in his bed, walks up and down with me,*
> *Puts on his pretty looks, repeats his words,*
> *Remembers me of all his gracious parts,*
> *Stuffs out his vacant garments with his form:*
> *Then have I reason to be fond of grief* (Enright, 1987, p. 288)

Mother's Day

On Sunday I was a mother for a little while.
With one final push the baby was out.
And everyone said how beautiful he was,
They let me hold him, and he really was beautiful.
He lay there motionless, dark hair like his father's,
One eye opened slightly as I shifted his position,
And closed again.
They weighed him and fingerprinted him and
took his picture.
They let me hold him again.
He seemed to be growing older and more wizened.
His arms and legs no longer felt warm to the
touch.
They left us alone with him for a long time, and
we sat and gazed at him.
Then they took him away.
Now, I'm a mother no longer, left only with a
brief moment, and an emptiness where I had
felt full before. (written by participant mother in Lauterbach, 1992)

Gilgamesh (Mason, 1970) is an epic narrative of similar importance and was used as an example of the phenomenon of death in creative literature; it was especially evocative of mothers' experience. The following passage from that work was included in the dissertation.

Like a hungry animal through empty lairs
In search of food. The only nourishment
He knew was grief, endless in its hidden source
Yet never ending hunger.
. . .
And,
All that is left to one who grieves
Is convalescence (p. 53).

Further, this creative narrative is reflective of the temporality in grief and loss and of the struggle to find meaning, to hold onto the memory of the friend who died. It is very similar to mothers' experience of infant death.

It has grown past conversion to a world
Few enter without tasting loss
In which one spends a long time waiting
For something to move one to proceed (p. 54)

Temporality as Seen Through Memorial and Mourning Art

The mourning and memorial art and jewelry used in the doctoral investigation provided other examples of the historical context and temporality of mourning. In the early 1970s, while living in the United Kingdom, the researcher discovered that memorial brasses were present in most English churches. Long before mourning became a topic of scholarship, many unusual brasses were rubbed with waxed crayon on paper and are now hanging in her home. Since the research began, a small collection of mourning art and materials has been initiated. While at a conference in 1996 and again while at a conference in England in 1999, the researcher revisited several of these churches in a search for infant memorials. In the Salisbury Cathedral, only one example of a perinatal death memorial was found dating from the 1700s.

The research methodology used for the doctoral investigation required that the researcher begin to pay attention to the existence of the phenomenon as it exists in the everyday human world. For several years, the trolley tracks in University City paralleled the road alongside Woodland Cemetery, near the University of Pennsylvania campus, where many beautiful examples of infant memorials were discovered as part of the existential investigation of the research. This route was taken daily by the researcher to teach at La Salle University.

Interestingly, the La Salle University campus is located on the former estate of the artist Charles Wilson Peale, whose oil painting *Rachel Weeping* was discovered by the researcher in the course of the existential investigation. This painting is discussed in Pike and Armstrong's (1980) *A Time to Mourn*. It is a particularly good example of an artistic depiction of a mother's lived experience with death of a child. The painting depicts a young child who had died and is laid out in her burial dress. As was discovered, the artist's first wife, Rachel, and their daughter, Margaret, contracted smallpox in 1772, and only Rachel recovered. That same year, the artist painted the image of the child and, in 1776, the image of his mourning wife was added. Rachel is looking upward and has a sad expression with tears on her cheeks. The painting was never displayed publicly but was hung in his studio, behind a curtain to which he attached a note, "Before you draw this curtain Consider whether you will afflict a Mother or Father that has lost a Child" (p. 128). Obviously, the child's mother experienced a long period of grief and mourning.

The custom of celebratory gatherings and walking through cemeteries was discovered to have existed since the beginning of cemetery burials. In Philadelphia, in the 1800s, a typical family outing was to travel by boat up the Schulykil River for a Sunday picnic in Laurel Hill Cemetery. At that time, Laurel Hill Cemetery was outside the urban area; now, it is within the city.

The American Association of Nursing History Web site has pictures of grave sites of nursing leaders and historical figures. Cemetery visitations are common rituals celebrating Nurses' Week in May, when the annual cemetery walk-about visits the graves of nursing leaders who are buried there. This cemetery, Woodland Cemetery in University City, is adjacent to the campus of the University of Philadelphia. It was also adjacent to Blockley Hospital, later named and known as Philadelphia General Hospital, which was finally demolished in 1978, 4 years after the researcher moved to that neighborhood and lived for 23 years, until 1996. While living in the University City neighborhood, the researcher's young family was begun, and it was home to the family during and after Amy's death.

Even though the researcher lived in University City, it was not until she was engaged in the existential investigation of perinatal bereavement that cemetery visitations to several Victorian "dead" cemeteries and modern "live" cemeteries began in Philadelphia. (Dead cemeteries are those not accepting new graves; live cemeteries accept new graves.) There are some particularly beautiful examples of memorial art in babies' graves in the Woodland Cemetery and in Laurel Hill Cemetery, discovered when the research first began. One family plot in Woodland Cemetery contains eight babies' graves. Babies' graves are sized according to age of the child, a common practice now and in early times. In the Arlington Cemetery in Lansdowne, a Philadelphia suburb, is a section called "Babyland." Modern babies' graves are in a particular area and are less expensive than family plots. This cemetery, which began in the 1700s, then in a rural area, is now across from a hospital. In Laurel Hill Cemetery is a family plot with three graves, each with a baby in a cradle engraved into the headstone. A beautiful example of infant memorial art in Woodland Cemetery is the child "Donnie." Another infant memorial has the inscription "To live in the hearts, is not to die." On the other side is engraved "The best little boy in the world." Lambs, cradles, hearts and flower motifs, and poetry adorn babies' memorials and graves. These examples of memorial art validated themes of mothers' experience in the research. Themes of *life and death*, present in the original stories of mothers, were validated in cemetery investigation. A mother's collection of angels, memorabilia of her baby's life and death, reflected the tremendous valuing and importance of the particular child who died.

Since completion of the doctoral inquiry, this researcher has continued to investigate and follow the phenomenon within human sciences. In the many presentations and discussions and in the existential journey to mourning artifacts, museums, and cemeteries, and in collecting narratives and essences of conversation with people who had some experience or knowledge of the phenomenon, the investigation has been dictated by the phenomenology of the phenomenon. The need for a continuing investigation was thus dictated by the phenomenon and the dimension of temporality. The focusing over time enabled a development of a fuller understanding of the phenomenon. In the original conversations with participant mothers and in subsequent contact with participant mothers, a follow-up investigation was assumed to be a necessity.

Cemetery investigations have continued to cemeteries in northern Florida, where the researcher's family were early settlers, and in the past 4 years in Mississippi, where the researcher lived. Interestingly, cemetery visits have revealed some regional differences in the burial of infants and children. In the southern Mississippi town of Hattiesburg, where the researcher moved in 1996, Oaklawn Cemetery has several beautiful exemplars of memorial art. In this cemetery, infants and young children were often buried between the parents, with the memorial statue also placed in between. There are several examples, including an especially beautiful grave and memorial statue in memory of a toddler who died at the age of 3. Several other southern cemeteries, including the Oak Ridge Cemetery in Madison, Florida, have similar memorials.

Emergence of Longitudinal Phenomenology: Investigating Meanings in Mothers' Experience of Death of a Wished-for Baby over Time— Etic and Emic Perspectives

Mothers who participated in the original research were enthusiastic about the opportunity to participate in a follow-up inquiry. Five years later, all five mothers agreed to participate and were interviewed. At that time, they agreed to continue to provide experiential data in continuing inquiry and described their continuing integration of mourning into their family and personal lives. In fact, mothers' said that the original participation in research validated their mourning, and continued, even without contact from the researcher, to exert validation and support of a continuation of reflective activities focused on their experiences. They described the continuing effects on work, creative writing, and attention to anniversary reminders as an opportunity to continue processing and reflecting on the original experience. In addition, they described how they included and incorporated anniversaries into their family rituals and experiences.

The researcher's own personal experience, now 19 years after the death of her second twin daughter, continues to inform and guide the exploration of perinatal loss. The researcher has had an etic and emic view of the phenomenon. In addition, the continuing formal investigation over time has guided the development of the longitudinal perspective with this particular phenomenon. On the basis of the emergence of the longitudinal perspective, women's stories, and the personal experience described herein, the researcher is currently developing a new investigation focusing on an elder women's retrospective investigation. The same methodology will be used with women who experienced infant death many years earlier. In this investigation, the longitudinal perspective will guide the retrospective investigation. It is hoped that women's experiences and narratives will again narrate a fuller understanding of the phenomenon, while at the same time affording an opportunity to assess the potential usefulness of the longitudinal methodology guiding research.

In the last few years of the researcher's maternal grandmother's life, the grandmother was preoccupied with her own mother's experience of having a baby die. The events surrounding this baby's death being revisited during life review is also common in stories told of perinatal loss. This grandmother described how her "mother called out for her baby as she lay dying." Although the grandmother had not experienced the death of her own child, she was the oldest sister of the infant who died. She had a brother 2 years older than she, and the infant who died followed her. Then, 10 years separated her birth and the birth of other siblings. In the course of the 10-year gap and perhaps responsible for it, a baby brother died in infancy.

Similar to patterns in rural southern families, this grandmother became the primary caretaker of the younger three children, two of whom were twins. Before her own death, the grandmother had located the cemetery and grave site of her baby brother in the Madison County community of Pineland. There had been a Presbyterian Church there which no longer stands, but the small cemetery still exists. A headstone and marble slab were placed to identify the grave of "Baby Millinor." In the last few years before her death, the grandmother visited the grave of her baby brother each time she went to town.

In stories and discussions with elder women, there appears to be a phenomenon where daughters (and other women in the family) whose mothers experience perinatal death continue to feel responsibility for, to remember and "care" for, graves and memories. The grandmother in the preceding story also experienced the death of her second child, at the age of 19, due to pneumonia. Within a couple of years after the death, a foster son was brought into their home.

In the original research, the importance of the perspective of the researcher was described through discussion of emic and etic views. These two vantages of perspective continue to be important. The continuing research reflects a continuing relation between the two, between inside the phenomenon and outside the phenomenon of mothers' experiences with perinatal death of wished-for babies. When investigating human phenomena, of which the researcher has personal experience, there is a tension and relation between emic and etic views of the phenomenon under investigation. Further, over time, through using a longitudinal perspective, there is a balancing of imperatives between the original research imperative and an emergence of a therapeutic imperative. Over time, there may emerge an increasingly present caring imperative within the research, which has resulted in a shifting and balancing of imperatives between research, therapeutic, and caring perspectives. Such was the case with this research.

A narration of personal experiences and research was the subject of a chapter (Lauterbach, 1995) in Munhall's (1995) book, *In Women's Experiences, Volume 1*. More recently, in a new text (Munhall, 2000), this author provides a continuing narrative of her experiences in becoming a mother. Like the participants in her research, continuation of phenomenological reflection has become a process of integration of mourning (through research and scholarship, in addition to personal activities) into continuing life experience.

In ending, this quotation from one mother describes her mourning:

There was nothing I could do about it. I had no choice. I just moved through it day by day. Time seemed suspended. I had my pictures, my privacy, and my memories. I could close my

eyes and see the experience all over again. I could be pregnant
. . . before it all came crashing down. I was afraid I'd forget what
he looked like. And in time it became more and more OK.

A poem by the researcher's son, Jared, who cried about his pinkest
flower being buried, is reflective of his continued thinking about and
mourning his baby sister's death.

> *Earth encapsulates chrome reflection*
> *Selected pink flowers tossed.*
> *Terrestrial soiled dreams.*
> *Ultra-Violet rays no longer lavishing in polychromatic petals.*
> *Precipitation falling from grieving fingers.*
> *Life from death, Joy in grief,*
> *The willow whispers.*
> *Life echoing from jagged cliffs.*
> *Reverberating to Shady Groves.*
> *Bereavement belong to chiseled faces*
> *Tears tearing cheeks,*
> *Saline feeling weeping roots.*
> *Shoveling seared souls.*
> *Grounding my pinkest flower.*
> *Here lies Amy Liv,*
> *Etched in foiled reflection.*

> —*Jared Walter Lauterbach,*
> *written in spring 2000*
> *He was 22 when this was written*

And, lastly, a quotation from the ancient Sumerian epic *Gilgamesh*
(Mason, 1970):

> *In time he recognized this loss*
> *As the end of his journey*
> *And returned to Uruk.*
>
> *Perhaps, he feared*
> *His people would not share*
> *The sorrow that he knew.*
>
> *He entered the city and asked a blind man*
> *If he had ever heard the name Enkidu,*
> *And the old man shrugged and shook his head,*

Then turned away,
As if to say it is impossible
To keep the names of friends
Whom we have lost.

Gilgamesh said nothing more
To force his sorrow on another.
He looked at the walls,
Awed at the heights
His people had achieved
And for a moment—just a moment—
All that lay behind him
Passed from view (p. 92).

SUMMARY

At this time, after 12 years spent investigating the phenomenon of mothers' experiences with death of a wished-for baby, the author has begun to describe the phenomenology of maternal mourning. Currently, the elder women's investigation of perinatal loss experienced many years earlier has received Institutional Review Board approval, and data collection is in progress. The purpose of the series of investigations is to explicate meanings in mothers' experience and to continue the explication, articulation, and validation of women's experiences through research and human science investigations into the creative arts and literature. The hope is that these investigations will continue to contribute to knowledge and understanding of the phenomenon, not only for nursing, human science disciplines, and the public, but for participant mothers and their families, and for those who are yet to experience the death of a wished-for baby.

REFERENCES

Becker, E. (1973). *The denial of death.* New York: Basic Books.

Chute, M. (1962). *Shakespeare of London.* London: The New English Library.

De Spelder, L., & Strickland, A. (1996). *The last dance.* Mayfield, CA: Mayfield.

Eliot, T. (1936). *Collected poems 1909–1962.* New York: Harcourt, Brace, & World.

Enright, D. (Ed.). (1987). *The Oxford book of death.* Oxford: Oxford University Press.

Heidegger, M. (1962). *Being and time* (J. Macquarrie & E. Robinson, Trans.). New York: Harper & Row.

Hughes, M. (Ed.) (1957). *John Milton: complete poems and major prose*. Indianapolis: Odessey Press.

Klaus, M., & Kennell, J. (1980). *Parent-infant bonding*. St. Louis: Mosby.

Lauterbach, S. (1992). In another world: A phenomenological perspective and discovery of meaning in mothers' experience of death of a wished-for baby. Unpublished dissertation. Teachers College Columbia University, New York, NY.

Lauterbach, S. (1993). In another world: a phenomenological perspective and discovery of meaning in mothers' experience with death of a wished-for baby: Doing phenomenology. In P. Munhall (Ed.), *Nursing research: A qualitative perspective*. New York: National League for Nursing.

Lauterbach, S. (1995). In another world: Essences of mothers' mourning experience. In P. Munhall (Ed.), *In women's experiences* (Vol. 1). New York: National League for Nursing Press.

Lauterbach, S. (2001). Reflections of a mother: Becoming and being-a-mother. In P. Munhall, and V. Fitzsimons (Eds.), *The emergence of family into the 21st century*. Boston: Jones and Bartlett.

Lauterbach, S. (1998). In another world: Five years later. Presentation at Sigma Theta Tau International Biennial Convention, Scientific Sessions, Indianapolis, December 1–6, 1998.

Lauterbach, S. (1999). From time present and time past to time future. Presentation at International Qualitative Methodology Conference, Edmonton, CA. February, 1999.

Lauterbach, S. (1999). From time present and time past to time future: Five year follow up investigation of maternal mourning. Presentation at Sigma Theta Tau International Research Congress, London, June 28, 1999.

Lewis, C. (1976). *A grief observed*. Toronto: Bantam Books. (Originally published in 1961.)

Mason, H. (1970). *Gilgamesh: A verse narrative*. New York: Houghton Mifflin.

Mason, H. (1997). The memory of death. In J. Young-Mason (Ed.), *The patient's voice: Experiences of illness*. Philadelphia: F. A. Davis.

Morse, J. (1989). *Qualitative nursing research: A contemporary dialogue*. Rockville: Aspen.

Munhall, P. (1992). Holding the Mississippi River in place and other implications for qualitative research. *Nursing Outlook*, 40(6), 257–262.

Pike, M., & Armstrong, J. (1980). *A time to mourn: Expressions of grief in nineteenth century America*. Stony Brook: The Museums of Stony Brook.

Prelinger, E., & Parke-Taylor, M. (1996). *The symbolist prints of Edward Munch*. New Haven: Yale University Press.

Untermeyer, L. (1964). *Robert Frost's poems*. New York: Washington Square Press.

U.S. Department of Health and Human Services. (1989). *Monthly Vital Statistics Report*. 39(3).

van Manen, M. (1990). *Researching lived experience*. New York: SUNY Press.

Young-Mason, J. (1997). *The patient's voice: Experiences of illness*. Philadelphia: F. A. Davis.

in the empirical data themselves. Speculative theory, in contrast, originates and develops in the researcher's mind and uses empirical phenomena to confirm or refute theoretical notions.

Grounded theories may be formal or substantive. Formal theories address a more encompassing and conceptual level of inquiry, such as status passage, socialization, stigma, or illness (Morse & Johnson, 1992). Substantive theories are generated for a specific, circumscribed, and empirical area of inquiry, such as quality of life in advanced AIDS (Wilson, Hutchinson, & Holzemer, 1997), recognizing and responding to alcohol problems among lesbians (Hall, 1994), or dying patients (Glaser & Strauss, 1968). Substantive theories, also called middle-range theories, can be used to build formal theories.

Barney Glaser and Anselm Strauss, two sociologists at the University of California, San Francisco School of Nursing, developed the grounded-theory method in the 1960s. Trained at Columbia University and the University of Chicago, respectively, Glaser and Strauss embarked on a study of dying. Their research resulted in two classic books, *Awareness of Dying* (1965) and *Time for Dying* (1968), and a book on method, *The Discovery of Grounded Theory* (1967). Their student Jeanne Quint Benoliel, a nurse sociologist, became the first nurse to do both collaborative and individual work in grounded theory. Her book titled *The Nurse and the Dying Patient* (1967) and her many articles on research and cancer nursing reflect the years she spent with Glaser and Strauss.

Since their seminal book on the method for discovering grounded theory, published in 1967, the work of grounded theory's originators has evolved into differing versions referred to by some as the Glaserian and the Straussian iterations. In attempts to provide more precise and rigorous refinements on the method, Glaser published *Theoretical Sensitivity* in 1978; and, with former student and colleague Juliet Corbin, Strauss published *Basics of Qualitative Research* in 1990. A debate arose concerning which version captured the true essence of the grounded-theory method. Glaser viewed the Strauss and Corbin iteration as a departure from the original that he terms "full conceptual description" and views as "forcing" rather than "emergence" (1992, p. 2). Strauss and Corbin (1990) view their iteration as offering a straightforward, step-by-step procedure for analyzing data by using what they continue to believe is a refinement of the grounded-theory approach. It is beyond the scope of this chapter to elaborate on the debate between grounded theory's originators and the respective merits of each of their refinements and restatements. Instead, this chapter presents the basics of the grounded-theory method in its original form and as we have employed it in our own research over the past two decades. In the context of the perceived departure from the original by Strauss and Corbin, this chapter's methods most likely reflect a present-day Glaserian iteration.

Research methodology is not a haphazard bag of tricks. Rather, each research method is linked to a perspective on a philosophy of science. Symbolic interactionism, described by social psychologists George Herbert Mead (1934) and Herbert Blumer (1969), provides the philosophical foundations for grounded theory and guides the research questions, interview questions, data-collection strategies, and methods of data analysis. Social psychologist George Herbert Mead is credited with teaching the basic tenets of a theory about human conduct, later named symbolic interactionism by Herbert Blumer, one of Mead's students. Mead postulated that human beings come to define themselves through social interaction with others in the forms of social roles, expectations, and learned perspectives. Blumer's concept of self was similar to Mead's, but his emphasis was on the premise that human beings who associate with each other are engaged in processes of interpretive interaction. Social life is expressed through symbols or language, according to Blumer. His ideas are captured in three classic premises (1969): (1) human beings act toward things (objects, institutions, situations, other people) on the basis of the meaning that the things have for them; (2) the meaning of things in life arises out of the social interaction that a person has with others; and (3) meanings are modified through an interpretive process in which people engage when they deal with things that they encounter.

Stern, Allen, and Moxley (1982) summarized these ideas in the following statement:

> Symbolic interactionism posits that humans act and interact on the basis of symbols, which have meaning and value for the actors. Examples of symbols include words for an object rather than the object itself, body language which communicates messages to others with or without words. (p. 203)

How people dress, how they speak, and the artifacts that they use all contribute to their presentation of self to the world. Both the behavioral or interactional level and the symbolic level of behavior are important to symbolic interactions (Chenitz & Swanson, 1986). From these philosophic notions in the social sciences came what Annells (1996, p. 382) characterized as "a new argument in regard to the nature, purpose and development of theory." The specific techniques of a research process based on these underpinnings were developed and refined as stated previously by sociologists Barney Glaser and Anselm Strauss in their book *The Discovery of Grounded Theory* (1967). Grounded-theory research is aimed at understanding how a group of people defines, through social interactions, their reality (Stern et al., 1982). The purpose of this chapter is to present the method of grounded theory that is aimed toward this goal of accurately perceiving and presenting another's world.

The generation of grounded theory relies on the inquiring, analytical minds of its researchers/theorists. Their task is to discover and conceptualize the essence of complex interactional processes. The resulting theory emerges as an entirely new way of understanding the observations from which it is generated. This understanding permits the development of relevant and innovative interventions in the social environment under consideration.

Denzin (1970) makes the point that all data, qualitative or quantitative, serve four basic functions for theory: to initiate new theory and to reformulate, refocus, and clarify existing theory. The grounded-theory method serves each of these functions well. If little is known about a topic and few adequate theories exist to explain or predict a group's behavior, the grounded-theory method is especially useful. The grounded-theory method can also offer a new approach to an old problem (Stern, 1980). Interventions resulting from grounded theory may result in the improvement of patient care (Glaser & Strauss, 1965, 1968; Morse & Johnson, 1992; Wilson, 1989; Strauss & Corbin, 1997) or curriculum enrichment (Glaser & Strauss, 1965, 1968; Hutchinson, 1992). Because of its practical implications, grounded-theory research can be classified as applied research.

VERIFICATIONAL RESEARCH

It is useful for the reader to understand some differences between verificational research and grounded-theory generation. In verificational research, the researcher chooses an existing theory or conceptual framework and formulates hypotheses, which are then tested in a specific population. Verificational research is linear; the researcher delineates a problem, selects a theoretical framework, develops hypotheses, collects data, tests the hypotheses, and reports the results. On a continuum, verificational research is more deductive, whereas grounded-theory research is more inductive. Verificational research moves from a general theory to a specific situation, whereas grounded theorists aim for the development of a more inclusive, general theory through the analysis of specific social phenomena.

It is not unusual for nurses to apply research instruments or theories indiscriminately in a variety of settings. Uncritical reliance on preexisting research instruments precludes even a preliminary exploration of the research problem and results in limited conceptualization, premature closure, and doubtful utility. Likewise, the misapplication or untimely use of theories from other disciplines produces only a superficial fit between theory and reality and does not adequately explain observed variations in behavior.

A researcher using an existing theory approaches the problem from the top down (from theory to practice) rather than from the ground up (from practice to theory). Grounded theory employs an inductive, from-the-ground-up approach using everyday behaviors or organizational patterns to generate a theoretical explanation. Such a theory is inherently relevant to the practice world from which it emerges, whereas the relevance of verificational research varies widely.

NURSING RESEARCH: A HISTORICAL PERSPECTIVE

From its inception, the focus of nursing research has been on theory testing—that is, verificational research. This bias is evidenced in nursing research journals, funded research, research presented at conferences, and the curriculum content in colleges of nursing. The excessive respect automatically accorded to quantitative methods indicates a premature rigor and misplaced emphasis in nursing research. An exclusive focus on verificational research also creates a false dichotomy between theory building and theory testing.

Nursing research in the past two decades has evidenced a trend toward some appreciation of the contributions of qualitative research, yet far too many critics continue to bring the canons of empirical science to bear on qualitative proposals. An increasing number of grounded-theory studies, and studies using other qualitative methods, have been published in leading nursing research journals such as *Nursing Research, Image, Advances in Nursing Science, Research in Nursing and Health,* and *Western Journal of Nursing Research.* Nurse researchers who have expertise in qualitative methods review grant proposals at the National Institute for Nursing Research (NINR) and other National Institutes of Health, and they also review manuscripts for research and clinical journals. These nurse researchers are responsible for altering the research climate so that grounded-theory studies, as well as studies using other qualitative methods, are more likely to be funded and published. The caliber of qualitative studies is rapidly improving, giving credibility to the method and the product.

ASSUMPTIONS OF GROUNDED THEORY

Grounded theories are guided by the assumption that people do, in fact, order and make sense of their environment, although their world may appear disordered or nonsensical to observers. Reality is a social construct, or, as Berger and Luckmann (1967) described it:

> The world of everyday life is not only taken for granted as reality by the ordinary members of society in the subjectively meaningful conduct of their lives. It is a world that originates in their thoughts and actions, and is maintained as real by these. (pp. 19–20)

People sharing common circumstances, such as people living with advanced AIDS or pregnant women addicted to crack cocaine (Kearney, Murphy, Irwin, & Rosenbaum, 1995), experience common meanings and behaviors that constitute the substance of grounded theory. Grounded theorists base their research on the assumption that each such group has in common a specific social psychological problem that is not necessarily articulated. This fundamental problem is resolved by means of social psychological processes. After spending a few months interviewing people with advanced HIV infection, the authors discovered that the study participants' unarticulated problem was one of living with dying. This problem was addressed through a basic social psychological process of salvaging quality of life in which informants progress through stages of first sustaining their previous quality of life, then preserving selected aspects of their quality of life, and ultimately surrendering quality of life concerns to concerns about the quality of their dying (Wilson et al., 1997). In an earlier study of family caregivers for relatives with Alzheimer's dementia, Wilson (1989) discovered that the unarticulated problem for the caregivers was "coping with negative choices" because all the possible alternatives were undesirable. The resulting process, "surviving on the brink," describes a "consciously examined, self-reflective, strategic, and difficult means of surviving on a day-to-day, if not moment-to-moment, basis under conditions of initial uncertainty and unpredictability, pressing demands with a paucity of support, and a dreaded future" (p. 95).

When a previously unarticulated problem and its resultant basic social psychological process are uncovered and conceptualized, one can explain and predict behavioral variation in a group. Glaser and Strauss advocated the search for social psychological problems and processes, viewing them as central to an understanding of people's behavior. Thus, research questions for grounded-theory studies focus on discovering social processes. The research question for the research on late-stage AIDS patients was, "What are the social processes involved in defining quality of life" for people who are living with dying? The research question for Wilson's Alzheimer's cargiving study (1989) was: "What is the process of family caregiving for elderly relatives with Alzheimer's dementia as experienced from the perspective of the caregiver?"

DATA GATHERING

In grounded-theory research, data gathering generally follows the pattern of field research. The field-research method has been traditionally practiced by anthropologists and sociologists, who, in fact, lived in the field. After the researcher/theorist has chosen a group or a setting to study, he or she becomes immersed in that social environment. Initial observations are used to understand and describe the typical social structure and observed patterns of behavior in this environment. Some experts refer to the social structure and behavioral patterns as the conditions in the analysis. Chenitz and Swanson (1986) noted:

> The focus of observation is on the interaction since it is in both verbal and nonverbal behavior that the symbolic meaning of the event is transmitted. The analysis of interaction includes participants' self-definitions and shared meaning. Observation focuses on the interaction in a situation and analysis focuses on the symbolic meaning that is transmitted via action. Analysis focuses on interaction, patterns of interaction, and their consequences. (p. 6)

Observations form the matrix from which the basic social psychological problem and process are derived. Initially, the researcher's observations are tentative and become focused only after a problem and basic social psychological process emerge.

Because grounded-theory research requires interpersonal interaction, the researcher is inevitably part of his or her daily observations. Therefore, one must become aware of personal preconceptions, values, and beliefs and how they might influence the data. Only through self-awareness of mind-set can the researcher begin to search out and understand another's world. Such understanding is critical to field research, as Berger and Kellner (1981) reminded us:

> If such bracketing (of values) is not done, the scientific enterprise collapses, and what the [researcher] then believes to perceive is nothing but a mirror image of his own hopes and fears, wishes, resentments or other psychic needs; what he will then not perceive is anything that can reasonably be called social reality. (p. 52)

A daily journal or diary in which the researcher can express personal feelings and reflections while the study is actively in progress is often helpful in sustaining this heightened level of awareness. Because subjectivity is inevitable in qualitative research, personal notes (PNs) written in the course of data collection and analysis enable researchers to become aware of how their subjectivity may be shaping their inquiries and analyses. Reflexivity in grounded-theory research requires that investigators observe themselves in a focused way and report to their readers how and why methodological decisions were made and how conclusions were drawn. Procedurally these decisions can be tracked by using methodological notes (MNs) and theoretical notes (TNs) as well as PNs in the course of making observational notes (ONs) (Schatzman & Strauss, 1973). Such self-awareness is particularly important when research is conducted from feminist or critical social theory perspectives where certain values inform the goals of the study from the outset.

As a participant in the social scene, the researcher begins to make observations. Interviews, generally informal in nature, augment these observations and serve to clarify the meanings attributed by the participants themselves to a given situation. For example, in the study of people living with advanced AIDS, the researchers noticed that monolingual Hispanic patients were not asked to participate in decisions about their care. We assumed this was an oversight until we asked their nurses about what we had observed. They explained that the patients and their families had chosen to place their care in the hands of God and preferred to relinquish control over health care decisions, focusing instead on their spiritual condition. We had observed nurses honoring and respecting their wishes with respect to involvement in decision making. Had we not asked (informal interview), we might have misunderstood what we saw. Interviews help the researcher understand a problem through the eyes of the participants. The observer searches for their concepts of meaningfulness rather than viewing a situation from his or her own perspective or that of any other group. The human touch—the capacity to empathize with these participants—is essential for this type of research.

Single or multiple formal, semistructured interviews are also foundational for grounded-theory research and, in certain studies, may be the only source of data. For example, in studies of past experiences such as incest, rape, or illegal drug abuse, interviews may be the only way to capture the participants' feelings and experiences. Matters of time and access may preclude fieldwork with people or groups currently experiencing similar situations.

Formal interviews take place at a time and a place acceptable to the participant, generally last from 1 to 2 hours, and may be repeated over time; multiple interviews facilitate the discovery of process and add depth and breadth to the analysis. The researcher aims to generate a theory that accounts for all behavioral variation within a group. To accomplish this goal, a diversity of perspectives is necessary. In the same setting, people who are of varying ages, socioeconomic groups, educational status, and cultures may be interviewed. Participants are chosen purposefully because they are knowledgeable about the area of study.

Interview questions move from the general to the particular; ultimately, they elicit information fundamental to grounded-theory studies, such as dimensions, phases, properties, strategies, consequences, and contexts of behavior. For example, a beginning general question in the quality of life in advanced AIDS study was: "Tell me what it is like to be living with your illness." A specific question much later in the research process was: "What would you like the last week of your life to be like?" The researcher asks different participants different questions as the theory evolves; interview questions are guided by the emerging analysis.

Additional data might include focus groups, patient medical records, hospice policies, newspaper and television coverage, and fictional and anecdotal descriptions that expand and further substantiate the database from which the theory emerges. AIDS patients shared diaries, letters, and poems. One woman shared editorials that she had written for the newspaper. Such diverse "slices of data" (Glaser & Strauss, 1967, p. 66) ensure density and provide multiple perspectives for illuminating social phenomena. Deliberately seeking out different slices of data has been termed data triangulation. Triangulation is a survey and navigation term for the taking of different measurements to ensure accuracy of the location of a point. However as Sandelowski (1995a, p. 569) pointed out, the term triangulation suffers from "definitional drift" and has come to refer to all devices that researcher's combine to grasp the complexity of human phenomena. Dense data, on the other hand, refer to data that contain numerous examples of specific incidents and behaviors. Too few examples yield an inadequate, incomplete, and even inaccurate theory. A dense theory has numerous propositions that are indicative of complexity, and such a theory cannot be easily simplified.

STRATEGIES FOR ENHANCING TRUTH VALUE OF GROUNDED THEORY

Researchers should and do ask the question, Does such an eclectic array of data accurately reflect the milieu, problems, and processes under study? Quantitative researchers frequently describe qualitative research as "too subjective" and inherently unreliable and invalid. They regard the presence of the field researcher as an intrusive factor that inevitably influences the behavior of the participants. They also maintain that, in both informal and formal interviews, these participants may lie, distort the truth, or withhold critical information, in which case the researcher is misled by incomplete, inaccurate, or biased data.

A rebuttal to such assertions would propose that, although a participant observer may initially influence the setting, social and organizational constraints will invariably neutralize this effect. Participants will become more concerned with meeting the demands of their own situations than with paying attention to, pleasing, or playing games with the researcher (Becker, 1970). In hospice care, for example, late-stage AIDS patients must be cared for in spite of the researcher's presence.

The temporal reality of fieldwork provides an additional check on the data. Grounded-theory research is conducted in the field and/or through interviews over a protracted period of time. The researcher continually formulates hypotheses and rejects them if they do not seem accurate. A grounded theorist looks for contradictory data by searching out and investigating unusual circumstances or occurrences. If such data do not fit what has already been found, they will not be discarded but will contribute to the richness of the theory in process. Data are compared and contrasted again and again, thus providing a check on their validity. Distortions or lies generated by the participants will gradually be revealed and the lying itself viewed as additional data. The multiple methods of data collection used in grounded-theory research—direct observation, interviews, focus groups, and documents—prevent undue bias by increasing the wealth of information available to the researcher. It must be remembered, however, that qualitative researchers value "engagement rather than detachment from the things to be known in the interest of truth" (Sandelowski, 1986, p 34).

Can a theory generated in a specific context be generalized to a larger group? Can a theory of people with advanced HIV infection in California be relevant to AIDS patients in another state or geographic area? A substantive theory is said to be valid only for the studied population. A quality theory, however, will inevitably identify a basic process that is also relevant to people in general.

One of the criticisms of grounded theory is that the purposeful sampling strategy does not meet the requirements for statistical generalizability. However, the concern in qualitative research is with analytic generalizability, not statistical generalizability. Analytic generalizability refers to the utility of the concepts/constructs to explain a given situation. To assess analytic generalizability, one might ask: Is the theory with its concepts/constructs useful in understanding particular social phenomena? In the area under study and/or in other related areas? For example, the basic social psychological process of salvaging quality of life was generated in a San Francisco Bay area population, yet HIV-infected persons consulted in other areas acknowledged that it was relevant to them. People may use the process of salvaging quality of life at difficult times in their lives (e.g., divorce, death of a loved one), but it may not be one of their basic processes. Further research into key processes should establish their validity in other areas and with other populations.

Another question might be: Is grounded-theory research replicable? The answer is: Probably not. Grounded-theory process depends on the interaction between the data and the creative processes of the researcher. It is highly unlikely that two people would generate the same theory. Berger and Kellner (1981) noted:

> The social location, the psychological constitution and the cognitive peculiarities of an interpreter are inevitably involved in the act of interpretation, and all of them will affect the interpretation. (p. 48)

The question of replicability is not especially relevant, because the point of theory generation is to offer a new perspective on a given situation and good and useful ways of looking at a certain world. Honigman (1976) pointed out:

> [Data are] not reflections of facts or relationships, existing independently of the observer. In the process of knowing, external facts are sensorially perceived and immediately transformed into conceptualized experience, the observer being an active factor in the creation of knowledge, not a passive recipient or register. (p. 245)

The question of reliability, or the consistency of data over time, is taken care of in part by the duration of field research. Investigators typically spend a substantial amount of time in the field collecting data. Observations, interviews, focus groups, and reviews of medical records for the quality of life in advanced AIDS study required more than 1 year of data collection. Because a theory is modifiable, changes in relevant variables can be accounted for by modifying the emerging theory to incorporate and account for such changes.

Lincoln and Guba (1985) suggested that criteria other than validity and reliability are more in keeping with the nature of qualitative research. These criteria include credibility (truth value), transferability, dependability, auditability (the ability to follow a researcher's decision trail), and confirmability of the findings themselves rather than neutrality of the investigator. In their book *Naturalistic Inquiry*, Lincoln and Guba provided detailed strategies that enhance these qualities. It is important that researchers using grounded-theory methods address the issues of believability and rigor in their work. A more detailed discussion of these matters appears later in this chapter in connection with the evaluation of grounded theories.

DATA RECORDING

The immediate recording of data is critical to the success of grounded-theory generation. Researchers rely on taped interviews and/or written notes combined with their memory before using a word-processing or qualitative analysis program. Field notes are typed double-spaced, with page numbers and identifying headings (place, date, and time). (See Table 7–1.) Wide left and right margins facilitate working with and coding the text. Computer word-processing programs provide specific instructions about formatting the files (ASCII or DOS text files) so that they are retrievable for data analysis. Qualitative research computer software programs such as Ethnograph, QUALOG, and NUD*IST (nonnumerical unstructured data indexing, searching and theory building) (Richards & Richards, 1991) have been developed explicitly for the purpose of interpretive analysis with the use of data that consist of narrative text. The main difference between the programs is that some have been designed for descriptive/interpretive analysis and others, particularly NUD*IST, have been designed for theory building (Tesch, 1990). Such software programs are rapidly replacing the scissors, glue, index cards, and multicolored pens historically used as data-analysis tools by

TABLE 7–1   Field Notes: Support Group Meeting Notes and Notes From Phone Calls

A common saying for bipolar clients that comes up repeatedly in group is: "Life is a Roller Coaster."

Regarding being hospitalized at the Mental Health Center, a common question is, "How can we be expected to act normal in an abnormal environment?" People went on to describe how other patients were hallucinating and acting more "insane" than they felt they were acting. However, in other situations, clients were very open about how crazy they were acting, how out of control they felt.

Nov. 28, 1991. After the group meeting, P called me and said "I'm slightly bubbling . . ." (referring to his state of mania). He proceeded to tell me how he felt other people were doing, which he has done repeatedly because of his role as group facilitator. He takes a great interest in all the clients and talks with many of them throughout the week between meetings. He also talked with me about his problems with alcohol and pot, which he uses to mediate his bipolar symptoms of mania and depression, along with his prescribed meds. He said he thought that C was doing well because of the support of his girlfriend and wishes that he had one. He said that there are many "bipolars" out there "drinking their little hearts away." Meaning bipolar disorders are covered up by booze and drugs.

---

grounded theorists. Computer software programs for descriptive/interpretive analysis perform two basic functions: they allow you to attach codes to segments of text and they will, according to your instructions, search through your data for the segments that were coded in a certain way and retrieve them. NUD*IST has advanced from the simple assembly of coded segments to the development of organizing systems called "indexing." Descriptive/interpretive programs create lists of codes, whereas NUD*IST can place categories and their related text segments into an inverted treelike structure. NUD*IST also lets the researcher create an entire database of memoranda about the original data that can be linked to files and organized.

The type of research setting and the skills of the researcher are variables that influence the choice of the data-recording method. The researcher must be sensitive to the social environment before making this choice. For example, the use of a tape recorder in a hospital that had recently experienced a grand jury investigation inspired an understandable fear on the part of the interviewees. Even the unobtrusive use of pen and paper can be offensive to participants in highly stressful settings, such as disciplinary hearings for hospital employees or at the bedside of a dying AIDS patient. In such cases, dictating notes after the proceedings/interactions is the most reliable method.

THE METHOD OF THEORY GENERATION

The Discovery of a Core Variable or Basic Social Psychological Process

The discovery of a core variable is an essential requirement for a quality grounded theory. Continuous reference to the data, combined with rigorous analytical thinking, will eventually yield such a variable. The researcher undertakes the quest for this essential element of the theory, which illuminates the "main theme" of the actors in the setting and explicates "what is going on in the data" (Glaser, 1978, p. 94). The core variable has six essential characteristics:

1. It recurs frequently in the data.
2. It links the various data together.
3. Because it is central, it explains much of the variation in the data.
4. It has implications for a more general or formal theory.
5. As it becomes more detailed, the theory moves forward.
6. It permits maximum variation in analysis (Strauss, 1987, p. 36).

The core variable becomes the basis for the generation of the theory. The categories, properties, phases, and dimensions of the theory are inextricably related to the core variable. The integration and density of the theory are dependent on the discovery of a significant core variable.

Basic social psychological processes (BSPs) are core variables that illustrate social processes as they continue over time, regardless of varying conditions (Glaser, 1978, 1992). Another kind of core variable is called a basic social structural process (BSSP) (Glaser, 1978, 1992; Glaser & Strauss, 1967). Strauss (1987) advocated searching for both interactional/processural and structural conditions and linking the two together. Most commonly, grounded-theory studies are either one or the other. Most of the grounded-theory studies in nursing focus on the microanalysis of social processes (see Chapter 8 and Wilson, 1989) and do not address the relevant macroanalysis of structural processes. However, with further data collection and analysis, relevant structural processes can be discovered and woven into the theory. Fagerhaugh and Strauss (1977), in *The Politics of Pain Management*, provided a good example of the interrelation of social structural and social psychological processes. They analyzed the organizational settings in which pain occurs, along with staff–patient interaction concerning pain.

In her Alzheimer's caregiving study, Wilson (1989) discovered surviving on the brink as a BSP that was a response to the problem of coping with negative choices. This process unfolds in stages, and these stages, with the individual properties and conditions, form the structure of the theory. Surviving on the brink may not be the only BSP of theoretical importance in family caregiving for Alzheimer's dementia patients, but it explains much of the behavioral variation in the data.

Once a BSP or BSSP emerges, the researcher selectively codes only those data that relate to it (coding is considered in the next section). Thus, the BSP becomes a guide for further data collection and analysis. With selective coding, many codes emerge either as separate categories or as conditions, strategies, or phases of categories. For example, "taking it on technically" was initially a substantive code; on further analysis, it became a first stage in surviving on the brink.

BSPs evidenced in the social organization of a particular group may be found in other groups and settings. Surviving on the brink as a process for coping with negative choices is not specific to Alzheimer's dementia family caregiving but may also be discovered in other interactional situations such as caring for a severely developmentally disabled child. As a basic social process, it is independent of the structural unit in which it was discovered and may explain other situations characterized by conditions similar to those under which it was discovered.

Several steps precede the identification of the BSP. These steps include different levels of coding, memoing, theoretical sampling, and sorting. (Table 7–2 helps set the theory generation process into a linear pattern.)

Coding

The process of doing grounded theory is both systematic and intense (Strauss, 1987) because it requires that the researcher simultaneously collect, code, and analyze the data, beginning with the first interview and/or the first day in the field. The method is circular, allowing the researcher to change focus and pursue leads revealed by the ongoing data analysis. A month of observation and informal interviews in a

TABLE 7–2 GROUNDED THEORY

PROCESS	PRODUCT
Primary literature review	Discovery of sensitizing concepts, gaps in knowledge
Data collection: interviews, observations, documents	Masses of narrative data
Coding: coding paradigm, axial coding, constant comparative method	Level 1 codes—called in vivo or substantive
	Level II codes—called categories
	Level III codes—called theoretical constructs
Memoing	Theoretical and methodological ideas
Theoretical sampling	Dense data that lead to the illumination and expansion of theoretical constructs
Sorting	Basic social psychological problem and/or process (BSP)—a central theme and/or
	Basic social structural process (BSSP)—a central theme
Selective coding based on BSP, BSSP	Theory delimited to a few theoretical constructs, their categories, and properties
Saturation of codes, categories, and constructs	A dense, parsimonious theory covering behavioral variation; a sense of closure
Secondary literature review	Discovery of literature that supports, illuminates, or extends proposed theory
Writing the theory	A piece of publishable research

medical intensive care unit (MICU) yielded little relevant information on nonprofessional behavior, the focus of a prior study conducted by Hutchinson, first author of this chapter.

"If I (Hutchinson) had not been reading and questioning my data regularly, I would have lost my focus by not recognizing the paucity of relevant information in my field notes. I concluded that, because I lacked a frame of reference with which to identify nonprofessional behavior, it was difficult to see what was going on. Consequently, I decided to move to a psychiatric unit, where I shared common meanings and was known to some of the nurses. In this setting, it was easier for me to ask direct questions about nonprofessional behavior and to perceive such behavior when it took place. I began to identify categories of nonprofessional behavior and planned to explore their relevance in the MICU. For example, if rough and insensitive treatment of a patient on a psychiatric unit is nonprofessional, are there similar (or different) kinds of nonprofessional behaviors in an MICU? Preliminary experiences from the psychiatric unit observations guided my focus into other, less familiar areas (personal/methodological note)."

Level I coding begins with words that describe the action in the setting. Such codes are the in vivo or substantive codes and may be the exact words that the actors use. As such, they tend to be catchy and meaningful. Examples of early substantive coding in the quality of life in advanced AIDS research were "feeling alone with my disease," "giving AIDS a name and a face," "feeling disrespected," "giving up the fight," "tuning into my body," and so on (Wilson et al., 1997). Substantive coding based only on the language in the data prevents the researcher from imposing preconceived impressions.

Open coding refers to the coding of each sentence and each incident into as many codes as possible, to ensure full theoretical coverage. For example, an incident may be coded as both "monitoring" and "being vigilant." All data must be coded or the emerging theory will not fit the data and explain behavioral variations. For example, if the advanced AIDS patients spend much time complaining about fighting for treatment, these data must be coded as well as the data that indicate how they experience and define their quality of life.

Level I codes break the data into small pieces; later, level II and level III codes elevate the data to more abstract levels. Level II codes can also be called "categories" and may result from the condensing of level I codes; that is, some level I codes may be subsumed in a larger category. In the process, some data may be discarded if they seem irrelevant. Decisions about categories are made by asking the following questions of the data: What does this incident indicate? Each incident is then compared with other incidents. What category would include these similar incidents? Finally, the emerging categories are compared with each other to ensure that they are mutually exclusive and cover the behavioral variations.

Level III codes, or theoretical constructs, are derived from a combination of academic and clinical knowledge. The constructs contribute theoretical meaning and scope to the theory (Glaser, 1978, 1992). Salvaging quality of life is a theoretical construct from the AIDS study, whereas developing personal sovereignty is the main theoretical construct from Redfern-Vance and Hutchinson's (1995) study of the social psychological processes of women who begin to change their behavior after contracting sexually transmitted diseases. These theoretical codes may or may not be BSPs, depending on the amount of behavioral variation for which they account. Theoretical constructs conceptualize the relation among the three levels of codes, "weaving the fractured data back together again" (Glaser, 1978 p. 116). This comprehensive pattern is, in fact, the theory. The theoretical constructs are grounded in substantive or categorical codes, precluding the possibility of unfounded, abstract theorizing.

Families of Theoretical Codes

Grounded theorists use a repertoire of theoretical coding families that suggest the posing of certain questions during coding. The questions enable the researcher to grasp the data more easily and to establish theoretical codes for the empirical indicators. The aim is to saturate the properties of the concept/construct. Some questions that Wilson asked about her data involved "the six Cs" coding family: causes, contexts, contingencies, consequences, covariances, and conditions. For example, what is the cause of AIDS patients' decision to self-deliver? Wilson learned that patients who suffered the loss of their dignity around basic bodily functions considered self-deliverance, or suicide. Patients who felt "stalked by death" considered self-deliverance. Patients who resolved their own spiritual issues and came to believe that their death was part of a grander scheme of things also considered self-deliverance. The context refers to the environment or setting in which the behavior occurs. Some patients chose to share their decision with others who could bear witness to their experience. Others contemplated the decision in private. Patients who believed their nurses and/or family members would honor their decision and not judge them felt that their social environment was safe to discuss their plan for self-deliverance out loud.

Other questions include: What is this behavior contingent on? For example, "redeeming quality of life," the final stage in the salvaging process was contingent on making the transition from fighting the disease to surrendering to their impending death. What are the consequences (for patients, families, nurses, physicians) of deciding to self-deliver? Patients who decide to self-deliver prematurely are unable to preserve and sustain selected aspects of their quality of life despite living with their illness. Family members may be unable to achieve closure with their relative and may experience prolonged guilt and grief reactions. Finally, health professionals may become embroiled in ethical if not legal issues.

Covariances generally have not proved relevant to nursing studies. Conditions or qualifiers (Glaser, 1978,1992) refer to those factors essential for the actualization of the social psychological processes under study. For example, nurses who bend the rules for the sake of their patients (Hutchinson, 1990) have knowledge, an ideology, and experience. They have knowledge about the patient's disease process, about the rules that the nurse bends, and about how the patient will respond to the rule bending. They share an ideology about patient care that involves patient advocacy; their experience helps them to assess the patient adequately and to anticipate the consequences for the patient when the rules are bent. All these conditions are prerequisite for their knowing how and when to bend the rules to benefit the patient.

Other coding families include the degree family, the dimension family (for an example of dimensional analysis, see Bowers, 1987), the type family, the strategy family, the cutting point family, and so on (Glaser, 1978,1992). The use of these families of codes enhances theoretical sensitivity. Glaser (1978) pointed out that every study is "of" one of these codes; the researcher must recognize which one "infuses the study theoretically while broadening its perspective" (p. 77).

In recent work published two decades after the original discovery of grounded theory, Strauss (1987) and Strauss and Corbin (1990) advocated the use of a coding paradigm (specific families of codes that encourage the development not only of categories but also of subcategories that are present in the context). The coding paradigm involves asking pertinent questions about each category in order to assess conditions, interactions, strategies/tactics, and consequences. Such questions provide a structured way to analyze the data. Strauss (1987) believed that, "without inclusion of the paradigm items, coding is not coding" (p. 28).

It is important to think of the codes as provisional and not to censor ideas during the initial open-coding phase. Further analysis and delineation of codes will yield codes that fit the data. Remaining open to theoretical ideas is essential to generating theory that is abstract enough to be interpretive rather than merely descriptive.

Axial coding refers to the use of paradigm coding around one category or concept at a time. The analysis revolves around the axis of the category and is necessary to ensure dense data. For example, coveting time was a category in the study of quality of life in advanced AIDS. When looking at coveting time as a code, Wilson asked: "What are the conditions for coveting time? What are the strategies/tactics for coveting time? What are the consequences of coveting time?" This intense focus on each category helps to show the relation among data, such as what specific conditions fit with what specific interactions, strategies, and consequences (Strauss, 1987, p. 78). Strauss also emphasized the need to "analyze the data minutely" (1987, p. 31). Line-by-line coding with the coding paradigm and the use of axial coding with each category facilitate the generation of a dense theory that covers all behavioral variation.

Questions asked during coding should emphasize both interaction and structure, in an effort to link one with the other. For example, when examining medication adherence among HIV-infected persons, the researcher should ask what effect the economic resources or living situation structure has on their adherence or nonadherence. If I have discovered a social structural process that is relevant, I might question how nurse–patient interaction affects the structural process.

As mentioned earlier, the fundamental aim of coding is to discover a BSP and its related properties. Selective coding refers to coding that aims to generate the BSP and all the codes that relate to it. The researcher searches for the BSP, the conditions of the BSP, the phases of the BSP, the consequences of the BSP, and so on. Certain questions asked of the data, while coding, aid the generation process:

1. What is going on in the data?
2. What are these data a study of?
3. What is the basic social psychological problem with which these people must deal?
4. What basic social psychological process helps them cope with the problem and how does it work?

These questions force the researcher to transcend the descriptive nature of the data and to think in theoretical terms.

Good theories are both dense and parsimonious. A parsimonious theory—one that is comprehensive without being unwieldy—consists of a few theoretical codes, a greater number of categorical codes, and a majority of in vivo or substantive codes. The researcher returns to the field and interviews repeatedly throughout the research process; coding takes place until the final draft of the paper is begun.

Constant Comparative Method

The constant comparative method is the fundamental method of data analysis in grounded-theory generation. The aim of this method is the generation of theoretical constructs that, along with substantive codes and categories and their properties, form a theory that encompasses and explains as much behavioral variation as possible. The proposed theory is molecular in structure rather than causal or linear.

While coding and analyzing the data, the researcher looks for patterns. He or she compares incident with incident, incident with category, and, finally, category with category or construct with construct. Using this method, the analyst distinguishes similarities and differences of incidents. By a comparison of similar incidents, the basic properties of a category or construct are defined; certain differences between incidents establish boundaries; relations among categories are gradually clarified. Comparative analysis forces the researcher to expand or "tease out" the emerging category/construct by searching for its structure, temporality, cause, context, dimensions, consequences, and relation to other categories. An in-depth examination of these properties is likely to yield a dense theory that also accounts for behavioral variation.

In addition to incidents, the researcher compares the behavior patterns of different groups within the substantive area. Eventually, categories and their related properties emerge. This process of categorization yields groups of categories/constructs that encompass smaller categories. Thus, major processes or clusters are revealed. Subgroup comparisons maximize differences and variation and thus yield a more dense theory. In the AIDS research, Wilson compared stories of patients with those of significant others, patients with experienced nurse clinicians in AIDS care, Hispanic patients with Anglo patients, and patients with different risk factors (intravenous drug users versus those who had been infected through sexual contact). Wilson found, for example, that Hispanic patients had difficulty with disclosure of their conditions to family members and friends who were present as their source of social support. A number of the gay white men interviewed had internalized their illness and believed that it was part of their "work" to educate others about it, thus speaking openly and even in public about dying of AIDS. Such comparisons contributed substantially to the richness of the theory.

Memoing

To generate a quality theory, the descriptions of empirical events must be elevated to a theoretical level. Memoing is a critical part of this process. On index cards, in a journal, or on a computer, the researcher quickly and spontaneously records his or her ideas to capture the initially elusive and shifting connections between the data. Memos on memos accumulate. Memos may be long or short and can be written without concern for style or formal punctuation. The emphasis is on capturing ideas. One ends up with hundreds of memos documenting the thinking process. The ideas are retrievable because the code or codes that it describes identify each memo. With the use of certain computer software such as NUD*IST, memos can be shifted around to check the relation with other codes. Irrelevant codes can be discarded and core codes retained. The emerging theory is, therefore, always modifiable.

While memoing, the researcher asks what relation one code has to another. Are they separate codes? Is one code a property or a phase in another? Is one event the cause of another or the consequence? What are the conditions that influence the codes? The intent of the questioning is to freely develop codes that can be sorted and compared again and again. Through repetitive questioning, the theory evolves. The basic social psychological process emerges, and its properties become integrated. The rapid generation of linkages occurs throughout the research process. Even during the writing phase, new insights may occur.

During the memoing phase, the thinking process is both inductive and deductive. One conceptualizes (inductive) when coding and memoing and then assesses (deductive) how the concepts fit together. Repetitive examination of the data, combined with theoretical sensitivity, aids both processes.

Memoing is a regular and critical part of the grounded-theory process, beginning with data analysis after the first interview, focus group, or observation. Strauss (1987) described changes in memoing during the analytic process that yield different types of memos. Among them are: initial, orienting memos; preliminary memos; memo sparks; memos that open attacks on new phenomena; memos on new categories; initial discovery memos; memos distinguishing between two or more categories; memos extending the implications of a borrowed concept (pp. 138, 139). Other memos or notes (Schatzman & Strauss, 1973) may include methodological memos that focus on strategies for data collecting and personal memos that illuminate the researcher's introspective process. In a methodological memo that Wilson wrote for the quality of life in AIDS study, she reminded herself to ask expert nurse clinicians in focus groups whether they observed differences in the meaning of quality of life in patients from different cultures. In a personal memo in the same study, she documented her varied and changing feelings about specific people and their situations and compared and contrasted them with feelings of both family members and professional nurse health care providers. Memos of all types leave an audit trail (Koch, 1994; Rodgers & Cowles, 1993) for the analytic decisions and may provide data for presentations, publications, and/or additional research.

Theoretical Sampling

Experimental research compares predetermined groups on specified variables. The groups are selected and presumed to be similar or matched on all points except one, the treatment variable. In grounded theory, sampling decisions are made purposively to advance the theory during the entire research process. One gathers information from any group that may be a meaningful source of relevant data. Relevance is determined by the requirements for generating, delimiting, and saturating the theoretical codes. Saturation of codes refers to their completeness; a code is saturated if the researcher can use the data to answer questions regarding the cause, context, consequences, and so on, of the particular code. One can see how the code fits in the theory. One engages in a constant dialogue with the data to establish direction for further sampling. For example, studying quality of life in advanced AIDS patients could lead us to study quality of life in patients with breast cancer or quality of life in patients with schizophrenia. If we wanted to develop a formal theory of quality of life with chronic illness, we would study these and other groups. The substantive theory of salvaging quality of life in advanced AIDS was generated, in contrast, by sampling the subgroups (patients, family members/significant others, expert nurses) with knowledge about that particular experience.

Diversity in sampling ensures extensive data that cover the wide ranges of behavior in varied situations. Hutchinson's study of bipolar patients (Hutchinson, 1993) revealed that they required different amounts of time to accept (to "own") their diagnosis and illness. Hutchinson began to collect more data from people with bipolar disorder to assess the conditions that influenced the different acceptance rates. A patient's symptoms, the time of diagnosis, the method of treatment, and personal illness history all affect when and how the patient owns his or her diagnosis. Theoretical sampling allows the significant variables to become apparent through the expansion and elaboration of the developing codes.

Sorting

Salvaging quality of life as a core variable (and BSP) in the late-stage AIDS research was discovered during the memo-sorting phase. Once codes are plentiful and memos are accumulating rapidly, sorting begins. One first decides on a core variable that explains most of the behavioral variation in the data. This BSP offers focus and direction to the sorting process. One then attempts to discover the relation of the different levels of codes to the BSP. Gradually, an outline emerges from the sorted memos that provides the structure for writing the theory. While sorting to produce an outline, one may draw and redraw integrative diagrams (see Figure 7–1), including

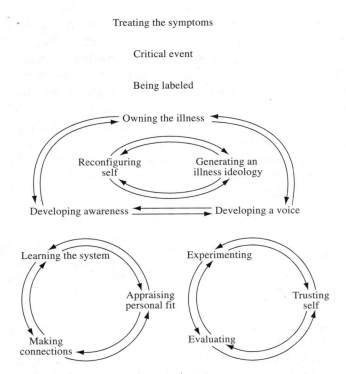

Figure 7–1 The quest for equanimity: theoretical codes for bipolar research.

logic diagrams that illuminate categories and their relations. [See also Strauss (1987) and Strauss & Corbin (1990) for more detail about diagrams.] These diagrams are very helpful in setting forth the developing theory.

The object of the sorting is to put the fractured data (Glaser, 1978, 1992) together into a coherent and workable whole. Sorting the memos facilitates the generation of a theoretical outline that integrates the main ideas. The mechanics of sorting require the researcher to separate all memos by code, delineating the causes, conditions, contexts, strategies, and dimensions of his or her theoretical constructs. As the codes become saturated, their boundaries are defined. The relation among these individual codes and their collective relation to the basic social psychological process become the framework of the theory. The researcher strives for a "parsimonious set of integrated concepts" (Glaser, 1978, p. 120).

Saturation

Saturation refers to the completeness of all levels of codes when no new conceptual information is available to indicate the need for new codes or the expansion of existing ones. Although new descriptive data may be added, the information will not be useful unless the theoretical codes need to be altered. When all the data fit into the established categories, interactional and organizational patterns are visible, behavioral variation is described, and behavior can be predicted. The researcher, by repeatedly checking and asking questions of the data, ultimately achieves a sense of closure.

Review of the Literature

In both verificational research—for example, hypotheses-testing studies—and grounded-theory studies, a literature review is written before data collection and analysis. Existing theoretical and methodological literature is used to build a case or rationale for the proposed research. Because the literature used in grounded-theory studies can provide only sensitizing concepts and an awareness of the gaps in knowledge, grounded theorists turn to an entirely new body of literature after generating their theories. This second literature review links extant research and theory with the concepts, constructs, and properties of the new theory. Literature that illuminates, supports, or extends the proposed theory is interwoven with the empirical data. Through its correspondence with the real world, literature establishes an essential connection between theory and reality.

WRITING THE THEORY

Smith and Pohland (1976) wrote:

> Really knowing not only means having it conceptualized, but also being able to describe its day-to-day working as well as, if not better than, the man who is actually living and working in the setting. (p. 269)

After the theoretical sorting and saturation, the researcher begins writing the conceptualization of the substantive theory, with the BSP as its central focus. The phases of the BSP (or any other theoretical coding family) serve as subheadings for the explanation of the categories. At this point, as Glaser (1978) wrote, the theory "freezes the on-going for the moment" in a "fixed conceptual description" (p. 129).

Both during and after the initial writing, the researcher continues to write memos and to reconceptualize parts of the theory. Through constant dialogue with the data, the theory emerges, complete with properties, conditions, strategies, and consequences. During the reworking of the draft, relevant literature is incorporated into the theory.

TEMPORAL CONSIDERATIONS

The grounded-theory method requires a time orientation that differs from that of traditional verificational research. Because the time frame of verificational research is linear, the researcher can generally estimate the time required to accomplish each phase of the research process. The generation of grounded theory is inherently circular in nature with data collection and analysis taking place concurrently. Consequently, it is difficult to estimate a specific amount of time for full conceptualization to occur.

During the process of grounded-theory generation, the researcher experiences alternating periods of confusion and enlightenment. Recognizing this fact enables the researcher to realistically approach this difficult but exciting method of research.

THE EVALUATION OF GROUNDED THEORIES

Because the methods and aims of grounded-theory research are substantially different from those of verificational research, the criteria for evaluation differ accordingly. In *The Discovery of Grounded Theory* (Glaser & Strauss, 1967) and *Basics of Qualitative Research* (Strauss & Corbin, 1990), the authors listed the significant criteria for evaluation. A quality grounded theory has codes that fit the data and the practice area from which it is derived. Data fall into place naturally; the researcher does not force them into a code where there is only a marginal fit. Readers of quality theories can actually sense or feel this fit. A quality theory must work; it will explain the major behavioral and interactional variations of the substantive area. Such a theory can predict what will happen under certain conditions or given certain variables. A quality theory must possess relevance related to the core variable and its ability to explain the ongoing social processes in the action scene. If the actors in the setting immediately recognize the researcher's constructs

("Wow, that's it!"), he or she can be confident that the theory possesses relevance or "grab." Relevance is dependent on the researcher's theoretical sensitivity in enabling the BSP to emerge from the data without imposing his or her own preconceived notions or ideas.

Social life is not static, and a quality theory must be able to capture its constantly fluctuating nature. A theory must be modifiable; for example, if values or related variables differ, a theory can be modified to fit the setting. As new data surface, new categories must be constructed or current categories must be modified to incorporate them. Flexibility is required for theoretical relevance.

Density and integration are additional criteria for assessing the quality of a theory. A quality theory is dense: it possesses a few key theoretical constructs and a substantial number of properties and categories. Good integration ensures that the propositions are systematically related to one another into a tight theoretical framework (Glaser & Strauss, 1968).

The evaluation criteria discussed in the preceding paragraphs were originally termed fit, understanding (grab), generality, and control by grounded theory's originators Glaser and Strauss in 1967 (pp. 237–250). Some authorities who are attempting to raise the level of discourse about what grounded theory ought to be have additionally changed the terminology for evaluating internal validity to credibility, external validity to fittingness across contexts, reliability to auditability, and objectivity to confirmability (Lincoln & Guba, 1985). Others have added criteria including the coherence and clarity of the theory's structure and its generalizability and pragmatic utility (Morse, 1997). Still others have examined issues around grounded theory's ability to explain and the credibility of its proffered explanations (Miller & Fredericks, 1999).

Although such discussions, analyses and epistemological debates are critically important to sustain the viability of grounded theory as a prominent methodology for human science research, the authors of the present chapter conclude that the overarching criteria for judging a grounded theory can be summarized in the following two statements: (1) a quality theory meets all the preceding criteria, providing an explanation of relevant social processes that describe the social psychological interaction in a given setting or group; and (2) by virtue of their abstract nature, these processes cover the major behavioral variations of the participating people.

In their work, Strauss and Corbin (1990, p. 253) proposed the following questions as guidelines or a specific evaluative framework for judging the adequacy of the grounded-theory research process as reported in a research presentation or publication:

1. How was the original sample selected? On what grounds?
2. What major categories emerged?
3. What were some of the events, incidents, and actions that pointed to some of these major categories?
4. On the basis of what categories did theoretical sampling proceed? How did theoretical sampling guide the data collection? How representative are the categories?
5. What were some of the hypotheses pertaining to conceptual relations among categories, and on what grounds were they formulated and tested?
6. Were there instances when hypotheses did not hold up against what was actually seen? How were these discrepancies accounted for? How did they affect the hypotheses?
7. How and why was the core category selected? Was it sudden or gradual, difficult or easy?

This set of seven questions can also provide an outline for conducting an audit trail (Koch, 1994; Rodgers & Cowles, 1993) by an independent researcher who is invited to scrutinize the decision trail in a piece of research and support a grounded-theory study's auditability.

The following additional questions (Strauss & Corbin, 1990, pp. 254–257) suggest criteria concerning the empirical grounding of the study:

1. Are concepts generated?
2. Are the concepts systematically related?
3. Are there many conceptual linkages and are the categories well developed? Do they have conceptual density?
4. Is much variation built into the theory?
5. Are the broader conditions that affect the phenomenon under study built into its explanation?
6. Has process been taken into account?
7. Do the theoretical findings seem significant? To what extent?

The next section of this chapter identifies the pitfalls that can detract from the integrity of grounded-theory research. In view of the trend among nursing students, faculty, and clinicians to jump on the grounded-theory bandwagon because they feel a kinship with its "no numbers" approach to scientific research and emphasis on human experience, criteria to evaluate grounded-theory research are of paramount importance to the consumer and investigator (Wilson & Hutchinson, 1996).

THE PITFALLS OF GROUNDED-THEORY RESEARCH

Certain pitfalls, which strongly influence the quality of the proposed theory, may confront a budding grounded theorist. Most pitfalls can be avoided with an awareness of them and their implications for risking the quality of the research.

Premature closure will cause the theory to be incomplete, to lack density, and to inadequately cover the behavioral variations. If a researcher is under time constraints, premature closure may be necessary. (The study of salvaging quality of life in advanced AIDS had to be completed within the 2-year funding period.) The core variable and major phases were clear, but some of the theoretical codes and categories, as well as the memoing and sorting, were incomplete, particularly with regard to the monolingual Hispanic subgroup. The researcher then has the choice of completing the study at a later time or settling for a partial theory. Premature closure often occurs with theses and dissertations under the time constraints and reporting requirements of extramural funding.

The failure of a BSP or core variable to surface is a significant pitfall. Because a BSP is the conceptual basis of a grounded theory, there simply is no theory without it. The question then becomes, How can the study be salvaged? However tempting the remedy, a core variable cannot be imposed on the data. Reporting the research as a descriptive study or a case study may be a worthwhile endeavor. If key concepts have emerged, they can be used as headings for the presentation of the research. Although the study terminates at a rich conceptual descriptive rather than an interpretive level, it may offer a foundation for future theory-building research.

A third potential pitfall concerns the researcher personally. The choice of research question is a highly personal decision. The method that one chooses to solve the problem also is a matter of personal preference. A researcher who thinks predominantly in the deductive mode has more difficulty generating a grounded theory than does one who is skilled in abstract and inductive thinking. The abstract thinker may have less interest in and more difficulty doing verificational research. The choice of method should be made carefully. Good grounded theories have great appeal and may seduce the unaware into underestimating their challenges. To generate a grounded theory, one must be a conceptual thinker and able to discover ideas in data.

Recognition of the requirements for generating a quality theory should be of use to researchers considering the grounded-theory method. The grounded-theory process is always rigorous and, at many stages, exciting. The lengthy time commitment and the necessity for original thinking, however, are equally essential parts of the process. The generation of a quality theory makes this investment worthwhile for many of us.

GROUNDED THEORY, POSTMODERNISMS, CRITICAL SOCIAL THEORY, AND FEMINISMS

For theories to be relevant, they must offer direction for the context of our rapidly changing sociopolitical and economic environment—what is called, by some, the postmodern condition. Postmodernism is "a widely ranging cultural movement which adopts a skeptical attitude toward many of the principles and assumptions that have underpinned Western thought and social life for the past few centuries" (Sim, 1998, p. 339). According to Sim, the central tenet of postmodernism is the notion that there is no firm truth on which to base any philosophical principles or research methodologies. Any ideology that is presented as a truth is open to challenge. People are left to construct meaning in specific situations. Instead of emphasizing central tendencies, the notion of ever-changing, complex, unfolding differences is emphasized in postmodernist thinking. Truth is thus multiple, shifting, and a reflection of the social construction of reality (Anderson, 1998). Because of this fluidity, "reality" cannot be represented (Hall, 1999). These ideas contrast with Glaser's assumption that there is a real truth that is to be discovered in the data. Yet, rather than conclude that grounded theory is not a relevant methodology in postmodern thought based on Glaser's "critical realist view" (Annells, 1996), it is more useful to consider how grounded theory can and does contribute to grasping the multiple, evolving meanings that characterize modern social life in the new millenium.

Critical social theory and feminism are contemporary philosophical movements that address the postmodern condition and challenge grounded theory to respect the subjective and social construction of reality. Feminist assumptions, goals, and values emphasize the world of women in a male-dominated society and the lived experience and history as the basis for knowing. Im and Meleis (1999) summarize critical social theory:

Critical social theory holds that all research and theory are sociopolitical constructions, that human societies are inherently
oppressive, and that all interpretations, including mythical, religious, and scientific . . . are open to criticism. (p. 15)

Clearly, feminist and critical social theory perspectives posit that
philosophical viewpoints should guide and direct theory development, research strategies, and the uses to which knowledge is put.
Many of the ways in which grounded theories have been used in nursing reflect exactly such a position (Benoliel, 1996; Liehr & Smith, 1999).

GROUNDED THEORY'S RELEVANCE FOR NURSING

Grounded theory has established itself firmly over the past three
decades as relevant to the evolution of nursing science. Grounded theory offers systematic, legitimate methods to study the richness and diversity of human experience, interaction, and meanings and to generate
relevant, plausible theory that can be used to understand the contextual
reality of problems and processes. Nurses have used grounded theory
to develop assessment guides. For example, Morse, Hutchinson, and
Penrod (1998) described the method that they used to develop patient
assessment guides from grounded theories of bipolar disorders and
hope. Wilson, Hutchinson, and Holzemer (1997) developed and then
validated a quality of life in AIDS assessment scale based on their salvaging theory. Grounded theory has been used to apprehend the nature
of nursing's phenomena of concern. In 1991, Morse and Johnson published *The Illness Experience: Dimensions of Suffering*. Sandelowski (1995b) reported a formal theory of the transition to parenthood by infertile couples, and Kearney (1998) used the constant comparative method to
develop a formal theory of women's recovery from addiction. DeJoseph
and colleagues (DeJoseph, Norbeck, Smith, & Miller, 1996) reported on
a social support intervention with lower-income, socially isolated African
American women that was derived from qualitative research. In short,
grounded theory can help nurses better understand their own world—
people in changing, complex social situations.

In an era of quality assurance and outcomes-oriented care, grounded-
theory methods also can be used for evaluation of any aspect of
our work. Instead of the exclusive use of the traditional statistical methods for evaluation, grounded theory offers us a qualitative approach to

evaluation that takes into account people's sociocultural contexts and the meaning of their experience. Sandelowski (1996) takes qualitative evaluation research into the realm of hard science by suggesting that "qualitative methods can be used to enhance the significance and harness the benefits of clinical trials, and to further describe and explain subject variation on outcome variables" (pp. 359–64).

Nurse scientists have begun to develop progressive programs of qualitative research conceived not in linear, quantitative, and financial terms but in more expansive ones. Programs of research can be organized around real-world clinical problems such as recovery after certain illnesses, around conceptual problems such as suffering, comfort, or caring, around substantive domains such as Alzheimer's dementia, and even around methodological domains where the scientist aims to refine research methodology (Sandelowski,1997). "It is up to us," as Goldman (1980) urged, "to accept the challenge of strange and difficult ideas and to abandon the complacency of converting all that is novel into cliches of the familiar" (p. 14).

REFERENCES

Anderson, T. (1998). Postmodern person. *Noetic Sciences Review, 45*, 28–33.

Annells, M. (1996). Grounded theory method: Philosophical perspectives, paradigm of inquiry, and postmodernism. *Qualitative Health Research, 6*, 379–393.

Becker, H. (1970). *Sociological work*. Chicago: Aldine.

Benoliel, J. Q. (1967). *The nurse and the dying patient*. New York: Macmillan.

Benoliel, J. Q. (1996). Grounded theory and nursing knowledge. *Qualitative Health Research, 6*, 406–428.

Berger, P., & Kellner, H. (1981). *Sociology reinterpreted*. New York: Anchor Books.

Berger, P., & Luckmann, C. (1967). *The social construction of reality*. New York: Anchor Books.

Blumer, H. (1969). *Symbolic interactionism: Perspective and method*. Englewood Cliffs, NJ: Prentice-Hall.

Bowers, B. (1987). Intergenerational caregiving: Adult caregivers and their aging parents. *Advances in Nursing Science, 9*(2), 20–31.

Chenitz, C., & Swanson, J. (1986). *From practice to grounded theory*. Menlo Park, CA: Addison-Wesley.

DeJoseph, J., Norbeck, J., Smith, R., & Miller, S. (1996). The development of a social support intervention among African American women. *Qualitative Health Research, 6*, 283–297.

Denzin, N. (1970). *The research act: A theoretical introduction to sociological methods.* Chicago: Aldine.

Fagerhough, S., & Strauss, A. (1977). *The politics of pain management: Staff-patient interaction.* Menlo Park, CA: Addison-Wesley.

Glaser, B. (1978). *Theoretical sensitivity.* Mill Valley, CA: Sociology Press.

Glaser, B. (1992). *Basics of grounded theory analysis: emergence vs. forcing.* Mill Valley, CA: Sociology Press.

Glaser, B., & Strauss, A. (1965). *Awareness of dying.* Chicago: Aldine.

Glaser, B., & Strauss, A. (1967). *The discovery of grounded theory.* Chicago: Aldine.

Glaser, B., & Strauss, A. (1968). *Time for dying.* Chicago: Aldine.

Goldman, I. (1980). Boas on the Kwakiutl: The ethnographic tradition. *Sara Lawrence College—Essays from the Faculty,* 3(4), 5–23.

Hall, J. (1994). How lesbians recognize and respond to alcohol problems: A theoretical model of problematization. *Advances in Nursing Science,* 16(3), 46–63.

Hall, J. (1999). Marginalization revisited: Critical, postmodern, and liberation perspectives. *Advances in Nursing Science,* 22(2), 88–102.

Honigman, J. (1976). The personal approach in cultural anthropological research. *Current Anthropology,* 17, 243–261.

Hutchinson, S. (1990). Responsible subversion: A study of rule bending among nurses. *Scholarly Inquiry for Nursing Practice,* 4, 3–17.

Hutchinson, S. (1992). Nurses who violate the Nurse Practice Act: Transformation of professional identity. *Image: The Journal of Nursing Scholarship,* 24(2), 133–139.

Hutchinson, S. (1993). People with bipolar disorders quest for equanimity: Doing grounded theory. In P. Munhall & C. Oiler Boyd (Eds.), *Nursing research: A qualitative perspective* (2nd ed., pp. 213–236). New York: National League for Nursing.

Im, E., & Meleis, A. (1999). Situation-specific theories: Philosophical roots, properties, and approach. *Advances in Nursing Science,* 22(2), 11–24.

Kearney, M. (1998). Ready to wear: Doing grounded formal theory. *Research in Nursing & Health,* 21(2), 179–186.

Kearney, M., Murphy, S., Irwin, K., & Rosenbaum, M. (1995). Salvaging self: A grounded theory of pregnancy on crack cocaine. *Nursing Research,* 44 (4), 208–213.

Koch, T.(1994). Establishing rigour in qualitative research: The decision trail. *Journal of Advanced Nursing,* 19, 976–986.

Liehr, P., & Smith, M. J. (1999). Middle range theory: Spinning research and practice to create knowledge for the new millennium. *Advances in Nursing Science,* 21(4), 81–91.

Lincoln, Y., & Guba, E. (1985). *Naturalistic inquiry.* Newbury Park, CA: Sage.

Mead, G. H. (1934). *Mind, self and society.* Chicago: University of Chicago Press.

Miller, S., & Fredericks, M. (1999). How does grounded theory explain? *Qualitative Health Research, 9*, 538–551.

Morse, J. (1997). Considering theory derived from qualitative research. In J. M. Morse (Ed.), *Completing a qualitative project: Details and dialogue* (pp. 163–188). Thousand Oaks, CA.: Sage.

Morse, J., & Johnson, J. (1992). *The illness experience: Dimensions of suffering.* Newbury Park, CA: Sage.

Morse, J., Hutchinson, S., & Penrod, J. (1998). From theory to practice: The development of assessment guides from qualitatively derived theory. *Qualitative Health Research, 8*, 329–340.

Redfern-Vance, N., & Hutchinson, S. (1995). The process of developing personal sovereignty in women who repeatedly acquire sexually transmitted diseases. *Qualitative Health Research, 5*, 222–236.

Richards, T., & Richards, L. (1991). The NUD.IST qualitative data analysis system. *Qualitative Sociology, 14*, 307–324.

Rodgers, B., & Cowles, K. (1993). The qualitative research audit trail: A complex collection of documentation. *Research in Nursing & Health, 16*, 219–226.

Sandelowski, M. (1986).The problem of rigor in qualitative research. *Advances in Nursing Science, 8*(3), 27–37.

Sandelowski, M.(1995a). Triangles and crystals: On the geometry of qualitative research. *Research in Nursing & Health, 18*, 569–574.

Sandelowski, M. (1995b). A theory of the transition to parenthood of infertile couples. *Research in Nursing & Health, 18*, 123–132.

Sandelowski, M. (1996). Using qualitative methods in intervention studies. *Research in Nursing & Health, 19*, 359–364.

Sandelowski, M. (1997). Programmatic qualitative research. In J. Morse (Ed.), *Completing a qualitative project: Details and dialogue* (pp. 210–225). Newbury Park, CA: Sage.

Schatzman, L., & Strauss, A. (1973). *Field research: Strategies for a natural sociology.* Englewood Cliffs, NJ: Prentice-Hall.

Sim, S. (1998). *The Icon critical dictionary of postmodern thought.* London: Icon Books.

Smith, L., & Pohland, P. (1976). Grounded theory and educational ethnography: Methodological analysis and critique. In J. Roberts & S. Akinsanya (Eds.), *Educational patterns and cultural configurations* (pp. 254–278). New York: David McKay.

Stern, P. (1980). Grounded theory methodology: Its uses and processes. *Image: The Journal of Nursing Scholarship, 12*, 20–23.

Stern, P., Allen, L., & Moxley, P. (1982). The nurse as grounded theorist: History, process and uses. *The Review Journal of Philosophy and Social Science, 7*(1, 2), 200–215.

Strauss, A. (1987). *Qualitative analysis for social scientists.* New York: Cambridge University Press.

Strauss, A., & Corbin, J. (1990). *Basics of qualitative research*. Newbury Park, CA: Sage.

Strauss, A., & Corbin, J. (1997). *Grounded theory in practice*. Thousand Oaks, CA: Sage.

Tesch, R. (1990). *Qualitative research: Analysis types and software tools*. New York: Falmer Press.

Warshaft, S. (Ed.). (1965). *Francis Bacon: A selection of his works*. New York: Odyssey.

Wilson, H. (1989). Family caregiving for a relative with Alzheimer's dementia: Coping with negative choices. *Nursing Research*, 38(2), 94–98.

Wilson, H., & Hutchinson, S. (1996). Methodologic mistakes in grounded theory. *Nursing Research*, 45(2), 122–124.

Wilson, H., Hutchinson, S., & Holzemer, W. (1997). Salvaging quality of life in ethnically diverse patients with advanced HIV/AIDS. *Qualitative Health Research*, 7, 75–97.

Wuest, J. (1995). Feminist grounded theory: An exploration of the congruency and tensions between two traditions in knowledge discovery. *Qualitative Health Research*, 5, 125–137.

8

Understanding Clients' Health Care Decisions
A Grounded-Theory Approach

JoAnne Weiss
Sally A. Hutchinson

Diabetes and hypertension, two prevalent chronic illnesses, affect millions of Americans. When these diseases coexist and other confounding factors, such as dyslipidemia and obesity, are present, the risks of cardiovascular, cerebrovascular, and renal diseases increase significantly. Clients frequently feel minimal effects from these diseases and often fail to appreciate these risks until complications occur. Health care professionals believe that it is essential to optimal disease management and complication prevention for clients to follow recommended health directives regarding proper use of medications, diet, exercise, weight loss, and smoking cessation. Because health care providers usually see the potential long-term consequences of these diseases from an "outsiders" view, their perspectives about client self-care decision making often are quite different from the views of clients.

Typical management of clients with diabetes and hypertension requires the development of strategies, primarily by health care providers, with the expectation that clients will follow them. Professionals label clients who do not follow directions as noncompliant or nonadherent. Health care providers and clients themselves often struggle with the seeming inability of so many to consistently follow the recommendations known to prevent or delay complications. Compliance and adherence research indicates that, with or without labeling, consistently following health care directives is extremely difficult.

The intent of the research was to study how clients with diabetes and hypertension think about their health and behavior regarding these diseases, including their adherence or lack of adherence to health care directives.[1] Research questions included:

1. What is the basic social psychological problem faced by persons with diabetes and hypertension?
2. What basic social psychological process do persons use to deal with this problem? Subquestions included:
   a. How do persons with diabetes and hypertension explain the causes of their diseases and related health problems?
   b. How do these persons think about preventive health behaviors suggested by health care providers such as dietary restrictions, regular exercise, limited alcohol use, and smoking cessation, as well as pharmacological interventions? How to they think about the consequences of their own health behavior choices?
3. How do these persons think relationships with family and friends affect and are affected by these diseases?
4. What contextual conditions (professional, familial, and social) influence the thinking and behavior of persons with diabetes and hypertension?
5. What contextual interactions (professional, familial, and social) occur around problems of diabetes and hypertension?

The grounded-theory method was chosen for this research because it is based on a symbolic interactionist view of human behavior. Symbolic interactionism emphasizes the importance of interaction with self and others in how people think about, live with, and make decisions about a given situation—in this case, diabetes and hypertension. The grounded-theory method provides a systematic way of generating theoretical constructs and/or concepts that illuminate human behavior and the social world (Chenitz & Swanson, 1986). In this method, peo-

---

[1]The discussion of the model of self-care decision making presented in this chapter is an expanded version of JoAnne Weiss's "Self-care decision making in clients with diabetes," in S. Funk et al (Eds.), Key aspects of preventing and managing chronic illness. © 2000, Springer Publishing Company, Inc., New York 10012. Adapted with permission.

ple who have problems in common are believed to have a basic social problem in common that is often unarticulated. It is the interpretive researcher's work to discover and articulate the problem from the clients' perspective (Hutchinson & Wilson, Chapter 7). In this grounded-theory study, we found that clients with diabetes and hypertension are bombarded with warnings alerting them to their vulnerability (Weiss & Hutchinson, 2000). We interpreted these warnings, which may be external or internal, as the basic social psychological problem that these clients have in common. In response to this "problem" of warnings and before making self-care choices, clients engage in a process called personal theorizing. Personal theorizing is a generally unrecognized analytical process in which clients consider the costs and benefits, the influence of social interactions, their past histories, and their future risks related to various choices that they might make. On the basis of this personal theorizing, clients make self-care decisions. A model of self-care decision making (Weiss, 2000) illustrates the process of personal theorizing that takes place in response to the problem of warning (Figure 8–1). Understanding this model, which illustrates how self-care decisions were made in this population, provides an opportunity to expand our standard thinking.

BACKGROUND

The control of diabetes and hypertension is a national concern, as well as a personal concern for clients. Control of diabetes- and hypertension-related morbidity and mortality is included in *Healthy People* 2000 objectives (U.S. Department of Health and Human Services, 1990) and reiterated in *Healthy People* 2010. On the basis of the ever-evolving body of research, these goals are readily attainable, but little real progress is being made.

Theoretically, the management of diabetes and hypertension is quite straightforward. Lifestyle changes, the backbone of effective treatment for both diabetes (Butler, Rubenstein, Gracia, & Zweig, 1998) and hypertension include diet, exercise, smoking cessation, and weight loss if needed. These changes, coupled with appropriate use of medication, are the ingredients of success; however, many clients find consistent implementation of these strategies extremely difficult. For example, although researchers have shown that achieving and maintaining tight glycemic control decreases complications, Greenfield and colleagues (Greenfield, Rogers, Mangotich, Carney, & Tarlov, 1995) found that more than half of those in their study with adult-onset diabetes maintained

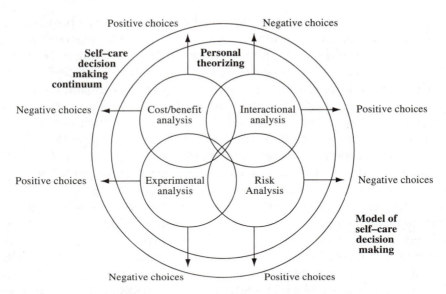

Figure 8–1 The Model of Self-Care Decision Making illustrates the process of personal theorizing, involving cost-benefit analysis, interactional analysis, experiential analysis and/or risk analysis, which leads to self-care decision making.

glycosolated hemoglobin levels greater than 9.5% (7.0% is the recommended upper level). Perhaps maintaining tight control is difficult because many clients are asymptomatic, making it difficult to believe that they truly are at risk for serious complications when they seem to have "no problems" (Butler et al., 1998). Encouraging clients to strive for greater levels of adherence does not seem to be working. In fact, the results of many adherence research projects have been inconclusive or even contradictory (Pfister-Minogue, 1993; Schatz, 1988).

Adherence, defined as the extent to which a person's behavior coincides with medical or health advice (Haynes, Taylor, & Sackett, 1979), has been a prevalent concept in the treatment standards of people with diabetes and/or hypertension. Early work regarding adherence, then called compliance, indicated that clients should always follow directives and were expected to do so. This view of compliance may have been tied to the dominance of medicine in which failure to comply with "orders" was portrayed as deviant behavior blamed primarily on clients (Donovan & Blake, 1992). According to Squyres (1986), the term adherence refers to a transition from client obedience to a therapeutic partnership in which clients adhere to treatment plans developed with their participation. But is this definition really different from expecting obedience to the rules?

According to the U.S. Preventive Services Task Force (1996), clinicians must assist clients to assume greater responsibility for their own health, and decision making should be a shared process between health care providers and clients. In reality, clients must assume full responsibility for their health and their health-related choices. The term "self-care," in regard to decision making, suggests a trend in this direction. Unfortunately, though this term is used in the professional literature, the view of advocating client responsibility for health rather than expecting obedience is far from common.

In the course of the research, it became apparent that the original focus on adherence to health care directives was too narrow, and a focus on how clients make self-care decisions better captured the data. Although very aware of the health directives given to them by providers, clients are concerned about their own self-care decision making. The subtle difference between adherence and self-care decision making, though a matter of perception, is significant. Adherence, the perspective of providers, suggests following the rules. Self-care decision making, the perspective of clients, suggests making decisions based not only on the rules, but also on many other, often more influential, factors. Rather than using the terms adherence and nonadherence, we refer to positive and negative self-care choices throughout the remainder of this chapter. Positive choices promote health and often coincide with health directives, making them adherent choices. Negative choices are those that violate health; they usually are nonadherent. It is important to understand that, when clients make positive choices, their intent is not simply to follow someone else's rules but rather to make choices that benefit their own health. To be effective providers, we must grasp this subtle difference and come to see the matter from the perspective of the client. Focusing on adherence alone does not work. For this reason, it is also important to change our thinking and terminology from adherence to self-care decision making.

Literature reviewed in the dissertation included not only research on adherence and self-care, but also a discussion and critique of numerous theoretical models potentially relevant to the problem. These models included the Health Belief Model (Bedworth & Bedworth, 1992), the Theory of Reasoned Action and Theory of Planned Behavior (Ajzen & Fishbein, 1980), Social Learning and Social Cognitive Theory (Bandura, 1986), Relapse Prevention Model (Williams & Gorski, 1997), Transtheoretical Model (Hotz, Allston, Birkett, Baskerville, & Dunkley, 1995), and the Health Promotion Model (Pender, 1996). Although these models have been helpful in understanding clients' views of health and illness, they have not been effective in bringing about behavior change. Perhaps this ineffectiveness is because the models were developed from the perspective of researchers and providers rather than from the perspective of clients. Many models consider the influence of client perceptions on adherence but do not address how such perceptions are formed. This study approached the issue from a new perspective, aiming to help fill the identified gaps in the literature by the development of a theory that explains the health choices and behaviors of clients with diabetes and hypertension.

METHOD

After university institutional review board approval, English-speaking adults diagnosed with both diabetes and hypertension were sought for this research. Participants were identified through networking with health care providers, acquaintances, and ministers, particularly of African American churches. In addition, invitations to participate in the study were placed in health care providers' offices and churches.

The first author interviewed a purposive sample of 21 clients. Demographics of the sample are shown in Table 8–1. Many of these participants experienced complications associated with diabetes and hypertension: three participants had known cardiovascular disease, four were aware of renal disease, one had received a kidney transplant, and one was on dialysis hoping to improve enough for a future kidney transplant. In addition, one participant had had both lower extremities amputated, and another one had lost several toes. Some participants had experienced episodes of transient visual loss, but none were blind. To add a broader perspective to this research, three health care

TABLE 8–1 PARTICIPANT DEMOGRAPHICS

13 females	11 Caucasian	2 African American
8 males	6 Caucasian	2 African American
Age	24–74 years	
Socioeconomic	Indigent to affluent	
	Medications	
Hypertension	Antihypertensives: all participants	
Diabetes	Insulin:	7 females	4 males
	Oral:	9 participants	
	Diet only:		1 male

providers—two primary care nurse practitioners and one physician (nephrologist)—who care for clients with diabetes and hypertension provided interviews.

Data collection entailed conducting unstructured interviews lasting from 1 to 2 hours that were audiorecorded and transcribed verbatim with the use of Word Perfect computer software. Most interviews took place in clients' homes; interviews with providers took place in their offices. Follow-up interviews to confirm and expand the initial interviews were with three participants and two health care providers.

In keeping with the grounded-theory method, data were jointly collected, coded, and analyzed; the ongoing analysis guided decisions about further data collection and analysis. Theoretical sampling, memoing, and selective coding, with the use of the constant comparative method, were continued until the point of data saturation.

Credibility for this research was enhanced by discussing the findings with colleagues (peer review) and study participants (member checks) (Lincoln & Guba, 1985). Dependability was facilitated by providing a clear audit trail describing decision making during data analysis (Beck, 1993).

FINDINGS

Basic Social Problem: Warnings of Vulnerability

Clients in this study reported being bombarded with warnings of vulnerability alerting them to their diseases and, more importantly, their present and future vulnerability.[2] The context of warnings, in this research, is broader than the traditional sense of directly urging caution (Weiss & Hutchinson, 2000). Often physical symptoms as well as verbal messages in the form of instructions constituted warnings to these clients. Warnings often preceded the time of diagnosis and generally continued throughout the rest of their lives. External warnings came from outsiders, such as health care providers, family, friends, and/or the media; internal warnings originated within the client. These warnings, often not consciously recognized as such, were of variable intensity.

Physical signs that presented as *objective* evidence detected by health care providers inspired external warnings from the providers. These warnings came in the form of instructions, admonitions, and

---

[2]A more elaborate discussion of warnings can be found in an article by J. Weiss and S. Hutchinson (2000).

occasionally threats. Initially warnings from health care providers usually were given in the form of instructions. The most common instruction/warnings centered on the need for proper use of prescribed medications, a healthy diet, smoking cessation, weight loss, and regular exercise. Admonitions and threats were more likely when previous instructions were not heeded. The client's health status usually determined the quantity and quality of these external warnings. Because diabetes and hypertension generally did not cause any symptoms until complications arose, warnings had variable effect.

> I feel so good. Why do I feel so good, and you tell me I'm so sick? Okay, that's what it basically comes down to. . . . They'll [doctors] say, "Well, how do you feel?" I say, "I feel great but I'm sure that damn lab work's gonna be bad. . . . He says, "Yeah, you're right."

Internal warnings are messages that originated from within the client, usually in the form of physical symptoms. Because they could actually feel these bodily changes, clients tended to pay more attention to internal warnings. Clients generally sought both initial and follow-up treatment because of these symptoms/warnings. The most dramatic symptoms experienced by clients were related to diabetes—in particular, blood sugar highs and lows.

> I've been out and all of a sudden start getting the shakes. And I've been in the supermarket where I've had to have something to eat right now because I thought I was gonna lose it. And people could see my physical condition that there was something wrong and wanted to get me help. . . .

Other symptoms included visual losses and neuropathic pain related to complications from these diseases. Symptoms related to high blood pressure were more vague. Because internal warnings were self-generated, they tended to have more effect on clients in promoting positive self-care choices. "That [visual loss] scared the hell out of me to be perfectly blunt. Boy, I walked, I did everything, watched my diet, took my food, cut it in half, lost weight." For this participant, the warning was "an out and out siren! I don't want to go blind."

Basic Social Process: Personal Theorizing

Clients responded to warnings by examining and evaluating them for meaning and relevance by using a process that we call "personal theorizing." This complex process took place subsequent and in relation to the warnings that clients received. They used personal theorizing to understand their health and to determine (consciously or unconsciously) their self-care choices. Listen to the personal theorizing of client X:

> I didn't take it [diabetes] serious because I didn't feel anything was wrong. I thought they [doctors] were just kidding at how serious it could be. . . . I knew . . . that you probably can lose your eyes, and you probably can lose your legs but I feel great; it's not happening to me. But you take advantage of it; you eat the sugar.

An understanding of clients' unique personal theories of disease causation and treatment is often a key to understanding their self-care decision making. Clients often are willing to share their personal theories during routine health care visits. Frequently, however, these beliefs are not elicited, are not heard, or are ignored or dismissed by health care providers, perhaps because of the unusual nature of some theories: "I thought maybe I could outgrow it [hypertension], or . . . eat right and . . . you know, try to lose it."

Uncertainty.   A context of uncertainty influences personal theorizing. Because clients are so often asymptomatic until complications develop, they are seldom certain about their disease status and the effectiveness of treatment, including their self-care choices. One participant remembered her attitude when she was younger and free from complications:

> Oh, I don't need a needle to live. . . . I can eat what I want, I feel just fine. I don't feel like I'm going blind, I don't feel like I'm losing my legs, I pee just fine, my kidney's aren't going.

The uncertainty of not knowing whether these diseases, particularly diabetes, are controlled or not can be very frustrating.

> Diabetes is very hard to live with. Now I know with my heart if I take my medicine, and I watch what I do, I'm fine. So . . . I have no worries about my heart at all because I know when I'm not feeling good and if I have a chest pain, I know I better go sit down. Now the sugar don't tell you anything. Because I've been in a state with this diabetes for the last five, six years that everyday is the same. And I don't feel any different from one day to the next, it's always the same.

Several participants referred to diabetes as "a mystery" to live with or understand. Uncertainties about disease status, about the accuracy of home blood sugar and blood pressure monitoring equipment, about treatment protocols that require multiple medications, and about provider–client relations influence the self-care decisions that clients make. Recognizing this broad context of uncertainty is helpful for understanding the struggles of clients with diabetes and hypertension and the process of personal theorizing.

MODEL OF SELF-CARE DECISION MAKING

The Model of Self-Care Decision Making (Weiss, 2000) illustrates the process of personal theorizing developed from the research. This model has four components: cost–benefit analysis, interactional analysis, experiential analysis, and risk analysis. When clients received warnings, they examined the data by using one or more of these analytical means. They considered the costs and benefits of various choices (cost–benefit analysis), the influence of other people (interactional analysis), the effects of previous experiences (experiential analysis), and/or the risks that they might encounter owing to their choices (risk analysis). At times, analysis was focused predominantly on one component; at other times, analysis was of multiple components. Self-care decisions resulted from these analytical processes.

Cost–Benefit Analysis

Cost–benefit analysis is one means used by clients to determine which self-care choices to make. In response to the numerous warnings that they received, clients weighed the costs and benefits of various choices. This process was unique for each client, though there were some common features. Most external warnings centered on choices about diet, exercise, body size, medication use, blood sugar testing, and smoking cessation. When clients weighed the costs and benefits of these choices, they frequently determined that the costs of consistently making health-promoting decisions were quite high. These costs were physical, psychological, social, financial, and temporal.

The most obvious cost of making positive, or health-promoting, choices was the need to live with restrictions requiring self-vigilance. Because diet often plays such a major role in diabetes and hypertension control, restrictions of food and drink are a cornerstone of most management plans. For some participants, the cost of these restrictions frequently was too great:

I love fruit, and if I eat any fruit at all my sugar goes sky high. In a matter of minutes it goes sky high. And to restrict yourself from all these here pleasures of different foods is, it's hard to live with.

Various choices were often weighed in relation to various self-care choices:

When I look at a piece of dessert, yea I think about diabetes, but . . . I finally gave up desserts after my first 150 diets that I was on, and so, sweets I've been able to say no to, finally. . . . I say no I don't want that, I shouldn't have that. And I can say no to dessert . . . but a second helping of pasta, then I'm probably not able to resist, which I know I should say no to also.

Sugar and salt replacements offered poor substitutes when weighing dietary choices:

I love salt and I'm not cautious one bit with salt. I tried for a while; I bought all these different little salt substitutes and you can hang that up. That's awful. Just terrible. Don't tell me you can't tell the difference cause I'll tell you the difference.

In addition to dietary limitations, the costs of positive self-care decision making often included restrictions in other areas, such as smoking. For some clients, these costs were just too high. "If I gotta throw the cigarettes away, you might as well take me out here and shoot me. Because I've got nothing left. I don't eat as it is."

Exercise, which can significantly improve diabetes and hypertension control, often was at a cost that seemed too great: "A lot of times I just want to get up and walk and I just don't have the energy to do it." Physical ailments also played a role, as one husband explained about his wife's painful diabetic neuropathy: "I would try to take her out to get exercise and her legs would lock up. . . . She can walk a little ways but then have to quit."

Social costs were another area of concern: "A lot of people have said to me, 'Well we didn't invite you cause I didn't know what to cook for you.'. . . And then other people just don't invite you anymore." At times, social engagements were "costly" when they interfered with meal and medication scheduling: "I used to always avoid going to people's houses because you go there and they'll say, 'Well we'll eat at six o'clock.' Well, then, when you don't eat until nine o'clock, that's a big difference for me."

Financial costs influenced self-care decision making, often decreasing health-promoting self-care decision making. "You get to the point sometimes when you don't have the medication and you don't have the money to buy it and you're worried about that. It's just one thing right after another."

Making positive self-care choices often required additional time, another cost of making positive choices: "Time is a very, very big thing. It takes time to eat properly, to prepare . . . it takes time."

In this research, it became apparent that whether or not clients followed health care directives, they had usually weighed the costs and benefits of their choices. Some clients accepted these costs and made positive choices. Often they did so because they recognized the physical and/or psychological benefits: "Basically, if I can maintain the weight . . . that I'm supposed to, eat, you know, like three meals a day . . . and stay on my diet, I don't have any problem."

Some could see the long-term benefits of positive choices more clearly than others:

> I figure if . . . the less medication I take for anything, I feel as though my body's better off. So I figure if I eat and drink properly I won't have to take the medication . . . so that's good. . . . If I understand Dr. Smith right, he said eventually, might be five years, ten years, two years down the road, you'll have to go on insulin, so I figure, the longer I put it off [insulin use] the better off I'd be. Cause I think it must be a pain.

Cost–benefit analysis is an important component of personal theorizing, the precursor of self-care decision making. Although clients often do not articulate or even recognize this process, they frequently weigh the costs and benefits of various choices before making them.

Interactional Analysis

Interactional analysis occurred as clients evaluated their social interactions with health care providers, significant others, acquaintances, and strangers. External warnings derived from social interaction with these persons. When social interaction was relevant for self-care decision making, clients evaluated it in a manner similar to that in which they weighed costs and benefits. They analyzed interactions to determine their meaning, value, and influence. They reflected not only on what was said to them, but also on how they felt about what was said and who was speaking. At times, self-care choices were based solely on interactional analysis, whereas, at other times, this analysis included other types of analysis as well (cost–benefit analysis, experiential analysis, or risk analysis).

Interactions with Health Care Providers.   The most significant interactions in terms of personal theorizing and self-care decision making took place between clients and health care providers and/or clients

TABLE 8–2   INFLUENCE OF OTHER PERSON IN INTERACTION

		++ Positive Influence	00 No Influence	–– Negative Influence
Importance of Interaction to Client	++ Important	++/++	00/++	––/++
	00 Neither Important nor Unimportant	++/00	00/00	––/00
	–– Not Important	++/––	00/––	––/––

and significant others. The purpose, needs, and expectations of interactions between health care providers and clients were quite different from those between clients and significant others. In client analysis of interactions with health care providers, two factors affected self-care decision making: (1) the influence of the provider on the client and (2) the importance of the interaction to the client. An overview of the significance of these factors is illustrated in Table 8–2.

Table 8–2 illustrates that, in interactional analysis, health care providers had a positive influence (++), no influence (00), or a negative influence (––) on clients and, therefore, self-care decision making. Also significant was the importance of the interaction to the client. The interaction was important (++), neither important nor unimportant (00), or unimportant (––). The greatest likelihood for interactional analysis to have a positive influence on self-care decision making occurred when both the influence of the provider was positive and the interaction itself was important to the client. In all other instances, any positive effect of the interaction was diminished, owing either to the negative influence of the other person in the interaction or to the decreased importance of the interaction to the client. For this reason, interactions often had a variable influence on self-care decision making, sometimes being noncontributory or defeating rather than empowering for positive self-care decision making.

Provider Influence.   Health care providers often assume that their input is particularly influential in client self-care decision-making processes. However, their influence may be less significant than assumed: "I hate doctors. I'm sorry. I'm not comfortable with doctors, I don't know why. I don't think too many people are." In this research, participants expressed feeling more negative influences from physicians than positive ones. For example, being told to lose weight by an obese provider may not be taken seriously as one obese participant's comment suggested: "He's like me, he's got a big belly, too." Providers may be unaware of their influence on clients, especially if it is not positive.

Four factors—mutual respect, trust, a feeling of collegiality, and style of presentation of health care information—determined the influence of health care providers on clients during interactional analysis. During provider–client interaction, a positive influence was more likely when clients perceived mutual respect:

> It's important to me that they respect me. . . . That's how they get my respect, by respecting me, just like I get their respect by respecting them. And if they're not willing to do that, then, I'm not interested in participating.

As evidenced in other research (Lorenc & Branthwaite, 1993), long waits before scheduled appointments decrease positive self-care decision making. Long waits suggest little respect for clients' time:

> I've always felt that I was a professional and I felt that I was on a same level as any doctor, and that my time was just as valuable as theirs, and there's nothing I hate more than going to an office and waiting . . . when I have an appointment. If they [doctors] don't have any respect for me and my time, I don't have any respect for what they have to tell me.

When trust is present, the health care provider is more influential and positive self-care decisions are more likely: "If I have a lot of faith in that person, I'm more likely to adhere."

Trust differs from respect in that mutuality is not a necessity for trust to be influential. Trust is more personal, often based on a specific occurrence that built trust in the provider.

> I'm very comfortable with him [my doctor]. I have all the confidence in the world with him. And he's straightforward with me, you know. He doesn't beat around the bush, he tells me like it is and he doesn't use big fancy words . . . he talks like I can understand him.

When providers did not remember previous therapies that they recommended, trust diminished. "They [doctors] don't know what the hell they're talking about. I've found that out more than once because they don't even remember what they gave me."

Although not as significant as mutual respect or trust, a feeling of collegiality with a health care provider increased the influence of the provider: "I probably have a tendency to listen to him [my doctor] more as being a friend as well as being a patient, as the doctor relationship." The influence of comfortable relationships may be more sustaining than is often realized. Often, however, this feeling of closeness was not the case, with clients feeling as one participant stated, "Doctors don't want you to know that they're human."

In addition to respect, trust, and collegiality, the style in which health care providers presented information, instructions, and admonitions affected the influence of interactions. One participant, when asked why she denied her diabetes for years, gave this explanation:

> I think it was the way it was presented to me. I mean I was all ready to leave the hospital waiting for him [husband] to come and the doctor came in and, you know, blank, "You got diabetes." And I mean, you could do that with some people but not very many. I mean you have to work into it and I just thought, huh, he's out of his mind.

Importance of Interactions. In addition to the influence of health care providers, the importance of interactions to clients affected self-care choices. Three factors influenced the importance of interactions for clients: the timing of interactions, clients' awareness of the need for input from providers, and clients' desire to please providers. At times, interactions were not as significant to clients as health care providers assumed. For example, when a client came only to get prescriptions renewed, the interaction was only minimally important: "My doctors here are to get me . . . the medicine legally cause I have to have them [doctors] to keep on giving the prescriptions. Otherwise, I wouldn't even see the doctors anymore." Canceled or forgotten appointments suggest that these interactions are unimportant to clients.

The timing of interactions had a significant effect on the importance of interactions to some clients. If the interaction took place amid of other competing or distracting concerns, the interaction was less important. One participant told of being discharged from the hospital following complications, only to find that her brother had been killed that day. Most competing circumstances were far less dramatic but still affected the importance of interactions.

Clients sometimes felt that they needed the input of providers because of the status of their health, of possible complications, or they had questions: "If I got a problem [with my health] I gotta let somebody know about it. . . . I try not to let it get in my way, but I know it's there." When clients did not feel a need, interactions were less important, and positive self-care decision making assumed less importance. One participant in renal failure reflected:

> The doctors talked to me. . . . I never knew diabetes was this serious. I did not know that it was actually a life-threatening disease. I knew that, yeah, you can die from it if you let your sugar [get] out of control. But all of this other stuff, I didn't listen.

The desire of clients to please their health care providers also helped determine the importance of interactions.

> When I go for my check-up to Dr. Jones, it makes me feel good just to see when he reads the reports and he looks at them, just to hear him say how good I'm doing and knowing that I'm doing what he's telling me to do. Makes me see and feel that much better.

Interactions with Significant Others. In addition to health care providers, significant others (whether spouses, parents, children, or friends) have an important influence on clients with diabetes and hypertension. As with other research (Wysocki et al., 1996), this project demonstrated that social support positively affected self-care decision making in chronic illnesses. Data from this research also suggested that the absence of such support was significant.

Relationships with significant others were more complicated than those with health care providers, because the goals were different and more time and energy was required to build the relationships. During the interactional analysis phase of personal theorizing, clients evaluated the support that they received from significant others. If clients felt supported by significant others, positive self-care decision making was more likely: "Without support of family and friends I don't think 'stick with it' will happen." If clients did not feel supported, positive choices were less likely:

> I don't want to put any blame on her [wife] because of diet or anything, you know, and it's pretty hard for me to do this because I forget. Trying to deal with everything else and I'll forget; I'll get a lot on my mind and I'll forget to take my shots and stuff like that. . . . I'm not gonna lay any guilt on her. This is not her problem, really. But I know that if she didn't have to work or whatever . . . she would be preparing my meals and weighing my stuff out for me.

Rather than experiencing support from significant others, some clients described feeling criticized:

> My family always tells me I got to take my medicine and I gotta watch what I eat. My husband is always on me, telling me I need to lose weight, you know. It's not good for me and I know that. . . . They're always on my case. I need to get out of the house, I need to do this, I need to do that; but it's easier said than done.

At times significant others had distracting effects on clients, which impeded positive decision making:

> I care about my family, I care about doing things that make them happy and a lot of times I put them before my own health . . . and I know that's bad. If I can't help my family then I feel like I have failed in some kind of way, that I'm not there for them to help them with things and it takes effect on me. . . . Because a lot of times I worry about them and don't think about myself.

Experiential Analysis

Experiential analysis occurred as clients reviewed their previous experiences to derive meaning from them, to explain their present health status, and to provide direction for their future choices. During the interviews, clients often told personal "stories," indicating that they spent a great deal of time in this analytical process. They formed and revised personal theories about health, illness, and appropriate treatment. They considered previous warnings, responses to those warnings, actions taken, and outcomes:

> I feel that if I haven't come . . . close to a coma or had an experience with a coma that I'm not as brittle as . . . the other diabetics are. . . . I've had my days when I've had my binges . . . whether it be a dessert or liquor or whatever, and I've never come close.

In this process, clients examined their experiences in several ways. In historical analysis, clients reviewed relevant personal history. By analyzing personal historical data, clients developed explanations for their present health status on the basis of what had happened in the past.

> When I was working . . . the stress and strain of working that I was under, that kept my pressure high all the time and, of course, then, when I would be under pressure or nervous or anything, I used to eat and drink and gain weight . . . and at one time . . .

> I weighed . . . over 220 and that was just from being nervous and
> everything and then the foods I ate aggravated the blood pres-
> sure and made it that much higher.

From the historical review, clients often identified previous experiences that provided direction for self-care choices:

> I believe I was really at death's door at that point [health crisis]
> because I was really sick and I think that played a big part in my
> really adjusting to the diabetes and the high blood . . . with me
> being as sick as I was . . . and to know that I was brought out of
> the condition without being totally blind altogether.

At times, however, historical analysis did not result in connections between health status and personal choices:

> I got real sick here, I ended up with kidney stones which liked to
> kill me. I ended up, they couldn't control my blood sugar. They
> said stress will raise it. . . . I was in the hospital because of the
> kidney stone and they had to go in and surgically remove it. And
> they put a shunt in me and sent me home and I was sick be-
> cause I couldn't eat, was nauseated all the time, I was throwing
> up . . . when I went home I still had that shunt in me and I ended
> up taking it out. And that was a mistake and I ended up back in
> the hospital that night . . . because I decided to have something
> to eat and I was living off tapioca pudding. . . . I ended up having
> five ulcers and a gastrated [sic] esophagus, so I was back in the
> hospital again for another two weeks. I was out just a couple
> days and ended up right back in again. Now I know that proba-
> bly wouldn't have happened if I wouldn't have been a diabetic.

In personality analysis, clients looked at themselves, assessing their
strengths and weaknesses: ". . . willpower. If it wasn't the willpower, then
I could eliminate all of that [struggle] as far as eating things I shouldn't
eat . . . keepin' up the weight and stuff like that." Often self-care choices
were related to personality analysis. After a dramatic warning, one participant realized that it was time for an attitude change: "It was deciding I was
gonna do it [make positive changes] . . . mental attitude . . . it was time."

Finally, in comparative analysis, clients compared their previous
personal experiences with the experiences of others.

> I have an elderly neighbor who will be real good and then all of
> a sudden she'll call me and she says, "Martha, I just ate a whole
> box of Eskimo pies and a pound of fudge. And my blood sugar's

going sky high, I'm gonna take more insulin." And I'll say, "Jane, that's not gonna help. Why didn't we eat just one piece." And she says, "Oh, I can't do just one." But you know in seeing how she allows herself to suffer sometimes because she can't accept the lifestyle I think helps me. I learn from other people.

Clients used these three categories of experiential analysis—historical, personal, and comparative—to evaluate warnings, to explain their present health status, and to determine future choices. When clients made strong connections among their choices, their previous experiences, and their present health problems, health-promoting decisions were more likely.

Risk Analysis. In risk analysis, clients considered potential risks to their health due to diabetes and hypertension. In cost–benefit analysis and interactional analysis, clients analyzed their *present* circumstances to determine appropriate self-care choices. In experiential analysis, they evaluated their *past* experiences and their relevance to decision making. In risk analysis, clients considered their *future* health as a determinant of self-care choices. In this component of personal theorizing, they considered various choices based on projections of what might happen in the future: "Understanding what diabetes will do to you if you don't try to take care of it, I see that that . . . could be a very bad future."

In risk analysis, clients analyzed their potential for future losses:

Being a diabetic . . . you got a risk of having kidney failure, so that's something you're going to have to worry about and then, by being hypertensive, you have a risk of having a stroke or a heart attack, that's something to worry about. . . . If I don't take my insulin I can go in a coma and if I don't take my pressure pills, [I can have] strokes and stuff and, being the problems with diabetes. I worry about that.

The risks of most concern to clients were couched in terms of personal losses—loss of present health status, loss of independence, as well as loss of life: "I worry about . . . the future . . . to the extent of my legs. It all boils down to the legs because if [I lose them] . . . who's gonna take care of me?" Health care providers often see these risks more impersonally in terms of increased morbidity and mortality.

Responses to risks varied from client to client and, within each client, from time to time. Responses to risks were based on client analysis of the likelihood that loss would occur. If they were convinced that loss was a great possibility, they feared the risks. One participant, who was bluntly told at the time of his diagnosis that he would be blind in 15 years, was strongly motivated by this fearful prospect:

> I was scared. You know, the thought of losing my sight . . . within a matter of a week they gave us all that literature and we read it, Mary [wife] and I . . . read every darn thing they gave us and then we went to their meetings they recommended and we went to additional ones over at the local hospital. And so we got to know the disease very early on, what it was like.

When loss seemed less likely, risks were understood but not feared. In this case, clients still realized that their choices would determine their future health status:

> It's like a fork in the road and you have to choose. If you want to keep barreling down the one you were on and end up right back in the hospital and not live to see your grandchildren grow up, that's what'll happen. If you want to continue and be healthy and survive to see 75 and retirement, you've got to make changes.

At other times, risks were completely disregarded: "They had a diabetes group over at the hospital, we went a couple of times but we have not been conscientious about following up. I guess it can be labeled as careless . . . or dangerous . . . disregard." A few clients in this study felt overwhelmed during risk analysis, which had a similar result:

> I would love to be able to get to see 83 and I would love to see my health improve but sometimes I just don't care. . . . By being a diabetic, you got to watch yourself, about the cuts and the bruises, it's just something else . . . and I wouldn't wish it on my worst enemy—being a diabetic or hypertension or anything. . . . It's just like a weight that's weighing you down. That's the way I see it. . . . It's just the idea of knowing that it's [illness] there and there's nothing that you can do about it.

Positive or health-promoting self-care choices were most likely when risks were feared and least likely when risks were ignored or considered overwhelming:

> I used to be a great chocolate eater, beer, a little scotch now and then . . . and I gave most of that up. . . . I just cut it out altogether knowing that I was in danger of possibly even losing my life.

DISCOURSE RATIONALES FOR NEGATIVE CHOICES

Subsequent to cost–benefit, interactional, experiential, and/or risk analysis, clients make health care decisions every day. Some are consistent with health care recommendations, whereas others are not. For example, some clients choose to take their insulin correctly but do not follow a recommended dietary plan. In this research, three different discourse rationales reveal how clients think about, talk about, and justify negative decisions. These rationales include balancing, bargaining, and neutralizing.

Balancing

Balancing is a rationale used by clients to achieve what they consider to be a reasonable compromise between acceptable and unacceptable choices. Balancing justifies negative choices in an effort to maintain stability in the face of living with multiple restrictions:

> If I can govern my own life, that's a form of freedom. And it's like I'm a prisoner with my daily living because of this diabetes. . . . I'm only allowed certain liberties. I can't . . . go out and eat a half a cherry pie and a scoop of ice cream. I can't do that. I know that. So I have to put some restrictions on myself but I'm not, I can't put 'em all on.

Balancing explains, in part, the active rather than the static nature of self-care decision making. On the one hand is the realization of the need for positive choices: "I know that my diabetes, if I keep it under control, . . . and watch my diet, the same way with high blood pressure, then . . . I would be fine. Be great." On the other hand is the difficulty of doing just that: "You really have to be strong to go through this, I feel. Because I mean, I could give up really because . . . it's something that I wasn't prepared for." By balancing, clients consider various choices and determine which ones they can accept and execute. Often clients compromise as they try to balance pleasurable choices with restrictive, health-promoting choices.

Nyhlin (1991), in a grounded-theory study, also identified balancing as a significant factor in the lives of insulin-dependent diabetics. Important in Nyhlin's research was the realization that the entire life of most clients with diabetes is dominated not only by the necessity of maintaining metabolic balance, but also by the need to find an equilibrium in other areas. "Walking a fine line" was identified as the core category and most important for understanding the meaning and management of diabetes.

In this research, maintaining an acceptable balance was often a daily process:

> One day I care and the next day I say, "I don't care." . . . I try to psych myself out . . . but sometimes it works and sometimes it don't. . . . Some mornings I say, well I'm gonna go on and take my insulin 'cause I know it's gonna help. And then some mornings I say, Well, shoot, I'm taking insulin and it ain't helping me now, 'cause my sugar's still up.

Bargaining

When balancing was difficult, clients bargained with themselves to justify their more dramatic ups and downs in making health care decisions. With bargaining, there was a sense of "giving up" something to justify an overindulgence.

> Once my sight came back, it didn't come back 100%, but it came back a lot better than what I thought it would, I wasn't afraid anymore and I knew that with diabetes [control is possible] if you don't eat sugar, and that I could give up, I could give up the sugar. . . . I know the sugar's harmful but I say to myself the carbs [carbohydrates] aren't as harmful as sugar is. So I can fudge on those, I can do a little more on those. Those won't kill me.

Bargaining usually entailed making some health-promoting choices in an effort to counteract the effect of negative ones.

> I was raised with a skillet in one hand and the grease in the other. This is very difficult. And then I find myself craving the fried chicken and the cornbread, things like that. . . . I eat it. . . . I . . . know I shouldn't, but I do. But then I try to compensate and at other times I try to be more careful.

Dietary bargaining often includes making negative decisions at one point but with plans for more positive choices in the future: "I just . . . got a glazed donut yesterday at the grocery store. So that was my dessert yesterday. Now I probably won't eat another one for a week or two, if then."

Sometimes clients rationalized by bargaining for smaller quantities rather than accepting restrictions or substitutes. The bargaining rationale may help clients feel better about themselves but often results in poor self-care choices.

I've eaten hot fudge sundaes but I found it was better to go eat a small one than to deny myself and eat all the dietetic candies that I didn't want to begin with. . . . I find the dietetic foods that they put out, a lot of them are good, but they don't fill you or your desire, you know, like when you want a piece of chocolate, you want a good piece of chocolate, you don't want the cheap stuff . . . so . . . I'll go get Russell Stover's, a box of chocolates, a small one . . . 'cause I'm picky about that, too. But, if I want chocolate . . . I'm better off doing it that way than to go eat everything else and add all those calories 'cause dietetic food doesn't mean lower calories. . . . I find, I can stick to my diet better if I do it that way.

Bargaining may result in positive, though costly, choices.

I'd like to weigh a little bit more, I'd like to put [on] about ten more pounds. . . . And I can't do that. I just cannot do that. If I eat, you know, to the extent that I start to gain the weight, the blood sugar's gonna go up. I know that. . . . Am I willing to do that? No, I'm not. . . . So, I've had to buy new clothes.

Neutralizing

The neutralizing rationalization differs from balancing and bargaining by negating the need for positive choices. Clients "neutralized" when the need for positive self-care choices was identified in one kind of analysis (e.g., risk analysis), but the significance of that need was decreased by analysis in another component (e.g., experiential analysis). Neutralizing often resulted in negative self-care choices. In the following example, the participant used her experience of never having been in a diabetic coma to neutralize the known risks of her disease.

I guess the . . . major thing with the diabetes is . . . I've never been in a coma no matter what I've done, whatever in the world I've decided to eat on any given moment in time. I've never even come close to a coma . . . never ever, whether I've had too much or too little. So, in my own mind I justify that maybe my problem's not that bad.

In some, neutralizing permits clients to feel that they are doing "all right" despite the potential risks of loss. In these cases, acceptance of the need for positive self-care choices was minimized:

One of the problems [I had] was cirrhosis of the liver, I quit, totally quit drinking for three years and slowly drifted back on wine. . . . So, actually, you know, I'm not as worried about cirrhosis as I used to be.

In other cases, neutralizing suggested that, despite efforts to improve health by positive self-care decision making, these diseases and the related risks of loss were nearly impossible to control:

> I really was watching my diet but it didn't help. I was watching the diet and everything and . . . my sugar steady was going up. So that's when I said, "Well, what's the heck if it's gonna go up, there's no use in me not eating what I want to eat." That the way I felt.

Whether the need for positive choices was minimized or the diseases and related risks were considered uncontrollable due to neutralizing, the result—poor self-care choices—was similar.

DISCUSSION

Clients with diabetes and hypertension are bombarded by far more warnings than health care providers may realize. It is important to appreciate the vast quantity of warnings, both external and internal, that clients receive in a single day. Owing to the vast number of warnings that clients receive related to diabetes, hypertension, and health in general, they are usually aware of their vulnerability (Weiss & Hutchinson, 2000). Appreciating the magnitude and significance of this process from a client's perspective can be a source of insight into the struggles that clients face. For example, saying "no" to a bowl of ice cream may be a significant positive choice for a client, whereas providers may see only their own narrow view of the client's consistently elevated blood sugar. These warnings (interpreted as the basic social psychological problem common to these clients) are not disregarded, as may be assumed, but instead are processed through personal theorizing.

A Model of Self-Care Decision Making explains this basic social psychological process of personal theorizing. This model suggests that self-care decision making is far more complex than simple adherence to rules. Understanding this process, which may or may not result in health-promoting choices, broadens the perspective from the limited provider view of adherence (following the rules) to the broader client view of responsibility for self-care (determining the rules). This understanding can facilitate client empowerment by providing a comprehensive basis for client education and the foundation for developing effective interventions originating from the client's perspective.

The Model of Self-Care Decision Making has some similarities to, as well as some distinct differences from, traditional behavior-change models. Although able to stand alone, the Model of Self-Care Decision Making can be a helpful adjunct to these models, serving as a source of insight into client reasoning, perceptions, and actual decision making. When applied, it can be useful for behavior prediction. Because the model was derived from the grounded-theory method, it is based on client-provided data and the interpretative analysis of that data by using an inductive, from-the-ground-up approach. As with most grounded-theory work, this theory provides an explanatory model for understanding human behavior(Chenitz & Swanson, 1986).

Traditional models of behavior change are used to predict behavior on the basis of the perceptions of clients. Significant client perceptions include those related to health, illness, the environment, and expectations of others, as well as personal capabilities, benefits, and barriers to action. Appreciating the presence and significance of these perceptions can be beneficial in predicting behavioral choices. Unfortunately, though these models identify influential perceptions, they are not sources of insight into how these perceptions are formed. An advantage of the Model of Self-Care Decision Making is the enlightenment that it provides regarding the origins and reasons for various client perceptions. For example, perceptions of benefits and barriers are often determined in cost–benefit analysis, whereas perceptions of personal capabilities or self-efficacy are often formed in historical and/or personality assessments during experiential analysis.

The domain of behavior-change models is frequently broad, often directed at outside factors, including "concerned others," such as health educators and providers, and how behavior can be changed or even manipulated by them. The focus of the Model of Self-Care Decision Making is solely on the cognitive and affective processes that clients use in determining self-care choices. The aim of most nursing models, particularly Orem's Self-Care Deficit Theory of Nursing (Foster & Bennett, 1995) is to provide a conceptual framework for nursing. These models are focused much more on the role of nursing in relation to the needs of clients and are more relevant for determining the timing and type of nursing care. As with behavioral models, these models are focused on the decision-making process of health care professionals, whereas the Model of Self-Care Decision Making considers the decision-making process from the perspective of clients.

The model provides a new perspective for understanding clients' self-care decision making. It identifies the analytic processes that clients use to assist them with decision making–cost–benefit, interactional, experiential, and risk analysis—and the rationales that they use when they talk about why they make negative choices. By understanding clients' thinking and subsequent behavior, we are in a better position to develop more effective clinical and research strategies.

RECOMMENDATIONS

Self-care decision making begins with but is not determined by the warnings that clients receive, as we often assume. Instead, the generally unrecognized process of personal theorizing takes place in response to the warnings as a determinant of these decisions. Living with diabetes and hypertension requires numerous self-care choices each day, most often related to diet, exercise, and medications. On the basis of personal theorizing, clients make the choices that they determine are best for them at any given time. At times, clients may view their decisions as health promoting, although their health care providers do not. Often providers make assumptions or judge clients on the basis of physical findings without recognizing the complex decision-making processes that resulted in those findings. We suggest that emphasizing client empowerment, rather than adherence, is the key to positive self-care choices.

The concept of empowerment is becoming more and more prevalent in the professional literature. According to Wallerstein (1992), through the process of empowerment clients gain increased control over their lives, and this increased self-efficacy results in better health and social outcomes. There is encouraging research on behavioral contributions to diabetes management, such as empowerment and self-management, however, the findings frequently are not incorporated into practice (Glasgow et al., 1999). Discovering how to empower clients is a difficult task.

Often, clients do not follow health care directives that they *are given*. Actively including them as partners in assessing their current health status and in developing and monitoring their own health maintenance plans is much more effective (Westberg & Jason, 1996). However, some providers trained in authoritarian, interventionalist models find this approach difficult because it requires significant changes in practice (Westberg & Jason, 1996). According to Byrne (1999), little work has been done to determine how health professionals move into an empowering role. Apparently this shift requires striving to understand the meanings that clients give to their lives as well as acknowledging and reducing the imbalance of power between providers and clients (Bryne, 1999).

Throughout the world, those taking part in the formation of health policy struggle with the problems of meeting and funding the ever-increasing health care demands while containing costs. Segal (1998) suggests that the answer may be in client empowerment. Not only do clients need more information, but they also need confidence and competence to act on that information and the capacity to influence the available health services. As well as understanding their health and available options, clients must accept responsibility for decisions about their health. In situations where clients are supported and encouraged to assume responsibility for their own health and to take a greater role in their own and/or their families' health care decisions, well-being is enhanced (Segal, 1998). This empowerment may be due to a greater sense of control, leading to improved self-care practices and changes in the utilization of health services (Segal, 1998).

Before trying to empower clients to be proactive health care decision makers, providers and clients themselves must understand how personal self-care decisions actually are made. The Model of Self-Care Decision Making can be a source of insight by identifying the components of the process: cost–benefit, interactional, experiential, and risk analysis. We suggest that more effective means of empowering clients and encouraging positive self-care decision making requires influencing the analytical process in one or more of these components.

In cost–benefit analysis, clients evaluate the costs and benefits of various self-care choices. If benefits seem greater than costs, clients are more likely to make health-promoting choices. More often, however, from clients' perspectives, costs outweigh benefits. There is great potential for vast differences between client and provider perspectives regarding cost–benefit analysis because clients often see and experience costs quite clearly, whereas providers focus only on benefits. To empower clients and promote positive self-care decision making, it is important to listen carefully and appropriately address client concerns regarding costs, whether physical, psychological, social, or financial. Although emphasizing benefits may be helpful, exploring with clients both costs and benefits from their perspective should increase efficacy. Then, rather than devising plans for clients, they can be asked to seek solutions and formulate their own plans. The provider assumes the role of consultant/advisor in self-care plan development.

Awareness of how clients analyze interactions with health care providers and important others is helpful in understanding how they make self-care decisions. Here again, great potential exists for different client and provider views regarding the significance of such interactions. As providers, we often assume that our input has maximal influence on client decision making. In this research, we learned that often this is not the case. How providers treat clients (mutual respect and trust) and the importance of the interaction to the client may be as significant in encouraging healthy choices as the information that clients receive. Sensitivity to client responses to warnings during provider–client interactions is an essential but often neglected component of health care. The importance of social support also is significant in this population. For this reason, significant family members may need to be encouraged to participate in client health care planning.

In experiential analysis, clients review their previous histories, often including personality appraisals. They may also perform a comparative analysis of their experiences with those of others. In this process, they develop explanations, find direction for self-care choices, and make connections between past experiences and present reality. The outcome of this analytical process generally leads them to or discourages them from health-promoting choices. Often providers are unaware of the influence of clients' previous experiences. Becoming aware of this component of personal theorizing may be essential to understanding how clients make decisions and an important step in encouraging them to make health-promoting choices. For example, if clients believe that, because they have never been in a diabetic coma, their disease is not serious (as several in this study did), their choices become more understandable. Also, if clients do not associate serious infections and the loss of toes, feet, and limbs with their diabetes (as several in this study did not), health care providers need to explain the connection between these problems clearly. Perhaps the development of statistical and/or graphic examples—not as fear-generating warnings but as instructional interventions—may be effective tools. Likewise, inquiring about clients' previous experiences and making note of them provide important background information.

Using risk analysis, clients examine future health expectations when contemplating present self-care choices. In this phase of personal theorizing, risks of concern include loss of present health status, independence, and/or life. These risks may be feared, appreciated but not feared, ignored, or considered overwhelming. Often, out of frustration, health care providers resort to fear tactics with the hope of promoting adherence to their directives. Clients in this study viewed these tactics as more a hindrance than a help. To be effective change agents, professionals should understand the process of risk analysis. Reviewing the risks of the future with clients (e.g., microvascular and macrovascular complications) is probably not enough to encourage health-promoting decision making, because providers see risks in broader, less-personal terms. Assisting clients to connect *their* present choices with *their* future risks without condemnation but with the potential for decreasing those risks is probably more beneficial. Rather than emphasizing only their own analysis of risks, providers need to ask clients about their expectations for the future and what risks concern them. If the risk of loss of independence is of greater concern than the risk of loss of life, fear of falling may inhibit exercise and therefore weight-loss choices. If risks are overwhelming to clients, an underlying depression may need attention in addition to diabetes and hypertension management. Examining risks *with* clients in regard to potential personal loss may be more helpful than trying to instill fear by threatening warnings. Providing personal accurate information that clients can use in risk analysis and health-plan formation should be beneficial.

To understand self-care decision making, it is imperative to listen to clients more carefully and to strive to understand this process from their perspectives. To be effective, providers must elicit conversations with clients in an effort to understand not only their choices, but also how they think about or determine those choices. With the right questions, clients will share their thinking about the influence of costs and benefits, social interactions, past experiences, and/or risks on their self-care actions—positive or negative. When they decide not to make the recommended positive choices, they may also provide rationales that reveal how they balance, bargain, or neutralize. Awareness of these rationalizations permits opportunities for discussion.

Client education is an essential part of health care particularly for persons with diabetes and hypertension. However, perhaps it is time for a shift in client education. The provider–client relationship must include more than a forum for providers to dump information on clients. Because self-care decision making is actually the responsibility of clients, our educational focus must change to reflect this fact. For too long, providers have tried to shoulder this responsibility, teaching clients to follow prescribed plans of care and becoming frustrated when clients do not follow their instructions. Results suggest that this tactic generally is ineffective. Understanding the Model of Self-Care Decision Making provides an opportunity to promote client responsibility for personal health, thus promoting positive self-care decision making.

A change is needed in the focus of client education. Assistance from other professionals may be a helpful adjunct in making this transition. As health care providers, our focus is on provision of care, which includes client education. However, assistance from health educators with fresh perspectives and creative ideas could change this ineffective system, because their sole focus is education. Critical information usually transmitted verbally in the course of client interactions can be presented in well-designed, simple, clearly written explanations. Ancillary staff can also be trained to facilitate client learning in this important aspect of health care.

Several participants in this study with a long-term history of diabetes and serious complications longed to share their experiences with others, particularly with young people still in a position to prevent such complications. New educational strategies utilizing such volunteers can be designed to emphasize the relationships between present self-care choices and future health.

REFERENCES

Ajzen, I., & Fishbein, M. (1980). *Understanding attitudes and predicting social behavior.* Englewood Cliffs, NJ: Prentice-Hall.

Bandura, A. (1986). *Social foundations of thought and action.* Englewood Cliffs, NJ: Prentice-Hall.

Bedworth, A. E., & Bedworth, D. A. (1992). *The profession and practice of health education.* Dubuque, IA: Wm. C. Brown.

Beck, C. T. (1993). Qualitative research: The evaluation of its creditability, fittingness, and auditability. *Western Journal of Nursing Research, 15,* 263–266.

Butler, R. N., Rubenstein, A. H., Gracia, A. M., & Zweig, S. C. (1998). Type 2 diabetes: Patient education and home blood glucose monitoring. *Geriatrics, 53*(5), 63–67.

Bryne, C. (1999). Facilitating empowerment groups: Dismantling professional boundaries. *Issues in Mental Health Nursing, 20,* 55–71.

Chenitz, W. C., & Swanson, J. M. (1986). Qualitative research using grounded theory. In W. C. Chenitz & J. M. Swanson (Eds.), *From practice to grounded theory.* Menlo Park, CA.: Addison-Wesley.

Donovan, J. L., & Blake, D. R. (1992). Patient non-compliance: Deviance or reasoned decision-making? *Social Science and Medicine, 34,* 507–513.

Foster, P. C., & Bennett, A. M. (1995). Dorothea E. Orem. In J. B. George (Ed.), *Nursing Theories: The Base for Professional Nursing Practice* (4th ed., pp. 99–123). Norwalk, CT: Appleton & Lange.

Glasgow, R. E., Fisher, E. B., Anderson, B. J., LaGreca, A., Marrero, D., Johnson, S. B., Rubin, R. R., & Cox, D. J. (1999). Behavioral science in diabetes: Contributions and opportunities. *Diabetes Care, 22,* 832–843.

Greenfield, S., Rogers, W., Mangotich, M., Carney, M. F., & Tarlov, A. R. (1995). Outcomes of patients with hypertension and non-insulin-diabetes mellitus treated by different systems and specialities: Results from the Medical Outcomes Study. *Journal of the American Medical Association, 274,* 1436–1444.

Haynes, R. B., Taylor, D. W., & Sackett, D. L. (Eds.). (1979). *Compliance in health care*. Baltimore: Johns Hopkins University Press.

Hutchinson, S., & Wilson, H. (2001). In P. Munhall (Ed.), *Nursing research: A qualitative perspective*. (3rd ed.). Boston: Jones and Bartlett.

Hotz, S. B., Allston, J. A., Birkett, N. J., Baskerville, B., & Dunkley, G. (1995). Fat-related dietary behavior: Behavioral science concepts for public health practice. *Canadian Journal of Public Health, 86*, 114–118.

Lincoln, Y., & Guba, E. (1985). *Naturalistic inquiry*. Newbury Park: Sage.

Lorenc, L., & Branthwaite, A. (1993). Are older adults less compliant with prescribed medication than younger adults? *British Journal of Clinical Psychology, 32*, 485–492.

Nyhlin, K. T. (1991). The fine balancing act of managing diabetes. *Scandinavian Journal of Caring Science, 5*(4), 187–194.

Pender, N. J. (1996). *Health promotion in nursing practice* (3rd ed.). Stamford, CT: Appleton & Lange.

Pfister-Minogue, K. (1993). Enhancing patient compliance: A guide for nurses. *Geriatric Nursing, 14*(3), 124–132.

Schatz, P. E. (1988). An evaluation of the components of compliance in patients with diabetes. *Journal of the American Dietetic Association, 88*, 708–712.

Segal, L. (1998). The importance of patient empowerment in health system reform. *Health Policy, 44*, 31–44.

Squyres, W. D. (1986). *Patient education and health promotion in medical care*. Palo Alto, CA: Mayfield.

U.S. Department of Health and Human Services, Public Health Service. (1990). *Healthy People 2000: National Health Promotion and Disease Prevention Objectives*.

U.S. Preventive Services Task Force. (1996). *Guide to clinical preventive services* (2nd ed.). Baltimore: Williams & Wilkins.

Wallerstein, N. (1992). Powerlessness, empowerment and health: Implications for health promotion programs. *American Journal of Health Promotion, 6*(3), 197–205.

Weiss, J. (2000). Self-care decision-making in clients with diabetes and hypertension. In S. Funk, E. M. Tornquist & J. Leeman (Eds.), *Key aspects of preventing and managing chronic illness*. New York: Springer.

Weiss, J., & Hutchinson, S. (2000). Adherence and warnings of vulnerability in clients with diabetes and hypertension. *Qualitative Health Research, 10*, 521–537.

Westberg, J., & Jason, H. (1996). Fostering healthy behavior. In S. H. Woolf, S. Jonas, & R. S. Lawrence (Eds.), *Health promotion and disease prevention in clinical practice* (pp. 145–162). Baltimore: Williams & Wilkins.

Williams, G. C., Freedman, Z. R., & Deci, E. L. (1998). Supporting autonomy to motivate patients with diabetes for glucose control. *Diabetes Care, 21*, 1644–1651.

Williams, R., & Gorski, T. T. (1997). *Relapse prevention counseling for African Americans: A culturally specific model.* Baltimore: Herald.

Wysocki, T., Taylor, A., Hough, B. S., Linscheid, T. R., Yeates, K. O., Naglieri, J. A. (1996). Deviation from developmentally appropriate self-care autonomy. Association with diabetes outcomes. *Diabetes Care, 19,* 119–125.

9

Ethnography
The Method

Carol P. Germain

Ethnography is a body of knowledge of cultural descriptions and theory, as well as research product and process. As a qualitative research process, traditional ethnography is the systematic description, analysis, and interpretation of cultures or subcultural groups. In the United States, ethnography originated as the tradition of inquiry of cultural anthropology in the early twentieth century with the work of discoverers such as Margaret Mead. In ensuing decades, this tradition of inquiry was adopted or adapted by other anthropologies that deal with living people (social, educational), as well as by other disciplines including sociology, political science, social psychology, and nursing. Ethnography was associated traditionally with the study of remote, foreign, or primitive cultures. One purpose for studying such cultures was to enable the researcher to acquire a perspective broadened beyond her or his ethnocentric one so that later cultural analyses of the home society could be accomplished more objectively. Over time, the emphasis in ethnography has shifted from the study of foreign or exotic cultures to the importance of obtaining cultural knowledge of the often unexamined, taken-for-granted realities of life in the subcultures or cultures of the researcher's own society. Ethnography, as a research product or outcome, and subsequently through cross-cultural comparisons, provides knowledge (theory) and understanding that can be used as a basis for planned culture change. "Doing fieldwork," or dwelling with people in their natural settings over a prolonged period of time, is a hallmark of ethnography, as is a central and explicit cultural focus.

Qualitative ethnography also has certain general characteristics of interpretive paradigm research, namely a holistic perspective—that is, an attempt to describe as much as possible about a culture or subcultural group, context preservation rather than context control, high value on the emic perspective of cultural insiders, an interactive approach that recognizes members of the culture-sharing group as coparticipants in the research process, and a dominantly inductive approach to data analysis and theory development.

Through the essential data collection methods of participant observation in selected cultural activities and in-depth interviewing of the members of the subculture, as well as supplementary methods, the researcher learns from informants the meanings that they attach to their activities, events, behaviors, knowledge, rituals, and other aspects of their lives. Gehring (1973) described ethnography as:

> . . . the art and discipline of watching and listening and of trying to inductively derive meaning from behaviors initiated by others. One must see the general in the rich, particularizing detail of good ethnography. To watch and to listen must come before interpretation and analysis. (p. 1223)

Valuable information about cultures and subcultures has also been obtained from the works of novelists, journalists, and missionaries, as well as from students whose ethnographic learning experience includes brief excursions to the field. However, the differences between these ethnographic accounts and ethnography are in the rigor of the research process and in the goal, which for traditional ethnography is a contribution to science through emphasis on theory development.

Patton (1990) stated that every human group that is together for a period of time will evolve a culture. Culture, broadly defined, is the learned social behavior or way of life of a particular group of people. Culture-sharing groups in American society may be found in rural and urban ethnic and/or racial enclaves; in nonethnic/nonracial groups such as those situated in prisons, bars, factories, or complex organizations; in the social institutions of education including academe; in the military and on military bases; in health care institutions such as assisted-living facilities, nursing homes, hospitals, or shelters for the homeless or the abused; in community-based groups of various types such as street gangs, motorcycle clubs, and volunteer organizations; in high-school groups such as jocks, skinheads, geeks, and nerds; in religious communities; and in professional disciplines such as nursing and medicine. Thus, for example, nursing is a professional culture, a hospital is a sociocultural institution, and a unit of a hospital can be viewed as a subculture.

Cultural groups have characteristics such as beliefs and values (e.g., health and illness beliefs and caring practices), ideals, norms (rules of behavior), controls and sanctions for social deviance, language, interaction patterns, dress, rituals, artifacts (technology), music and art, sociopolitical systems and processes, structure and function, and many others. Structure refers to social structure or configuration, such as the organizational structure of a modern corporation or the kinship structure of a tribal group. Function refers to the patterns of social relations among members of a group that influence behaviors of the members.

PHILOSOPHICAL PERSPECTIVES

All research proceeds from philosophy, articulated or not. The assumptions of the philosophy inform the conceptualization of the study, the research design and methods, the interpretation of findings, and the evaluation of scientific merit or trustworthiness of the research. Thus, there must be consistency in ontology (what is there to be known), epistemology (how knowledge is acquired), and methodology (how knowledge products are created) in any ethnographic study. Traditional or classical or conventional ethnography is in the tradition of natural science at the descriptive and relational levels of inquiry (Diers, 1979), as will be described later. In the late decades of the twentieth century, development of and refinements in postmodern philosophies such as critical theory and the feminisms have widened the utility of ethnography for answering cultural questions or addressing cultural problems. For example, critical ethnography or participatory ethnography is distinguished from conventional approaches by its focus on issues of injustice or social oppression. Although theory is developed from analysis of data, emphasis is also placed on participant activity in a more activist research project with a political purpose of aiding emancipatory or empowerment goals (Thomas, 1993; Denzin, 1997).

PARADIGMS (WORLD VIEWS)

The most fully developed theoretical model for cultural studies in nursing is that developed by Leininger, a nurse anthropologist (1985). Her ethnonursing research method, derived partly from ethnography, focuses on nursing phenomena from a cross-cultural perspective. The concepts of Leininger's Sunrise Model are interactive with care expressions, patterns, and practices and the holistic health or well-being of individuals, families, groups, communities, and institutions in diverse health systems. The latter would include generic or folk systems, nursing systems, and other professional health systems. Other nursing paradigms can be used to raise cultural questions for ethnographic research. For example, in Orem's Self-Care Framework (Orem, 1995), culture is one of the basic conditioning factors that the nurse must address in an assessment of the patient. In the Neuman Systems Model (Neuman, 1995), the sociocultural variable is one of five that make up the client–client system. When such conceptual models of nursing lead to cultural questions for inductive research, the ethnographer must bracket, or suspend (identify and set aside), the etic world view of the model during the period of data collection and analysis so as not to impose the framework on the culture and so that the emic perspective of culture members can be preserved. The researcher can then return to address the model during the final analysis and interpretive phases of the study. An example of this approach is found in Villaruel's (1995) ethnographic study of pain in Mexican Americans in which the Orem Self-Care Framework was used. In addition to the research findings of this focused ethnography, Villaruel and Denyes (1997) provided a qualitative test of the nursing model.

Anthropologic ethnographic paradigms in which culture is variously defined have been used by some nurse researchers to provide a foundation for a much needed body of cultural knowledge for nursing. These paradigms include the holistic (classic or traditional) paradigm that views cultures as wholes with interacting component groups (Jacob, 1988). The semiotic view, associated with ethnoscience ethnography, is also called componential analysis, or cognitive anthropology. This view looks at culture as located in the minds of people—that is, their ideas, beliefs, and knowledge that are expressed in the group's language and semantic system (ideational culture)—and is analyzed in domains of cultural knowledge (Spradley, 1979; Werner and Schoepfle, 1987a, 1987b; Morse, 1991). In symbolic anthropology, culture is viewed as a symbolic system made up of shared, identifiable symbols and meanings, embedded in thick description provided by members of a culture. This view is represented in the interpretive work of Clifford Geertz (1973) and others. Another world view is associated with cultural ecology and cultural materialism in which culture is viewed as an adaptive system and is considered in terms of a group's observable patterns of behavior, customs, and way of life (materialist culture). Fetterman (1998) noted that ethnographers need to know about aspects of both cultural behavior and ideational culture to describe a culture or subculture adequately. Ethnographers in the field listen to what people say (ideational culture), observe what people do (material culture), and what they make and use (artifacts). Anthropologic paradigms are in a continuous state of refinement (Sanday, 1983; Lett, 1987). Lett pointed out that, when problems overlap between paradigms, a purposeful and deliberate kind of eclecticism can offer complementary explanations.

ETHNOGRAPHY AND THEORY DEVELOPMENT

Ethnography contributes descriptive and explanatory theories of culture and cultural behaviors and meanings. Each ethnography is itself a descriptive theory of culture, broad in scope. Within the ethnography may be identified other middle-range theories such as typologies and hypotheses for further study. Successive levels of explanatory theory generated from holist research are presented by Reason (1981) as derived from Diesing (1971). In this pattern model of explanation, fieldwork data are analyzed and resultant themes are connected empirically in a network or pattern that, in turn, explains the human system in its context. The ethnographic account, then, describes and explains the kind of relations that the various parts have with each other.

One alternative model of theory development is Dier's (1979) presentation of levels of scientific inquiry. Ethnoscience ethnography can yield descriptive theory in the form of taxonomic analyses of particular domains of meaning or other types of classification theory. This type of research answers the question, What is this? It is at the factor-searching level of inquiry (level I) as are phase theories or staging theories. Exploratory, descriptive, relation-searching studies, such as holistic ethnography, are at the second level of scientific inquiry (level II) and answer the question, What's happening here (i.e., in this culture)? The search for themes or patterns through the study of the parts of a culture, the relationship of the parts to one another, and the relationship of the parts to the whole cultural context would result in descriptive and explanatory (factor-relating) theory. Traditional or conventional ethnography generally incorporates both these levels of inquiry, but its mode of relation-searching is qualitative rather than quantitative.

Thus, qualitative ethnography is theory generating and in the context of discovery, in contrast with studies that are theory testing and in the context of verification. The theory produced is grounded theory in that it is grounded in or derived from the empirical data of cultural description.

CLASSIFICATIONS OF ETHNOGRAPHY

Ethnography is difficult to classify owing to all the types and possible subtypes and the cross-cutting of classificatory principles. Werner and Schoepfle (1987a), proponents of ethnoscience, devised and reported a classification system for ethnography. In more common usage, some ethnographies are classified according to the discipline of origin, to an anthropological paradigm or theory such as cultural materialism, or to symbolic or cognitive anthropology (ethnoscience). Binary classifications include conventional or critical, urban or rural; narrative or visual (film or photographic); classic (holistic and usually book length) or focused (referring to time-limited exploratory studies within a fairly discrete community or organization and usually published as journal articles); and Leininger's (1985) mini and maxi types. Still others are classified according to the group participating, such as street drug dealers, the aged in day care, or African Americans; the space occupied or geographic setting, such as a village, a school, or a nursing practice center; the knowledge system or cognitive domain, such as how people define medical emergencies (Evaneshko and Kay, 1982); and the time, or temporal, unit such as life history or life health history. Some ethnographies would fall into multiple categories.

ETHICAL AND LEGAL CONSIDERATIONS

Possessing a nursing license may give greater access to a health care setting as a participant-observer to a nurse ethnographer than to other social scientists, but a nursing license also carries particular ethical and legal obligations. The ethical principles of respect for persons, beneficence, and justice, which are incorporated in *The Belmont Report* (Department of Health, Education and Welfare, 1979), must be adhered to in all research involving human subjects. However, the application of these principles is necessarily different in each ethnography, because the ethnographer interacts as a participant with live persons in constantly evolving, unpredictable human situations. Ethical issues and conflicts will undoubtedly arise. Although general issues may be surmised in advance, one does not know the specific issues before immersion in the culture. In general, ethical considerations in ethnography by nurse researchers require:

1. Obtaining initial informed consent from informants and renegotiating consent throughout the period of fieldwork. Specific written permission is usually required for tape-recording (audio and visual) and photographs. Recent laws in some states related to the HIV and AIDS epidemic require explicit permission to read patients' records and to speak to patients' visitors. Finding out about such rules from the institution's research review board or an equivalent is essential.
2. The protection of privacy, anonymity, and confidentiality of members of the subculture during the period of data collection and at the time of publication of the report while maintaining scientific integrity of the report.
3. Objectivity versus subjectivity with regard to selection, recording, and reporting phenomena.
4. Decisions regarding intervention versus nonintervention in the activities of the subculture.
5. Professional accountability for the legal and ethical components of the assumed participant-observer activities. This sometimes means walking a tightrope with regard to weighing the potential long-range benefits of the research vis-a-vis potential early termination from the setting if issues surrounding the protection of human subjects arise that cannot be resolved.
6. Potential use of findings due to power relations among various levels of the study population.

Germain (1985), Tilden (1980), and Munhall (in Chapter 19 of this book) offer further sources for examination of ethical issues in ethnography and other empirical, qualitative research.

With regard to legal aspects, the nurse ethnographer planning field research in a clinical setting should check to see that her or his professional liability policy applies in a nursing research role. The potential ethnographer is advised that field data in some jurisdictions are subject to subpoena. Thus, notes and tape recordings must be safeguarded, and the anonymity of the subjects and locations must be provided for through the use of pseudonyms in field notes and the final report. On the other hand, in some jurisdictions, one's scholarly status as a researcher makes some data legally privileged.

THE RESEARCH PROCESS

Basic components of the traditional ethnographic research process, modified for contemporary ethnography and modifiable for postmodern paradigms, have some general characteristics in common with interpretive paradigm research. However, certain distinctions are important for those who wish to do or to critique ethnography.

Aims

People's cultural knowledge is often unknown to them or taken for granted, and they do not have an opportunity to stand back from the exigencies of everyday life and examine pertinent aspects. Ethnographers seek answers to significant research questions that are aimed at explicating aspects of culture in context. The answers eventuate in cultural theory grounded in the knowledge that people use to organize their behavior and interpret their experience. Thus, ethnography aims to get at the implicit or latent (backstage) culture in addition to the explicit, public, or manifest (front-stage) aspects of culture.

The Research Problem

The cultural problem may be one about which little is known or about which there is disagreement, but one that requires context preservation for its understanding. Research questions are posed (rather than hypotheses for testing) that can best be addressed through descriptive analysis and interpretation of a particular culture or subcultural group. The researcher will be guided initially by broad questions addressing the ethnographic focus. These questions will take the general form of "What is this?" or "What's happening here in this subculture?" The direction of the research and the research questions are not as fixed ahead of time as they are with the more linear quantitative research designs. As the ethnographer becomes immersed in the culture, participants may provide data that lead to new, more meaningful questions for cultural understanding or to revisions of initial questions.

Review of the Literature

Because ethnography entails exploration, an extensive data-based literature is not expected to be available on the particular research focus. As Spradley (1979) stated, "Ethnography starts with a conscious attitude of almost complete ignorance" (p. 4). However, a critical review of sources that led to the selection of the problem to be studied at this exploratory level should be provided, although this literature may be largely conceptual rather than data based. The pulling together of threads or themes from a number of diverse sources may provide the theoretical perspective or framework for examining the complex human situations for which ethnography is most appropriate. In the final analysis and interpretation phases of the study, another literature review is conducted for comparison of findings with existing or new literature.

The Setting

For nursing, the setting for ethnography can be wherever there are people and activities that give rise to cultural questions related to nursing and health care that need to be addressed in a holistic context, including people's homes. The researcher must have the means to know and make the effort to know that significant data are obtainable in a particular setting but need not have prior experience in the setting. In fact, studying a familiar setting or one's own work setting poses significant risks to the integrity of the study.

Pilot studies are not characteristic of ethnography, because meanings are emphasized rather than surface data and trust needs to be built over time with informants to get meaningful data in context. Entering the field as a reflective stranger and learner who has identified and set aside theoretical and experiential knowledge reduces the risk of bias and improves trustworthiness of the study. Fetterman (1998) advised that the ethnographer should go to the field with an open mind but not an empty head!

The ethnographer needs to understand and allow for the possibility of a degree of culture shock even when the culture is not entirely unfamiliar. Culture-shock is a stress reaction brought on by a person's inability to understand or control a new cultural situation, accompanied by the loss of usual social supports. In moderation, culture shock is not negative, because it allows the ethnographer to get the feel as well as the facts and subsides as skills appropriate to the new environment or situation are acquired.

Participants or Informants

Either of these terms is used rather than the term "subjects," which is not part of the language of interpretive research. All who provide data are informants. However, in ethnography, the term informant does not carry the sometimes pejorative connotation of the common use of the term. Key informants and other informants are culture bearers and participants who are very much a part of the research process. Primary informants are those who are directly associated with the focus of the research in a major way. Secondary informants make significant contributions to the sociocultural context but may be peripherally associated with the focus of the study. Because the ethnographer is interested in peoples' perceptions of their own situations, members of the subculture who provide such data are viewed as coparticipants in the research process. These people are selected because they know their community well, including its members, language, history, rituals, and backstage data, and can teach the researcher about them. It is essential to get as much informant description as possible, to cross-validate informants' perceptions, and for the researcher to validate his or her own perceptions with key informants.

Informants have various motivations for participating in a research enterprise that requires a time commitment and possibly some risks. These motivations may include pride in sharing aspects of one's culture, curiosity, commitment to science as an enterprise, the opportunity to share feelings and concerns, or a break from the routine aspects of the cultural scene. Some informants may turn out to have a personal agenda that leads to embellishment of information or a need to tell the ethnographer what they think the ethnographer wants to hear. This is one reason why cross-checking and validation of perceptions with multiple informants is necessary.

Gaining Access

It is very helpful to know at least one insider or facilitator who can provide initial access to the research setting. However, several levels of clearance and consent may be required before an ethnographer can enter a subculture or culture to initiate field study. The prefieldwork phase is time consuming but essential so that the members of the subculture can become aware of, and supportive of, the primacy of the research role of this stranger to their setting. Access rules, such as the frequency and hours of coming and going, the means of identification of the ethnographer, permission to take photographs or use technical recording devices, and determination of what data sources are absolutely off limits must be worked out in advance insofar as possible. A private place, however small, to which the ethnographer can withdraw to write field notes should be sought. Role negotiation regarding the expected type of participant-observation activities are especially important when the ethnographer is a nurse in a health care setting.

A liaison person, or key informant, may be identified at this time to guide the researcher's entry and orientation to aspects of the culture, to fulfill the gatekeeper role for the duration of the study, and to introduce the researcher to other key informants who can serve as guides and provide crucial data. A key informant can also assure members of the culture that the researcher is safe to have around.

Sampling

No ethnography is ever a complete picture of a subculture. The sample is that part of the reality that is observed and recorded. Sampling is done of events, activities, informants, documents, and other data sources. Because the best cultural informants are sought, that is, those who can "tell it like it is," random sampling or systematic sampling of informants is not appropriate. The sampling principle is based not on numbers of interviews or events but rather on the richness of the data—that is, how accurately the data portray the full context of the culture as well as answers to the research questions. These research questions provide direction for the ethnographer's selection and involvement in the scenes of the subculture.

Informant sampling and event sampling are initially purposive and opportunistic. Time sampling may be appropriate in some situations. The ethnographer seeks out persons, events, places, documents, and other sources that provide the greatest opportunities to gather the most relevant data. Fetterman (1998) calls this type of sampling stratified judgment sampling. Sampling becomes, however, increasingly theoretical—that is, directed by ongoing data analysis, logic, and aim.

Data Collection

Participant-observation (see next subsection) is the major data-collection method of ethnography, and, because actively participating in some way in the experience and actions of others to find meaning necessitates interpersonal and group interaction, interviewing members of the subculture is likewise an essential component. Thus, the ethnographer is the primary research instrument. The ethnographer seeks *emic*, or insider, answers to research questions and aims to capture the cultural context in rich, particularizing detail by observing and participating in the events of the culture or subculture. With the help of the group's members, the ethnographer looks for patterns, connections, relationships, and themes related to the research focus that have meaning for the people.

Although all ethnography entails participant-observation, not all research called participant-observation research aims at producing ethnography. Likewise, although all ethnography deals with culture, not all cultural research need be, or is, ethnography. The adjective "ethnographic" refers to culture in a general sense, including the gathering of cultural data in very brief encounters with individuals or communities. "Doing ethnography" refers to prolonged, systematic, in-depth field study.

Other methods of data collection such as documentary analysis and oral history may supplement these major methods. This triangulation of data-collection methods and data sources enables the researcher to obtain the widest range of perspectives on issues as well as to obtain a complete data set.

Although some ethnographers may choose to employ closed-ended measurement tools such as questionnaires or personality inventories, there are limitations to the use of these tools when a sole researcher studies a complex part of society. A team of ethnographers would facilitate intercoder reliability and mutual support, but teams are expensive, and with a team, there is also the risk of loss of the intimate, trusting relationships built up over time that are an essential part of the ethnographic process. Moreover, the essence of ethnography is the discovery of the way of life and the meaning of events and relationships to the people, from their point of view, rather than through the use of tools developed from a priori assumptions. Quantitative measures are associated with empiricist paradigm research, not with the paradigm of ethnographer as instrument. When such design and methodological triangulation is used, the principle is to remain consistent to the paradigm assumptions of each component.

Because the ethnographer accumulates a very large data set, it is wise to seek funding for the study, if only for the transcription of tape-recorded data. A laptop computer taken to the field would eliminate the need for transcription and its costs. Another pragmatic consideration is the selection of a qualitative software package for data management. This selection should be done in the preparatory period for an extensive field study so that some skill in its use can be achieved by the time data collection starts. Additionally, a labeling system should be devised for all data sources—that is, participant-observations, interviews, oral histories, and field notes. Data should be paginated and identified by date, time, place (by pseudonym), event or activity, pseudonym of person(s), and brief focus.

Participant-observation.   Participant-observation means immersion of the researcher in the cultural data of the field. The ethnographer must work out a participant role that enhances data collection and blends in with the life of the people being studied. The researcher attempts to become a part of the culture or subculture by participating in a low-keyed manner so as to induce as little change as possible. The stance is one of a listener and learner. Participant-observation allows the researcher to look beyond statements of ideal behavior (cognitive conceptualization of culture) to observe behaviors directly (behavioral conceptualization of culture) so that the correspondence or the discrepancy between the real and ideal cultural statements can be described, assessed, and explained.

Data obtained through participant-observation are recorded as close to verbatim as possible and in specific, concrete, and particularistic detail. If a laptop computer is not available or cannot be used and if taking notes during an event is impossible or inappropriate, brief notes may be jotted down (condensed notes) and, as soon as possible, expanded to include a full description of the participant-observation or interview experience, taking care not to rephrase the local language or to move to higher levels of abstraction.

Junker (1960, pp. 35–38) described a continuum of participant-observation and noted that the practicing fieldworker oscillates through this range in the course of the study. Major points on the continuum, adapted from Junker on the basis of the author's experiences as a nurse ethnographer, are:

- *Complete observer*: In this role, the fieldworker may be visible but does not interact with those being observed, for example, in a meeting of a board of directors, when only consent to observe has been given or when professionally "hanging around" (nonparticipant observation). Invisible observation may be accomplished through a one-way window or a hidden vantage point (the potted palm technique) or through the use of cameras, ethics permitting. Sometimes it is necessary for a nurse ethnographer to figuratively sit on her hands so as to not intervene when only observation is in order. On the other hand, to continue to use only observation without interaction or participation assumes that the researcher can interpret the experiences of others without their input.

- *Observer as participant*: The research role of the observer is publicly known at the outset and the research is intentionally not kept under wraps. This role may provide access to a wide range of information, and even secrets (or back-region data) may be made available when the researcher becomes known for guarding confidential information. The researcher can be selective with regard to observation and participation and has the flexibility to move about opportunistically as the research demands.
- *Participant as observer*: The research role is not wholly concealed, but the research activities are subordinated to the person's primary role in the setting, which may be as an employee. Because of job responsibilities, this role may limit the researcher's flexibility in movement to events that maximize data collection and may also limit access to certain kinds of information, especially backstage or back-region information, which fellow workers might be reluctant to share.
- *Complete participant*: When this role is deliberate, the participant-observer's identity as a researcher is intentionally concealed as he or she attempts to become a full-fledged member of the group under study. In today's research scene, a deliberately deceptive role is considered to be unethical, because it violates the principle of informed consent of study participants. However, this role is sometimes inadvertent, such as when some noncentral and anonymous persons in an isolated event or activity in the subculture do not realize that a study is being conducted and when it is not wise to interrupt such activities to explain the study. It may also be used when the participants' identities are not in jeopardy, as, for example, in a study of gambling behavior when no individual person and no specifics about the location are made known.

Leininger (1985) and Spradley (1980) provided variations of the preceding version of the participant-observation continuum.

The ongoing analysis of data guides movement on the continuum of participant-observation, which is also influenced by the design of the study, the research purpose and problem(s), the aspect of the culture being studied, and the background and ability of the ethnographer to assume tasks that are a natural part of the subculture. Bruyn (1966), a sociologist, pointed out that, whereas the traditional research scientist's role is:

. . . that of a neutral observer who remains unmoved, unchanged, and untouched in his examination of phenomena, the role of the participant-observer requires sharing the sentiments of people in social situations; as a consequence he himself is changed as well as changing to some degree the situation in which he is a participant. (p. 14)

For the researcher, the important point is to record these changes and use them as part of the data being analyzed.

Field Journal

Engaging in the activities of another culture or subculture through participant-observation and trying to find meaning in the behaviors of others demand considerable introspection on the part of the ethnographer, who, by the accumulation of education and life experiences, brings his or her own cultural perspectives (*etic*) to the field. Quint (1968), a nurse sociologist, emphasized that, when doing participant-observation, it is necessary "to use one's inner conflicts and biases as an essential part of the data being collected" (p. 12). Thus, in addition to the record of participant observations, field notes, and written or transcribed records of interviews, it is recommended that participant-observers keep a record of feelings, reactions, biases, and other results of introspection. This process is sometimes referred to as reflexivity. Different sections of the overall field journal can be dedicated to memoranda related to theoretical insights, ideas for theoretical sampling, ethical issues, and the fieldworker's reflective responses to the experience. Agar (1986) stated that "ethnography is neither 'subjective' nor 'objective.' It is interpretive, mediating two worlds through a third" (p. 19).

Interviewing

In-depth interviewing, formal and informal, structured, semistructured, and unstructured, of individual or group informants is essential to grasp the native's point of view, as well as to clarify discrepancies among members of the subculture or between the researcher's perceptions and a member's perceptions. Formal interviews have purpose, structure, and appointed times. Probes are used to get responses to specific questions, to encourage the sharing of detailed information about specific events, and to obtain further clarification on certain topics. Often qualitative (ethnographic) interviews contain less structure than is contained in the use of formalized open-ended questions. As Evaneshko and Kay (1982) noted, "Ethnographic inquiry is different from openended interviews in that the latter [are] structured to stay within preestablished general guidelines, while the former is more free roaming and pursues promising avenues of cultural knowledge suggested by the informant's remarks" (p. 53). This type of inquiry not only permits the researcher to get essential questions answered, but also allows for unexpected data. One device that can be used to ensure that the ethnographer's essential questions or issues are addressed is to list them on a card, unobtrusively glance at the list periodically, and use gentle probes if the interviewee does not address a topic spontaneously. Fieldwork often dictates that many interviews are "on the hoof"; that is, questioning of informants takes place while the ethnographer accompanies them in the natural course of cultural activities.

Supplementary Data Sources

Because ethnography frequently embraces change over time and across situations, past events may require analysis to determine their influence on current behaviors. Thus, archival data, oral life histories, and personal diaries or other written narratives may be used. Qualitative content analysis of such documents as minutes of meetings, policies and procedures, newsletters, newspaper articles, or patient records (including relevant numeric data) also may provide important information. Examining formal hierarchical or kinship structures, linguistics, cultural artifacts (technology), photographs, or films may add to an understanding of the culture under study.

Reciprocity

Good fieldwork relationships call for some kind of reciprocity on the part of the ethnographer. This reciprocity can take many forms, such as being a volunteer driver for a community shelter's residents where research is being conducted or providing printed literature when technical information resources are not available to participants. Role reciprocity enhances data collection and need not interfere with objectivity if change induced by the researcher is minimal.

Phases of Fieldwork

Being in the field may mean that a researcher actually lives for a period of time with the people being studied or spends a certain amount of time in the subculture as a participant-observer on a regular basis over a prolonged period of time such as 2 or 3 hours, three times a week, with flexibility in scheduling to maximize data collection. For studies done in people's homes or in schools, flexibility may be limited, but arrangements must be made to have access to crucial events.

During the initial phase of fieldwork, the ethnographer learns about the culture by asking questions and seeking clarification and explanations from cultural informants. She or he obtains a broad overview of the situation, writing detailed field notes or descriptive accounts of what, in general, goes on there. Some demographic data are collected as well to describe relevant characteristics of the primary members of the subculture. A system of pseudonyms for persons and places is initiated. What people say, how they act, their cultural artifacts, and available information about the structure, function, and sociopolitical system of the group are recorded. The setting is mapped, and spatial, physical, and other characteristics of the environment are recorded. Historical data may be relevant to the current context, thus accessing archival data may be necessary.

Building trusting relationships is essential during this initial period so that, over the long term, quality data may be obtained. It has been suggested that ethnographers might distort events by their mere presence, because people may act guarded and reserved, but the experience of ethnographers has been that after a few days the people of the subculture must focus their energy and attention on the usual events of the culture. The ethnographer who acts in the agreed-upon participant-observer role competently and provides appropriate reciprocity tends to blend into the background, so to speak. After this initial period of general observation and involvement in the activities of the subculture, the researcher may note the need for refining or revising the research questions.

Subsequent to this initial phase, data collection often continues to be exciting and intriguing, and fieldworkers, especially those who like clinical nursing situations, are attracted to spending considerable time in the field. However, Berg (1989) noted that 2 hours of data collection may require as long as 8 hours to expand into comprehensive field notes. Thus, trips to the field should be goal oriented. The researcher samples the total scene or population of data, depending on the research focus, which is guided by the research questions and ongoing data analysis. The occurrence of significant cultural events and the amount of time demanding the researcher's presence to obtain a valid sample of the scene are very important considerations in planning time in the field. For example, an ethnography with a focus on registered nurse role behavior in the subculture of a hospital acute care unit would necessitate sampling all three shifts probably over at least a 1-year period because there are notable seasonal variations in hospital life.

The actual length of time in the fieldwork phase of a study varies according to the research questions, the complexity of the subculture, the building of relationships with key informants, the access to significant data, and the seasonal or cyclic variations that influence the subculture. Generally, 1 year in the field is the rule of thumb for holistic ethnography. It is considered a reasonable time in which to be accepted by persons in a relatively complex subculture, to learn its manifest and latent aspects, to attend to a wide variety of the subculture's activities, to see members in various contexts, to conduct theoretical sampling, and to follow certain events to their conclusions. In-depth knowledge of the subculture rather than surface familiarity with it is the goal. In school nursing studies, the academic year would be the rule of thumb. Shorter time in the field would be appropriate for less-complex cultures or focused ethnography or for studies of seasonal employees, for example.

Collection of data and preliminary data analysis proceed simultaneously. This process of data collection and analysis in ethnography has been described as dialectical or cyclical, compared with the linear model of hypothetico-deductive studies. As coding of data and categorization proceed (see next two sections), persons, events, and other sources are more deliberately chosen (theoretical sampling) on the basis of the data analysis. Although some general descriptive observations may continue until the end of the study, deliberate or focused sampling is necessary to validate or compare data, to cover the entire range of the phenomena under study, to fill in gaps in the data, and to seek negative cases—that is, those that do not support or that refute the developing theory. The ethnographer's cultural inferences, formed through observing, participating, listening, and analyzing, are working hypotheses that must be tested repeatedly until there is validation that people have in common a particular system of meanings.

There is a search for patterns, gradually discovered, and then interrelated with other patterns. When no new data add to the emergent themes or patterns and no new dimensions or insights are identified that can shed light on the research questions—that is, the point of data saturation or theory saturation has been reached—the active fieldwork phase ends.

Although the study of complex cultures could go on and on, pragmatic considerations may be determining factors in the cessation of data collection. Pragmatic considerations carry the risk of lessening the theoretical value of the study. Finances, the demands of other types of work or life activities, the end of a sabbatical, or a dissertation deadline are examples of such pragmatic considerations.

Role disengagement must be incorporated into the final phase. Termination of fieldwork means terminating relationships built over a long period of time. The members of the subculture, as well as the fieldworker, need preparation for this departure. Whenever possible, arrangements should be made by the researcher to continue contact in some way with informants or to make forays back into the field during the final analysis and writing period for clarification, verification, validation, or closure on certain issues. The members of the subculture and the ethnographer also need to develop a plan for sharing the outcomes of the study.

Data Management

All data from all sources make up the ethnographic journal or record. Processing the data immediately after each visit is time consuming but important because it allows for ongoing review of data and assists the researcher in establishing goals for subsequent visits. The time-consuming and tedious tasks of storing codes, cutting, sorting, indexing, cross-referencing, filing, retrieval, and other aspects of data management can be greatly reduced with computer technology (Weitzman, 1999), including qualitative data management software. But it must be understood that, although software can facilitate data management, data analysis is done in the mind of the researcher.

As soon as possible, it is wise for the fieldworker to type field data not already on diskette into a word processor (or to have an assistant do it) and to store one hard copy in a confidential but secure and separate location to guard against loss. Another intact set provides a working copy. Typing field notes double-spaced on one-half or three-quarters of the horizontal measure of a page leaves room in the wide margin for codes and for jotting down notes or questions. Transcribed data must be reviewed with the original recording. Each page of data should be numbered and labeled with the critical identifiers previously described (pp. 288–289).

If a computer software package for qualitative data management (Weitzman, 1999), such as THE ETHNOGRAPH (Seidel, 1998), is not used for enhanced data management, additional copies of data are necessary for cutting and sorting into file folders or some other convenient cross-referencing system after coding and categorizing of data have been done. Ethnographers who are computer skilled can also develop their own data management systems.

Several graphic display devices presented by Miles and Huberman (1994) may aid data reduction, analysis, and conceptualization.

Data Analysis

The entire ethnographic record or field journal is subjected to analysis. The ethnographer uses primarily qualitative content analysis to inductively derive patterns or themes from the data. Although there is no single way to conduct qualitative content analysis, there are basic steps and guidelines.

Coding of data from the seemingly immense volume of qualitative information contained in field notes and interviews is the first step in the analysis process and is essential for moving from the concrete raw data to higher levels of abstraction. Codes are labels assigned to units of meaning. These units will vary with the type of data. A meaningful unit may appear in a line (especially with dense interview data), a sentence, a paragraph, or a larger section of data. Initial codes are succinct but in the language of the raw data itself. Coding is critical because it provides the direct link with the concrete data of the cultural reality. There may be overcoding in the early stages of analysis in an effort to retain as much relevant information as possible. Recoding may be necessary as data accumulate and comparisons of new codes with early codes are made.

Codes are compared, and similar codes are grouped into categories. Categories might be, for example, responses of a particular type, systems of relationships, stages of a process, the varieties of a behavior such as gestures of deference, and so on. Although the phrase, "categories emerged from the data," is often used with regard to the outcomes of qualitative analysis, in fact, categories do not emerge spontaneously. They are identified and worked out by a careful mental process of logical analysis of content from all data sources. Categories are then compared and clustered. Care must be taken not to leap to codes or from codes to categories or from categories to clusters on the basis of the etic knowledge of the researcher.

The processed data are reviewed periodically for emergent concepts, typifications, themes, and patterns. Theoretical memoranda, kept in the field journal, assist this movement from the concrete to higher levels of abstraction. Variations that are recurrent but atypical must be accounted for as well. Every culture has occasional aberrations that may prove to have future relevance.

Qualitative researchers resist imposing a priori theoretical schema on the data, because this imposition violates the principles of induction. Nevertheless, an alternative analysis system using the codes of the Human Relations Area Files (HRAF; Lagace, 1974) has been used by some ethnographers. The HRAF comprises both a major cultural data archive or ethnographic data bank and a system for the rapid and accurate retrieval of data on specific cultures and topics. More than 310 cultural units are represented in files arranged according to a special subject-classification system consisting of more than 700 numbered subject categories grouped into 79 major topical selections. The HRAF is located at several major universities throughout the United States. The recent process of transferring these files from written text to CD-ROM enhances accessibility of this ethnographic source.

Although the process of coding, categorizing, and questioning the data takes place throughout the data-collection phase, the major work of analysis and interpretation takes place after leaving the field and is guided by the assumptions and research questions. As long a period of time may be needed for the final intensive analysis, synthesis, and writing of the ethnography as was spent in the field. Werner and Schoepfle (1987b) estimated that a one-year ethnographic field study may generate 3000 pages of transcription, and an ethnography drawn from this database may have 300 pages, or a 1:10 data reduction.

Comparing, contrasting, analyzing, and synthesizing take time and considerable mental effort. Subjective meanings of members of the subculture, verified through the observer's work, serve as a basis for the drawing of cultural inferences, which, it should be remembered, are the researcher's meanings of the meanings communicated by informants. That is, although the descriptive data are provided by members of the subculture and can be validated by them, the final analysis and conclusions are the researcher's, guided by his or her own theoretical (etic) perspectives.

In the course of the final analysis, comparisons with existing ethnographies and other midrange theories are made. Existing theories may be supported or refuted and new midrange theories, in addition to the descriptive and explanatory theory of culture (the ethnography), may be induced.

Writing the Ethnography

Because of the value of context preservation, ethnographies are lengthy and are often presented as books or monographs or on film or videotape. Journal articles may provide a condensed summary of a holistic ethnography, or they may report a focused ethnography. These reports can be found in such journals as *Western Journal of Nursing Research*, *Research in Nursing and Health*, *Journal of Transcultural Nursing*, *Human*

Organization, Journal of Contemporary Ethnography, Biomedical Anthropology, Qualitative Health Research, and *Sociology of Health and Illness.*

Liebow's (1967) *Tally's Corner,* Gans's (1962) *The Urban Villagers,* and Fadiman's (1997) *The Spirit Catches You and You Fall Down,* are examples of ethnographies of subcultures of American society. Examples of nursing ethnographies in books are: Germain's (1979) *The Cancer Unit: An Ethnography;* Kayser-Jones's (1981) *Old, Alone, and Neglected,* a comparative study of a nursing home in Scotland and one in the United States; Wolf's (1988) *Nurses' Work, The Sacred and the Profane,* a study of nursing rituals in a large, urban hospital; and Street's *Inside Nursing,* a critical ethnography of clinical nursing practice in Australia. Kay (1982) edited a book containing multiple ethnographies of human birth. Morse (1992) edited a book containing several examples of traditional and ethnoscience ethnography.

Ethnography is usually reported in narrative, literary style to preserve the flavor and nuances of the cultural scene. This style allows an expression of the world of meaning. Each ethnography contains multiple levels of abstraction, ranging from raw data providing evidence of the native's point of view to constructed taxonomies, cultural inferences, analysis, conclusions, and problems or hypotheses for further study. Maps, diagrams, and tables of demographic data may be included to enhance the narrative.

Styles of reporting ethnography vary, as do styles of doing ethnography. Some analysis, for example, may be incorporated within the thick description and more completely emphasized in a separate, final section. This opportunity for creativity and the flexibility in reporting style compared with the usual style of quantitative reports is what makes ethnography challenging to write and, if well written, easy to read. If an ethnography is easily read, it is not because the study and the writing of the report were easy to do; rather, it is a mark of the ethnographer's ability to synthesize and write in a style that facilitates reading while preserving scientific adequacy. Bruyn (1966) suggested that "the participant-observer must remain a scientist with the insights of a Shakespearean dramatist" (p. 253). The well-done ethnography draws the reader into the feeling as well as the facts of the culture.

The nature of the final report is affected not only by the background and style of the ethnographer and the group described, but also by the intended audience. The ethnographer must decide, for example, if the ethnography is intended primarily for other scientists, a dissertation committee, an employer who commissions a study, the educated lay public, or a combination of several or all of them. In addition to the descriptive analysis and interpretation of the culture, each presentation of an ethnography should include a description of the methodology as well as changes that the ethnographer underwent as a result of the research enterprise.

Ethnographers may intend to make a contribution to knowledge for its own sake. In this case, making recommendations for culture change within the report may be inappropriate. However, applied ethnographers or action ethnographers may not only aim to make a theory contribution to cultural understanding, but will also ask themselves how this knowledge advances the cause or serves the needs of humankind (Spradley, 1980, p. 19). Thus, some ethnographies may contain the researcher's recommendations for change, but some ethnographers may actually engage with participants in a cultural change project. Informed by ethnographic findings, they will make preassessments, apply an intervention, collect data throughout, take postmeasures, evaluate outcomes, and include them in the ethnographic report. This has been done, for example, in fishing and farming communities to increase local productivity. Although these studies are intervention studies, they are not causal hypothesis-testing studies in the empiricist tradition. Rather they are in the tradition of postmodernist participatory ethnography, using the diverse perspectives of participatory action research, action research, or participatory research (Thomas, 1993, Chap. 2). Research using these perspectives is certainly relevant to nursing's advocacy mission, particularly in community-based settings.

Criteria for Scientific Adequacy

Ethnographers are as concerned as other scientists that their work meet criteria for scientific merit, or trustworthiness, appropriate to the level and type of inquiry. Explicit standards for assessing scientific adequacy of ethnography have changed over time. For example, Bruyn (1966, pp. 180–185) cited six criteria of subjective adequacy for making interpretations in community studies. These criteria are: (1) the time that a researcher spends with a group; (2) place, or actual observation of subjects in their everyday lives; (3) social circumstances, or the variety of social settings, roles, and activities witnessed; (4) language, or the understanding of different connotations, phrasings, and sentence structures in daily use; (5) intimacy of the encounters; and (6) consensus, or "confirmation in the context" that the meanings interpreted by the observer are correct. Germain (1979), in her ethnographic study of a cancer unit, provided an example of how these criteria were addressed.

Traditional criteria for ethnography include validity and reliability. In the following treatment, traditional criteria are presented first and are followed by a fusion of traditional criteria with the more contemporary generic criteria for naturalistic inquiries of Lincoln and Guba (1985), as modified by nurse authors Catanzaro and Olshansky (1988) and Sandelowski (1986).

Validity.   Validity is the primary criterion of good ethnography. The test of validity in ethnography is how accurately the instrument (the researcher) captures (measures) the observed reality and portrays this reality in the research report. *Face validity* is established by the assumption that members selected as informants to represent the subculture have expert knowledge in certain cultural components. *Content validity* is established through verification with as many cultural informants as possible.

Sample selection bias, observer bias, accuracy in recording field notes, analytical accuracy, and bias in reporting affect internal validity, as do historical and maturation factors. In the course of a study, for example, the motives of informants may change, their positions or statuses may be altered, and commitment to the project may wane.

External validity, or *generalizability*, of ethnography is sometimes criticized by those who regard its contribution to be a study of a single case. A response to this criticism is that an in-depth study of a situation over a long period of time is more generative of insights than are broad surveys or the experimental study of variables in isolation from meaningful context. Burgess (1966), cited in Denzin (1978), explained that, in the sense that a single specimen is representative of its kind or species and is typical (belonging to a type), a case may be made for some degree of generalization to other specimens of a similar type or class of units. Benoliel (1984) noted that two important assumptions underlying the qualitative paradigm are the importance of understanding the situation from the participants themselves and believing that truth ultimately rests on the direct experience of individuals.

External validity, or *transferability*, or "fittingness" is obtained when findings fit other contexts as judged by readers or when readers find the report meaningful in regard to their own experience. Thick description and verbatim quotations in the report increase transferability.

Internal validity, *credibility*, or *truth value* is enhanced by the ethnographer's direct and repeated involvement in the scenes of the culture, the selection of key informants who have cultural expertise, the testing of inferences (working hypotheses) until there is validation that meanings are common to all, and the verification of information with as many informants as possible. Validity can be affected by the researcher's sample-selection bias, observer bias, accuracy in recording field notes, bias in selecting what to report, and ability to assess that informants are accurate portrayers of their culture. The researcher's field journal is examined by an auditor for evidence of biases made explicit. In addition to prolonged engagement and persistent observation in the field, validity, credibility, or truth value is established through triangulation processes, through peer or colleague debriefing whereby the ethnographer's analyses and interpretations can be challenged and the soundness of working hypotheses and future plans can be assessed, and through negative case analysis in which there is testing and refining of working hypotheses until the final version is consistent with all observations of the phenomenon without exception. Referential adequacy is accomplished by storing a selection of raw data and then later retrieving it so that it can be analyzed and compared with similar data previously analyzed.

Reliability. Reliability traditionally pertains to the consistency of both the sources of data, including participants and the researcher, and the methods of data collection. One cannot literally replicate an ethnography, because there is no way to capture time, but a good ethnography presents what can be expected to occur. Frake (cited in Spradley, 1980) stated that the adequacy of ethnography is to be evaluated "by the ability of a stranger to the culture (who may be the ethnographer) to use the ethnographer's statements as instructions for appropriately anticipating the scenes of the society" (p. 10).

Reliability, dependability, consistency, or *auditibility* is enhanced by asking the same questions of different informants over a long period of time and in different circumstances, obtaining repeatability of data over time from each key informant, carefully matching what informants say with their observed behavior, and seeking explanations for discrepancies. In interviewing, the researcher purposely varies approaches with individual informants to enhance credibility of data. Reliability, dependability, or consistency is also established through peer debriefing and through referential adequacy as above.

Inquiry audits—formal assessments of all processes by an expert—may be conducted on all components of the field journal, as well as the products of analysis at several points in the data-collection and analysis stages. Confirmability audits are conducted when the project is nearing completion and at its completion to determine if the findings and conclusions are supported by the data. Guidelines for inquiry and confirmability audits were presented by Lincoln and Guba (1985).

Preparation for Ethnography

Researchers contemplating ethnography must like to learn about the culture and life style of others and be comfortable in the learner's role of asking many questions in settings where the action is, such as in the real worlds of clinical nursing practice. It helps to have a high tolerance for uncertainty and ambiguity as well as the ability to withstand the cultural shock, including actual symptoms of illness, that occurs to some degree when entering a new territory. A nurse standing back and observing the cultural scenes of nursing practice is not immune to culture shock. A somewhat laid-back personality that enables one to develop and maintain a stance of detached involvement—that is, being authentic and identifying with the community but still maintaining professional distance from it—is crucial. Flexibility and a sense of time appropriateness in regard to asking questions of individuals or rescheduling interviews are essential to obtaining significant data. Obviously, the ethnographer must be able to build trusting relationships with informants by keeping data confidential. And after the excitement of data collection in the field, patience is essential for the lengthy and often tedious final analytic process. The ethnographer must not only like to collect and process data, but have the ability and interest in writing a research document in a stylistic literary fashion—that is, primarily in word symbols rather than numeric symbols.

Doing ethnography is often a lonely though very rich and growth-producing experience. There are threats to physical safety, as well as physiological, emotional, and potentially legal and ethical risks. Informants in the field may be friendly and helpful, but they cannot provide the necessary kind of ongoing support that is helpful on such a journey. A personal and collegial support system outside the field, a sense of humor, and a great deal of work space in one's home or office for stacks of field notes and resource materials are necessary. To prepare for such a peak adventure one can use course work, supervised fieldwork exercises, peer/colleague support, an experienced ethnographer adviser, and a habit of reading ethnographies. From the plethora of methods texts, selecting a few favored guides for the journey is important. The Council on Nursing and Anthropology (CONAA) is a support group for qualitative nurse researchers in addition to its primary scientific mission. Many of the current members are ethnographers.

Being a nurse ethnographer in a health care setting has advantages: it enables the capturing of nuances and the selection of data that might be missed or deemed insignificant by a nonnurse ethnographer. Nurse ethnographers also have the advantage of having been trained in interviewing skills, being accustomed to entering different subcultures for clinical experiences, knowing the language of health care, and having a degree of comfort in health care situations that may ease though not entirely eliminate cultural shock.

RELEVANCE FOR NURSING

Besides contributing descriptive and explanatory theory and possibly hypotheses for further study, ethnographic research of nursing practice can be a source of insights useful for promoting cultural change to improve nursing practice systems, for presenting health care and nursing practice realities to the scientific and lay communities, for influencing health policy, and for addressing a wide range of human problems in our society and its health care systems. Additionally, multiple, comparative, transcultural ethnographies of nursing situations having a similar focus would contribute to a worldwide ethnology of nursing. And each ethnography of nursing, with its vivid detailed description, becomes a piece of nursing history.

REFERENCES

Agar, M. (1986). *Speaking of ethnography*. Newbury Park, CA: Sage.

Benoliel, J. Q. (1984). Advancing nursing science: Qualitative approaches. *Western Journal of Nursing Research, 6*(3), 1–8.

Berg, G. (1989). *Qualitative research methods for the social sciences*. Boston: Allyn & Bacon.

Bruyn, S. (1966). *The human perspective in sociology*. Englewood Cliffs, NJ: Prentice-Hall.

Burgess, E. (1966). "Discussion." In C. Shaw (Ed.), *The jack roller* (pp. 185–197). Chicago: University of Chicago Press.

Catanzaro, M., & Olshansky, E. (1988). Evaluating research reports. In N.F. Woods & M. Catanzaro (Eds.), *Nursing research: Theory and practice* (pp. 469–478). St. Louis: Mosby.

Denzin, N. (1978). *The research act* (2nd ed.). New York: McGraw-Hill.

Denzin, N. (1997). *Interpretive ethnography: Ethnographic practices for the 21st century.* Thousand Oaks, CA: Sage.

Department of Health, Education, and Welfare. (1979). *The Belmont report: Ethical principles and guidelines for the protection of human subjects of research* (GPO 887-809). Washington, DC: U.S. Government Printing Office.

Diers, D. (1979). *Research in nursing practice.* Philadelphia: Lippincott.

Diesing, P. (1971). *Patterns of discovery in the social sciences.* New York: Aldine.

Evaneshko, V., & Kay, M. (1982). The ethnoscience research technique. *Western Journal of Nursing Research, 4,* 49–64.

Fadiman, A. (1997). *The spirit catches you and you fall down: A Hmong child, her American doctors and the collision of two cultures.* New York: Farrar, Straus & Giroux.

Fetterman, D. (1998). *Ethnography: Step by step* (2nd ed.). Thousand Oaks, CA: Sage.

Frake, C. (1964). Structural description of Subanum religious behavior. In W. Goodenough (Ed.), *Explorations in cultural anthropology* (pp. 111–130). New York: McGraw-Hill.

Gans, H. (1962). *The urban villagers.* New York: Free Press.

Geertz, C. (1973). *The interpretation of cultures.* New York: Basic Books.

Gehring, F. (1973). Anthropology and education. In J. Honigman (Ed.), *Handbook of social and cultural anthropology.* Chicago: Rand McNally.

Germain, C. (1979/1982). *The cancer unit: An ethnography.* Wakefield, MA: Nursing Resources, Inc.; Rockville, MD: Aspen.

Germain, C. (1985). Ethical considerations for the nurse ethnographer doing field research in clinical settings. In A. Carmi (Ed.), *Medicolegal library: Vol. 4. Nursing law and ethics.* Heidelberg: Springer Verlag.

Jacob, E. (1988). Clarifying qualitative research: A focus on traditions. *Educational Researcher, 17,* 16–24.

Junker, B. (1960). *Field work.* Chicago: University of Chicago Press.

Kay, M. (Ed.). (1982). *Anthropology of human birth.* Philadelphia: F. A. Davis.

Kayser-Jones, J. (1981). *Old, alone, and neglected.* Los Angeles: University of California Press.

Keesing, R. (1974). Theories of culture. *Annual Review of Anthropology, 3,* 73–98.

Lagace, R. (1974). *Nature and use of the HRAF files.* New Haven, CT: Human Relations Area Files Inc.

Leininger, M. (1985). Ethnography and ethnonursing: Models and modes of qualitative data analysis. In M. Leininger (Ed.), *Qualitative research methods in nursing* (pp. 33–69). Orlando, FL: Grune & Stratton.

Lett, J. (1987). *The human enterprise: A critical introduction to anthropological theory.* Boulder, CO: Westview Press.

Liebow, E. (1967). *Tally's corner.* Boston: Little, Brown.

Lincoln, Y., & Guba, E. (1985). *Naturalistic inquiry.* Beverly Hills, CA: Sage.

Miles, M., & Huberman, A. M. (1994). *Qualitative data analysis* (2nd ed.). Beverly Hills, CA: Sage.

Morse, J. (1991). The structure and function of gift giving in the patient-nurse relationship. *Western Journal of Nursing Research,* 13, 597–615.

Morse, J. (1992). *Qualitative health research.* Newbury Park, CA: Sage.

Orem, D. E. (1995). *Nursing: Concepts of practice* (5th ed.). St. Louis: Mosby.

Neuman, B. (1995). *The Neuman systems model* (3rd ed.). Norwalk, CT: Appleton & Lange.

Patton, M. (1990). *Qualitative evaluation and research methods* (2nd ed.). Newbury Park, CA: Sage.

Quint, J. (1968). Role models and the professional nurse identity. *Journal of Nursing Education,* 6(2), 11–16.

Reason, P. (1981). Patterns of discovery in the social sciences. In R. Reason & J. Rowan (Eds.), *Human inquiry* (pp. 183–189). New York: Wiley.

Sanday, P. (1983). The ethnographic paradigm(s). In J. Van Maanen (Ed.), *Qualitative methodology* (pp. 19–36). Beverly Hills, CA: Sage.

Sandelowski, M. (1986). The problem of rigor in qualitative research. *Advances in Nursing Science,* 8(3), 27–37.

Seidel, J. (1998). *The ethnograph* (Version 5.06). *Salt Lake City:* Qualis Research Associates. (*Thousand Oaks, CA: Scolari, Sage Publications, distributor*).

Spradley, J. (1979). The ethnographic interview. New York: Holt, Rinehart & Winston.

Spradley, J. (1980). *Participant observation.* New York: Holt, Rinehart & Winston, 1980.

Street, A. (1992). *Inside nursing: A critical ethnography of clinical nursing practice.* Albany: State University of New York Press.

Thomas, J. (1993). *Doing critical ethnography.* Newbury Park, CA: Sage.

Tilden, V. (1980). Qualitative research: A new frontier for nursing. In A. Davis & J. Krueger (Eds.), *Patients, nurses, ethics* (pp. 73–83). New York: American Journal of Nursing Co.

Villaruel, A. (1995). Mexican-American cultural meanings, expressions, self-care and dependent-care actions associated with experiences of pain. *Research in Nursing and Health,* 18, 427–436.

Villaruel, A., & Denyes, M. (1997). Testing Orem's theory with Mexican Americans. *Image: Journal of Nursing Scholarship, 29,* 283–288.

Werner, O., & Schoepfle, G. (1987a). *Systematic fieldwork: Foundations of ethnography and interviewing* (Vol. 1). Newbury Park, CA: Sage.

Werner, O., & Schoepfle, G. (1987b). *Systematic fieldwork: Ethnographic analysis and data management* (Vol. 2). Newbury Park, CA: Sage.

Weitzman, E. (1999). Analyzing qualitative data with computer software. HSR (*Health Services Research*), 34, Part II (special supplement, Qualitative Methods in Health Services Research), 1241–1263.

Wolf, Z. (1988). *Nurses' work: The sacred and the profane.* Philadelphia: University of Pennsylvania Press.

Cardiac Patients' Hospitalization for An Acute Episode and Their Symptom Management
An Ethnography

Zane Robinson Wolf

This ethnographic study was conducted to: (1) describe chronically ill cardiac patients' experience during hospitalization for an acute illness; (2) describe nursing staff's concurrent caregiving experiences; (3) compare patients' and nurses' experiences; (4) describe the symptoms that chronically ill patients report during their hospitalization; and, (5) position these descriptions in the social world and physical context of Core 3, a medical unit of a large, urban hospital. The investigation was carried out over a period of 2 years.

Core 3 (C3) was situated in a 600+-bed teaching hospital located in a decayed section of a large city. The nursing service organization of the hospital was known in the region for its progressiveness. The hospital had successfully navigated Diagnostic Related Groups, "right sizing," a flattened organizational structure, and health care reform.

I used participant observation, semistructured interviewing, event analysis, and document analysis, including focus notes, progress notes, admission forms, and posted literature on C3 bulletin boards, as sources of data. Primary informants included 17 members of the nursing staff and

40 chronically ill cardiac patients, 20 men and 20 women. Patients had long-term cardiac disease. Most suffered from other chronic conditions such as diabetes and hypertension. Many patients were admitted to C3 because they had anginal pain and agreed to have diagnostic cardiac catheterizations, percutaneous transluminal angioplasties (PTCAs), and coronary artery bypass graft surgery (CABG). However, there were other reasons for admission, such as myocardial infarction, dysrhythmia, pulmonary embolus, and congestive heart failure.

C3 had a long history as a medical unit; during the study, it became a designated cardiac floor with most patients admitted with cardiac disease. Toward the end of the study, beds on the east and west side of the unit were wired for telemetry with monitors situated at the nurses' stations. The nurses worked out of two nurses' stations, focal points of nursing activity. The bed count ranged from 41 to 49; on weekends, the census often dropped so that either the east or the west side of the unit was closed until more patients were admitted.

Nursing staff assigned to C3 routinely cared for patients on both sides and were often aware of what was happening on the other side on a given day. Most patients occupied two-bed rooms with door and window designations, but some stayed in private rooms. The nursing staff worked well together. They covered for one another, giving medications, letting patients know that they were not ignored, and attending to their needs. They asked one another for advice and tried different approaches when solving patients' problems. The nurses answered many questions posed by patients and family members, balanced laboratory study results and medications, and knew their patients' stories. They saw how patients fit in the context of their personal and family resources.

Two sections of the study have been condensed. What follows is the experience of men and women with chronic cardiac disease who were admitted to C3 as a result of crises defined by them, their physicians, or the Emergency Unit staff.

Chronically Ill Women's Hospitalization Experience and Symptom Management

Life History
A woman with a history of heart disease who is admitted to the hospital places her current crisis in the context of her history. She brings

her story with her. The episode that supplies the reason for admission is just another circumstance that fits into a larger pattern of life experiences.

Living with her chronic illness has taught the woman to pace herself when working in or outside the home. She has told herself to "simmer down" and to understand that she is unable to do many of the things that she did before. She is more patient and knows that things around the house will get done. And, if they do not get done, "Whoever doesn't like to look at it doesn't have to look at it."

The present crisis, whether signified by chest pain or shortness of breath, makes the woman review her past. She acknowledges previous crises and compares them with the current one. A woman recalls her difficult life: "I went through hell since I was a little girl." Another comments:

> My father was killed in the mines. I buried a baby, a girl. Everything was shouldered on me all my life, really. I just helped all the kids out and I was working. I was skimping myself to help them out a lot of times. . . . I'm a widow for forty years. But I didn't have a good marriage. It was a very, very bad marriage. And finally one Christmas he died.

A woman's social history has nourished her sense of independence in spite of how life's difficulties burdened her. She learns to depend solely on herself as she accepts her husband's alcoholism. She finds work in a leather factory in the city and eventually buys her own home.

Later in life as she ages and heart disease limits her easy movement in the world outside her house, she yearns for her independence. She is disgusted by her dependence on her children for transportation for food shopping, doctors' appointments, and other errands. She tells a story of recently navigating her neighborhood in the northeast section of her city one last time, alone, without her children. Her determination brings back her independence, temporarily: she is victorious.

> One day I got so disgusted about them taking me, I said, "I have the ability; I'm determined." Then I talk to myself. "I'm going out there if it kills me. I'm not sitting here any more." So I get dressed and walk three blocks to the bus. I get up to the corner and the man that gives me communion says, "Where are you going?" See he didn't think I went out, and I didn't. But I was bold enough to get on that bus and get off. After I got up there, I went in and out of the five and dime. I need some panties and I went in and got that. I'm getting a little tired, I'd better go home again

and I get on the bus and headed home again. I get off the bus again and walk the three blocks. I stopped twice on people's steps and rested. When I get home I thought to myself, I was smart but I'm ready for the undertaker. I was so exhausted. But I made it.

The chronically ill woman recognizes how her disease has confined her as her circles of interaction with others have constricted. She compares herself with younger acquaintances and takes pride in being a survivor who has lived more than 80 years and still does ". . . everything even for my age." At the same time, she is very aware of her dependence and relies on her family, a daughter or a son, for appointments and errands.

Disease History

In the Center of Heart Disease.   Women with chronic cardiac disease are so consumed with this element of their lives that it is inseparable from the way in which they see themselves. It is a focus of their lives whether they accept it or not. Coronary artery disease has encroached on them everyday and changed patterns. They take regularly prescribed medications and are frequently admitted to the hospital.

A woman earns her well-established history of heart disease. It is built by the every-1-to-3-month admissions to the hospital, the often frightening experience of heart attack, the invasion of diagnostic procedures such as cardiac catheterizations, and the treatments including percutaneous transluminal angioplasties and coronary artery bypass grafts. Or, if she is relatively new to having heart disease at the time of admission to the hospital, the patient discovers that she has had a "silent" myocardial infarction. Perhaps she has a history of dysrhythmia: "I had a rapid heart beat and I got sick. My heart was beating 150 per minute and my blood pressure was 80 over 65."

Women describe their experience with heart disease in various ways, depending on the problem and how they lived through it: "My first heart attack, I was really sick. A lot of pain." "When I first come in here last month with a slight heart attack, they found my arteries blocked a little bit. So, this time when I come in they wanted to do this catheterization." Subsequent experiences with chest pain and shortness of breath are compared with others. These and other experiences create her "known" cardiac history.

Having Other Health Problems.   Menopause might not have even phased the woman; nor did a fractured patella or the possibility of breast cancer, especially when the biopsy was negative. But cardiac and other sometimes related diseases mark a woman's body. Up to this point, she has considered herself healthy. Heart disease changes that. Other problems that go along with heart disease appear, such as fatigue and chest pain.

Other major chronic conditions add to the threat of heart disease. She has a stroke history, carotid occlusion, arterial insufficiency, chronic bronchitis, hypothyroidism, or ulcerative colitis. She discovers that she has diabetes mellitus when suffering a heart attack.

Preceding the Present Admission

Minimizing and Denying Symptoms.   Being chronically ill has brought the woman a tolerance for symptoms. She lives with them but hesitates to bring them to the attention of her physician. Symptoms are part of the fabric of everyday life, are woven into it. So, when she experiences symptoms, she delays seeking a physician's help. She refuses to face the fact that she is acutely ill. She is frightened. For her, having a cardiac diagnosis is equated with death.

One patient had two heart attacks. She denies how serious her situation is. "No I wasn't having any pain. I thought nothing was going on." Another ignores symptoms for weeks as cardiac symptoms worsen daily. She reflects:

> Sometimes I would have a bad day, and I also took nitro pills that day; it was mostly numbness in my arm and my hand especially.

The woman endures the symptoms before seeking help. "I waited all day with this numbness and then finally around six o'clock, it stopped. Then I decided to go to the emergency room, thinking they'd send me home. They kept me for 4 hours and told me they were going to keep me 24 hours for observation."

Another patient's denial of her symptoms is fueled by a previous misdiagnosis. Chest pain is interpreted as costochondritis by her physician. She carefully follows his directions to take Motrin. She has the pain several times after that and takes the Motrin. Finally the pain does not stop and she is at higher risk for heart attack.

On the other hand, the patient may not perceive the symptoms to be present. "I feel like I always feel." Whether denial or failure to perceive symptoms, such as chest pain and shortness of breath, are operating, the reality is that the woman is not getting the attention that she needs.

Having Symptoms Before Admission.   Whereas some women report experiencing no symptoms before being admitted to the hospital for acute distress, others evince convincing accounts of heart disease and other problems. For example, a woman is scheduled for a carotid endarterectomy after undergoing an MRI (magnetic resonance imaging) that confirmed carotid stenosis. Her lightheadedness caught her physician's attention. But, during her visit with the anesthesiologist at her preadmission testing work-up, the anesthesiologist is worried about her heart disease. Surgery is canceled and additional testing is scheduled. She is considered a poor surgical risk.

Another's symptoms are classic for heart attack. Her symptoms are dramatic:

> And I guess I was asleep about a half an hour and the pain woke
> me up. I had pains in my chest like somebody was pressing
> down real hard and I couldn't breathe and my left arm was numb
> and everything was blurry.

In contrast, an elderly woman has symptoms of heart disease and impending stroke. Although her current admission is for cardiovascular disease, she is unable to separate the difference between stroke and cardiac symptoms. She experiences them as the same.

> When I blacked out, my nose was very sore. Four years ago I had
> the same experience. I got out of bed at home and felt very
> dizzy. I thought, "Oh I'd better sit down before I fall." If I lie down
> it would maybe not have happened. I sat down on the edge of
> the bed and blacked out. The next thing I remember when my
> face crashed on my floor.

Still others go on as before, working inside or outside the home. They resist admitting the seriousness of the evidence. "The last 4 days that I worked were hard, especially the one day because I had chest pains. There was more numbness than I had all day long. I also took nitro pills." Hours later they decide to go to the emergency unit of a hospital, after their families beg them to do so.

Realization That Her Illness Would Disrupt Family Balance

For the woman with adult children, grandchildren, or a husband and younger children at home, the unmistakable possibility of a hospital admission is very threatening. She plays a key role in keeping the family together. She takes care of her grandchildren, keeps her husband intact, anchors her children, prays for her son in jail, and worries about a sick daughter. Taking her out of the picture through hospitalization, even for a short time, can threaten the stability of her support system.

Support System Helps Legitimize Crisis

It may take minutes, hours, or days for the patient to seek help from a physician or emergency room. She is mindful enough of her symptoms and makes certain that a physician, family member, or other supportive person agrees that the symptoms are worthy of attention from other professionals at the hospital.

Her daughter, husband, or neighbor may not fully comprehend how serious her condition is, but they try to help and encourage her. They acknowledge how sick she is by driving her to the hospital as fast as they can or by lending her their oxygen tank to help ease her dyspnea. "I reached over and called my sister and told her to bring her oxygen tank over, and so she did that, and I put the oxygen on and I was throwing up bile. I said, 'Let's go, I'm going to the hospital.' So he (son) rushed me over." She may tell her son that she is not herself and does not know what is happening to her or she tells her husband that she is going to die. They respond to her request and in so doing grant an aura of respectability to the symptoms, whether or not they are legitimized as important ones by the professionals who assess her later. Some who are close to her understand her situation better than others, "My daughter understands what I'm saying."

This affirmation of family and friends helps her to make the decision to call or visit her physician or go to the emergency unit (EU). "That morning I just couldn't breathe, so I got on the phone right away and he (doctor) knew what was happening."

Physicians may or may not sanction the patient's symptoms as worthy of attention. Sometimes the woman confronts this fact, realizing that she is not being taken seriously.

We had to start over at square one again because I changed doctors. That's been a big problem, too. He was more than my doctor, he was my friend, I kept going for tests, tests, and every time I'd go and have all these tests done (previous doctor). He'd never make any changes and the heart problem had been there and the diabetes was there too. He'd say, "You look wonderful," and I'd say, "I'm tired of you telling me I look wonderful." Because I wasn't wonderful. I think that was the big thing for me to get over was the fact that he was my friend and he didn't go into this as fully as he should have done. It is very hard to pick up again (with another physician).

It is comforting to be cared for by a physician who knows her story rather than by a new one who does not. It is also comforting to be taken seriously, to be believed, to be carefully evaluated, and to be respected regardless of the extent of her present problem.

In the Emergency Unit

Whether brought to the hospital by family members, friends, neighbors, or a rescue service, the woman is finally seen by EU staff. "I told them that I was having chest pain. They examined me and I had to be admitted. I have a lot of stress and had a heart attack before." The staff learn the patient's story through a series of questions and by collecting additional corroborating data. "They all question me, naturally. I had to repeat several times. But that's important to them."

The emergency unit is often the first of many stops for a cardiac patient in the hospital. The woman often leaves the EU to go to the cardiac care unit, or what she calls the ICU (intensive care unit), or a telemetry unit may be the next place she sees.

> They stopped me at the admissions desk in the emergency ward. They ask you all these questions and somebody else asks a question so they can do work on you. So, by the time I got done, they took me back and the doctors worked on me right away. I always holler for my heart specialist. Something went wrong and they had to wind up zapping (cardioverting) me. I remember somebody saying something and then I remember my body jumping. Because after that I was fine.

The nurses in the emergency unit rapidly connect her to leads attached to a monitor. They start an intravenous solution and measure vital signs and listen to her heart and lung sounds. At the same time, they take an electrocardiogram and give her nitroglycerin. If she has congestive heart failure, the EU staff gives her diuretics. "As soon as they treated me down in emergency, it did ease up a lot. I guess they gave me a lot of Lasix to get rid of the fluid."

The woman waits while the physician deliberates about whether to admit her to the hospital. Sometimes the stay in the EU lasts many hours. The doctor tells her that an electrocardiogram does not always show that she had a heart attack. The team of emergency unit physicians rules out other diagnoses.

Other Reasons for Admission to the Hospital

There are elective reasons for which women are admitted to the hospital because of their heart disease. Some of these reasons include percutaneous transluminal coronary angioplasties, coronary artery bypass grafts, and cardiac catheterizations.

A physician could see his patient during an office visit and decide that a cardiac catheterization is warranted.

> There was more, a circulation problem, and he also discovered that there were a couple of silent heart attacks which we were not aware of because of the diabetes. The doctor says that diabetes covers up for any indication that you are having a heart attack.

Her next step was a cardiac catheterization. The referring physician could have performed the catheterization in the community hospital or referred her to another cardiologist in the tertiary care hospital where the patient was finally admitted. The physician scheduled other interventions such as PTCA or CABG.

Next Stops After the Emergency Unit

After evaluation in the EU, a woman's next step could be admission to the critical care unit (CCU) where she is stabilized before anything else is planned for her. "I finally was admitted to the ICU; I have no ideas what the nurses did; I don't remember going up there; I don't remember anything about that first day in the hospital until over to the next day." She may stay in the ICU or CCU for longer or shorter time periods. She notices the difference in the critical care unit compared with a unit with less staff. "When you are in intensive care, you get nothing but help."

As the woman undergoes treatment, she is anxious about what is happening to her. She meets many people in the course of her stay, including cardiologists, residents, physician's assistants, and nurses. She appreciates the staff's expertise or she critiques it. She says, "Let's face it, this is a better hospital than anywhere I've been; first of all, they're more on the ball. The nurses want to help you." Or she realizes some shortcomings: "When I first came in, the first day or the second, they had all the records and they spelled my name wrong."

As soon as the woman stabilizes and is transferred to what she considers a regular room, she relaxes a bit. Next comes additional diagnostic studies and other components of the plan of care.

Being Supported During Hospitalization

Family and friends keep a watch on what is happening to their loved one during the hospitalization. Many of them are alert to the nature of her problems and actually transport her to the hospital. The patient is an integral part of their lives. Her illness upsets them. They contact her by telephone after she is admitted to the hospital and often share her worries and fears about the uncertainty of heart disease and what is going on at home. The memory of seeing her with chest pain, seriously ill, sharpens their concern.

Often daughters, sisters, sons, and husband consult with her about decisions to have PTCAs or CABG surgery: "They had quite a few opinions before they decided what they thought, if I should go through it or not go through it." When she has chest pain or experiences another crisis while in the hospital, the family wonders about what is happening to her and needs information from the physicians and nurses about her status. Many are mobilized to help her through the time in the hospital.

The woman puts her trust in God. She has already reconciled her life, given that she has already been widowed and lives alone. She is convinced that God is with her no matter what. She meditates, prays, receives communion, or reads her Bible, and finally sets her troubles aside. Her personal philosophy carries her through the problems with her heart.

> I don't carry anything with me, and I feel that things could be a lot worse. I have a neighbor and I say, "How are you?" I get a resumé this big. And I always say, that's not good, you have to look at things on the brighter side: I was a very lucky person to have had nothing but nice memories. You have to accept your blessings.

She is not afraid of dying, because of her faith. Her fatalism about death speaks for itself, "If I'm going to die, I'm going to die."

Confronting Her Heart Disease

When a woman's physician tells her that her heart is failing, she has had a heart attack, or her artery is blocked, she begins to see her situation more clearly. Before this, she failed to pay attention to some of her chronic symptoms, whether by denying them or just living with them every day. "I never gave it a thought, about the heart failure or anything else. You never think of those things."

Another woman has considered her heart disease carefully, so that confirmation of the heart disease is not a surprise; rather, the extent of her pathology is: "The doctor said that the catheterization was wonderful. But the bad news is, all my arteries are closed. I knew even before that I have hardening of the arteries; so everything is clogged."

Undergoing Diagnostic Tests and Treatment

First, she agrees to have a stress test to determine the boundaries of her chest pain or whether there is "more damage to my heart." Or she may have a thallium perfusion test by which the blood flow in her heart is evaluated. She may have a bone scan that is related not to her heart disease but, rather, to her physician's suspicions about her fatigue and possible cancer. If the results of a diagnostic test are temporarily mislaid or if she has to wait a long time for the physician to convey the findings, she becomes more anxious than she already is.

Plans for a cardiac catheterization become more real as the cardiologist explains the procedures. She begins to understand that the procedure shows the physician how many arteries are "stopped." If she has other major problems, such as kidney disease, she understands that the procedure is riskier. The physician explains that it is better for her to have the test taken to find out whether something is wrong, if an artery is "clogged or not, blocked or not." He goes on to try to convince her that more treatments can be planned as soon as the extent of cardiac damage is discovered. "He said my heart was more important than my kidneys, but I was scared." She is afraid that she will die during the procedure.

> I wasn't going to have it done, because I would never have it done, because they hurt and everything. My husband was fighting with me and crying; they (family) want me to have it done. I don't want to die myself, I got too much to live for. I have two adopted, two foster children, two step children, and two regular children and I have two beautiful grandchildren.

Finally, she undergoes the catheterization. "They found blockages. The doctor suggested an angioplasty."

Some women do not remember having the procedure, whereas others recall the details. The percutaneous puncture that enables the physician to get to her femoral artery may be painful for her. The medication to "to make me be on cloud nine" does not work as promised. She feels more pain than she would like to.

Getting in Touch with Her Personal Agenda

> The fact is that I want to get well, that is one thing, and being taken care of. I don't know what else there is to expect from the hospital.

A woman with heart disease reflects on her treatment options in the context of her life. Hospitalization brings thoughts of the way that she wishes herself to be in the future. She prefers that the angioplasty works, opening her arteries so that she avoids chest pain and heart surgery. She hopes that her physician is able to get her arteries open "just a little bit more. That is all that it needs." In the event that she does need an operation, she looks forward to a future that is framed by short time, "At my age I take one day at a time."

She hopes that she still "keeps on going. I've always been a very active person all my life." This dreamed-for level of activity includes being able to keep house independently or return to work.

The woman plans to change her ways, "I hope that this time that I can stick to my diet and lose the weight that I have to lose." "I'm going to behave myself." She plans to take care of herself and to try to reduce stress in her life: "I haven't been walking for a while, but I'm getting back to it again and it really makes a difference."

But, above all, she wants to return to normalcy again where she is home, living with her disease, yet feeling much better. "I got a lot to live for and I love life. I don't want to die but I'm so scared. They hurt me down there (cardiac catheterization laboratory) bad." In fact, she hopes to live, she hopes that "I come out all right."

Getting back to what is for her considered normal is desirable. It is better to have less-severe symptoms or none at all and for life to return to its typical, everyday patterns—that is, without crises and without the evidence of disease forcing itself on her. She wants to get back to when "I really feel good, and I'm happy most of the time and don't dwell on my illness."

Having Symptoms

Managing Symptoms at Home and Work.   The woman with chronic heart disease lives with many symptoms and learns to manage them herself. A large part of her strategies include resting until the symptoms ease and resuming usual activity when they abate.

> I have that problem (lightheadedness). I try to sit down then. I think where I notice that where it really bothered me the most

was when I would stand in church to sing a hymn or something, then it bothered me to have to stand for a long length of time. I was OK if I sat down, but when I had to stand that's when it would bother me.

But if she has chest pain, she takes nitroglycerin: "Every little pain I get, I take it, and I can tell if it helps, it's fast."

Before this hospital admission, the woman with cardiac disease may have noticed that she was feeling very tired as she worked her part-time job. She may have ignored this symptom only to become concerned when more evidence presented. When her fatigue was followed by chest pain, it prompted her to call her daughter and get to the EU. Because she had had a heart attack previously, she knew to take the chest pain seriously.

Often, a woman has lived for a while with heart disease and other problems, such as diabetes, and has allowed the diseases to become part of her life. Although the manifestations of the diseases are part of her daily experience, she may or may not have accommodated herself to them by changing her life very much. For example, a diabetic admits that she has not kept her blood sugar under control:

I'm a diabetic. I didn't follow their advice that I eat properly and so forth. I probably would have been really great if I would have done the things that I was told to do, but I just didn't do any of those things. I know that with my own weight it's hard. The blood sugar level is a little bit high. I do take my own sugar. I have a kit and do keep up on that a little bit. It's not what it should be. It should be lower than what it is. That's my problem. It has been 170 something, 200 something too frequently.

Or she may have had a false alarm and was embarrassed at "crying wolf." One woman was traveling to New Jersey by car when she felt her heart skip a couple of beats. She became very excited and admits that she is "highly excitable." She interrupted her trip, went to her physician's office, and was sent by his office staff to the hospital. As she approached the hospital, she started having chest pain, which she reports as a "ten" (on a 10-point scale). But, as soon as she got to the hospital, it stopped. After evaluating her, the hospital staff told her that it "certainly was not a heart attack." So she drove herself home. The next time that she thinks she may have a heart problem, she may be slow to seek help.

But most often symptoms are put off if they are not interpreted as being critical. A woman's fatigue is dealt with but does not improve: "I would go to the sink and try to make a little oatmeal. I had to sit down;

my legs came out and I had to sit down for 5 minutes, get up, stand up for about 2 or 3 minutes and sit down again." She may grow accustomed to having pain: "I manage my pain at home by walking, rocking, and taking Motrin. I would sit on the side of the bed and rock a little bit, and go to the bathroom and come back and sit back on the bed for a while; I was kind of afraid to lie down because I didn't know how I was going to get up again." Some feel better on their feet, walking, but most prefer resting and sitting or lying down.

Heartburn and nausea are treated with over-the-counter drugs such as Tums or Alka Seltzer. Most of the time, the symptoms go away. High-blood-pressure symptoms, such as headache, do not bother her often. If she notices a headache, she takes Excedrin and drinks a little Pepsi. If her self-remedies fail and her symptoms persist, she weighs whether or not to call her physician or go to the hospital. She trusts that hospital staff will know whether it is serious or not.

The woman with a known history of heart disease is very accustomed to taking nitroglycerin for chest pain. She does not hesitate to take it, because the chest pain goes away. Other heart medications, such as Isordil and Procardia, are prescribed by her doctor, so she takes them routinely for many years. Aspirin or Coumadin may also be taken to keep her blood "thin."

The Presence of Symptoms.

Taking Prescribed Medications. Except for taking nitroglycerin for chest pain, a woman does not connect her regularly prescribed medications with symptom management. She pretty much takes them according to the doctor's prescriptions. "The medication I was on was Procardia, Isordil was the other thing. I've been taking the Procardia and Isordil for 5 or 6 years." She takes Coumadin "for the heart" or she takes Mevacor for hypercholesterolemia. Some of her concerns about the cost of health care are connected to the cost of prescribed medications: "I give my doctor a hundred dollars a year, and I'm on PACE [Pharmaceutical Assistance Contract for the Elderly] for medicine; it was good when it was four, now it's six, and I think they're going to go higher and higher."

Medications may give her other symptoms. She is watchful for symptoms when she fills her prescriptions for new medications, such as Isordil: "It was giving me awful headaches." Nevertheless, she appreciates the efficacy of medications and is happy that there are medications that help to control her blood pressure, decrease her chest pain, and lower her lipids by 100 points. But she does not make the connection between shortness of breath, as a symptom, and her heart disease right away. She learns about this connection as she experiences a crisis.

Dyspnea. Common symptoms that women with heart disease live with and mentioned when asked are shortness of breath and chest pain. In particular, shortness of breath is not always interpreted as a cardiac symptom. Instead a woman attributes it to possibly having pleurisy or simply having occasional "trouble" breathing. If her heart disease is showing itself in other than the typical way, which is chest pain, she may be completely unaware of the significance of the symptom: "I never gave it a thought that it could be that (my heart) or even my lungs filling with fluid. I had no idea that was even happening. The way I was gasping he (doctor) must have known what was going on."

Not being able to catch her breath is disturbing, but she describes it most in relation to how it affects everyday function: "I have a little bit of shortness of breath. If I made a bed I would be a little short of breath and when I walk very fast, I slow up; I take deep breaths and I sit down." She compares this experience with that in which her shortness of breath improves after taking medication or undergoing other treatment. She says, "I'm now able to walk without having to slow up." She knows the difference.

At times, the shortness of breath is experienced as a slow crescendo, increasing over several days as congestive heart failure grows worse:

> I was a little out of touch, but I didn't think anything of it because I thought it's the aftermath of the heart attack. I've been awful tired though since I came out from that heart attack. The next day it started a little bit more. I'd walk a little bit and I could hardly get my breath. The next day in the morning when I got up, I just couldn't breathe. It was terrible.

The shortness of breath that goes along with congestive heart failure is not as upsetting to her as having chest pains: "That experience with fluid on the lungs before, it's not as scary as those heart attack pains. It's much different." The difference lies in her perception of the severity of both symptoms. Shortness of breath, while frightening and not as severe at the time, is not as upsetting as chest pain. For some women, dyspnea often occurs concurrently with chest pain: "I couldn't breathe with the chest pain." Slowly she learns that taking nitroglycerin helps her to breathe.

She can also have other conditions that complicate shortness of breath caused by heart disease. The wheezing from asthma can be augmented by shortness of breath due to heart failure or the pressure felt with chest pain. Furthermore, she can have a cold or pneumonia. Both of these conditions can add to the severity of the symptom and her confusion about what is causing it.

Chest Pain. She interprets chest pain as serious and worthy of attention, or not. The pain can be more dramatic than the first time she had it a few years ago: "I've never had this in my life. A knife went across all the way here (points to chest), and my hands went up and my eyes burned. I told my daughter, 'I got something to tell you; I think I'm going to die.' Here we go again."

That chest pain frequently accompanies coronary artery disease is undeniable. This time her chest pain is classic heart attack pain and signals a potential myocardial infarction:

> I was having pain in the center of my chest and pain down my left arm and about that time I had started some sweating, I was sweating. Well, I knew what the symptoms were. I don't think that I was particularly happy. It was funny, because when I had the heart attack, I knew it wasn't angina, because the pains were so severe that I called the rescue squad right away.

She knows the difference between angina and crushing chest pain because she has felt both: "Over the years I had angina pains, but they were nothing like the heart attack pains, very different." Another explains, "The pain in my arm was greater than the pain in my chest; rather uncomfortable. I explained to the doctor that I had been hurting. It wasn't that the pain was getting worse, it was at that time I was just tired." Or, "The pain was not crushing and I wasn't nauseous. The sweating was not profuse, so the things that I would normally be looking for weren't there." Other women describe the pain as they are having a heart attack:

> Then it (pain) went up higher into my throat. It was the worst I ever had in my life. First off it's sort of a wheezing feeling and then it felt like my throat is hurting. I didn't say anything right away, then I asked the nurse to call the doctor.

But she may not be certain, as her chest pain begins, whether she is having a heart attack or not. She notices that it is not that severe. Furthermore, she may not describe it in the way that another would, because she perceives it differently. One woman describes her experience: "There wasn't any pain; it was all numbness like in my chest, my arm, and everything; my right arm, my left one, and my chest, and across my shoulders." She could consider it "a tightness," as if you are holding something tightly in your hand. Another woman states, "The angina to me sometimes felt like heartburn." One woman reveals her fear as she has anginal pain:

> I got a feeling like somebody had their arms around my waist and squeezed it so tight I couldn't move. I thought, "Am I going out of my mind?" I thought, "There's nobody in here." I thought, "I'm strong." And I tried to pull away and I was throwing my back in the chair just as hard and I laid there.

But for some women, being more aware of their symptoms, such as symptoms of heart failure, helps to sensitize them for the next experience, if it occurs, so that they are more responsive to the severity.

Some women experience no pain or chest pressure. The physicians and nurses are surprised at their accounts, given that they have evidence of old heart attacks or silent myocardial infarctions. "Even with my heart attack, I keep telling them, no pain. And they say, 'You come in with chest pain.' I say, 'I didn't have any pain.' I told them for 4, 5 years and they still don't believe me." This woman learns that her chest pain is not severe but that she must pay attention to it. "My chest pain is not even mild, not even that."

Indigestion, Nausea, Vomiting, Anorexia, Decreased Appetite.

> (I had) 2 days of the pain, but certain days even drinking a glass of water did not interest me. Part of my symptoms was throwing up. I threw up about eight times, and I was too sore and I didn't want to eat.

The symptoms of nausea, vomiting, and heartburn or indigestion, anorexia, and decreased appetite are well recognized as indicators of heart disease and thus potentially serious. But the patient does not always connect these common gastrointestinal symptoms to heart disease. Rather she thinks that she is having gas, a little tight feeling, or heartburn. It aggravates her somewhere over her "breastbone." She uses an antacid or Alka Seltzer.

> I started having something like gas. I thought I had the heartburn. I told my daughter to run to the AM and go and get me some Alka Seltzer. So she got me two packs of Alka Seltzer and I took one pack. Then I felt really good but then I got this little tight feeling like gas.

She notices that every now and then when she feels sick she burps a lot and experiences a "really upset stomach." The nausea that she experiences can be mild or "unbelievable." In particular, when her heart disease reaches a crisis, she suffers repeated bouts of nausea. Her appetite decreases, so she does not eat as much as formerly. She is unable to make herself eat and relates that she does not want to. The woman becomes more concerned if she almost vomits or actually does vomit.

Fatigue. The patient often lives in a state of chronic fatigue; she might call it exhaustion. She admits that "tiredness is my name." She pushes herself in order to be able to accomplish daily activities. She blames her fatigue on the heat and humidity, not on her heart. Although she does not have chest pain, she does have shortness of breath. If she is the kind of woman to push herself to the limits of endurance, she admits that she might be wrong to do that. She may be afraid of hurting herself or of being embarrassed that she does not know that fatigue and heart disease go together.

She feels that her energy is drained and wonders if she needs to take vitamins. She may also experience weakness and try to manage her fatigue and weakness by sitting down. Her exhaustion becomes so severe that she prefers not going into details to describe what is happening to her, because the telling takes too much energy.

Cough. Although a woman with cardiac disease initially attributes a cough to a cold or bronchitis, she later learns that coughing is a symptoms of heart failure: "I have had coughing in the past. I have just had a bout of retention of water and had a very bad cough then. I was on Lasix and that's (fluid retention) been relieved. I lost that right before I came in. I couldn't understand why he (doctor) wasn't concerned about it. He wasn't concerned about the cough because he knew I was retaining the water."

Because her heart disease does not go away, owing to its chronic nature, she begins to accept alternate explanations for her occasional coughing spells. One woman was surprised that her physician was not as concerned as she was, because she knew that it was an ominous sign. Given that many women with heart disease are elderly, it is not surprising that they have symptoms of other diseases.

Insomnia. Being in the hospital brings about insomnia for some women. However, those who have been living with chronic congestive heart failure frequently have difficulty sleeping and may sleep in a recliner chair at home so that they can breathe better. Sleeplessness may get worse as a woman gets sicker.

At home she takes a Tylenol PM or a prescribed sleeping pill. Her worries add to her reasons for sleeplessness. If she starts to think about her illness, past history, or a crisis in her family, she gets little sleep. "Sometimes I stay awake until maybe three/four o'clock. I just toss and turn."

Anxiety, Depression, and Denial. That the woman is anxious about her present situation is unquestionable. Not only is she worried about her family, especially those who rely on her support (e.g., a daughter and grandchildren), but she is concerned about the extent of her heart disease and how her illness will affect her life.

She may lose sleep. She admits that she is a regular worrywart. Her worry and outward nervousness are heightened and yet explained by her concern about what the physicians will find and whether medications and treatments will decrease her symptoms and extend her life.

On the surface, her anxiety relates to news of the extent of her heart disease, "what they are going to find". But beneath the surface lies fear of suffering and dying. Finding out "what's what and the corrective action" helps her to consider her options.

Although she may embrace the philosophy of taking each day as it comes, she is also burdened by sometimes almost insurmountable problems such as a sick daughter and two sons in jail. She relies on God to help her with her burdens and fears.

At times, denial of the realities of her present situation enables her not to think about the connection between her inability to "get my breath" and heart failure: "I never gave it a thought. You never think of those things." Rather, foremost in her mind is not being able to get her breath, not that shortness of breath means heart disease. Perhaps her fear of heart disease causes her to be greatly concerned—so concerned that acknowledging it is more than she can handle.

Those women who live in a state of complete dependence on others, such as one elderly woman residing in a nursing home, are so depressed by their circumstances that they cry about it. Fear that nursing home staff will ignore her shortness of breath or other symptoms when she is discharged from the hospital, just as they did before she was admitted, leaves her hopeless. There is no one on earth who will fight for her and protect her. She considers this as she contemplates discharge and returning to the nursing home: "I get kind of droopy. I've noticed that once or twice I've really gotten drippy, the tears just run." Her depressive symptoms are rooted in her lack of a support system and the realities of her heart disease. (The patient was ignored by a nurse; she had a breathing problem and feared suffocating and dying alone.) She relates her story about the nursing home before this admission.

> They sent for this big oxygen tank and they gave me oxygen and had me on this small inhaler. I rang for the nurse and she came in, whoever she was, and she's giving me instructions on how to take care of myself, to sit up and what not. I did that but that didn't seem to help. Then the wheezing got worse. And I rang again for her. At the time, whatever she was doing, I seem to be disturbing her. She said to someone else, "She (patient) keeps ringing the bell," like I was disturbing her. So when I go back to the nursing home I want to report this to the board. When I go back I'll need this care and I'll need people to answer the bell.

Fear of Dying

Having survived the chest pain, imminent heart attack, or heart failure, the patient considers how she should feel, that is, somewhat relieved at having lived and not died. Nevertheless, the reassurances that she is doing fairly well provided by the hospital staff do not necessarily make her feel very happy: "It's just when I think back to that morning I get a little nervous still, just thinking of what could have happened and I get a little upset." She was very afraid that she was going to die at that time of crisis.

She is very afraid of being alone and having chest pain or difficulty breathing. She fears dying: "I'm very, very scared now. I don't remember anything but the oxygen; I was just frightened to death." Her fear is heightened as she realizes that she survived cardiopulmonary resuscitation: "Four nights that I couldn't sleep, day or night; every time I tried to close my eyes, I guess my body jumped all the time."

Her concern about dying also comes from what she has heard about the mortality statistics from bypass graft surgery: "I heard all about it on television that there are too many heart operations for people and nine out of ten die and nine out of ten are women and it's got to stop." In contrast, her fear arises from another crisis, that of bleeding profusely after returning to her bed on the unit after cardiac catheterization: "I don't know what I was thinking (during post-catheterization bleeding). I was scared. At the time I didn't think about dying or nothing like that. They said I could go into a coma. I didn't want to go into a coma, I didn't want to do anything. I just wanted the pressure to get up."

Nurses Take Care of Her Symptoms

On the medical cardiology unit, when a woman complains of chest pain, the nurses pay careful attention to her report. One woman describes a nurse's reaction:

> The nurse is very, very good. She knew what to do. They asked, "Where do you have the pain?" And I showed them and they gave me two nitros. It took eight nitros before it passed over and meanwhile they brought other equipment (ECG) and attached it to my ankles. And he (physician) was telling her what to do and he was watching the cardiogram. After the six nitro, they kept questioning me "one to five" about the pain or "one to ten" on the pain. But in the beginning I said, "Nine." Then they took me to intensive care and put me in there for a couple days and then I came here.

If the woman is very independent, especially after she settles into life on C3, she helps herself, even though she finds the nurses very helpful. She sees a lot of what they do associated with the giving of medications.

On the other hand, when she is sicker, she admits that the nurses check on her, give her juice, and take care of her personal needs: "They turn your body, turn right, turn left, and they wash you and take care of your back and everything. Most of the time I was on the bedpan, but after that they walk you to the bathroom."

A woman sees that C3 nurses are even more attentive when she is in crisis and asks for help: "They came in right away; they took my blood pressure, my temperature, my pulse, they drew blood, and they come back and talk to me."

As she begins to feel better, she gets bored with the hospital routine and not being in her own home. She admits that she is tired of the hospital: "They're here to help you, but they wake you up at two, they wake you up at four. And if you can tell me how you can rest; you absolutely get no rest."

Nevertheless, women are hesitant to complain about hospital staff, preferring instead to say that the staff are "nice," that they can't complain, or that they have been on C3 only a few days.

Thinking About Symptom Management When Preparing for Discharge from the Hospital

Because of having survived the last crisis and her diagnostic testing during the current hospitalization, a woman has learned more about her heart disease. However, this experience does not necessarily prepare her for knowing when and how to interpret symptoms as serious ones.

> How do I determine whether it's the heart or something else?
> That's the terrible fear. To have to walk around everyday. If you
> get a little twinge, what do I do, wait, or do I run to the hospital?
> How do I handle it?

A certain degree of anxiety is associated with how to manage symptoms at home or work after discharge from the hospital. Although her physician and nurse will talk to her about taking nitroglycerin for chest pain, this information does not solve her problem or reduce her anxiety. Her fears are somewhat allayed by her physician's reassurances that he is not expecting problems during her recovery. However, it is still up to her to respond to chest pain and other symptoms appropriately, even if she does not have full knowledge of what the best and most appropriate response should be, short of taking nitroglycerin.

Self-Reflection: On Taking Care of Me

That her acute illness has intruded into her life is not to be denied. Such an intrusion compels her to consider her place in her family and her responsibility to those whom she loves. Her other- rather than self-direction is reassessed. But it is viewed in relation to the others in her life:

> I need to be here for me and to be here for them. So I'm hoping
> that I can make some changes. Some changes will help but it
> takes a long time and it's hard to get rid of things that you build
> up over the years.

Part of her hopes that she will exercise more and stop smoking:

> I will have a problem with smoking, but I'm going to try to master
> this. We've talked about it in our family, my daughter smokes
> but there won't be any smoking in my apartment. I want to make
> sure that everything is dumped clear, wiped up, put away before
> I go home. Nobody is going to buy me a cigarette. I'm hoping
> that by the time I get out that maybe the worst will be over.

Women hospitalized for an acute episode of their chronic cardiac disease live their lives in relation to others. For this reason, they delay seeking health care and minimize their symptoms. Disease exacerbations hamper their ability to care for others.

CHRONICALLY ILL MEN'S HOSPITALIZATION EXPERIENCE AND SYMPTOM MANAGEMENT

History: Work and War

Men with chronic cardiac conditions let you know that they have a past that is not disease connected. They considered themselves healthy up to this point; this is important and needs emphasis.

The men's present cardiac crisis makes them reassure themselves and you that they served the country as military personnel. Through this assertion, they remind you that they are strong, not weak, and have proved this before. They reminisce, reflecting on the time when they were younger and more vigorous:

> I was shot, badly wounded. I was three tours in Viet Nam, I was a sniper for 13 months with confirmed long range. That affected me a great deal because, since being out of that, I've developed a conscience which I never really had.

Other accounts are descriptions of being at work, performing hard, physical labor.

Much of their identity and self-esteem is linked with life at work, on the job. Moreover, the men are often proud that they have worked very hard. But the social expectations of the role played at work sometime contributes to the development of their heart disease:

> I am a mechanic. The time I'm around the guys, we're taking a coffee break or whatever and I get idle, I found out drinking coffee makes you want a cigarette. This is why I stopped drinking because I stopped smoking during that same period of time. I went to a union meeting one time and we're sitting around talking and what not, had a beer and that beer called for a cigarette.

Furthermore, the environmental hazards associated with the job may compromise his health further. Another man says, "Being up on a roof and breathing the different chemicals and dust from the slag, it was causing a lot of problems for me. I was spitting up black phlegm and everything."

Whether they are roofers turned barbers, machinists, carpenters, foremen for a cleaning service, or physicians, work continues to define the male cardiac patients. Their long tenure at work is a source of great pride.

After it becomes known at the patient's workplace that he has cardiac disease, his employer may seize the opportunity to change his job or to use the illness as a reason to lay him off:

> I'm laid off now. I'm pretty much around the house. I play video games, I do puzzles. Once in a while I help a friend. Before I went to see the doctor, I went to a friend's house and helped him by carrying some concrete blocks up and down a ladder. I almost passed out. I had trouble breathing, too, running up and down the ladder.

Before his recent hospitalization, this patient continued to perform as though he was still at his job. And in performing heavy labor he further compromised his status.

In contrast, another man talks his physician into giving him a note to go on light duty. The physician wanted to retire him and was told by his patient that he was not ready "for that."

Even though he sits in a hospital bed, his preference is definitely to continue working. The imperative to work and to be strong in spite of cardiac symptoms is illustrated by the man who does not go to his usual job, because of his heart disease, but instead agrees to help a friend build a brick chimney. He does so in spite of the fact that he has chest discomfort. He has to be busy, working at something, because that is what defines him as a man.

Being away from work may serve to make him more at risk for worsening heart disease. One man begins smoking again, even though he experiences burning chest pain. Another starts eating gummy bears.

> I had gotten gummy bears. I sat up in bed at night, looking at TV and I chew on gummy bears. I had stopped smoking and was eating a lot. I put on a couple of extra little pounds and got a little pot belly.

It is not surprising that work is so integral to his identity. Work becomes a part of men's life from childhood on. One elderly man's father made him responsible for everything that he had to do:

> As a little boy I do work that my father didn't have to do. My father would give me something to do that he wanted done, regardless of my age. I was responsible for everything my father had to do. But I worked for mine and got so I was unable to work because I started to suffer with arthritis.

Being sick, not being at work, and not being busy makes many men uncomfortable. They voice their concerns about jobs around the house needing attention, what they will do when they return to work, their volunteer jobs, and hobbies that they yearn for such as making furniture or repairing cars.

Illness causes them to reflect about the future and where they will be and how they will feel: "That really got me started thinking." They find it difficult to believe that they are not healthy any longer and that part of their history has been changed because of cardiac disease.

Cardiac Disease Rewrites Imagined History

Cardiac and other diseases get the man's attention. When he is "too bad and wind(s) up in the hospital," sometimes two or three times a month, he is aware of how his life has changed. Crises occur more frequently, assailing the formerly robust breadwinner.

Often he expresses the nature of the intrusion that his condition has caused in connection with his work: "By the time I get done a day's work, I'd feel like I'd worked for a whole week in one day." As he reflects on the future, he projects some limitations based on notable changes in his physical abilities: "I worked hard and in the back of my mind I think that I better not try to go up onto a roof and try to work hard again because something might happen to me."

The current hospital admission is a crisis in that he has to deal with the diagnosis and potential limitations. For example, he cannot have his second femoral-popliteal bypass graft surgery until he has a PTCA to improve his cardiac status. He has to have a cardiac catheterization to detect the extent of his heart disease before he is scheduled for a carotid endarterectomy. Or his heart condition must be stabilized so that an access for hemodialysis can be created surgically.

Some men are surprised at the extent to which their condition has changed their lives. And, as other problems are uncovered over time, they foresee a dramatically altered future. Not only does one man have diabetes, he also has chronic renal failure and a heart condition.

Having an indeterminate prognosis makes him insecure and uncertain and causes great anxiety. Not knowing the extent of his heart disease, he wants to understand his circumstances: "I know I would rather know exactly what it is," what exactly caused the current crisis, and what are the limits of his daily activities, because he wishes to know what he can and cannot do.

Different episodes of heart disease are part of the patient's history. For example, one man's nephrologists watch his heart murmur along with his kidney disease. Another man has an extensive history of rheumatic heart disease: "I had rheumatic heart disease and a valve replacement at 29. This experience started pretty early. I've been on medication off and on since I was 26." His long-time association with heart disease is accompanied with regrets: "You want to do the things you see other people doing." His life is undeniably altered.

Even though the patient has a history of angina and has more or less become accustomed to it, he is upset when additional cardiac disease is diagnosed: "This hospital stay is for something that I had hoped would never happen to me, a heart attack." One man reports having a heart attack while being hemodialyzed, and he is upset. Another is pleased that he avoided "a super heart attack" after receiving a thrombolytic agent in the emergency unit. Still another has had two heart attacks already and hopes that he does not have another one and that more problems are not discovered while he is hospitalized for his current crisis.

The man with diabetes mellitus knows the connection of this "sugar" disease with heart disease. He is very aware of the chronic nature of his health problems, having this fact confirmed daily by blood glucose monitoring and by once-a-month visits to the physician: "I'm diabetic but the sugar is OK. I feel like I lost all the energy in the organs."

Having a Family History of Heart Disease

Some men are not surprised at all by the fact that they have heart disease. They have noticed how it has struck different members of their families. They are almost fatalistic about its appearance: "Every member of my family, my mother, my father were patients for various serious illnesses (many of which were heart disease). There may be a hereditary factor here also." They see it in the living and the dead: "My mother has heart palpitations and my aunt had some heart attacks or I believe she died of heart attack."

Resisting Control and Dependency

The oftentimes life-threatening crisis that gets the man to the physician or the hospital positions him in a more dependent role than is typical. He is vulnerable. Although he tries to be a good patient, having been seen in the emergency unit or admitted to a cardiac floor, he is nevertheless aware that his family or friends helped him, as did hospital personnel. In fact, by using many arguments, his family may have prevailed on him to make the decision to seek help from others.

This is the time when he is most vulnerable, when he places his decision-making abilities and his life in the hands of others. The loss of personal control leaves him quite uneasy:

You know you think about that, about being in someone's hands. And out of control. I think that's a big deal. It just does take a while to get past it physically. I think you think about what has happened in a different way. It sort of makes you look at life a little bit differently. When I was laying up here, right down the hall, a lot of things went through my mind about life itself. I guess what a lot of people take for granted, that changes a little bit more, a little bit in my thoughts and this is even making me change more so, I say my God I made it through that first time, but will, will I be strong? Will my body be strong in the hospital, or will the doctor's hands be steady or sturdy enough to get me through this one?

The uncertainty of the present and the future causes him to be more insecure.

Some men explain their giving up control by capitulating to hospital rules: "I just made up my mind that I follow all the rules and regulations they got." Others look forward to the time when they will get better. They fight being dependent on anyone and fear becoming a burden: "I try to get better so that I won't have to call on them or anyone else." They are intolerant of dependency.

Restricting and Accessing Support from Friends and Family

Those men who are close-mouthed about having cardiac disease and what their worries are about the present crisis limit access to persons who are theoretically and actually there to support them. Whether it is done so that they are not thought of as being weak or to avoid worrying a relative with the upsetting facts, this behavior restricts potentially available emotional support. "I always try to play it (illness) down because people have the tendency to treat you differently. I tell them I'm in just for tests," relates one man. Another says, "I haven't to any great extent discussed the hospitalization with my mother."

Some patients fear that people will tend to feel sorry for them. Others prefer that friends and relatives not know the extent of their disease, because they will put their "two cents" in and tell them what they should and should not do. Still others do not believe that those who do not have the same disease will understand its implications, because "healthy people really don't understand."

The men who have been chronically ill for some time are afraid of wearing down the good will and strength of family and friends. They prefer not to notify loved ones, because they think, as this man does, that:

> I want them to just go on with their own routine unless something personally happens (crisis), then they'll be notified. It's really kind of depressing to go out of their way to come over here and sit with me when they'd really rather be doing something else.

Others read their wives' reactions and keep the details of chest pain and other problems to themselves, telling their wives that they are having problems but they are nothing to worry about. Some consider their wives' reactions to minimize the seriousness of their situation. A man who is secretive about the nature and extent of the illness and the planned treatments is occasionally found out by a spouse, who reacts angrily: "She (wife) got angry with me because I didn't say anything about the angioplasty." For whatever reason, the man who limits access to his illness, therapy, prognosis, and the events of the hospitalization is isolated from those most interested in his well-being.

Those men who more actively seek the support of family and friends talk about what is going on with them in greater or less detail. Some are very dependent on their families. Others have people very dependent on them, such as a chronically ill wife with esophageal varices, urinary tract infections, and a host of other problems.

The information given by a patient to those at home keeps the supportive person aware of the extent of his problem and what is going on in the hospital. At times it is a support person, such as a wife, who brings the patient's symptoms to the attention of a family doctor. She is the go-between who does what he cannot, admit that he is having a problem:

> My wife went to the doctor. The doctors says, "How's he doing?" She says, "He's having these attacks." And he said, "Well you have him come up here right away." She says, "The doctor wants to see you." So I go up to see the doctor and he said, "I'm going to send you to a cardiologist".

The patient fits into the world at home. This is evident as family and friends wait through the time that he is in the cardiac catheterization laboratory, call him on the telephone, and visit him in his room. Some patients are acutely aware that they are being cared for by strangers: "I just told 'um I gotta come and put in hospital and I was talk with strange people. I say for me, that's all."

Long-established relationships with loved ones continue. They keep in touch with the patient while he is in the hospital. One man tells of a cousin who also has heart disease: "I told my one cousin who had a rheumatic heart. We are really close. We know everything about each other. We grew up together."

The Nature of His Support

Family and friends provide a variety of supportive interventions for the patient. Some support precedes the hospital admission date, in that the wife, son, or others legitimize the seriousness of his problem. They listen to his complaints of chest pains and become concerned about him: "My children been telling me go and get it taken care of, and find out what the problem is, and get the problem eliminated, or at least be able to know exactly what the problem is and find some kind of solution." They put pressure on him to go to the doctor or hospital: "My wife would listen to me and she was caring. She didn't know what to tell me but just go and get examined."

In addition to this affirmation, family and friends call the attention of health care providers to his crisis: "My wife was worried. She called 911." Or, they transport him to the hospital themselves: "I called my mother and said, 'Can you come down and take me to the hospital, I can't breathe and I have these pains in my chest?' " Furthermore, they take care of him by finding the nitroglycerin that he has misplaced to treat his chest pain.

Many times, a wife has been concerned about her husband for some time. In fact, some men do not worry about themselves, because their wives do the worrying for them. Seeing him on a daily basis helps her to know the extent of his symptoms. Anticipating that something bad will probably happen, she exhorts him to see his physician and to stop smoking.

Moreover, family and friends continue to watch over him when he is admitted to the hospital. They check on how the physicians and nurses are taking care of him: "They ask me how my doctors are, am I able to ask them questions, do they explain enough what they're going to do, the rest that's involved, what it's going to cost, if any, if I got to pay for it you know." This maintains their already established connections with what is going on with him. In time, he tells them what is happening daily: "I tell her what the doctor told me. There's a block that's causing the pain." He also reassures his family and friends that the doctor will tell him what to do to get well. In turn, the support group tells him that he is looking better or shows their worry if he is not.

Those who are widowed or divorced find support in friends or from an animal: "I feed him and that dog loves me, too. I see that he gets plenty to eat." One widower was comforted by his memories. Having survived concentration camps and having had a wonderful marriage sustains him. Men who have accessible families, yet rely on friends more than family, keep some of their situation away from home, seeking support elsewhere:

> My friend, my supervisor, had gone through this. He had a balloon (PTCA) done. He went through the whole procedure, because he went through the same thing. He had that catheterization and then he had the balloon.

Help from family and friends comes in the form of advice about what work the patient should and should not do after discharge and how he should change his lifestyle. Whether his family and friends get all the information that he has received or not, it is clear to him that they depend on him and he on them. Although some of this interdependence looks as if it is based on work, it nonetheless holds a place for him.

Preceding Admission to the Hospital

That cardiac patients have had symptoms signaling something gone awry before admission is evidenced in their accounts of events preceding hospitalization. An elderly gentleman describes his symptoms: "I come with pain in the feet and my head. I have twice a day to take pain killers, but the pain killers is no good for the head. I am not a small child and I don't want to be dizzy." It is common for many men to treat the more acute symptoms with prescribed drugs for cardiac disease and over-the-counter medications. Because they have nitroglycerin on hand, they take it for chest discomfort. They also take aspirin, because they know its benefits for pain and for decreasing coagulability. However, not all of them are aware of the names of the drugs for which they have prescriptions or their indications: "I was taking three other (heart) medications. But I don't know the names." Another states, "I been on this high-technical medication, which is one baby aspirin."

Subsequently, if the drugs that he takes fail to make him feel better and the symptoms persist, he begins to consider an emergency unit visit. However, the time that it takes him to make up his mind varies, because the crisis can evolve slowly or happen rapidly before he decides to go to the hospital for care.

Antecedent to the Emergency Unit Visit

For one man, a motor vehicular accident resulted in chest pain that, he finally found out, was cardiac, not muscular, in origin: "I had a car accident and, as a result of that car accident, I had real bad chest pain. I went to go see the doctor, who started treatment of my chest pains." Another man was coming to see his physician about chest discomfort. The physician's office was located on the hospital campus. However, the patient and his family got turned around and had trouble locating the office suite. Helpful transport personnel found them, quickly assessed the patient's chest discomfort, and brought him to the emergency unit.

Yet another man had chest pain resulting from shoveling snow. He delayed the inevitable for some time, and, when finally deciding to seek treatment, drove himself to the hospital in indomitable style:

> I shoveled the snow. I rested in between. I felt sore, but I thought it was more muscular than anything. It didn't go away, and then about a week later I was in bed and I woke up. It wasn't a pain, but it was discomfort. I rolled over on the right side and it got a little worse, and I sat up in bed and I broke out in a heavy sweat and got a little light headed and so I went to the community hospital and the doctor said it was the heart. I just got in my car and got to the hospital.

Seeking Legitimization of a Serious Cardiac Event from Health Care Providers

It is not surprising that men eventually decide to seek professional help. Their chest discomfort is so persistent or the shortness of breath so annoying that they can no longer ignore it. They finally seek help from physicians and hospital staff to confirm the hypothesis that something serious is happening that has to do with the heart. "I went to the hospital to get it checked out because I was starting to get concerned. It turned out to be a heart attack."

If a man decides to make an appointment to see his physician, he may achieve a less dramatic entrance to the hospital. His physician prescribes nitroglycerin after administering it to take care of the chest pain, if the patient has not been taking it already. Next, the physician schedules a stress test to determine the extent of cardiac disease and to help direct the next step in the plans for treatment.

In both instances, the actuality of a cardiac crisis is confirmed by health care personnel. This helps to validate the patient's hunch that he is sick. He can now become authentically sick; he is really a patient.

Hypothesis Testing

Before going to the hospital, many men sort through their symptoms and test various treatments, hoping that the symptoms are not signals of serious disease. In this process of identifying treatment, trying treatments, and waiting for improvement, valuable time is lost for those men who end up with an actual myocardial infarction or severe congestive heart failure and pulmonary edema.

Even though the symptoms are alarming, the process of analyzing the symptoms goes on: "I've had times where I was just sitting there, watching TV, when all of a sudden I have serious and sharp chest pains. I took a deep breath and tried to figure out what just happened." Or, "I had an incident maybe 2 days before, but very, very mild (chest pain). It could have been muscle spasm, it could have been anything. I just relaxed and in a few seconds it was gone." For these men, skeletal muscle pain is hoped for, not cardiac muscle pain.

Whereas some men ignore their chest pain ("I didn't pay any attention to it"), others seek solutions to it. Chest pain is explained: "I got new dentures. I was having this indigestion so often, I figured my not having dentures (caused it). The teeth in the back were causing me to not chew my food up. I had heartburn, so I went out and got them (dentures)." One man lets his shortness of breath persist as he treats it:

> I'd go out and go around the corner to go to the store and have to stop four or five times and four or five times coming back because I couldn't get my breath. I read all the labels of the stuff that I had bought and all these medicines say if you have these conditions, high thyroid and enlarged prostate, you can't use this. So I stop using it and I figure that's why I'm feeling the way I'm feeling on account of the medication then and the medical problems.

Another man had burning in his chest for months. He explained it to himself as being incisional healing and waited patiently for it to go away. Finally, after he was admitted for a cardiac catheterization, his physicians located an aortic bulb aneurysm, a consequence of mitral valve repair surgery. However, his explanation and treatment with over-the-counter analgesics delayed diagnosis and treatment and further compromised his cardiopulmonary status. He knew that his chest pain was different from previous episodes of such pain, yet he found and employed his own solution, following a self-imposed course of treatment for months: "One never knows, but I thought it was something else (incisional healing)."

When a diagnosis that refutes his suspicions and diagnosis is finally confirmed, one man admits having premonitions that his heart disease was in evidence, had caught his attention, and was serious. His foreboding of an upcoming crisis was supported by his physicians and subsequent diagnostic tests: "I had a feeling. I didn't want to probably admit it to myself."

Some men rely on being lucky, explaining that the odds were in their favor that severe disease and death would pass them by. They were lucky to have avoided hemodialysis for years, to have responded to drug therapy rather than having to have had surgery, and to have avoided a heart attack: "I got here. It wasn't a super heart attack. They said we're going to give you TPA and I said OK and they did and it apparently worked well."

Emergency Unit Experience

If a man's own treatment fails to stop his chest pain, the next solution is to seek help from his physician or local hospital's emergency unit. After having taken his nitroglycerin twice, one man finally considered going to the hospital: "I expect to (go) to emergency because I'm not going to die."

Whether he rates his chest pain or other symptoms as severe or not, he knows that he has cause for concern or he would not have made such a decision to seek help: "I didn't feel real bad. Just because of the other heart attack, something's not right." Nevertheless, he is relieved when the physicians and nurses confirm his problem.

After finally arriving at the EU, he can be pleased or not with his emergency unit experience. He is impressed when the nursing and physician staff see him quickly, triage his problem, and then work on ruling in or ruling out a heart attack, congestive heart failure, or other serious conditions. His sense of satisfaction or dissatisfaction with emergency unit care relates to how much attention he receives and his judgment of how well the staff perform.

By definition, an emergency unit moves fast and can be extremely chaotic if many patients with serious conditions converge at the same time. If this happens, a patient very likely reacts, coming from the unique egocentrism of his cardiac crisis: "The only part I don't like is when I first came in. The doctors in the emergency room, that was the only bad part. There were a lot more people getting sick, plus serious injuries. I came in about 2:30 A.M. and was down there till six o'clock."

On the other hand, he can be reassured, and thus satisfied, with the knowledge and skill of the emergency unit staff: "They knew the problem (congestive heart failure and pulmonary edema) right away because they hit me with a couple of needles and gave me some intravenous. And within 4 hours I was able to actually lean back and be comfortable."

The men who are admitted to C3 often travel from the EU to the ICU, perhaps to the step-down unit, and finally to C3: "It was Emergency to ICU and they took me out of there into another room on the ICU floor and then they brought me over here." Being transferred from unit to unit makes it possible for the patient to meet a large number of hospital staff, many of whom are nurses. Generally, his physicians remain the same and travel to the room where he is located.

Trusting the Physician

Important to and inherent in a patient's experience in the hospital is the trust that he has in his physician or physician group. Because part of the group is made up of physician's assistants, here, again, the number of people to deal with can be many. Knowing that his physicians are on top of what is going on with him and communicate it to him helps to renew his sense of trust: "I feel much more confident. The way that I'm treated here is a plus. Anything that I would have to have done, there's no need to feel insecure about it."

That the physician displays interest in him as a person goes a long way to pave the way for a favorable experience in the hospital. This connection is made by some physicians before the patient is admitted. After calling in his symptoms and concerns about his condition to his doctor's office, a patient goes on to work. He is happy later that his physician returns his call in person: "I get a telephone call that night. 'You better get into the hospital, to the emergency, right away.' He takes a personal interest in me."

The physicians try to level with him by explaining the pathology of his problems in understandable terms. A physician describes one patient's problem during rounds and for the benefit of the patient, who is actively listening:

He's got this aneurysm in his aortic root adjacent. One of the complications of endocarditis is that you develop a root abscess in the healing process (after surgery). It can sort of become an aneurysm. This healed root abscess comes to the left main (coronary artery). You're compressing the origin of the left main, which in fact is producing blood buildup to the left side of the heart. What you have to do is go back in there and cut out the aneurysm. Every time your heart beats, it sort of is a block in the coronary artery.

The patient is able to explain the pathology, indicating a level of comprehension and acknowledging the fact that his physician explained it to him a few times.

Discharge instructions also provide evidence to men that physicians are interested in them as patients and as people: "They told me pretty much what I have to do and to improve myself when I get home."

Another patient felt so out of control by the worsening of his heart disease that he hopes that his physicians interfere in his life by setting strict limits on his behavior. He seeks external controls and does not feel confident in his ability to change his life style. He wishes to know just how much exercise and activity he is allowed and wants to be told which foods will help to reduce the future risk of having another heart attack. Additionally, he wishes to be told to stop smoking.

Nurses Manage Symptoms

In addition to comforting and caring for C3 patients, nurses manage symptoms. One patient appreciates how a nurse determined that he needed an order for Maalox after every meal for "heaviness." After eliminating a cardiac cause of his distress, the nurse obtained the order and helped him become more comfortable. The same patient noted that he was becoming congested. A nurse encouraged him to deep breathe in spite of his incisional pain after his bypass graft surgery.

They paid a lot of attention to my symptoms. When they first took my blood pressure after I was taken off the IV, and all of a sudden the pressure was 92/50, they contacted the resident and the cardiologist on call over the weekend, because they were very concerned when they see a blood pressure like that. They help me through the pain. Every time I've had pain, one of the first things that they started with me is, on a scale of zero to ten, what would I call the pain? Like if I called it "two," they know how to explain it to the doctor, because, in a lot of cases, the doctor is not going to come down, and I've seen this with the resident, a few times, "Oh, give him such and such." They (nurses) become the diagnostician.

Another describes how nurses help him to manage his pain:

> I don't like to say anything unless I really need something, but
> they can always tell. As long as I've been here, they always look
> out for you. They pop in every once in a while and ask if there is
> anything that I need. They know when I'm not feeling well and
> they take care of that. If I got a thing, within a few minutes they
> would know and ask me if I want something for pain. They're
> pretty good, they keep up on that. . . . It's not like they'll stop in
> here and go out and go to work and forget that I have a pain in
> the leg and come back a couple of hours later on and ask you if
> you want something. They ask if I'm comfortable; they're around.

They also take care of other problems:

> I was telling the nurse I had a headache. They were putting me
> on that Isordil. I took it and I had the worse headache I ever had
> in my life. It lasted for 3 days. She said, "Well try it one more
> time, I don't think it's that." She said this because I was taking
> the patches (nitroglycerin). So I took it; 20 minutes later, boy
> that thing started. I called the nurse and I told the doctor. He
> gave me two Tylenols.

Whether the solution works remains to be determined by the patient.
On the other hand, some men report that they "haven't told them
(nurses) anything" about their symptoms. Others have little knowledge
of what nurses actually do: "I guess they do what they're trained to do."
Some see what nurses do to be following the orders that the doctor
writes because "they can't prescribe anything on their own." Nurses
also alert physicians to symptoms that need to be managed.

Not every patient thought that what was going on with the nurses
provided the best for him. One patient criticized and was "nervous"
about the patient assignment system, in which "you have one nurse
then the other."

Fear of Dying

Uppermost in some patients' minds is the idea that they could die
while currently hospitalized. They recall the same sense of fear when
they were hospitalized previously for serious conditions. Such fears
are renewed as they confront upcoming cardiac catheterization procedures. Their hesitancy to go through the procedure is expressed as being "a little leery," not wanting "to go under the knife anymore," learning "how fallible the human body is," and wanting "to live." Some fears

of death are bluntly reinforced by health care providers' explanations of treatment alternatives:

> Aneurysms can rupture; you don't want that. All the blood that comes from your heart is going out your aorta. If your aorta ruptures in that area, you'd be dead. You won't survive it. That's why this is dangerous. Right now the aneurysm is compressing that artery, but it can rupture.

One man discusses his brush with death, as recognized after cardiac arrest accompanying his heart attack. Still others experience life-threatening dysrhythmias, postcardiac catheterization bleeding, or severe pulmonary edema. Such encounters allow each man the dubious pleasure of confronting his own mortality. He made it, survived a life-threatening event, and begins to come to terms with the limits of a life span while he is in the hospital. Up to this point in his life, he has felt fairly immortal:

> I never used to want to understand it and I've learned how fallible the human body is. It's going to happen to somebody else, but not me. Because I jog 2 miles a day and I smoked, and it happened. You're not infallible, not superman.

That he escaped this time is especially poignant for one man who had an out-of-body experience.

> I had an out-of-body experience, in the cardiac cath lab. It has changed my outlook on a lot of things. My heart went into ventricular fibrillation and they had to shock me. And I was actually from above myself, watching them work on me. And just prior to the last shot actually working, I had somebody from behind put their hand on my shoulder and told me it wasn't time yet, it wasn't my time yet. Next thing I know, I woke up from the last shock and it was a very profound experience. And I think that more people have, maybe not the same, but similar experiences, in a seriously ill setting and they're just afraid to relate it. Because the first time I told a few people, people told me I was a lunatic. You have to understand one thing. I'm a Jew, I'm an ex-Green Beret, a trained killer, a total skeptic, who, up to my incident, thought it was all bullshit. But now if you ask me, it's an altogether different thing and I have every intention of putting it into work on paper.

This patient found that, when he related this experience to others, he was met with either acceptance or skepticism. The nurse manager listened to him and arranged for a rabbi to visit him. This rabbi accepted what he had to say. Another rabbi told him it was "all nonsense." This made the patient turn to his religion after staying away for a long time.

Serious heart disease makes death seem imminent and no longer deniable.

Being Born Again: Promises to Reform His Life Style

Hospitalization helps the patient to see his part in the recurrence of cardiac disease. He blames himself for continuing old, harmful habits:

> I feel like it's my fault this time. I was drinking and smoking and it just kind of crept up on me. I knew I was doing wrong and I did it anyway. I feel guilty and mad at myself, whereas before I felt sorry for myself.

He realizes now that he has not taken care of himself. This lack of care is a failure of sorts and a denial that anything as serious as this disease could happen to him. For a while he is able to ignore the possibility that his heart disease could get worse. However, his current situation refutes this possibility.

Some men are so addicted to their lifestyles that they never change their harmful ways. They admit the addictions that make the heart disease worsen. One man admits that he feels the taste of cigarettes: "What stands out in my mind happens to be something said by my doctor. I have spent 25 to 30 years with what the taste of cigarettes is. I now have felt what cigarettes are! Felt the taste of cigarettes." Still another tries to quit only to leave the house to go to the local store to buy more.

Many admit that smoking is not good for them and attribute their heart disease to this addiction. Some are able to stop completely and find themselves unable to tolerate someone else's smoking. Others were not able to stop after their first cardiac crisis.

Self-Care Before, Self-Care After

It is not surprising that men with chronic heart disease have already learned to take care of themselves. Nevertheless, heart disease brings such self-care skills into a different focus. They have already managed indigestion with over-the-counter medications and other remedies. Therefore, it is not unusual that, given the symptom of indigestion, a man reaches for an antacid such as Maalox. Or he tries an old treatment: "I was taking baking soda (for indigestion)."

Often men find it easy to stop what they are doing when they experience some symptoms and rest: "When I had that pressure, I laid back and finally it just went away." Another says, "Finally I just sat down; the chest pains come and go. It comes out of nowhere. I'll be sitting, watching TV, and start getting it." Many times resting stops the symptoms and enables them to resume what they were doing. But merely staying still and resting will not make chest pain or shortness of breath go away all of the time:

> I got short of breath. But I'm all right when I sit down, take a couple of minutes and rest and the shortness goes away. The burning sensation lasts for a little while. Sometimes it lasted for a few hours.

They take care of the chest pain simply: "Most of the time I just laid in bed." Eventually, they may have to take a more aggressive approach and enlist the help of a health care professional.

Because they have preexisting heart disease, all of the men are familiar with medications prescribed specifically to treat their conditions. However, from months to years can have passed since their last crises, so they do not have all of their prescription medications with them at all times.

Taking nitroglycerin is a commonly used treatment for chest pain. A lot of men take it for chest pain, and some combine it with an antacid to get the most relief: "In my experience, I take a little pill under the mouth, and then if it no work it can mean something else. Then I take Maalox, I know it work."

Other men avoid taking the nitroglycerin if they do not think it is warranted. Still others avoid taking it because of the headaches that result: "I was taking medication, nitro patches, for chest pain and they didn't agree with me, because I always had headaches right above the eyes. So I was a little skeptical of taking them."

Additionally, they take other medications to treat chest pain, including aspirin, Tylenol, or Tylenol 3. One man admits that he realized that he may not have known what was going on with his heart and was worrying about more serious events. Sometimes a minor flareup of his heart condition makes him stop and think and go back to his regimen: "That got me started thinking and I started taking a little better care of myself. Around the middle of the year I started taking my medicine on a regular basis."

Taking care of themselves means for some that they need specific information about the pathophysiology of myocardial infarction. His nurses supply the facts: "It's great to say, well the right coronary artery was blocked with plaque. Well, that's great, it's a nice technical thing, how has this happened? So, they (nurses) explained this to me. I was learning what literally went on." This man needs more information in order to consider future changes in his life style. However, for other men, there are no guarantees that they will be cured of heart disease. Nonmalleable factors can very easily prevail in spite of changes: "I had slimmed down my bad habits to the point where I could say that I was actually being good; this snuck up on me."

Beginning the prescribed regimen, including taking and learning about medications, undergoing procedures to improve cardiac blood flow, eating meals incorporating dietary changes, performing physical therapy prescriptions, and the like, help the patient, if for a short time, practice the new treatment plan before he is discharged.

Personal Agenda

I'm thinking about myself right now. I'm taking this test because I want to go to work; that's it.

Being in the hospital transforms men into anxious, fearful people. They find hospitalization difficult because they are not ready to have a flareup of their heart disease or to experience all the testing and treatment that that the crisis entails. Worse than that, they fear being "tied down with treatments," which threatens their independence. Men characterize the fear of dependence with such statements as, "My mind is ready to go home," "I want to go home," or "Just getting out of here."

The uncertainty of not knowing what is wrong with them brings frustration. Many men seek the knowledge of what is going on with their hearts or other organs and look for a plan that will correct the problem: "I wanted what the doctor sent me for; I wanted my heart to be all right. I didn't want to play around, so I wanted to know what was going on." This man specifically wished to avoid PTCA and CABG surgery. Finding out the details of what is wrong and how to correct it helps the man to regain some measure of control and, therefore, independence.

Another wishes to avoid revisiting his recent crisis, which was caused by an incompetent mitral valve. Still another patient hopes that he can avoid bypass surgery and wishes for a medication to make his problem disappear.

Those who think more in the moment as they await cardiac catheterization desire a clean bill of health in the form of results that say everything is "OK." Having premonitions to the contrary, some realized before the catheterization that it was unlikely that cardiac catheterization results would be negative for plaque formation and serious cardiac narrowing. "I'm just hoping that, as a result of the catheterization, that we can come up with a solution that can eliminate both my smoking habit and chest pains and chest discomfort. I'd like to pick things up from there and move on from there." One solution is PTCA, which is understood as a way "to open up any blocked arteries." A man who recently had a PTCA states, "I hoped that they opened up the problem blood vessel and I hope it stays opened." Having seen the actual cardiac catheterization image, he is aware of three coronary occlusions and has connected them causally to his chest pain. He is also aware of the difficulty that his cardiologist had in keeping one of the vessels open during the procedure.

Having considered the strong possibility of death, another man looks forward to modifying his lifestyle so that he does not have another heart attack. His spirit of reform comes through:

> One of the things was being brought back to health has been done. Number two, is I wanted to be given, to be told, what foods I should eat that would help to reduce any risk or further risk, or future risk of another MI. I wanted to actually stop smoking.

Finally another man, readmitted many times, wistfully hopes for all of his cardiac disease to go away. His current admission and list of diagnoses illustrate how complex his heart disease is and how many complications he has experienced.

> I'd like to get as well as can be so I won't have any problems. It bothers me. I say, "Why am I having so much problems?" Because I had always been a healthy type of person. There was nothing wrong with me. I had never been on drugs or nothing. Why did this thing have to happen to me? And then when I had this valve replacement done last year. Why do I have a weak part in the back part of the heart?

Having Symptoms

Men report having symptoms before they are admitted to the hospital and in the course of their hospital stay. They learn quickly that some symptoms are caused by prescribed medications. They also deny having symptoms at any given time: "I feel fine this morning. I no have no pain or nothing." Furthermore, they often note that their symptoms have subsided since their first day of hospitalization. Pain abates, shortness of breath disappears, and they have more energy. They have found relief through rest, medications, and PTCA or CABG procedures. They often may not tell nurses and physicians about their symptoms, especially if they do not interpret the symptoms to be associated with cardiac disease. It is almost as though the physicians' and nurses' attention to cardiac symptoms lets the patient himself rule out others as being unworthy of mention.

Perhaps men with chronic cardiac disease become so accustomed to its symptoms that symptoms have to be new ones in order for them to attend to them. Whereas some pay little attention to symptoms that suggest heart disease, "I had an incident maybe two days before (admission) but very, very mild," others simply do not know the significance of the symptoms that they are experiencing. One man brushes off his chest pain even though "they get really bad at times." Rather, he explains the chest pain's origin to be from bronchiectasis, because he commonly has chest pain when he coughs. Another man explains his cardiac symptom to be caused by a cold. He tries various solutions before finally giving up and going to his physician.

> I have a little pain in my back and after that they go away. I call my doctor and it was like a little cold. So after 1 week, I have a little cold in the chest. So I take a little pill (nitroglycerin). Now the pain it no go away, so later on I take a Maalox, and the pain go away; so this happen two, three times in one week. So then I'm a little upset. I feel a little dry. So I went to my family doctor. I describe all these thing and she says she don't want me to take another chance and she wants to send me to my heart specialist. So I told the story to the doctor and he wants to make sure everything is all right and let's do it with the cardiac catheterization.

Having Chest Pain. Chest pain is not always described as chest pain. Sometimes it is called discomfort, back pain, or jaw pain. Because this pathognomonic symptom indicates heart disease for most health care providers, it is interesting that many patients do not describe their experience as described in the textbook. Furthermore, they are often unaware that their symptoms, of the other-than-textbook variety, may be generated by cardiac disease.

Chest Pain from Myocardial Infarction. One patient was unable to avoid having a heart attack. The heaviness that he felt in his chest continued for days before he was admitted. He lost track of how many days it went on. His wife reminded him that it lasted for 5 days before admission, down the arm and into the shoulder. The pain is so severe and so distressing that he is unable to comprehend it, and neither, he thinks, can anyone who has not suffered it understand its severity. He compares it to the other pains that he knows: "Now I've been shot, several times in Viet Nam, and this heart attack was worse than getting shot. This heart attack was worse than that."

Chest Pain from Being Defibrillated.   The same patient also sustains cardiac arrest. Residual chest pain results, and the treatment adds a variation of chest pain to his experience:

> When I was shocked with the defibrillator, I was shocked several times, and how I classify it is the experiments we do in biology with electricity. Getting shocked a couple of times has created a soreness in the muscle. And that soreness has to heal.

He is able to compare this different sensation with his previous experience of ischemic chest pain. He knows the difference, regrettably, between the pain of a heart attack and that of repeated chest-wall defibrillation.

Discomfort, Not Chest Pain.   Few new nurses and physicians are taught the differences in the language that patients use when they seek help for a heart problem. Instead of describing chest pain, patients complain of chest discomfort or merely discomfort. This description could serve to confuse new clinicians who could tend to minimize the symptom. Similarly, the use of the term discomfort could also work to help a patient minimize or even deny the potential of his discomfort, that of cardiac ischemia and the possibility of heart attack.

Patients insist on using their language in this way. That the discomfort reported means that he is strong, even macho, and will not complain of pain is but one simple explanation. Conversely, he could actually be experiencing a sensation of discomfort, not pain. One man gets his point across:

> When I take and stick myself with this point, that's pain. But to have something, say, annoying me, I call it discomfort. They keep asking about all these pains I was supposed to be having and I can't give them a straight answer because I don't (feel it). I accept pain, what I consider pain is being stuck, or cut, or hit, when I hit my hand with a hammer. I seldom, if ever, have pain.

Having Angina Before Being Admitted.   Sometimes men with cardiac disease experience chest pain when they are resting and other times when they are exerting themselves. In either case, the intensity of the pain helps them to decide whether to rest and wait for the pain to go away, take nitroglycerin or other drugs, such as aspirin, and see what happens next, or to alert family and friends that they want to see their physicians or go to the hospital as soon as possible.

> I woke up with tightness in my chest and, beings I had a heart attack before, I tried taking my nitro and couldn't find it, left it in another shirt, couldn't find it, so I took up my aspirin.

Mild. Patients judge their chest pain or discomfort before acting on the interpretation. They weigh how bad the symptom feels before deciding what to do. Mild pain is frequently ignored. Sometimes they take nitroglycerin; other times they stop and then resume whatever they were doing.

> It happened one morning when I was going to go fishing. I was taking my grandson fishing. I got up and sat on the bed and just that fast it hit me. I laid back for about 10 minutes and it went away. Then I got up and went fishing.

Moderate. Pain that is perceived to be more intense than mild pain gets the patient's attention; he tries to interpret what it could mean. He describes it as pressure, when trying to relate the sensations he feels: "I had pains in my chest, like pressure." His speech includes qualifying adjectives that clarify his rating of the chest pain. Thus, the word "some" is used to note an increase in severity and distress: "I had some pain, burning in my chest." He may locate the pain: "It's sharp chest pain in the heart area. Just like on the left side of the chest."

Those with a clear memory of earlier chest pain compare the current sensations with a symptom or sensation memory. So they estimate their pain to be at a moderate level, because the sensations are less distressing than the pain associated with their first heart attacks.

However, not all patients with chronic heart disease experience heart attack. In fact, some that do so have "silent" ones. Consequently, they possess little or no symptom memory. Those who had a heart attack and realized it have a basis for comparison. They remember, "It was more of a tightness. It's pretty hard to describe. It was a muscle tightness. And pressure. The first heart attack was like pressure. This was like a knot."

Moderate chest pain is often accompanied by other sensations. It is difficult to discern whether chest pressure and shortness of breath coincide or are distinct for some patients and whether chest pain and indigestion are the same or different symptoms. The men express it in various ways: "I can't breathe, I can't get my breath and I have these pains in my chest"; "It is just up and down my neck and shoulder and the middle of my chest"; "I had the pains in my chest, not pain discomfort. A little like indigestion, heartburn."

Those who have known what angina feels like are able to discriminate moderate from severe angina: "I had a couple of minor angina, some of it's caused by laying in bed. Like a sore shoulder. I haven't had any heart attack."

Severe. Severe angina does not go away. If it decreases after the patient takes nitroglycerin, it is certain to return. It signals that a serious cardiac crisis is present.

> Three times I had the pressure on the chest and that sensation in my arms. If it wasn't for my wife, that's when she called the doctor for a refill. It was *just* like an elephant, something heavy crushing on your chest. It's just no pain, just like pressure and your arms, they feel like they were just floating and you have no control over them, when they float around and you get like a dizziness.

Severe chest pain warns a patient to stay away from work for a day or so; it directs him to think about going to the doctor or emergency unit and to call the rescue service or a family member or friend to take him to the hospital. The pain is different from that of his usual angina.

Despite his decision to go to the hospital or to call his physician, he may not be diagnosed as being in imminent danger of heart attack. Rather, he is diagnosed as having a pulmonary problem or indigestion, not heart disease.

> The chest pains were just getting worst. I went back and I had to get chest x-rays and they found out that I had pleurisy. Towards the end of the first week, beginning of the second week they gave me some nitroglycerin and within 3 days I was back up on my feet.

If he takes his doctor's advice and takes an antacid, such as Mylanta, he may get temporary relief of his chest pain or indigestion. However, the chest pain returns and forces him to rest and decide not to go to work. His misery makes him able to nap only when sitting on the toilet. As his discomfort increases, he is unable to sleep, feels more fatigued, and finally goes to the hospital.

Having Chest Pain and Other Pain While in the Hospital.   Whether the patient is admitted to the hospital through the emergency unit, received by the CCU staff, or directly admitted to C3, he receives immediate attention when reporting chest pain. The emergency unit or cardiac nurses take his complaints seriously and begin to take an ECG and administer nitroglycerin.

Typically, complaints of chest pain are sorted out by the patient himself before bringing it to the nursing staff's attention. Additionally, the pain that is foremost in his thoughts while in the hospital can be related to other conditions, such as pain from osteoarthritis, fairly intense claudication from arterial disease, severe foot pain from the peripheral neuropathy resulting from diabetes mellitus, or headache pain from medications, such as Isordil. One man's leg pain was so severe that he was severely depressed as a result: "The last couple of months, I have pain. Pain I cannot take. I cannot take more pain. I have pain. I cry a lot. All day and night." With evaluation and treatment, his pain becomes less severe.

Shortness of Breath.   Often, chest pain or discomfort is accompanied by shortness of breath. In fact, many men frequently do not distinguish shortness of breath from chest pain: "I'm short of breath, but I'm not really. I don't know how to pinpoint it. I described it last night to one of the nurses as feeling like you want to belch, but there's no belch there." The perceptions are frequently integrated into a synthesis of symptoms.

Men admit that their shortness of breath is "slight," causing a little bit of trouble, or more serious, because they breathe harder, have difficulty getting their breath, or endure limitations on everyday activity. Some explain the dyspnea by attributing it to cigarette smoking or, later, when they learn that it was caused by congestive heart failure, to fluid retention.

When the shortness of breath is severe, they realize that they are not feeling well at all: "I felt lousy, really lousy. I couldn't get around, I couldn't breathe." Their anxiety increases as they become progressively more dyspneic.

Getting treated by a doctor or the hospital staff brings relief. Whether the source of dyspnea is related to chest pain and coronary heart disease or to congestive heart failure, many are happy that they breathe more easily.

Fatigue. In addition to dyspnea, fatigue is a frequent companion symptom for the man with chronic cardiac disease. He may admit feeling a little tired or occasionally tired before his admission or he could have felt exhausted most of the time: "I was very energetic. I feel the energy is gone; I always walk. I start to walk and stop. I walk with less energy because I know that I don't have to see I feel tired."

His fatigue limits his daily activities. Periodic tiredness finally makes him reduce the amount of work and entertainment that he pursues. On the other hand, he fights his limitations by doing major renovation work at home or by helping a friend with a construction project. But, eventually, exhaustion, chest pain, or shortness of breath bring him and his family and friends to the conclusion that he needs help.

Indigestion. That indigestion is a common symptom for the populace in general is reinforced by advertisers, physicians, and other health care providers. Moreover, many patients know that indigestion masks chest pain as the presenting symptom of coronary artery disease. They acquire most of this knowledge after they are admitted and receive cardiac diagnoses:

> The heartburn I associated with the chest pain. The heartburn is really super bad the whole time I had the real bad chest pain. Even after I had gotten better, I had a couple of times where it came on again, just before the chest pains, I got this severe heartburn. I used to pass it off.

In spite of the fact that vasodilators, such as nitroglycerin, treat the chest pain or discomfort associated with cardiac disease, antacids are often taken to relieve indigestion. Some men take antacids regularly.

Insomnia. Other symptoms often interrupt a patient's sleep. Chest pain wakes him up and shortness of breath makes it difficult for him to fall asleep. As his condition exacerbates, his sleeplessness worsens: "I felt bad during Friday night. I couldn't sleep, and I tried sitting up and I can't sleep when I'm sitting up."

Insomnia is related to how sad he is about losing his health to heart disease. He may be depressed because of the changes in life brought about by symptoms, medication, and not feeling whole. One man is afraid that he will be as depressed as he was "years ago." He describes his depression as "losing energy, walking with less energy, not wanting to be bothered about things, and being sorry that he retired because he has to feel busy."

Additionally, he loses other parts of his life. He may no longer be able to go on a 2-month vacation. Perhaps he cannot afford his apartment, because of losing his job. Because this happened with his last hospitalization, it could very likely happen again.

Denial

Some men deny that they have heart disease. One man stated that he never had heart disease, although he admitted having a prescription for nitroglycerin. Another had two coronary bypass surgeries. He admits, "I never felt like I had a problem. That's my problem. I never felt sick. I was up after the operation (CABG). I was up and down. I can't stand around and moan and groan. Once I got going, I wasn't sore."

They admit that denial of a serious problem is typical in that they do not get upset about anything. Their wives worry, but they do not. They are simply not worried.

What they do admit is concern about what may happen if the angioplasty fails to open partly occluded vessels. Not one of them looks forward to cardiac surgery. "I really wasn't worried; it didn't bother me coming in, just the result of what might happen if it (angioplasty) didn't work out."

Anxiety

Men acknowledge that they are anxious about having a cardiac catheterization or a percutaneuous transluminal angioplasty. If the angioplasty fails to open vessels, most likely the patient will have a coronary artery bypass graft. Some prepare for the worst, which is death.

Short of death, there are several options for those who have coronary artery disease and angina. The treatments available include medications, cardiac catheterization, and other diagnostic tests to identify the location and extent of the pathology, percutaneous transluminal angioplasties to open vessels, and coronary artery bypass grafts.

I have a lot more confidence than I did before I started. I was a little leery of having the catheterization done. Something is wrong. I'm anxious to know that we come up with a solution to resolve the problem. I know that I still have the blockages and I think psychologically that it affects me because I know I have chest pains and I know that there's a problem. Not knowing what that problem is kind of keeps me on edge. I felt a lot more peace of mind being that this procedure is over with. I'm one to think that something can be five times as worse as it actually is.

They are relieved when the catheterization and other procedures are over, even though the next step brings more risk. They are eager to get past the 8-hour time period in which they are required to lie immobile to protect the access site and return home. Or they hope that they get past the PTCA or CABG soon. A PTCA and a CABG are major events that have the potential to improve cardiac status and place men at greater risks. But the potential benefits outweigh the risks for some. A man describes his reactions after having undergone PTCA.

> I'm a little bit worried, because when he said he had trouble with the occlusion staying open, he said it might collapse, so I want to talk to him when he comes, what are the symptoms if it does collapse? What are the chances and how can I keep it from collapsing?

Chronic cardiac disease adds to present life stress. The most recent crisis throws a man into imbalance. He considers the possibility of death, suffering, and unfulfilled responsibilities to loved ones.

Anxieties increase for some men as they begin to realize what their symptoms mean and to understand the nature of their problems. Before one man had a heart attack, he did not understand what his symptoms meant. As a result of having a heart attack, he knows how to interpret what is happening to him. He begins to understand what a heart attack feels like:

> I go to my doctor because I'm really afraid now, because of the heart attack, because of what happened before. The heart attack before wasn't scary because in the beginning I didn't understand it was a heart attack.

Patients are afraid of dying and afraid of being treated: "I was scared to death when I first came in here. I expected and was wondering about what the results were going to be." One patient admits, "It's just an idea of being cut open again, I guess. And going through that agony again, the soreness and all of the other things."

Anger

Anger about a patient's situation may not often be expressed during the hospitalization. The number of days that the patient is hospitalized are few, especially if his catheterization is not followed by PTCA or CABG surgery. One man was angry when a mix-up occurred with his lunch. He had fasted in preparation for a diagnostic study and had to wait to eat until the second half of the test was completed. The nurses called the dietary department for his food tray, which was later left at the nurses' station unbeknown to his nurse, who was busy with other patients. He was ready to "kill" or "hit" someone. He finally went to the snack shop for lunch, only to find out later about his misplaced food.

Men with chronic cardiac disease reminisce about more robust times of their lives; they try to prove their strength in the face of the current hospitalization. They often deny being concerned about the current cardiac crisis. The detailed descriptions of chest pain and other symptoms belie this denial and may get them the attention of nurses and other health care providers.

This study attempted to address the experience of hospitalization and symptom management for patients with long-term cardiac disease in the context of an urban, tertiary care hospital. The immediate setting of the medical unit, or telemetry unit, and the caregiving of nurses were not presented in this abbreviated presentation.

Chronically ill patients are hospitalized for increasingly shorter hospital stays. Shorter hospitalizations are due to the focused attention of caregivers, including nurses and physicians, who determine the extent of their disease and treat the exacerbations that brought them to the hospital in the first place. Core 3 patients admitted for chest pain experienced hospitalization through a framework that included diagnostic studies that identified the extent of their cardiac disease. Consequently, the shape and pace of the hospital experience was determined largely by such studies and patients' need for immediate management of chest pain. Nurses provided the 24-hour continuous care that included teaching about diagnostic and therapeutic procedures, symptom management (chiefly that of chest pain), and recovery from cardiac catheterization, PTCA, and bypass surgery. Cardiologists carried out diagnostic and interventional procedures.

Before admission to the hospital for a heart problem, men and women managed their symptoms successfully at home. Many avoided seeking help from physicians and used nitroglycerin to decrease chest pain. But, if the chest pain did not disappear after two or more nitros, they eventually sought help at a doctor's office or the emergency unit of a community hospital or tertiary care hospital.

Women relied on their support systems more heavily than did men. Relatives and friends transported them to the hospital, checked in to find out what was happening during the hospitalization, and accompanied them home. Yet the women preferred not to become dependent on the people in their support systems. They realized that many family members relied on them to keep the family steady and that their hospitalization was going to disrupt the family.

Before they agreed to bring their symptoms to the attention of a health care provider, chronically ill women with heart disease asked that others, including friends and relatives, confirm the fact that they were sick enough to do so. By going to see a doctor or the staff of the hospital's emergency unit, the women acknowledged that they were sick. Such acceptance began the process of confronting the reality of their heart disease. Soon, diagnostic and treatment options were offered by cardiologists and other attending physicians and were then agreed to.

Hospitalization for acute cardiac problems stimulated women to think of the possibility of death. Their fear was not remote, because chest pain reminded them of death, as did other crises associated with cardiac disease. But surviving was important, especially as they interpreted their lives in relation to others, those they cared for at home.

Women tended to ignore their symptoms until they were unable to do so. Men with cardiac disease saw hospitalization as a threat to their masculinity, noting the intrusion of the latest hospital stopover into their lives at work. They discussed their service in the military and their work history. Such discussions emphasized their former strength and command.

The male patients were not very surprised to learn that they had heart disease, citing various members of their families who also had it. Furthermore, they were fairly comfortable in the hospital, especially if they reported having been treated well during previous hospitalizations.

On the other hand, being in the hospital represented a time of increased vulnerability for men that was characterized by their being uneasy. The men did not want to lose personal control. They maintained control by playing down the extent of the present illness with their loved ones. Rather than consulting family and friends to legitimize their symptoms as being serious, they sought sanctions from health care providers about how serious the situation was. Furthermore, they hypothesized about what their symptoms meant and speculated about the cause and severity of the present acute episode. Like the women, they were afraid of dying.

Men were hungry for the details about the events of hospitalization, including diagnostic studies and treatment. They were more aware than women of what nurses did as they managed chest pain. They also provided more detail about their chest pain compared with women.

The men interpreted the present cardiac crisis and hospitalization as an opportunity to reform their life styles. They requested that limits on their behavior be imposed by physicians and planned changes in their diets and activity levels. They were more committed than the women in the study to taking care of themselves.

That the experiences of women and men are so different is not surprising. However, the implications of the differences are important for health care providers to consider.

Perhaps nurses and others could reexamine the differences between male and female reports of symptoms, especially chest pain. Health care providers may tend to underestimate women's pain because women do not provide great detail when answering the questions posed by them. Men and women also differ in the amount of detail reported about the events of hospitalization, including cardiac catheterization and PTCAs. Perhaps this difference can be explained by the intuition that men require detailed information and retain it so as to regain some of the control over their situations that they perceive to have been lost as a consequence of illness.

Additionally, nurses might reexamine the fear that their patients experience as they endure a chest pain episode. Just being in the hospital for a flareup of their chronic heart disease stimulates fear. Both men and women fear death, and this fear warrants discussion if patients are open to it and nurses and other health care providers are primed for these reflections.

11

Case Study
The Method

Carla Mariano

In the world of science, the term *case study* is an enigma. As Lincoln and Guba (1985) noted:

> [W]hile the literature is replete with references to case studies and with examples of case study reports, there seems to be little agreement about what a case study is . . . there is no simple taxonomy within which various kinds of case studies might be classified. (pp. 360–361)

Case studies are variously described as a research strategy/design (Creswell, 1998); Kratochwill & Levin, 1992; Naumes & Naumes, 1999; Yin, 1994, a reporting mode (Lincoln & Guba, 1985), a teaching technique (Naumes & Naumes, 1999), and an evaluation method (Patton, 1990). The case study is used in a variety of settings—schools, health care, the military, business, and industry—and by numerous disciplines—psychology, sociology, anthropology, history, ethics, economics, medicine, psychiatry, law, nursing, education, social work, management, political science, and public administration, to name but a few. In addition, the unit of analysis varies greatly among case studies. The unit of analysis can be a person, family, group, community, organization, culture, event, movement, program, or process.

Case studies are conducted at "various levels of complexity—from a single, brief, trivial episode to a lengthy major life-event with multiple strands" (Bromley, 1986, p. 2). They also use differing levels of analysis: merely factual, interpretative, and evaluative/judgmental levels of analysis (Lincoln & Guba, 1985). Case studies can focus on a single case as the unit of analysis or on multiple cases that are then compared.

Within the research arena, case studies can be exploratory, descriptive, interpretative, or explanatory (Tesch, 1990; Yin, 1994). Designs range from purely qualitative naturalistic inquiries (Lincoln & Guba, 1985) to single-case experiments (Barlow & Hersen, 1985) and complex time series designs (Cryer, 1986). The case study approach can be used either for hypothesis/theory generation or for hypothesis/theory testing. An understanding of case study develops in one a genuine appreciation for a mainstay axiom of qualitative research: there are truly multiple realities.

Because the purpose of this book is the consideration of qualitative research approaches, the remainder of this chapter will focus on the case study method primarily within the naturalistic paradigm.

DEFINITIONS AND CHARACTERISTICS

A case study is an "intensive, systematic investigation of a single individual, group, community, or some other unit, typically conducted under naturalistic conditions, in which the investigator examines in-depth data related to background, current status, environmental characteristics and interactions" (Woods & Catanzaro, 1988, p. 553).

Bromley (1986) characterized a case study as "a general term widely used, especially in the social and behavioral sciences, to refer to the description and analysis of a particular entity. . . . Such singular entities are usually natural occurrences with definable boundaries, although they exist and function within a context of surrounding circumstances. Such entities also exist over a short period of time relative to that context" (p. 8). Bromley also contended that the case study method is a "basic form of scientific inquiry that underpins effective professional practice especially in relation to human problems" (p. 41).

Yin (1994) defined a case study as an empirical inquiry that "investigates a contemporary phenomenon within its real-life context; when the boundaries between phenomenon and context are not clearly evident" (p. 3). Additionally, multiple sources of evidence are used. Denny, as cited in Guba and Lincoln (1981), defined the case study as "an intensive or complete examination of a facet, an issue, or perhaps the events of a geographic setting over time" (p. 370). Tesch (1990) described a case study as an ". . . intensive and detailed study of one individual or of a group as an entity, through observation, self-reports, and other means" (p. 39). Creswell (1998) defines case study as the "study of a 'bounded system' with the focus being either the case or an issue that is illustrated by the case (or cases). A qualitative case study provides an in-depth study of this 'system,' based on a diverse array of data collection materials, and the researcher situates this system or case within its larger 'context' or setting" (p. 249).

Four elements typify case studies: context, boundaries, time, and intensity. Case studies are conducted in context. Bromley (1986) reminded us: "The proper focus of a case study is not so much a 'person' as a 'person in a situation'" (p. 25). This is equally true when studying an organization, an event, or a process. The case must be viewed in its "ecological context" (Bromley, 1986), that is, in its physical, social, cultural, and symbolic environment. Naturalistic ontology proposes that "realities are wholes that cannot be understood in isolation from their contexts, nor can they be fragmented for separate study of the parts" (Lincoln & Guba, 1985, p. 39). For thorough understanding to be achieved, the research must be conducted with the case in context. This is crucial for three reasons:

1. Because it must be determined whether the conclusions apply to other contexts;
2. Because of "the belief in complex mutual shaping rather than linear causation, which suggests that the phenomenon must be studied in its full-scale influence (force) field" (Lincoln & Guba, 1985, p. 39); and
3. Because values are an integral element of context, defining and influencing behavior.

Hinds, Chaves, and Cypess (1992) suggested that phenomena are always embedded within four layers of context:

1. The *immediate context*—the present, the here and now.
2. The *specific context*—one's unique and individual perspective, incorporating both the immediate past and the significant facets of the current situation.
3. The *general context*—a person's "general life frame of reference" (p. 38). The present situation is often interpreted in view of this context.
4. The *metacontext*—a social construction representing a shared social attitude and viewpoint.

Hinds and colleagues (1992) noted that meaning originates from interaction with these various contexts.

In a case study, the researcher defines the boundaries of the inquiry. Stake (1983) noted: "The case need not be a person or enterprise. It can be whatever *bounded system* (to use Louis Smith's term) is of interest" (p. 283). The investigator delineates the issues and reference points. This characteristic distinguishes the case study approach; that is, boundaries are continually kept in focus with the emphasis on what is and what is not the case:

> What is happening and deemed important within those boundaries (the emic) is considered vital and usually determines what the study is about, as contrasted with other kinds of studies where hypotheses or issues previously targeted by the investigators (the etic) usually determine the study. (Stake, 1983, p. 283)

Case studies are present oriented. They examine contemporary experience rather than historic events. Although the investigator may use "historical" data about the person or organization, the investigation focuses on the here and now. Case studies can be differentiated from life histories, which chronicle the links and connectedness of a person's or group's life occurrences.

Data collection over time is another important consideration in case study research. This topic is discussed in a later section.

Case studies employ an intensive orientation to the phenomenon under study. A very close association between the researcher and the participant(s) usually develops over a long period. The researcher immerses himself or herself in the setting or situation and collects extensive evidence to describe and/or explain the case. Understandings that develop as an outcome of the study are often powerful and profound.

PURPOSE AND RATIONALE

Case studies are conducted for several reasons. Guba and Lincoln (1981; Lincoln & Guba, 1985) identified four purposes of case studies:

1. To chronicle (recording facts or events temporally or in the order in which they occurred);
2. To render (describing, depicting, or characterizing);
3. To teach (instructing); and

4. To test (using a case to test particular theories or hypotheses or both).

Table 11–1 presents a typology of case studies and indicates the four purposes, the corresponding levels of analysis, and the product of each type of endeavor.

Stake (1994, 1995) identified three types of case studies:

1. *Intrinsic*—to better understand a "particular" case because, in its particularity and ordinariness, the case itself is of interest.
2. *Instrumental*—to serve as a source of insight into an issue, problem, or refinement of theory where the case is secondary, facilitating our understanding of something else.
3. *Collective*—to inquire into a phenomenon, population, or general condition by studying a number of cases jointly (p. 237).

Case studies are conducted when little is known about a phenomenon or situation or when the traits of a person, organization, or event are unusual. They are very useful in the exploratory phase of an investigation when:

1. There is little prior research in the area;
2. There is a need for preliminary data and information for planning larger research studies; and
3. The generation of hypotheses for further verification is desirable.

Another reason for using the case study approach is to illustrate, demonstrate, or test a theory; this was the goal with many of the psychoanalytic case studies. Yin (1981a) contended that, "although case studies indeed can be used for exploratory purposes, the approach also may be used for either descriptive or explanatory purposes as well—i.e., to describe a situation . . . or to test explanations for why specific events have occurred. In the explanatory function, the case study can therefore be used to make causal inferences" (p. 98).

However, Stake (1983) noted:

When explanations, propositional knowledge, and law are the aims of an inquiry, the case study will often be at a disadvantage. When the aims are understanding, extension of experience, and increase in conviction in that which is known, the disadvantage disappears. (p. 281)

Although case studies have been used by anthropologists, psychoanalysts and many others as a method of exploration

TABLE 11–1 CASE STUDY TYPES

Purpose of the Case Study	LEVELS OF THE CASE STUDY					
	Factual		Interpretive		Evaluative	
	Action	Product	Action	Product	Action	Product
Chronicle	Record	Register	Construe	History	Deliberate	Evidence
Render	Construct	Profile	Synthesize	Meanings	Epitomize	Portrayal
Teach	Present	Cognitions	Clarify	Understandings	Contrast	Discriminations
Test	Examine	Facts	Relate	Theory	Weigh	Judgments

Source: From *Effective Evaluation* by E. Guba and Y. Lincoln, 1981. San Francisco: Jossey-Bass Publishers. Reprinted by permission of Jossey-Bass Publishers.

preliminary to theory development, the characteristics of the method are usually more suited to expansionist than reductionist pursuits. Theory building is the search for essences, pervasive and determining ingredients, and the making of laws. The case study, however, proliferates rather than narrows. One is left with more to pay attention to rather than less. The case study attends to the idiosyncratic more than to the pervasive. The fact that it has been useful in theory building does not mean that is its best use. Its best use appears to be for adding to existing experience and humanistic understanding. Its characteristics match the "readiness" people have for added experience . . . intentionality and empathy are central to the comprehension of social problems, but so also is information that is holistic and episodic. The discourse of persons struggling to increase their understanding of social matters features and solicits these qualities. And these qualities match nicely the characteristics of the case study. (p. 284)

Case studies are also the approach of choice when a particular problem has arisen and necessitates a solution. Problematic decision making in an organization, cases of child abuse and neglect, substance abuse in families, and so on—all require exploration from a case study approach. The results/conclusions of this type of case study often take the form of policies or recommendations for remedial or therapeutic action (Denzin, 1989; Majchrzak, 1984).

Ideally, a case study attempts to integrate theory and practice by applying general concepts and knowledge to a particular situation in the real world. (Bromley, 1986, p. 42)

In all of these situations, the distinctive need for case studies arises out of the desire to understand complex social phenomena. In brief, the case study allows an investigation to retain the holistic and meaningful characteristics of real-life events. (Yin, 1989, p. 14)

CASE STUDY RESEARCH PROCESS

Strategies used in data collection and analysis in a case study are similar to some of the techniques used in other qualitative designs. There are, however, specifics related to collecting, organizing, and analyzing data in a case study.

The process of case study consists of the following elements:

- Identifying the purpose and questions of the study;
- Identifying the theoretical propositions if appropriate to the type of case study being conducted;
- Determining the unit of analysis;
- Developing a case study protocol (the guide for carrying out the case study);
- Deciding on the most appropriate design;
- Conducting the case study—collecting, analyzing, and interpreting the data; and
- Writing the case study report.

Purpose/Questions

The content, organization, duration, data-collection points, and type of evidence of a case study are dependent on the purpose of the inquiry. Therefore, the aims and goals of the study should be explicitly stated.

Research questions best answered by case studies are *what, how,* and *why* questions. Powers and Knapp (1990) indicated that case studies are concerned with "discovering what the relevant variables are that may explain, for example, why a study subject thinks and acts in certain ways, how a program was implemented, or how and why a particular event took place" (p. 18). *What* questions lead to exploratory/descriptive case studies and *how* or *why* questions convey an explanatory case study approach. Because the potential number of factors and amount of data in any case study can be enormous, defining the research question becomes one of the most important steps in this type of research.

Theory

A theoretical framework or theoretical propositions may guide the inquiry, depending on the purpose of the case study. These a priori propositions reflect the research questions, literature review, and researcher's intuitions. They focus attention on what should be explored in the study. In explanatory or theory-testing case studies, this theoretical orientation shapes the analysis and the examination of alternative interpretations. With exploratory/descriptive case studies, the theoretical propositions or framework usually evolve from the data themselves.

Regardless of the question being asked, the investigator should clearly examine and specify his or her *assumptions* about the phenomenon of interest at the outset of the study.

Unit of Analysis

The unit of analysis (e.g., individual, family, organization, event) and the context in which the unit exists must be clearly differentiated at the beginning of the inquiry. Clarity of focus is imperative to the appropriate collection of data.

Elucidating the unit of analysis also has implications for the study design. Case studies can be conducted as holistic or embedded case studies. A holistic design examines the phenomenon of interest as a totality, from a global perspective (a group as a whole). An embedded design examines multiple units or subunits within the case, even though the study may be about a single entity (individual members of a particular group). As one can see, the identification of the unit(s) of analysis would have many implications for whom to interview or what to observe.

Case Study Protocol

The case study protocol (Yin, 1994) serves as the researcher's guide in conducting the case study. It keeps the goal of the study in the forefront while defining the field procedures, the data-collection procedures, and the analytic procedures. The protocol identifies how entré will be gained, what resources may be necessary while in the field, a preliminary schedule for data-collection activities, and a consideration of unexpected happenings. It further defines what data need to be collected and why; the sources of information and evidence—for example, which people need to be interviewed, which documents need to be examined, and which observations must be done; and the data-collection strategies. Lastly, the study protocol identifies the beginning plans for the analysis and development of the case report. The protocol serves as a preliminary guide and may need to be modified as the research emerges. However, it does keep the investigator focused on the purpose of the investigation.

Design

Two basic designs are used when conducting case studies: the single-case design and the multiple-case design. Before data collection, it is important to decide which design will best answer the research question.

The Single-Case Design.   The single-case design is used when the case represents a typical case, a critical case, an extreme or unique case, or a revelatory case (Yin, 1994).

The use of a critical case is appropriate when the investigator wishes to test a well-formulated and pivotal theory. Theories specify interrelated constructs and circumstances in which these propositions are thought to be true. A critical case can be used to ascertain whether these propositions are accurate or whether there are competing explanations that are more apropos. In this way, the theory can be confirmed, extended, or challenged. Use of the critical case can contribute significantly to knowledge generation and theory building.

When a case is unique, extreme, or rare (such as when there has been no opportunity, in practice or research, to uncover and confirm common patterns), a single-case design is beneficial. It is used to document and analyze the precise nature of the phenomenon under investigation and to raise questions for further exploration.

A revelatory case is one in which the researcher is privy to a situation that heretofore had been unavailable to scientific inquiry. This inaccessibility can be due to the newness of a situation or it can occur when a phenomenon is common but scientists have not had the opportunity to access that particular event or population (such as certain subcultures). Revelatory case studies enlighten us about phenomena obscurely understood, if understood at all, and stimulate further research in the area.

Single-case studies are also used to illustrate typical or exemplary situations that are representative of larger groups or incidents.

The Multiple-Case Design.   In the multiple-case design, inferences and interpretations are drawn from a group of cases. This type of design is appropriate when the researcher is interested in exploring the same phenomenon in a diversity of situations or with a number of individuals. It is used when the investigator desires to establish whether a proposed explanation is confirmed across a number of cases. The multiple-case design is particularly applicable when generating theory through the constant comparative method of grounded theory (Strauss & Corbin, 1990).

Schultz and Kerr (1986) discussed the use of two strategies for conducting comparative case studies: the "most similar case" and the "most different systems" approaches. The most-similar-case technique analyzes findings and characteristics across similar or comparable cases. The most-different-systems technique is somewhat akin to the use of the "negative case," that is, actively seeking variation and difference to add depth to our understanding. These authors suggested that comparative case studies can be approached from either an idiographic or a nomothetic perspective. An idiographic perspective focuses on the particulars of the case, whereas the nomothetic orientation emphasizes generalizations based on laws or principles.

Data Collection

The case study approach requires the gathering of comprehensive, in-depth data about the case in point to describe the phenomenon or to explain the "case." Although the unit of analysis may be only one case or a small number of cases, the number of variables of interest in each case is usually large, and all must be examined. The information for each case must be as thorough as possible. And the researcher should choose the case from which she or he feels that she or he can learn the most (Stake, 1994).

The case study approach often uses both qualitative and quantitative evidence. This evidence may come from a variety of sources: fieldwork, focused and open-ended interviews, verbal reports, direct observation, participant observation, documents, questionnaires, measurement instruments, clinical or agency records, life profiles, pictures, "epiphanies . . . existentially problematic moments in the lives of individuals" (Denzin, 1989, p. 129), archival accounts, artifacts, or any combination of these sources. Case data also can include impressions and statements of others about the case—"in effect, all the information one has accumulated about each particular case goes into that case study" (Patton, 1990, p. 386).

Principles of Data Collection.   Three principles of data collection (Lincoln & Guba, 1985; Yin, 1994) are helpful in increasing the trustworthiness and quality of a case study:

1. Using multiple sources of evidence;
2. Establishing a case study base; and
3. Maintaining a chain of evidence.

The use of numerous sources of data provides for triangulation of data sources—multiple measures and appraisals of the same phenomenon. Triangulation can include comparing the perspectives of several participants, comparing interview with observational or documentary data, or comparing the consistency of responses over time. The technique of triangulating different data sources increases the accuracy and credibility (construct validity) of the findings. It facilitates the researcher's corroboration of the findings by using different but converging lines of investigation.

A case study database consists of observational field notes, audio- or videotapes, case logs, documents, and narratives. In case study research, the case study report often is not distinguished from the case study database. It is important that there be a retrievable database so that other researchers can examine the evidence without being restricted exclusively to the case report. This procedure substantially increases the dependability (reliability) of the entire project.

Maintaining a chain of evidence is similar to what Lincoln and Guba (1985) referred to as an audit trail. The principle is to permit an external viewer to follow the researcher's process and procedures from research question to evidence to conclusion and vice versa. This "chain of evidence" greatly enhances the confirmability (reliability) of the case.

An additional principle of good data collection is the gathering of evidence over time. The case study is considered by some to be a "slice of life." A particular quantitative approach is the one-time case study design. Nonetheless, the more appropriate precept in the naturalistic paradigm is prolonged engagement. The researcher needs sufficient time and opportunity to become familiar with and understand the context within which the person or event is embedded. A period of prolonged engagement promotes the researcher's understanding of the "culture" of the person or organization and the building of trust. It aids in recognizing and accounting for distortions of either the researcher or the participants. Prolonged engagement also provides the researcher with an opportunity to get to know the subtleties of the situation and have the time to "peel away" layers until the core of the phenomenon, the real meaning, emerges.

Persistence during observation focuses the researcher on details, characteristics, and factors that give relevance to the phenomenon being explored. "If prolonged engagement provides scope, persistent observation provides depth" (Lincoln & Guba, 1985, p. 304).

Analysis
Yin (1994) noted:

> [T]he analysis of case study evidence is one of the least developed and most difficult aspects of doing case studies. . . . Unlike statistical analysis, there are few fixed formulas . . . and the strategies and techniques have not been well defined. . . . Instead, much depends on an investigator's own style or rigorous thinking, along with sufficient presentation of evidence and careful consideration of alternative interpretations. (pp. 102–103)

Basically, there are two strategies for analyzing case study data:

1. Developing a case description (whether purely descriptive or exploratory); and

2. Employing the theoretical propositions on which the study is based to explain the case (Yin, 1989).

These two strategies are similar to Tesch's (1990) systems for interpretational qualitative analysis: creating an organizing scheme from the data themselves or creating an organizing scheme from the adopted theoretical framework that has directed the inquiry.

A third strategy, the quasijudicial (QJ) method (Bromley, 1986), combines features of the judicial and scientific methods. It is frequently used in psychological case studies. The QJ method attempts to solve scientific and practice problems by applying rigorous reasoning in the interpretation of empirical data that have been systematically collected.

Descriptions of each of these methods of analysis follow.

Exploratory/Descriptive Strategy.   The early scientists and practitioners who conducted case studies did not describe their techniques for analysis. "They interpreted their observations in the very basic sense of reflecting on their data until they achieved a better understanding of what they meant" (Tesch, 1990, p. 69). Those pioneers of the case study method produced enlightened portrayals of the people and events that they studied.

Today, however, there are many approaches for analyzing qualitative data for exploratory/descriptive case studies. These approaches include content analysis, analytic induction, constant comparison, and phenomenological analysis. (For details, the reader is referred to discussion of these approaches in other chapters.)

Although each of these modes of analysis is different, there are generic elements integral to all. Data analysis takes place simultaneously with data collection. In order for the investigator to determine whether evidence from various sources intersects on a particular set of facts, the researcher must integrate data collection with data analysis so that each informs the other.

The analysis is comprehensive and systematic but not inflexible. Data are divided into smaller units for analysis and then reintegrated into a conceptual whole. Various authors refer to this process as "de-contextualizing/re-contextualizing" (Seidel, Kjolseth, & Seymor, 1988); coding and categorizing/pattern, theme, and thesis development (Bogdan & Biklen, 1982); and extracting/clustering/exhaustive description (Colaizzi, 1978). The outcome of any of these analyses is "some type of higher-level synthesis. While much work in the analysis process consists of 'taking apart' (for instance, into smaller pieces), the final goal is the emergence of a larger, consolidated picture" (Tesch, 1990, p. 97).

Interpretation of the data is the expectation. Patton (1990) defined interpretation as "attaching significance to what was found, offering explanations, drawing conclusions, extrapolating lessons, making inferences, building linkages, attaching meanings, imposing order, and dealing with rival explanations, disconfirming cases and data irregularities as part of testing the viability of an interpretation" (p. 423). He furnished Schlechty and Noblit's (1982) description of the purposes of interpretation:

1. Making the obvious obvious;
2. Making the obvious dubious; and
3. Making the hidden obvious.

Stake (1995) contends that a major part of case study research is direct interpretation. Emphasis is on the researcher (interpreter) in the field observing the case, objectively recording what is happening and simultaneously examining its meaning and, when necessary, redirecting that observation to refine or substantiate those meanings.

There is an "interpenetration of data and analysis" (Lofland & Lofland, 1984, p. 146) or a "balance between description and interpretation" (Patton, 1990, p. 429). Interpretations and analytic text are directly supported (grounded) in description, documentary evidence, and direct quotations. A distinction is made between evidence and inference.

A variety of products emerges from these diverse analytic strategies (Tesch, 1990): a "composite summary" (Hycner, 1985); a description of "patterns and themes" (Patton, 1990); an "identification of the fundamental structure" of the phenomenon of interest (Colaizzi, 1978); a "creative synthesis" (Moustakas, 1990); a "personalized structure" (Denzin, 1983); a "provisional hypothesis" (Turner, 1981); assertions or conclusions (Stake, 1995); a policy for alleviating fundamental social problems (Majchrzak, 1984); or a "formal or substantive theory" (Strauss, 1987).

The investigator uses three dominant processes in analysis: reflection, comparison, and creativity. Reflection is both personal and data bound. By examining his or her own assumptions and intimate involvement with the case material, the researcher attempts to become aware of and suspend (bracket), to the extent possible, preconceived ideas. These preconceptions may unduly bias not only the investigation but also the understanding of the phenomenon. Through reflection on, dialoguing with, and critical appraisal of the data, the investigator develops a clarity of meaning and advances the descriptive evidence to a more conceptual level.

The case study researcher uses comparison in most phases of the analysis. From forming coding categories to designating data into specific categories to contrasting negative evidence, the investigator is attempting to discover conceptual similarities and differences. In cross-case analysis, the investigator conducts several individual case studies and compares their explanations to form a more general explanation. Case analysis also includes the development of themes and patterns within or across cases or sites. Association and contrast are the analytic processes utilized in both of these analytic strategies.

Creativity is the hallmark of qualitative analysis. Because there is no "one right way" to make meaning, the researcher must blend critical thinking and creative insight. The use of metaphor, analogy, and imagery is beneficial when generating this type of "creative scholarship" (Mariano, 1990). Patton (1990) provided some valuable advice for nurturing creative thinking:

> Be open; generate options; divergence before convergence; use multiple stimuli, side-track, zig-zag, and circumnavigate; change patterns, make linkages; trust yourself; work at it; and play at it. (pp. 434–435)

Theoretical Orientation Strategy.   In this approach, a predetermined theoretical perspective or framework guides the case analysis: the objective is the building and testing of an explanation. A variety of analytic modes is used (Yin, 1994).

Pattern matching is based on a procedure discussed by Campbell (1975). It compares an a priori predicted pattern derived from theory with an observed pattern to see whether the patterns conform. Another way to pattern match is to articulate a number of mutually exclusive rival theoretical propositions and then compare the observed pattern with each of these competing explanations.

Explanation building is very similar to the grounded-theory strategy. However, one again begins with an initial theoretical statement or proposition instead of developing the theory derived from the data themselves. This procedure seeks to explain a phenomenon through the development of a set of causal links. An iterative process (Yin, 1994) is used. Explanation building consists of identifying an initial proposition, comparing findings from the first case with the proposition, revising the proposition, recomparing the case with the revised proposition, comparing the subsequent revision with additional cases, and repeating the process as necessary until a solid, uncontended explanation evolves.

The foregoing strategies are analogous to the methods used by detectives in solving crimes. The goal is to achieve a single explanation for the crime by ruling out rival explanations. Yin (1981b) described this process as follows. The detective is presented with the crime scene, its context, and possible eyewitness reports. The detective must decide the relevance of various evidence. Some case facts will be unrelated; other clues, however, must be vigorously followed. "The adequate explanation for the crime then becomes a plausible rendition of a motive, opportunity, and method that more fully accounts for the facts than do alternative explanations" (p. 61).

When testing theory, it is important that the case be argued from different theoretical perspectives, thereby ruling out perspectives that fail to account for the available evidence (Bromley, 1986, p. 42).

Another technique, the time-series analytic strategy, compares changes or specific indicators of the case over time with a prespecified theoretically meaningful trend.

Miles and Huberman (1984) described two models for data analysis: the flow model and the interactive model. Each of these models requires the use of an extant conceptual framework before data collection. These models comprise four components: data collection, data reduction, data display, and conclusion drawing/verification. These authors placed great emphasis on the value of display as an integral aspect of analysis and a mode for understanding case material.

The Quasijudicial Strategy.   The first step in the quasijudicial method is to clearly state the problems or issues. Background information is gathered to provide the context within which the problem or phenomenon is to be understood. Prima facie explanations about the issue can usually be furnished on the basis of the background information alone. These rather obvious explanations should be examined first because they often guide the investigator's search for further evidence. If these original explanations do not correspond with the available evidence, alternative hypotheses are generated.

The investigator then collects sufficient evidence to eliminate as many of the proposed explanations as possible, continually looking for one that will account for all of the evidence and be countered by none of the evidence. The evidence, as well as its source, is closely scrutinized for explanatory power, relevance, and credibility.

A critical query is made into the internal congruity, logic, and validity of the entire argument that claims solution or explanation. Some lines of argument will be deficient and others will be convincing. The best interpretation compatible with the evidence is chosen. This process and its outcome should contribute to the "case law" (patterns of meaning or abstract and general principles explaining the phenomenon) of the discipline.

Whatever the approach to analysis, the ultimate aim is to "treat the evidence fairly, to produce compelling analytic conclusions, and to rule out alternative interpretations" (Yin, 1994, pp. 102–103). The goal is not to identify the "truth" but to eliminate erroneous interpretations so that one has the most feasible and compelling rendition of the case under study.

Reporting

Case study reports can be presented in written or verbal format or through more innovative means such as photographs or videotapes. Regardless of the format, the case report remains one of the most suitable means for relating the results of naturalistic inquiry. Because most case studies generate written products, I will focus on the written report.

It is not easy to articulate the methods for writing a case study report, because there are no rules or standardized procedures. At best, one can state that the researcher must become immersed in a process of composing and, often, of artistry. As Guba and Lincoln (1981) noted:

> Probably not much more can be said than that the usual principles of good composition—the writing of understandable prose—apply. (p. 375)

The audiences of the case study report must be identified. Different constituencies have different needs and interests in the case being presented. These diverse audiences may require of the report different emphases, particulars, compositional style, and length.

Lincoln and Guba (1985, p. 362) suggested the following elements as the content of a case study report:

* An explication of the problem or issue;
* A detailed description of the context/setting within which the phenomenon occurred;
* A complete delineation of the processes and transactions in the setting/context that are relevant to the focus of the inquiry; and
* A discussion of the results ("lessons to be learned") of the study that lend understanding to the phenomenon of interest.

In addition, they recommended a methodological section or appendix to detail the investigator's credentials, assumptions, and biases regarding the phenomenon of interest or the setting. This section would give an exact reporting of the data collection and analysis methods used in the study and it would furnish a precise account of the steps taken to ensure the quality and trustworthiness of the study.

There are several varieties of written case reports (Yin, 1994). One is the single-case study in which a lengthy narrative (often book length) is developed to describe or analyze the case. A variant of the single-case report is the multiple-case report. This form comprises multiple narratives (usually chapters) individually describing each of the cases in the study. One or more chapters then incorporates the cross-case analysis and findings (themes/patterns across cases). A third example of a written report describes or analyzes a single or multiple case; however, it does not use the customary narrative. This model incorporates a sequence of answers to a set of questions, usually those on which the study was based. A fourth type of written report is used exclusively with multiple-case studies. The entire report is about the cross-case analysis; no individual cases are reported. Specific chapters focus on specific cross-case issues or themes. Individual case information is interspersed throughout each issue chapter or is presented in highlighted vignettes.

EVALUATION OF CASE STUDIES

A number of criteria are used to evaluate case studies. They include criteria that establish the trustworthiness (Lincoln & Guba, 1985; Sandelowski, 1986) of the study as well as additional standards specific to case study.

Trustworthiness necessitates the achievement of four objectives: credibility, transferability, dependability, and confirmability. For credibility, techniques are used that ensure that plausible interpretations and constructions will be generated. The techniques include prolonged engagement, triangulation, peer debriefing, negative case analysis, and member or participant checking of the researcher's interpretations. Transferability allows someone to decide whether the conclusions or findings can be transferred to another context. It is accomplished by providing a detailed database and thick description of the phenomenon. Dependability, which permits another to follow the process and procedures of the inquiry, is accomplished by incorporating an audit procedure in the study. Confirmability attests that the findings, conclusions, and recommendations are supported by the data and that there is an internal congruity between interpretations and actual evidence. This, again, is accomplished by the use of an audit process.

Burns (1989) identified additional standards for the evaluation of qualitative research: descriptive vividness; methodological congruence (rigor in documentation, procedure, ethics, and auditability); analytical preciseness; theoretical connectedness; and heuristic relevance (intuitive recognition, relation to existing knowledge, applicability).

Yin (1994) identified what he regarded as the characteristics of an exemplary case study. Primarily, the case study should be significant. It should make a significant contribution to the understanding of an unknown phenomenon; or compare two or more pivotal but rival theories in a discipline to explain the case; or incorporate both discovery and theory construction in the case study.

The case study must be as complete as possible. The evidence collected should be extensive and relevant. Critical pieces of evidence ought to be given thorough attention. Not all data are relevant, so the investigator must present *meaningful* information. The researcher needs to stay in the field as long as necessary to achieve "completeness."

An explanatory case study must examine the evidence from varying perspectives and viewpoints or consider alternative propositions. The investigator should anticipate what these alternative interpretations are and be able to demonstrate how and why these rival explanations can be rejected on the basis of the facts of the case.

The case study report should present the most compelling data so that the reader can independently come to a conclusion regarding the worth of the inquiry. The report should instill in the reader a confidence that the investigator has truly acted with scholarly and professional ethics. Evidence must be presented in a truthful, objective manner and must include both supporting and challenging information. The researcher must be selective in the inclusion of evidence. However, that selectivity refers to the relevancy of the data—for example, to the most critical evidence or the fair treatment of all cases—and not to the exclusion of any data that do not support the researcher's conclusions.

Review and validation of the investigator's interpretations should be done by the study participants. This review minimizes bias in the presentation and ensures that the facts have not been misconstrued. In addition, it often gives the participants a better understanding of the whole phenomenon under investigation (Yin, 1981a).

Finally, it behooves the investigator to fashion the case study report in an engaging style. Through technique and form, it should captivate the audience and entice them to read or hear more. This requires an investigator who is enthusiastic about the study and strongly desires to communicate the findings of the inquiry.

ADVANTAGES OF CASE STUDY RESEARCH AND ITS ISSUES

Stake (1983) noted that case study will often be the favored method of inquiry because it is "epistemologically in harmony with the reader's experience" (p. 279) and therefore provides a basis for natural generalization. Guba and Lincoln (1981) identified a number of reasons for the choice of the case study. A case study produces "thick description," which lets others in different settings decide whether the entity studied is applicable to their own situations or contexts. The case study is grounded, thereby providing a perspective that evolves directly from experience instead of from a priori hypotheses, assumptions, or instruments. Case studies are "holistic and lifelike"; they paint realistic pictures of actual participants in their own language. A case study report integrates a large and often diverse amount of information in a unified, focused manner. Unlike statistical scientific reports, case studies communicate to their audience in such a way as to illuminate meaning and increase understanding.

Lastly, a case study builds on the reader's "tacit knowledge" or that which is implicitly understood. Case studies provide others with vicarious experiences:

> [P]laced in the actual situation, the reader of a case study would sense many things that he could not scientifically document but in which he would have a great deal of confidence. . . . We all know more than we can say; the case study provides a vehicle for the transference of that kind of wordless knowledge. (Guba & Lincoln, 1981, p. 377)

There are, however, several issues associated with case study research that need to be addressed. The problem of generalizability of case study findings is often raised as a disadvantage of this method of inquiry. "It is difficult to argue with certainty that what is learned from a single case is representative of patterns or trends in the entire population" (Skodal-Wilson, 1985, p. 137). The question frequently arises regarding "truth." Does "truth" lie in general axioms or in particulars?

Stake (1983) contended that valuable understanding can come from a complete and detailed knowledge of the particular. He considered this knowledge to be a type of generalization, albeit not a scientific generalization. He used the term "naturalistic generalization," emanating from a recognition of similarities of entities in and out of context, to define this knowledge:

> Naturalistic generalizations develop within a person as a product of experience. They derive from the tacit knowledge of how things are, why they are, how people feel about them, and how these things are likely to be later on in other places with which this person is familiar. They seldom take the form of predictions but lead regularly to expectation. They guide action, in fact they are inseparable from action. . . . (p. 282)

Stake (1995) notes that "Naturalistic generalizations are conclusions arrived at through personal engagement in life's affairs or by vicarious experience so well constructed that the person feels as if it happened to themselves. . . . A narrative account, a story, a chronological presentation, personalistic description, emphasis on time and place provide rich ingredients for vicarious experiences" (pp. 85–87).

Case studies have unique issues related to ethics. These ethical concerns can arise from inquiry "shaping" by the investigator, manipulation of the data, nonreporting of contradictory data, and bias in interpretations. Use of the techniques identified in the section on evaluation of case studies (utilizing an external auditor, member checking, grounding interpretations in evidence, and so on) will help to ensure the integrity of the case study.

Stake (1995) contends that case study researchers commonly make assertions on a rather small database. They have the privilege of asserting what they find meaningful as a result of the inquiry. But they also have a responsibility regarding interpretation: "Good case study is patient reflective, willing to see another view of the case. An ethic of caution is not contradictory to an ethic of interpretation" (p. 12).

Another ethical dilemma in the case study approach is the protection of the anonymity of the participant(s) or site(s) in the study. Assurance of anonymity is particularly problematic when the researcher is investigating a unique situation. Guba and Lincoln (1981) suggested following the principle that participants "own" the data that apply to them. Data will not be reported without explicit consent of the participants after being fully informed about expected use and potential risks.

RESEARCHER CHARACTERISTICS

A number of authors have expounded on the attributes and skills required of researchers who conduct qualitative research (Bromley, 1986; Mariano, 1990; Yin, 1994). These characteristics are equally applicable to the conduct of case study inquiry.

Case study investigators must be comfortable with ambiguity and flexible enough to deal with the unexpected as an opportunity rather than a menace. A willingness to comprehend meaning in context and to accept more than one "truth" enhances one's understanding and ability to conduct case studies.

The case study researcher must possess good communication skills. The art of listening and absorbing large amounts of data without bias, an aptitude for observing with an inquiring mind, and the facility for writing in an articulate and interesting style are imperative for quality case study research.

The case study researcher must be mature, introspective, and reflective. Awareness of one's assumptions, preconceptions, and values is especially important when making inferences and interpreting phenomena; otherwise, a case study can be misused to support the researcher's preconceived position.

The ability to conceptualize is essential for the case study researcher. With the use of the vast amount of data amassed, patterns must be identified, themes discovered, connections made, propositions developed, and meaning abstracted. Imagination coupled with discipline is necessary for the case study investigator to produce creative scholarship.

THE FUTURE OF CASE STUDY RESEARCH

Case studies will continue to be essential in investigating certain topics of interest to nursing. The case study method will be refined and will advance as investigators continue to analyze and share their own experiences with it. The usefulness of the case study approach for all facets of inquiry (description, exploration, and explanation) makes it an invaluable strategy for understanding and for increasing knowledge about the human condition.

REFERENCES

Barlow, D., & Hersen, M. (1985). *Single-case experimental designs: Strategies for studying behavior* (2nd ed.). New York: Pergamon.

Bogdan, R. C., & Biklen, S. K. (1982). *Qualitative research for education: An introduction to theory and methods.* Boston: Allyn & Bacon.

Bromley, D. B. (1986). *The case-study method in psychology and related disciplines.* Chichester, England: Wiley.

Burns, N. (1989). Standards for qualitative research. *Nursing Science Quarterly,* 2(1), 44–52.

Campbell, D. (1975, July). Degrees of freedom and the case study. *Comparative Political Studies,* 8, 178–193.

Christensen, C. R. (1987). *Teaching and the case method.* Boston: Harvard Business School.

Colaizzi, P. F. (1978). Psychological research as the phenomenologist views it. In R. Valle & M. King (Eds.), *Existential-phenomenological alternatives for psychology.* New York: Oxford University Press.

Creswell, J. (1998). *Qualitative inquiry and research design: Choosing among five traditions.* Thousand Oaks, CA: Sage.

Cryer, J. D. (1986). *Time series analysis.* Boston: Duxbury Press.

Denzin, N. K. (1983). Interpretive interactionism. In G. Morgan (Ed.), *Beyond method: Strategies for social work* (pp. 129–146). Newbury Park, CA: Sage.

Denzin, N. K. (1989). *Interpretive interactionism.* Newbury Park, CA: Sage.

Guba, E. G., & Lincoln, Y. S. (1981). *Effective evaluation.* San Francisco: Jossey-Bass.

Hinds, P., Chaves, D., & Cypess, S. (1992). Context as a source of meaning and understanding. In J. Morse (Ed.), *Qualitative health research* (pp. 31–42). Newbury Park, CA: Sage.

Hycner, R. H. (1985). Some guidelines for the phenomenological analysis of interview data. *Human Studies,* 8, 279–303.

Kratochwill, T. R., & Levin, J. R. (Eds.). (1992). *Single-case research design and analysis: New directions for psychology and education.* Hillsdale, NJ: Erlbaum.

Lincoln, Y. S., & Guba, E. G. (1985). *Naturalistic inquiry.* Beverly Hills, CA: Sage.

Lofland, J., & Lofland, L. H. (1984). *Analyzing social settings: A guide to qualitative observation and analysis* (2nd ed.). Belmont, CA: Wadsworth.

Majchrzak, A. (1984). *Methods for policy research.* Newbury Park, CA: Sage.

Mariano, C. (1990). Qualitative research: Instructional strategies and curricular considerations. *Nursing & Health Care,* 11, 354–359.

Miles, M. B., & Huberman, A. M. (1984). *Qualitative data analysis: A sourcebook of new methods.* Beverly Hills, CA: Sage.

Moustakas, C. (1990). *Heuristic research: Design, methodology, and applications.* Newbury Park, CA: Sage.

Naumes, W., & Naumes, M. (1999). *The craft of case study writing.* Thousand Oaks, CA: Sage.

Patton, M. Q. (1990). *Qualitative evaluation and research methods* (2nd ed.). Newbury Park, CA: Sage.

Powers, B. A., & Knapp, T. R. (1990). *A dictionary of nursing theory and research.* Newbury Park, CA: Sage.

Sandelowski, M. (1986). The problem of rigor in qualitative research. *Advances in Nursing Science,* 8 (3), 27–37.

Schlechty, P., & Noblit, G. (1982). Some uses of sociological theory in educational evaluation. In R. Corwin (Ed.), *Policy research.* Greenwich, CT: JAI Press.

Schultz, P. R., & Kerr, B. J. (1986). Comparative case study as a strategy for nursing research. In P. L. Chinn (Ed.), *Nursing research methodology: Issues and implementation* (pp. 195–220). Rockville, MD: Aspen.

Seidel, J., Kjolseth, R., & Seymor, E. (1988). *The ethnograph: A user's guide.* Littleton, CO: Qualis Research Associates.

Skodal-Wilson, H. (1985). *Research in nursing.* Menlo Park, CA: Addison-Wesley.

Stake, R. (1983). The case study method in social inquiry. In G. Madaus, M. Scriven, & D. Stufflebeam (Eds.), *Evaluation models: Viewpoints on educational and human services evaluation* (pp. 279–286). Boston: Bluwer-Nijhoff.

Stake, R. (1994). Case studies. In N. Denzin & Y. Lincoln (Eds.). *Handbook of qualitative research.* Thousand Oaks, CA: Sage.

Stake, R. (1995). *The art of case study research.* Thousand Oaks, CA: Sage.

Strauss, A. L. (1987). *Qualitative analysis for social scientists.* New York: Cambridge University Press.

Strauss, A. L., & Corbin, J. (1990). *Basics of qualitative research: Grounded theory procedures and techniques.* Newbury Park, CA: Sage.

Tesch, R. (1990). *Qualitative research: Analysis types and software tools.* Bristol, PA: Falmer Press.

Turner, B. A. (1981). Some practical aspects of qualitative data analysis: One way of organizing the cognitive process associated with the generation of grounded theory. *Quality and Quantity,* 15, 225–247.

Woods, N. F., & Catanzaro, M. (1988). *Nursing research: Theory and practice.* St. Louis, MO: Mosby.

Yin, R. K. (1981a). The case study as a serious research strategy. *Knowledge: Creation, Diffusion, Utilization, 3*(1), 97–114.

Yin, R. K. (1981b). The case study crisis: Some answers. *Administrative Science Quarterly, 26,* 58–65.

Yin, R. K. (1989). *Case study research: Design and methods* (rev. ed.). Newbury Park, CA: Sage.

Yin, R. (1994). *Case study research design and methods* (2nd ed.). Thousand Oaks, CA: Sage.

12

Drifting Without Consciousness
A Descriptive Case Study—Nina's Story

Mary Colvin

We see other alternatives when a new light falls on our pain and suffering and it becomes unbearable.
(adapted from Sartre, 1963, and Watson, 2000)

In July of 1998 a 65-year-old woman entered the health care system through the emergency room. She was a mother, a grandmother, a wife, and an accountant. But that does not define the person whom I came to know in a period of 36 hours.

Nina was special. Physically she was attractive and clearly cared about her appearance. Her wig, her nails, her clothes were perfect. But that did not distinguish Nina. Her sense of humor, her interest and caring for others, her wisdom, and her humanism were the qualities that drew others to her. When she spoke, it was with authority and clarity. When she smiled, her eyes watched yours. She sparkled.

Nina was diagnosed with ovarian cancer in 1996. Her pathology report named her cancer as adenocarcinoma, stage three. For 2 years, she experienced the effects of chemotherapy. In 1996, Nina retired. She and her husband were planning a long-awaited vacation and an enjoyable retirement together. That dream was never to be realized once she was diagnosed.

One morning she awakened and noted that her left arm was swollen. She wondered if this swelling was related to her central line. As the day progressed, the swelling became more pronounced and subsequently painful. It was midnight when she asked her husband of 45 years to take her to the emergency room, which is where her last journey in life began. What she and her husband perceived to be simple became complex and chaotic.

In July of 1998, Nina did not die of ovarian cancer. She died many hours later in an intensive care unit because those who cared for her drifted without consciousness. This is Nina's story as chronicled in the last 36 hours of her life and thereafter. It is disturbing and appalling. It is sad.

Dateline

July, 1998, Day One 7:15 A.M.	Nina is admitted to an oncology unit with r/o phlebitis of the left arm. She has spent most of the night in the emergency room. Nina is admitted under her primary care physician of 15 years. The emergency room physician consulted him about her status. Orders are written for an x-ray, a panel of laboratory work, and to begin anticoagulation by a heparin drip. These orders are implemented on her arrival in the oncology unit where I am supervising a group of students from a local University.
	I (as a clinical instructor) ask a senior student to complete her admission assessment. A rapport is established between the student and the client. Nina's central line is assessed for patency and determined to be functioning. Her vital signs are within a normal range. No temperature is noted.
8:00 A.M.	The student asks that I validate her admission assessment. It is clear that the student is establishing a relation with Nina and her husband, because the student is bilingual. When the oncology nurses become aware that Nina has been admitted, they visit her. It is like a family reunion. A special bond has developed between the nurses, Nina, and her husband.

9:00 A.M.	Nina settles into the room that she knows so well. She begins to have pain in her arm. Her husband asks when her physician (primary) will make rounds? The charge nurse calls the physicians service and leaves a message. Nina is taken by wheelchair for her x-ray.
10:00 A.M.	Nina trys to rest, but she is not feeling well. She is uncomfortable. The nurse calls the primary physician and leaves a message, again. The student remarks that, in the course of her admission assessment, Nina's husband expressed concern that they had spoken to the primary physician a week earlier. He had told them that he had a professional conflict with the oncologist and did not feel he could work with her. He asked the family to select another oncologist. They were upset because they liked and trusted the oncologist who had cared for Nina during this health crisis. They were not sure what to do and felt uncomfortable having to make a choice.
12:00 noon	Nina becomes anxious. She is in pain. Her husband calls the physician and leaves a message. He receives no response. He calls their oncologist and is informed that she is out of town. The service promises to inform the physician covering for her.
2:00 P.M.	Nina's vital signs change, her blood pressure drops, and she becomes tachycardic. Her belly is distended, but she is voiding and eating small amounts. Her temperature rises just one degree. She is restless in bed. She says, "I can't get comfortable." The wig is off and the makeup is not a concern for her now. She is short of breath, and oxygen through nasal cannula is administered.
3:00 P.M.	The student and I as her clinical instructor report our summary to her primary nurse,

July, 1998, Day Two
7:00 A.M.

emphasizing the change that was evolving
and the fact that she has not been seen by a
physician. We also consult with the social
worker who immediately begins to assess
the circumstance. We (the student and I)
leave for the day.

Nina's room is dark and she is weeping. Her
husband ask's why her "doctor" hasn't been
here. He leaves to call her primary physician, yet again. Now Nina has a temperature
of 103 and her belly is hugely distended.
She remains short of breath on oxygen. The
primary nurse, who is not a full-time staff
nurse, pours two aspirin for Nina. We question her judgment in light of the heparin
drip and ask her to please pull up Nina's last
coagulation times. She states that she does
not know how to use the computer. The unit
secretary helps to retrieve this laboratory
data, which reveal that Nina is not in a therapeutic range; she is in danger of bleeding. I
plead with the primary nurse to call the
physician and discontinue her heparin drip.
Because I do not trust that the nurse will do
so, I find the charge nurse who discontinued
the heparin but kept a line open and again
call the primary physician. I also ask to see
the nurse manager, but she is on vacation.
The sparkle in Nina's eyes is gone. Time
seems to be suspended, in slow motion. As
a nurse for 18 years, I know that Nina is in
serious trouble and feel impotent in trying
to create change, some movement to save
her life. I ask the student to stay with her,
and she recognizes the importance and
need to do so. The student bathes Nina,
changes her linen, and sits by her side. What
may seem so simple is so meaningful to
Nina; she keeps thanking the student.
Meanwhile her husband is on the telephone

again to the primary physician. Finally, the social worker calls the physician and, in Spanish, which I cannot understand, tells him to get to the unit. (The social worker also has a law degree. I know that she is concerned that trouble lies ahead.)

10:00 A.M.

Nina's primary physician arrives on the unit and visits her. He does not touch her. He addresses the husband, stating that he told them that he cannot work with the oncologist and asked them to make a decision. He will care for Nina if they "fire" the oncologist. They have to make a choice right now; him or the oncologist. The husband is crying and speaks to Nina, who wants to stay with her oncologist treating her ovarian cancer. The physician then says, "you have fired me. I am no longer on this case." He turns his back on people for whom he has cared for more than 15 years and leaves the room. The student is stunned; the patient and husband are speechless. The physician is angry, and I observe his behavior as he writes his note. "Patient discharges me, transfer to oncology group for all further care." Period. Orders; d/c heparin drip, give Percocet q 4–6 hours prn, give Tylenol grains × prn, fever, notify oncology group. His anger is clear in his writing, which leaves indentations five pages below. The chart is thrown on the desk toward the secretary. He marches off the unit in a flurry. Everyone looks at one another. The social worker heads toward the room while the charge nurse reviews the chart.

10:30 A.M.

Nina's husband is crying. He does not know what to do because of his HMO. Nina is more relaxed, owing to a narcotic, but she is clearly in big trouble. I go back to the charge nurse and express my concerns. She replies: "I know, I know, I am trying to call the covering physician." I ask her if the medical residents can be called. She says, "Only in an emergency. Let me talk to the covering M.D."

11:00 A.M. The charge nurse notes a renowned oncologist making rounds and asks if she would see Nina. This physician does so and writes a suggestion for a number of diagnostic tests but also writes "This is not my patient." This notation further confuses the patient and husband. However, there is a sense of relief that a physician has examined Nina.

1:00 P.M. Nina's blood pressure drops again. She is tachypneic and her pulse rate is accelerating. The student and I have been her consistent caregivers. Again I go to the charge nurse and, at this point, I plead with her to call the residents, call anyone, please do something. She states that she is waiting for a return call from the covering physician. I say, "I don't know that you can wait." She says, "I'll have the resident team see her on their second rounds."

2:00 P.M. The student bathes Nina. She does not want her wig or makeup. Her husband is still making telephone calls. He cannot find a doctor to come and see her. He cries a lot; he knows; she knows. Now Nina wants the room dark. She is in so much pain that she cannot stand any stimulation. The student remains at her bedside. Now, the prayers begin, and her husband calls the children.

3:00 P.M. The residents make rounds and are asked to visit her. While they are doing so, Nina goes into respiratory arrest. They are yelling, "Who is her doctor?" while they intubate her. All of the staff look at each other puzzled. She has no doctor who is available. Drifting without consciousness.

4:00 P.M. Nina is transferred to the ICU, ventilated and in organ failure. Her husband is still crying. He is asked about continuing life support. He refuses further resuscitative efforts.

July, 1998, Day Three
8:00 A.M.

We find Nina in the ICU with "spagetti" tubes everywhere. The student wants to stay with her. After a long discussion, I agree that she should be with her. She says that she can deal with the intensity and she wants to follow this through. I wonder, but agree with her. The critical care nurse calls the student and me out for a private discussion. She says, "How the hell did this happen?" We just stare at her; drifting without consciousness. Nina's husband takes me in his arms and thanks me for trying to help his wife, and I think I cannot bear this grief and pain. I lay my hands on Nina and say good-bye, and I note with relief that she has the best view; she is lying on her right side facing the bay. It is a beautiful day; it is a breathtaking vista of sun shimmering over the still water. I whisper "sleep well," because I know the outcome. The student takes watch at her side, stroking her forehead and talking to her in Spanish. It is peaceful. The ventilator is rhythmic and sighs, and sighs as Nina tries to find her own peace.

10:00 A.M.

I check on the student and Nina. There are few life signs. I know the outcome. I ask the student if she is sure that she should stay. She emphasizes again that she wants to see this through. The family has arrived.

1:00 P.M.

I return to the ICU to check on the student and Nina. Nina is working hard to breathe on the ventilator. The student is working hard to keep her composure. I take her to a private area and say that I need her to come back to the unit with me. She agrees and says her goodbye to Nina and her husband. I stand by her and am honored by her compassion. Finding the words comes easily to

	her. She retains her composure as we leave Nina and say our goodbyes.
3:00 P.M.	The students and I are waiting for an elevator by the ICU. Nina's family comes out to the waiting area where we are. They are not crying; they are sobbing. The wife, mother, and grandmother has died. We offer comfort that cannot be meaningful during this grieving. We come together as a group and offer a prayer(s) for Nina.
One week later	The student comes to see me in my office. She is very angry and wants to know why I "made her go to ICU." She states that she never wanted to go there and I encouraged her to. She expresses that I did not do enough for Nina, stating, "After all you are a nurse, not just a teacher."
Six months later	The same student comes to visit me. She looks physically different and more mature. She shares her clinical experiences with me. And we agree that, in the end, Nina taught us a lot. I say how to not drift without consciousness, and she says, "I'll think about that."

THEORETICAL BACKGROUND: CASE STUDY METHOD

Lincoln and Guba (1985) and Yin (1994) are the predominant authorities in the case study method. All come from a humanities background—specifically, social research. Lincoln and Guba prefaced their book *Naturalistic Inquiry* as follows:

> Every historical age has exhibited some characteristic way of answering the questions of what there is that can be known and how one can go about knowing it. Sometimes the answer is mystical, as in the case of the great Oriental religions. Sometimes it has been magical as Sir James Frazier pointed out long ago the primitive magic and modern science, in that both attempt to

control the universe for the benefit of humankind. (Lincoln &
Guba, 1985, p. 7)

In either a qualitative or a quantitative way, science seeks truth. I believe it is a quest of humankind and interfaces every aspect of life.
However, truth is a reflection of the world in which we live at any point
in time. What is considered hard science versus soft science is a use-
less debate. As the world changes, so follows scientific inquiry. Quantum theory, phenomenology, naturalistic theory, and consilience will
all try to explain the world and the human condition. All will seek the
truth. All will use tools to research and analyze particular phenomena.
And the theme will always be: the truth is out there.

POSITIVISM VERSUS NATURALISM

Mariano (1993) defined a case study as an "intensive, systematic investigation of a single individual, group, community or some other
unit." Yin (1994) stated that the case study method has been a weak
sibling among other methods of research in the field of social science.
In defense of this method, Yin states that the case study method is preferred when questions are posed where the investigator has little control over events and when the focus is on contemporary phenomena.
For example, as I finish this chapter, we have had a national election
that raises many questions of truth. A case study in any one particular
aspect would enlighten us about the value of understanding one another, such as in such a close historical election. Lincoln and Guba
(1985) differentiate positivism from naturalism. They do so by distinguishing the nature of reality, the relation of the knower to the known,
the possibility of generalization, a causal linkage, and the role of values. Positivists' and naturalists' ontological and epistemological interpretations are polar opposites. For example, if I told you that I broke
my foot today, the ontological positivist view would focus on the fact
that I slipped and fell. The ontology of the naturalist would raise more
questions: Were you stressed? Were you disabled? What led to this
event? The positivist would have no relation with the subject. The naturalist would have to have a relation to gain epistemology about the incident. A phenomenologist (Munhall, 1994) would want to find meaning and understanding in this human experience. Ergo the case study
method is a naturalistic, phenomenological, and qualitative research
method.

PHENOMENOLOGY

Phenomenology as a philosophical movement began in the nineteenth century and developed in the twentieth century as a credible approach to discourse about what it means to be human (Munhall, 1994). Phenomenology moved through different cultures and countries. Brentano named the movement, and it was further developed by German philosophers Husserl and Heidegger (who coined the existential thought of being with time); it then moved to France, where it was further explored by Marcel, Sartre, and Merlaue-Ponty. Phenomenology as a method of inquiry was advanced by Merlau-Ponty in the 1960s. Although the scientific community named this method of inquiry "soft science," it persisted as a formidable opponent to the "hard science" of the Aristolean, Kantian, almost Machiavellian way of thinking. The differences between the two are incredible. Quantitative research, or "quantity," refers to numbers and is more objectifiable. Qualitative research emphasizes the "quality" of the human experience. Whereas quantitative research reduces itself to numbers in making decisions, qualitative research constructs themes that correspond to a human experience at a given time. Together they contribute to an understanding of world phenomena. As human beings, we are objective and subjective. Objectivity is intertwined with subjectivity, making us unique, creative, and unpredictable.

This research reported herein is qualitative and uses the case study method to examine the meaning of abandonment, diffusion of responsibility, oppression, and desensitization. The goal is to look through a lens of change so that few will drift without consciousness.

TRANSPERSONAL NURSING: NURSING IN A POSTMODERN AGE

Dr. Jean Watson has publicly shared her journey through a difficult time when she lost an eye through an accident and subsequently lost her husband. These experiences underpin her new work *Postmodern Nursing and Beyond* (1999). She describes transpersonal nursing as a model for the new millennium. To do so, she identifies transpersonal nursing in three ways: as ontological archetype, artist, and architect. Her last chapter calls for nursing to "relight the lamp," a metaphor that honors Nightingale in a new millennium.

Nursing as archetype refers to the feminine nurturer and caring human being who was lost in the identification of the masculine archetype of the twentieth century in medicine described as paternalistic and authoritarian. Watson contends that, within this structure, nursing lost some of its identity. Blame is not laid, because that would not be healing. Rather, Watson calls to nurses to raise and hear their voices in regaining their roots as archetypal caregivers, healers, and nurturers in an environment that honors Western and Eastern medicine. Power and inequities between medicine and nursing are so institutionalized that they are accepted as norms (Watson, 1999). As a result, nurses have overvalued others and undervalued themselves. Transformational nursing will require a paradigm shift to valuing self and others equally.

The ontological shift to transpersonal caring and healing as artist finds meaning in the expression of self through self-awareness and the expression of self through many mediums. Artistry can be drawing, acting, music, writing—forms of expression that allow us to become aware of our authenticity and to share it with another. Nursing as an art and human science lends itself to gaining perspective and understanding of the human experience, which come in times of intimacy and crisis not characteristic of many other professions. An example of artistry in nursing is the idea promoted by Munhall (1997, 1999) of thinking "out of the box."

Transpersonal nursing as architect refers to how we structure the environment in which we practice and find meaning. Aspects of the environment touch the deepest core of our being and can assist in transcending illness, pain, and suffering, helping us to remember our common humanity (Watson, 1999). Nurses as architects, with an innate sense of others' needs, have created hospices and shelters—in essence, a sense of home where individuality is not lost. Architects of the hospital, who were, in part, physicians and bureaucrats, developed dormitories that could house many and functionally control the care/cure of an individual person.

Watson lists characteristics of transpersonal nursing, which are expressed as paths on which to embark:

- Path of awareness, of awakening the feminine archetype to re-balance conventional medicine with modern cultural mindset;
- Path of cultivation of higher/deeper self and consciousness, the transpersonal self;
- Path of honoring the sacred within and without;
- Path of acknowledging the metaphysical/spiritual level of existence;

- Path of acknowledging quantum concepts and phenomena such as caring/healing energy;
- Path of honoring connectedness of all, unitary consciousness;
- Path of honoring unity and the transcendence of the human being who is becoming;
- Path of reintegrating artistry into healing practices;
- Path of creating healing "space," healing architecture;
- Path of relational ontology open to new epistemologies; and
- Path of moving beyond postmodern and new thinking required for the next millenium. (Watson, 1999)

This case study reveals the need for change in systems of organization and communication. This is the functional lesson gleaned. The humanistic, more abstract lesson is to create and live in an environment where no person is left behind because we drift into the essence of unconsciousness. Nina would have preferred to die at home with her family and not at the expense of an HMO, a physician who vowed to do no harm. When we abdicate our rights to a bureaucratic system, we lose control of our very basic rights. No one person acted with malice toward Nina. They just drifted away from her and her well-being. Intentionality was lost and so followed Nina's life.

RESEARCH AIMS

1. To explore the meaning of drifting without consciousness in relation to nursing.
2. To identify implications for nursing.

Reason for Exploration

This case study was formally completed after the experience. Serendipitously, the author kept notes and wrote an informal study of this clinical case for a doctoral class. The purpose of this descriptive study is to gain perspective and understanding that the author can use in teaching nurses.

Data Collection

The methods of data collection included documentation, archival records, interviews, direct observations, and participant observation. These data-collection methods are identified by Yin (1994). From these data, particular themes were gleaned, which led to the essence of drifting without consciousness, acting with anesthesia, drifting in and out of consciousness, wondering what happened.

A description of each theme that Nina's story brought forth follows.

Oppression

In this study, and as reflected in the dateline, nurses became powerless. This is the overriding goal of an oppressor. Freire writes:

> While both humanization and dehumanization are real alternatives, only the first is the people's vocation. This vocation is constantly neglected, yet it is affirmed by that very negation. It is thwarted by injustice, exploitation and violence by the oppressors, it is affirmed by the oppressed for freedom and justice, and by their struggle to recover their lost humanity. (Freire, 1997)

No one consciously oppressed another. But, in reflection, the medical system oppressed nurses who tried to speak out, and in turn the nurses oppressed the client who was fighting for her life.

Nursing as a profession has entangled itself in a web of confusion. Nurses have been autonomous for years, but their actions have always been directed by the physician order. The notion of order summons the idea of authority. The authority has been the physician, legally accepted by our society. This system has worked until nursing began to find its voice and recognize that physicians are not all knowing. But the hangover effect of this perception will take time to change. Nurses and physicians have a common goal, and their practices are intertwined.

Oppression is manifested by power shifts, low self-esteem or self-concept, denial, and what Friere (1997) refers to as the submissive aggression syndrome. This means that the oppressed cannot express themselves to the oppressor, and so they oppress each other through many strategies, which only serves to give the oppressor more power. In this case, the nurses criticized each other. Blame was placed, and no nurse accepted responsibility for her actions as possibly contributing to this tragic outcome. Blame was laid at the feet of the physician but only after the nurses rigorously attacked one another. Part of this behavior was due to guilt related to not having cared in the best way for Nina and to the feeling of having disappointed her. After Nina's death, the nurses did not find solidarity in having advocated for Nina. Instead, they may have been embarrassed about the fact that a faculty member and a student had persisted in advocating for Nina and they had only partly listened. They had avoided the room and the issue when it was difficult, and there were no answers to give the family. And so they reacted with horizontal violence. Their frustrations and sorrow were turned toward each other and in fear they could not admit that they contributed to Nina's death. This led to other actions such as abandonment.

Abandonment

In this case, the entire health care system abandoned Nina. Her primary care physician acted in an unethical and angry manner. I do not know what led him to disavow himself from the oath to which he was sworn. I only know the perceptions of the abandoned victims in this debacle. Nina expressed this feeling when she said, "Where is the doctor? Why won't he come to see me?" The lack of response from the physician as evidenced by the numerous calls made and unreturned sent the message, "I am leaving you." The ultimate abandonment came when Nina was asked to make a choice between her physicians as she lay critically ill. Nurses abandoned Nina when they did not vigorously advocate for her and demand that their voices be heard. The health care system abandoned Nina when it could not help her to identify a new primary care physician within her managed plan of care. The only players in this drama who did not abandon Nina were the faculty member and the student. Because they were guests of the institution, their voices were not heard, a little muffled, a bit irritating. This leads to the next response or theme, diffusion of responsibility.

Diffusion of Responsibility

Advocacy is a fundamental responsibility of nurses and physicians. Voices raised and heard result in actions that promote life, health, and well-being. In Nina's case, telephone calls were made and unreturned and remade and unreturned. No strong voice resonated the emergent needs of Nina. The nurses diffused responsibility to the physician(s). The physician(s) did not respond and, when one of them did, he abdicated his responsibility. Both were equally complicit in diluting, or diffusing responsibility. Although actions were not implicitly negligent, I will never forget the student's words after Nina's death. She said, "This is murder, not intentional, but it is murder." I understood her anger. I also understood that it was not murder; it was, once again, drifting without consciousness.

Desensitization

Anesthesia renders us unconscious. Substances numb us from truth and reality. Denial as a protective mechanism helps to maintain our equilibrium, for a time. In this case, Nina pleaded for help. She knew that she was dying and stated, "I'm dying." No one believed Nina. Although her vital signs changed and there was objective evidence that she was whirling toward a crisis, her voice was not heard, in part, I believe, because she was not admitted for "ovarian cancer." Her difficulties were becoming out of the realm of cancer. Because her temperature remained elevated and her central line was not removed or antibiotics started, I believe Nina became septic and, already compromised, progressed rapidly to major organ failure.

Interviews with the nurses after Nina's death resulted in a common theme of rationalization and desensitization, as revealed by comments such as, "It is much better to die quickly; she would have had a long and painful death with her ovarian cancer; it is sad, but it's just better in the long run." The nurse manager whom I respect greatly had the same reaction. In addition, she stated, "I know my nurses did what they could; sometimes we can't control situations."

Implications for Nursing

This case has left me forever changed as a nurse and educator. I think about what more I could have done, and I truly cannot see anything differently. As a faculty member, I could not pick up the telephone and call physicians. I could not call the medical residents. I wonder: if I had been more vocal, more adamant, more expressive, would it have changed the outcome? I do not think it would have. I would have been perceived as instrusive, and my credibility would have been questioned. When I visit the unit where Nina died, I remember her and the nurses do not want to talk about her death. They are eager to talk about Nina, the person. They reminisce easily. I perceive that it is too painful and to what end? They have reconciled their experience and want me to "get over it." I will never "get over it." For months, I kept it inside because it was too painful to express. Now, I think I honor Nina in telling her story. I will never forget her. Even though I had just a few days with her, I realized her individuality and then I watched it slip away.

The implications for nursing are self-evident. We must break the cycle of oppression and raise our voices when the need is most critical, such as life or death. We must not abdicate our advocacy for others when their voices cannot be heard. We must not dilute or diffuse the essence of our profession illuminated by the light of Nightingale, who still resonates in our everyday practice and in education.

In addition, we must respect and care about each others' perceptions as meaningful and possibly significant. Students must be educated toward a transpersonal paradigm while giving all due respect to the empirical sciences as critical to understanding the totality of man or woman, of human beings.

Conclusion

Munhall and Van Manen's work have recently been conceptualized by Munhall (2001). Munhall states that the essence of phenomenology is to search for understanding of how another feels. Phenomenological research demands that we liberate ourselves from preconceptions (Munhall, 1994). Anecdotal descriptive expressions come to life when a singular experience compels you to study a phenomenon coming from out of nowhere (Munhall, 1994). Van Manen (2000) describes an anecdote as a very short and simple story, relating to one single incident, including several quotations, and having a "punch" ending.

This descriptive case study became more than an anecdote. Within it are human phenomena, complex situations, never-to-be-resolved issues, and themes derived from actual events that describe the protagonist and antagonist. This is Nina's story. This is a small case study that was not consciously pursued until a faculty member asked for a case study. That is when the unexpected becomes a case study, an experience from which others can learn. There is no scientific rigor to this study. It is a case study (story) about an unforgettable case in nursing. How not to drift without consciousness.

REFERENCES

Freire, P. (1997). *Pedagogy of the oppressed.* (*20th anniversary ed.*). New York: Continuum.

Lincoln, Y., & Guba, E. (1985). Naturalistic inquiry. Newbury Park, CA: Sage.

Morse, J. (1994). *Critical issues in qualitative research methods.* London: Sage.

Munhall, P. (1994). *Re-visioning phenomenology.* New York: National League for Nursing Press.

Munhall, P. (1997). Out of the box. Image, Journal of Nursing Scholarship. 29, 203.

Munhall, P. (1999). Image, Journal of Nursing Scholarship. 31(2). Second quarter 1999.

Munhall, P., & Boyd, C. O. (1993). *Nursing research*: A *qualitative perspective*. New York: National League of Nursing Press.

Munhall, P. (2001). *Nursing Research*: A *qualitative perspective*. (3rd edition). Sudbury, MA: Jones & Bartlett.

Roberts, S. J. (1983, July). Oppressed group behavior: Implications for nursing. *Advances in Nursing Science*, 21–30.

Sexton, T., & Griffin, B. (1997). *Constructivist thinking in counseling practice*: *Research and training*. New York: Teachers College Press.

Van Manen, M. (2000, March 2–3). Keynote address presented at phenomenology workshop at the Fifth Annual International Conference of the International Institute of Human Understanding, Miami.

Watson, J. (1999). *Postmodern nursing and beyond*. New York: Churchill Livingstone.

Yin, R. (1994). *Case study research*: *Design and methods*. Thousand Oaks, CA: Sage.

13

Historical Research
The Method

M. Louise Fitzpatrick

The purpose of this chapter is to introduce nurse scholars to the field of historical research in nursing. Specifically, the recent developments in historical inquiry as a scholarly pursuit, the objectives of historical research, and, most importantly, the methods, approaches, and procedures associated with historical investigation, analysis, and interpretation will be explored. Historical inquiry, by its very nature, implies a degree of subjectivity in the interpretation and narration of past events. However, the rigor of the research process, corroboration of facts, and comprehensive examination of available data serve to provide the objective evidence on which analysis and interpretative historical exposition rely. The balanced combination of objectivity and subjectivity in the process of the research distinguishes history from the chronicling of events at one extreme and unsupported anecdotal narrative at the other. Like all scholarly investigations, historical research requires careful attention to method and procedure and adequate training of investigators in both the method and the contextual background of the subjects that they select for study.

HISTORICAL INQUIRY IN NURSING

Historical inquiry in nursing, as a legitimate scholarly pursuit, received increased attention and interest in the past three decades. The renaissance of interest in the profession's heritage reflects the concern of a mature profession with its antecedents, not only as a means of informing itself, but to gain a backdrop for current and future directions. It also reflects a renewed concern with the role and contributions of nurses as part of important but more contemporary world events, such as World War II, and society's increased attention to historic events of the twentieth century at the time of the new millennium. History serves a pragmatic purpose as well as a contextual one. It connects us with a heritage and confers on us an identity, personally and professionally. Simultaneous with this heightened interest in nursing's roots has come an expansion of opportunities for doctoral study in nursing. Logically, some individuals found historical research an exciting and productive path to take as part of their doctoral studies and, ultimately, their preferred research agendas.

Understandably, there was resistance to this movement in some sectors. In some universities, there were no nurse historians prepared to guide students. In others, history departments were reluctant to guide students who had not had previous education and experience in historical research methods. In a majority of situations, there was documentation by nurse faculty who, understanding the need for greater research productivity in the field, emphasized the need for clinical research over all else and did not place a value on history or on scholarly attempts to interpret the profession's past.

Scholtfeldt (1975), in her classic article titled "Research in Nursing and Research Training for Nurses," encouraged history and the preparation of historiographers for nursing and commented on the dearth of prepared historiographers (p. 181). She contended that reasons might be the extent to which nursing history is presented to neophytes in ways that capture and nurture their interests and the unavailability of educational opportunities designed to prepare nurses for historical inquiry.

Persistence, administrative support in certain universities, and maintenance of a high standard of performance and rigor in the preparation of nurse historians provided catalysts for the renaissance in the 1970s. Finally, a revised opinion has developed of history's value and worth as a scholarly research endeavor among nurses prepared for such investigations.

From a small cadre of individuals, a growing community of nurse historiographers has emerged. Funding for historical research in the field is possible to obtain, and centers for nursing history and research have developed in selected universities where doctoral study in nursing history is encouraged. Additionally, organizations such as the American Association for the History of Nursing have evolved, thereby providing a network for colleagues in the field and a focus for programs, research conferences, and related activities concerning historical research in nursing. Increasingly, there are international conferences and opportunities for nurse historians to share the results of their research.

THE OBJECTIVES OF HISTORICAL RESEARCH

History, like philosophy, concerns itself with the thought side of human existence. As such, it has worth in and of itself. There is usually a tendency to justify historical research in professional fields such as nursing from the standpoint of its helping to inform future decisions and to avoid repeating past mistakes. Such arguments have only slight merit because they serve a reductionist belief that historical facts can be distilled with a formula. History, although its goal is the establishment of fact that leads us to truth, cannot be reduced to statistical proof. The historian views events as unique. Therefore, it is impossible to ensure that any set of variables, acting in concert, will arithmetically result in some outcome. In human affairs, there are always intervening variables that make it impossible to control or precisely predict destiny. In addition, as Tholfsen (1977) posited, there is danger in demythologizing everything, and an understanding of the limits imposed by the past is what makes liberation and revolution possible (p. 247).

Commager (1966) contended that the scientific historian studies the past because it is part of the evolutionary process and that this process is the key to solving problems (p. 10). Allen Nevins believed that history is to be enjoyed, not endured, and attempted to popularize the results of scholarly research without corrupting it (Billington, 1975, p. xxi). In a practice discipline, the sharing of the results of historical inquiry in ways that are interesting and useful to a majority of the profession's members is probably an important consideration. Narration, presentation, and connection of solid historical interpretation with current trends, issues, and areas of professional interest are the keys to the utilization of such research findings by the contemporary professional and to the education of students about their corporate heritage.

If one of the reasons for pursuing historical research is to build up the body of knowledge in nursing, it is also essential that ways be found to make findings useful to other historians and to the public. The relation of nursing's contributions and activities to the history of women, women's work, and women's studies needs to be strengthened. A related area is the public's perception and image of nursing. History, effectively used, can serve as the collective memory of nursing's accomplishments, not just its struggles; therefore, it can be a principal socializing agent for new members of the profession.

Increasingly, the products of historical research can be viewed in action-oriented dimensions. They can provide prototypes for the development of leaders, they can inform strategic plans of an organizational and political nature, and they can contribute to the development of clinical practice. The outcomes of the historical research process can provide useful analysis of the recent past, as well as an evaluation of events and circumstances that have been well-tempered by time. Without compromising the quality of scholarship, the products of historical research for public consumption can effectively shape the public's perception of nursing, by better informing others about the profession and its contributions.

Synthesizing the past and present through useful insights contributes to the work of those who are architects of the profession's future and brings historical research in nursing into an active and useful mode while continuing to expand the knowledge and understanding of the profession's genesis and evolution for more esoteric reasons. Although the value of historical inquiry needs no justification as a scholarly pursuit when it is applied within professional disciplines, those within the disciplines of both history and the professional fields may still require reassurances concerning the preparation and ability of the investigator, the rigor of the research method, and the utilization of findings. For these reasons, among others, maintaining high quality in the research process and in the narrative exposition is extremely important.

Increasingly, nurse scholar-historians, like other career-minded researchers, are embarking on a line or program of related research activity that they pursue throughout their careers. This effort has the net result of increasing their expertise, making a more sustained contribution to the field, and contributing in-depth substantive data to historical knowledge in the profession.

The development and evolution of nursing as an organized profession, a scholarly practice discipline, and a system of education provide a rich source of potential areas for study. Nursing's relation to world events also provides endless opportunities for study and research. Although valuable and credible historical surveys that highlighted major benchmarks in the profession's development were written as texts from the 1920s to contemporary times, more in-depth scholarly investigations and historical analyses about specific events, institutions, individuals, and changes in clinical practice have emerged in the past 30 years. During this more recent period of scholarship, foundational work has given way to more conceptual areas of study such as feminist themes and their relation to nursing's development.

THE NATURE OF HISTORICAL INQUIRY

Various schools of thought have influenced the field of historiography, just as they have affected all disciplines and professions. The extent to which investigators subscribe to or are influenced by their philosophical approaches to history has critical effects on the research activity and influences the products of the studies. Historical inquiry, like all research, has the discovery of truth as its objective. It is systematic in its method, and objective evidence is determined and judged by using tools of validity and reliability (commonly referred to as methods of internal and external criteria) in historical research.

Today, the schools of thought that traditionally influenced historians are rarely in evidence in their extremes. Rather, an eclectic use of approaches from several schools is generally operational among contemporary scholars. One example of a school of thought that has had both negative and positive influences on the course of historical research was the Positivist, or Neopositivist, school. In this reductionist approach, the historical method attempts to parallel empirical methods in the natural sciences. There is an attempt to reduce history to universal laws. Discovery, verification, and categorization of data are used to provide objective evidence that in and of themselves serve as the interpretation of past events. There is an effort to quantify, to show cause–effect relations, and to force interpretation of data through preexisting formulas, models, and generalizations. This school of thought concerns itself with conditions as predictors of outcomes, rather than attempting to discern what specific conditions caused the known outcome. This school of thought employs the use of hypotheses liberally.

The use of constructs and frameworks has a place in historical explanation, but there should not be an attempt to force the development of universal axioms to explain a unique phenomenon—the historical event. It is possible, however, to use some survey methods and statistical analyses commonly employed in the social sciences to enhance the presentation of objective evidence. This has been successfully accomplished in nursing by Kalisch (1981), in particular. These measures in and of themselves do not lend themselves to good historical interpretation but can support it.

Another school of thought that has had influence on contemporary history and interpretation is the Idealist school, which places procedure, intuition, and experience as ingredients for interpretation. This line of thinking posits that all events have an inside and outside view and that the historiographer must get inside the event and rethink the thought of the originator in the context of his or her time, place, and situation, to make adequate historical interpretations.

Today, historiography is influenced by elements of both schools. From the Positivist school have come attention to rigor in method, use of hypotheses, and instruments of statistical investigation and historical explanation. From the Idealist school have come an emphasis on making interpretations within an appropriate temporal and social context and the importance of viewing events as unique and diverse. From the Positivist school, we acknowledge the possibility of describing patterns that seem to exhibit themselves over time; this possibility is shared by the Idealists, who ascribe what is exhibited to unique and interrelated circumstances. Interconnectedness, or the relation of the parts to the whole, is necessary if coherent and meaningful historical explanation is to result from the research. Although the use of hypotheses is not common among inexperienced investigators, hypotheses can be used effectively in historical inquiry. The danger in their use is a tendency for the investigator to be attracted to a hypothesis and to therefore collect only data that will assist in upholding it while inadvertently ignoring other data. This potential bias in data collection can influence the analysis and interpretation of a historical study and is therefore discouraged for novice investigators.

The use of theoretical frameworks, models, or approaches in the conduct of historical studies and their interpretation requires familiarity with the framework and sophistication in the analysis and interpretation of history. The more common or popular frameworks and approaches used by historians include:

1. *Great person*: This approach focuses attention on individuals and their personal power within a social context. It is particularly useful when the objective of the research is a biographical study or there is a desire to emphasize the people who make changes, rather than the changes themselves.

2. *Deterministic*: This approach minimizes the importance and power of individuals in shaping history and relies primarily on predetermined moral/ethical or religious codes for making judgments and explaining historical phenomena.

3. *Sociological*: This approach emphasizes the primacy of social forces and their influence on people and groups as determinants of historical events. With such a framework, historical phenomena are explained through the use of social trends and cultural events as instruments for the interpretation of specific occurrences.

4. *Political/economic*: This approach may employ the use of an ideology as a framework for the interpretation of historical events and is frequently used in combination with the "great person" approach. The use of Marxism or other ideologies as a framework for explaining historical events is one example of this approach.

5. *Psychological*: This approach requires a solid grasp of psychology as well as facility in the historical method of research. It attempts to explain the thinking, motivations, and behaviors of individuals in a historical sense, using psychological theories as instruments for analysis and explanation. Erikson's biography *Young Man Luther* (1962) is an example of such an approach. Both historians and psychologists have frequently raised valid concerns about the adequacy of either group when it takes on such complex interpretation.

THE PROCESS OF HISTORICAL RESEARCH

The initial stages of development in a historical study are critical to the process and the successful production of the product. Selection of a topic should be considered carefully and in light of its value as a contribution to the field. Frequently, seminal work in an area can provide the foundation for a logical extension and expansion of research on a specific topic. The degree of preparation of the investigator in the historical research method, as well as the investigator's knowledge, history of the period under study, and background in nursing history, can considerably influence the ease of application of the research process and the confidence that can be placed on the result of the investigation. Frequently, the exposition of true interpretative history, in contrast with the development of chronicle, turns on these variables.

When a topic has been selected for study, the framing of the title becomes critical: the title takes on the same significance as the research question in other kinds of studies. Each word in the title is critical to communicating the thesis of the study and the relative emphasis that will be given to specific dimensions named in the title. Frequently, a time period will be specified, and words in the title will become devices to delimit the topic and determine the study's scope.

Early in the process, a thorough investigation and location of sources should ensue. It is possible that the most fascinating topics will become impossible research challenges unless, at the outset, the investigator can ensure the existence of sufficient data to study and research. Location of potential sources such as archives, libraries, and personal collections of individuals can be of great value in determining one's ability to execute the research and to further justify the study. In many instances, embarking on a historical study is like becoming a detective who leaves no stone unturned. Written sources and individuals can be of significant assistance in locating data and ensuring its adequacy for the investigation. Location of sources logically leads to an initial inventory of items that become helpful in shaping the process of the study and collecting data later.

The importance of taking sufficient time to craft the study design systematically, to consider the appropriateness of using or not using hypotheses or specific constructs, and to develop a plan and system that facilitate data collection and analysis cannot be minimized. Although data collection in such research tends to be time consuming, additional time spent in preliminary steps will ensure more ease of analysis, interpretation, and exposition when the study develops beyond the data-collection phase. Developing topical and chronological classification systems can be extremely helpful for filing collected data in ways that make it possible to retrieve them and to read notes in a variety of configurations preliminary to analysis and interpretation.

Sources of Evidence

Contemporary scholars generally agree that a variety of relevant sources, both primary and secondary, are valuable in providing data for historical investigations. Primary sources, either written or in the form of individual verbal responses, provide a firsthand account of an event by one who was present. Examples of primary sources include official documentary material, such as verbatim minutes and proceedings, and interviews with individuals who were present at an event. Although recollection can be faulty and some documents may reflect the subjectivity of the recorder, in general, these primary sources are considered to provide strength to the discovery of truth and establishment of fact.

Secondary sources also can provide rich data. These data are accounts of events at least once removed. They are not hearsay; they are data that can be accepted with confidence despite the fact that they are interpretative reports of events. Some of these sources may include articles written about an event, notes taken at a meeting or summaries of meetings, or narrative descriptions of events by individuals who were not present at the occurrence. Reliability of sources is not related to a particular category. Frequently, a secondary source may be more reliable than a primary one, such as an interview, which may be colored by egocentrism, hyperbole, and selective memory. Guiding and important principles in selecting and collecting available data are: (1) take measures to ensure balance when sources disagree, and (2) include sufficient amounts of available data to establish reliability.

The data-collection stage, the longest stage of the historical research process, can be tedious and isolating. To guide data collection, it is helpful to develop a research outline that raises pertinent questions under each topic or time period. This outline serves to guide the investigator and maps the area of exploration that needs to be addressed through the process of data collection. The outline, though usually broad, should help to focus the investigator and sharpen the parameters of the study in relation to the thesis contained in the title. Ideally, it leads to the articulation of specific questions to be asked of the data. The advent of the electronic age and changes in patterns of communication constitute a formidable challenge to historians. Although the presentation of materials is more sophisticated, human communications are frequently conducted through the use of the computer, and the identification and presentation of existing data become more difficult. The effect of the computer age on the retrieval of historical data as well as the presentation of contemporary documents has both positive and negative aspects.

Establishing Fact from Objective Evidence

Two important elements in the research process are measures of validity and reliability that form the basis for establishing fact. In historical inquiry, validity takes on the form of external criticism of the data. Questions may be raised about authenticity, origin, and originality of documents. Techniques to verify the authenticity of an author's handwriting, and the composition of paper at various time periods, also may be expressed in more elaborate studies. Reliability is the primary means by which fact is established. The strength of the data leading to conclusions that result in the determination of fact depends on tests of reliability. When absolute fact cannot be established, probability and possibility become alternatives. Corroboration of data becomes the critical element in the process. In contrast with validity, reliability is related to the internal criticism of data. Therefore, a correct understanding of language, which itself evolves and changes over the decades, is important. Because parlance changes over time, accurate interpretation of the meaning of words in their particular social and temporal milieu becomes essential. Related to this type of interpretation is the adequacy of understanding the customs of a time period, which may be reflected through the language. Placing both words and events within an appropriate context is a basic ingredient for good analogies and interpretation.

Although there is resistance today to the use of formulas for the determination of historical fact, the following guidelines may be helpful to the investigator when setting out the requirements for establishing fact. Two independent primary sources that corroborate one another establish fact, as does one primary source corroborated by an independent secondary source that contains no substantial contrary evidences. When this guideline cannot be followed, probability can be the goal. This goal requires data from one primary source with no substantial contradictory evidence or data from two or more primary sources that disagree only in some minor aspects. If neither fact nor probability can be established or if corroboration is from only secondary sources, possibility can be established by using data from a primary source that cannot be critically evaluated. In short, reliability in historical research is an attempt to establish truth. Validity and reliability become critical elements in the conduct of the research and in the critique of the quality of a completed study. Historical evidence and proof are cited in references and footnotes. Frequently, multiple references are used to reflect the process of corroboration. Content footnotes that further explain information in the text also are useful devices for the historiographer.

Interviews, whether they are primary or secondary source materials, are usually best conducted after data collection from documents has taken place. This sequence provides an opportunity for further clarification and corroboration of written material. Frequently, anecdotal material provided in interviews helps to connect disparate pieces of already collected data and assists the historiographer in interpreting the evolution and pattern of events.

When all known data have been reviewed and collected, the investigator usually becomes aware of a repetition that emerges in further data collection and is able to complete the process, confident that essential information has been gathered.

Development of the Interpretative Report

The next phase of the study, sometimes taking weeks, comprises careful review, reading, and analysis of the collected data. Simultaneous with this process is the construction of a highly specific writing outline. The more detailed the outline, the easier it becomes to engage in the interpretative and narrative phase of the investigation. A good writing outline helps to form the gestalt. The particular and unique are viewed in relation to the whole without losing their integrity. In addition, careful reading of the data provides an understanding of the interconnectedness of events and moves the process from analysis to synthesis and, finally, to interpretation. Perhaps synthesis is the most difficult of the processes, development of the narrative the most creative, and giving meaning to facts through interpretation the most critical. Historical explanation expressed through the use of a unifying construct or framework or narration based on the predetermined topical or chronological outline emerges through expository writing. At this point, subjectivity plays an essential part in bringing the research process to its logical conclusion. Subjectivity in the interpretation of objective evidence is central to the historical research process and distinguishes history from chronicle; researcher bias in the collection and selection of data must be carefully avoided. In the search for truth, objective evidence and facts provide the foundation for understanding the past; but interpretation by the individual investigator provides the perspectives and views that fill out our understanding of the past and raise new questions for study.

SUMMARY

The use of the historical research process in nursing is a valuable approach to expanding nursing's understanding of itself, as well as for interpreting the field and its contributions to others. It provides a scholarly means of connecting the field to the whole of human experience. Its liberating and liberalizing quality assists the profession to further define its identity through an understanding of its heritage and to provide direction for its future. As a research method, it links nurse scholars with their colleagues in the humanities. As a scholarly pursuit within the professional field, historical inquiry, properly executed, has become essential to the refinement of nursing's understanding of itself.

REFERENCES

Billington, R. (Ed.). (1975). *Allan Nevins on history.* New York: Scribner's.

Commager, H. S. (1966). *The study of history.* Columbus, OH: Merrill.

Erikson, E. (1962). *Young man Luther: A study in psychoanalysis and history.* New York: Norton.

Kalisch, P. (1981). Communicating clinical nursing issues through the newspaper. *Nursing Research,* 30(3), 132–138.

Lusk, B. (1997). Historical methodology for nursing research. *Image: Journal of Nursing Scholarship,* 29, 355–359.

Russel, R. L. (1998). Historiography: A methodology for nurse researchers [Guest editorial]. *Australian Journal of Advanced Nursing,* 16, 5–6.

Scholtfeldt, R. (1975). Research in nursing and research training for nurses: Retrospect and prospect. *Nursing Research,* 24(3), 177–183.

Tholfsen, T. (1977). The ambitious virtues of the study of history. *Teachers College Record,* 79(2), 245–257.

ADDITIONAL REFERENCES

Fealy, G. M. (1999). Historical research: A legitimate methodology for nursing research. *Nursing Review (Ireland),* 17(1/2), 24–29.

Hewitt, L. C. (1997). Historical research in nursing: Standards for research and evaluation. *Journal of the New York State Nurses Association,* 28(3), 16–19.

Rafael, A. R. F. (1999). From rhetoric to reality: The changing face of public health nursing in southern Ontario. *Public Health Nursing,* 16, 50–59.

Szabunia, M., & Buhler, W. K. (1998). Nursing history: Repositories and the Web—historical methodology for nursing research. *Image: Journal of Nursing Scholarship*, 30(2), 109–110.

Turner, C., & Lawler, J. (1999). Mouth care practices in nursing and research-based education: An historical analysis of instructional nursing texts. *International History of Nursing Journal*, 4(3), 29–35.

14

"Constant and Relentless"
The Nursing Care of Patients in Iron Lungs, 1928–1955

Lynne Dunphy

> Polio had not left Mother lying prettily against fluffed white pillows, but palsied, in a torpor. A rubber collar separated her head from her body, her brown hair was matted from perspiration and fell back from her face, her long, slender neck was marred by a raw, shrunken hole and a metal fixture holding a rubber tube.
> Kathryn Black, *In the Shadow of Polio,* 1996

Although methods of manual artificial respiration were in existence, the development of the iron lung in 1928 heralded the first time that a machine kept a human being alive. And who was it who cared for the patient in the machine? Well, nurses, of course! The arduous care required by these patients, both "constant and relentless," has received little examination. Given the innovation of this technology, the complicated associated nursing care, and the need for nurses to straddle the domains of scientific and technological advances in the care of suffering human beings, this examination is warranted.

As noted in M. Louise Fitzpatrick's excellent chapter titled, "Historical Research: The Method," historical inquiry ". . . has worth in and of itself." Additionally, as stated by Allen Nevins, history is to be ". . . enjoyed, not endured" (Billington, 1975, p. xxi). Noted historian Barbara

Tuchman, in an interview conducted by Bill Moyer, was asked about the "why" of history. She responded (with characteristic aplomb), "Why a Beethoven symphony?" In other words, the "thing" has value in and of itself. And, she noted, "It is frightfully interesting."

It is in this spirit that this chapter is written. The intent is to interest the reader in a frightening time in American history, that of the polio epidemics of the first half of the twentieth century. The development of a new, unique technology, the iron lung, will be explored in the context of the epidemics and the scientific thought of the day. The unique contributions of the nurses of that time will be examined, specifically, the "constant and relentless" care required by patients in iron lungs. The time frame delineated is from the time of the development of the lung and its initial use (1929) through the end of the epidemics (1955) with the advent of mass immunization against the virus.

It is theorized that nursing's unique contributions to the care of patients subjected to emerging technologies—in this case, the iron lung—provides a particularly vivid and fascinating example of disparate nursing worlds, one dominated by science, the other by humanism. The tension between these two domains highlights struggles that still exist for nurses in current practice and much that will compose our future. Historical investigation of clinical practice in nursing and its evolution is relatively new and provides significant uncharted territory. It is up to emerging nurse historians to map this important ground, with new and critical insights, providing direction for a meaningful future.

METHODOLOGY

Primary source data, both textual and visual (photographs, drawings, procedures), were drawn from procedural pamphlets from the March of Dimes and American Red Cross used to train and educate nurses in the use of the technology of the iron lung, from old brochures and instructions available from the companies that manufactured the lungs, and from scientific articles and first-person accounts. Photographs and first-person accounts were striking, horrifying, and visionary. A treasure-trove of information was discovered, interestingly, on the Internet. My research assistant and I knew that we had hit "pay dirt" when we discovered the "Virtual Museum of the Iron Lung" web site, filled with all kinds of information as well as first-person accounts of people who had been in lungs during the epidemics, some who to this day are still lung dependent. The web site fostered communication, and many wrote their hitherto unpublished accounts of their experiences.

Archival evidence was located in a number of places. The March of Dimes Birth Defects Foundation headquarters in White Plains, New York, is a rich source of both visual and audiovisual information but does not possess a significant amount of other material. A historical archive exists at Warm Springs, Georgia, and the university archive at Tuskegee, Alabama, contains important documents pertaining to the treatment of Black Americans with polio at the institute there. The Franklin D. Roosevelt Library in Hyde Park, New York, contains voluminous biographical information on Franklin D. Roosevelt, the 32nd president of the United States, and a victim of polio himself. President Roosevelt established the National Foundation for Infantile Paralysis (NFIP, later the March of Dimes), as well as an early treatment center located in Warm Springs, Georgia, where original documents pertaining to these activities are located.

Aspects of the early history of polio in the United States are housed in the Library of the Philosophical Society in Philadelphia, Pennsylvania, including the papers of Simon Flexner, a pioneer in the study of the polio virus. The National Library of Medicine in Washington, DC, contains a variety of original source material related to polio; the archive of the Sister Kenny Institute in Minneapolis is a rich source of data on the controversial Australian nurse and her American years, as well as documents from the Sister Kenny Foundation. The office of the Gazette International Networking Institute in St. Louis, Missouri, has a large collection of polio- and disability-related books, as well as back issues of the Institute's publications, such as the *Polio Network News*.

First-person accounts and memoirs are plentiful and frequently heartbreaking (Bates & Pellow, 1964; Black, 1996; Beisser, 1989; Gould, 1995; Grinnell, 1989; Hall, 1990; Hawkins & Lomask, 1957; Hobson, 1978; James, 1961; Kriegel, 1991; Le Comte, 1957; Marshall, 1955; Marshall, 1962, 1964; Milam, 1984; Murphy, 1987; Opie, 1957; Plagemann, 1949; Purdy, 1953a; Roosevelt, 1949; Roosevelt, 1937, 1962; Roosevelt & Brough, 1974; Strauss, 1979; Woods, 1994). For this specific study, polio survivors were contacted and a small number (two) were interviewed as a supplement to the first-person accounts surveyed. Their recollections of their experiences, with special emphasis on the nursing care, were gathered. Five nurse informants were interviewed about their experiences in caring for patients in iron lungs as well as their recollections of working with this technology.

Secondary sources also were widely and easily available and included numerous medical and nursing texts of the time as well as scientific articles and media accounts, such a newspapers and magazine articles. This type of evidence provides corroboration and helps the historian contextualize the primary source data. To prevent the isolation of nursing from the many surrounding forces that affect practice, the times and other factors that influence care were broadly examined, especially the scientific thinking of the day (much of which was proved wrong). Leading polio researcher, and thus "insider," Dr. John R. Paul of Yale University wrote the riveting A *History of Poliomyelitis* (Paul, 1971). A variety of other histories and studies of the times, as well as biographies, also were used (Benison, 1967; Berg, 1948; Bigland, 1956; Bowen, 1970; Carter, 1966; Cohn, 1955, 1975; Cook, 1992; Davis, 1963; De Kruif, 1926, 1962; Dowling, 1977; Draper, 1916, 1935; Farrell, 1965; Fisher, 1967; Freidel, 1954; Gould, 1995; Lash, 1972; Levine, 1954; Lippmann, 1977; Morgan, 1985; Rogers, 1992; Smith, 1990; Ward, 1989).

Data analysis and synthesis, as discussed in Chapter 13, are subjective and creative interpretive processes ". . . distinguish(ing) history from chronicle." The richness and previously unexplored nature of the material made these processes particularly exciting.

THE MECHANICAL MONSTERS

By the last part of the nineteenth century, the idea of extending life through some means of mechanical ventilation seemed within reach. An early ventilatory device was made by Alexander Graham Bell, inventor of the telephone, on a trip to England 1882. He constructed a "vacuum jacket" consisting of a rigid shell in two halves with a soft lining, which was strapped around the chest, with a connecting bellows providing the negative pressure. Sketches of this device survive, and in 1892 Bell continued to perfect it; however, no documentation of its actual use exists.[1]

The first effective use of artificial ventilatory assistance is traced to 1928, with the use of the first "iron lungs" developed by Phillip Drinker.[2] The Drinker tale is a great one of dedication and scientific discovery (Paul, 1971; Dunphy, 2001; Drinker, 1929; Bowen, 1970). The following description is taken from "Memoirs of the Respirator":

> The first patient was a little girl treated in a tank with household vaccuum cleaners as pumps. One could hear it running for a

---

[1] Others achieved some modest success in experimentation with various devices, notably Woillez, in France, and Sueret, in South Africa in 1918.

[2] According to Paul (1971, 316), this name was given to the machine by a newspaper reporter; it stuck.

quarter of a mile away because it was summer and the windows were all open. (Wilson, quoted in Paul, 1971, p. 318)

Although the little girl died less than a week later, she had survived a week longer than she would have without the machine. A newer machine was successfully used on a young man shortly thereafter. In less than a year he recovered enough to breathe on his own and was able to walk with the assistance of braces on his legs and a cane. Dr. Wilson, who assisted with his care, remembers that this case demonstrated several things. Most importantly, the man survived, providing justification for use of the respirator, and he led a quite useful life despite the residual handicaps. Additionally,

> He seemed almost totally paralyzed and the use of the respirator demonstrated several things. One, the great difficulty of caring for a big man. The thing was closed with multiple clamps on a hard rubber gasket so there was no access to the man's body to clean him or do anything to him. (Wilson, quoted in Paul, 1971, p. 328)

Dr. Wilson noted that to bathe him took a heroic effort with six men and nurses in an organized team. This led Wilson, on the advice of Philip Drinker, to buy some portholes made for boats and have them welded on to the machine so that they could be opened. They then fitted the portholes with rubber collars through which hands could be inserted to "manipulate" the patient without taking him out of the tank and disrupting his respirations. The work of nursing care was clearly laid out.

THE SHIFTING SANDS OF SCIENTIFIC THOUGHT

Poliomyelitis is an acute generalized disease caused by a virus. Formerly, it was the most common form of viral infection of the nervous system. Before 1956, from approximately 25,000 to 50,000 cases of poliomyelitis were reported annually in the United States (Muldar, 1998). The disease occurred in sporadic endemic or epidemic form, most commonly in late summer and fall. The number of cases followed an irregular curve, reaching epidemic proportions at intervals. The epidemics were random and local, and the geographic site of highest incidence varied from year to year.

The diagnosis of poliomyelitis was made on the basis of a flaccid paralysis that occurred during an acute febrile illness. Confirmation of diagnosis was made by examination of the cerebrospinal fluid. Early in onset, there would be an increase in cerebrospinal pressure and increase in cell count, initially polymorphonuclear cells; but, after a few days, lymphocytes would predominate. Protein count increased especially in patients with paralytic polio. Only as the epidemics were winding down did specific viral studies become readily available.

Paralysis is reported to occur in fewer than 1 in 100 patients infected; even among those paralyzed, many had only limited and transient weakness. These cases were often overlooked; thus it can be concluded that the total number of patients infected with the polio virus during the epidemics was far higher than reported. The disease was most common in infants and children (hence, the term *infantile paralysis*), although it could and did strike adults. By the 1940s and 1950s, more and more young adults and adults were stricken.

In cases of spinal polio, the virus attacked the motor nerves of the spinal cord. Damage could range from weakness in one set of muscles to quadripligia. When it attacked the respiratory muscles, the intercostals, and the diaphragm, as many as 50 percent of patients would die. Patients affected by this type of viral attack were helped by the iron lung. When the virus attacked the bulbar cells of the central nervous system, however, it posed additional threats: it could attack the cranial nerves that control chewing; more commonly, and more ominously, however, the virus could attack the cranial nerves operating the pharnyx, larynx, and soft palate, making swallowing, talking, and breathing difficult or, in some cases, impossible. These patients had a poor chance of survival, even in the iron lung. When patients suffered from both types of polio—bulbar and respiratory—dilemmas were posed.

Treatment for the two types of paralysis conflicted. Patients with bulbar polio—specifically, paralysis of the pharynx—were not helped by the iron lung; flat on their backs, they choked on their own secretions if not carefully tended. Some thought that tracheostomies were the most effective way to treat these patients. Others felt that, enough tilting of the machine, careful aspiration of the throat, patient cooperation was enough. Sometimes this functional pharyngeal paralysis lasted only a few days. Additionally, it was often impossible to distinguish between the two types. Some patients ended up having tracheostomies and being in the lung. Sixty percent of patients with bulbar-respiratory polio died.

Kathryn Black, whose mother was stricken with bulbar-respiratory polio as a young woman of 28 years of age in 1952, described her visit to the hospital to see her mother during the acute phase of her illness: "Wards of tank respirators looked something like the boiler rooms of giant ships, with the blur of gauges, tubes, latches, and dials. The six-foot metal cylinder[s] that breathed for patients lay like coffins. . . . Intravenous bottles hung from aluminum poles next to respirators, and at one end of each [tank respirator] lay a head" (Black, 1996, p. 14). She goes on to describe how her grandmother brought a gift for her mother on her first visit to the hospital: a white quilted bathrobe with white velvet ribbons. However,

> At the sight of her daughter's gaunt face protruding from the massive iron cylinder, (she) gasped, then paled, as she reeled with dizziness. A nurse took her arm and led her to a chair, commanding that she lower her head. Time was almost up when my grandmother felt steady enough to cross the room to see Mother. (Black, 1996, p. 14)

The source of infection was the subject of much debate in the early part of the twentieth century. Initially, the virus was believed to gain entry into the nervous system through the olfactory nerves. On the basis of this theory, in the 1930s there was an attempt to block children's noses with chemicals such as zinc sulfate and picric acid. This measure had been thought to have worked with monkeys; it was, however, a dismal failure in human beings (Gould, 1995).

Without accurate identification of the reservoir of infection and portal of entry or of the virus itself, it was impossible to really understand how long patients were contagious and the proper sanitation measures to implement. As late as 1948, Dr. W. H. Bradley, Senior Health Officer of the Ministry of Health in London, summed up our approaches to the problem of polio in three words: "Ignorance, impotence, and insecurity" (Gould, 1995).

Whoosh-whoosh-whoosh

Then there was the characteristic "hospital symphony," the rhythmic cacophony of the lung as its bellows inflated and deflated, a mechanized, wheezing sound. Others described the ". . . loud whine of the motor" (Bowen, 1970, p. 150). The lungs functioned on the principle of negative pressure body ventilation. The respirator was equipped with a motor that drove some form of blower, or "bellows," as they came to be called, which is what accounted for the **whoosh-whoosh-whoosh** sound. A patient's entire body was surrounded in an airtight chamber with the head protruding through an airtight collar at one end.

The following poem, "The Man in the Iron Lung," was composed by Mark O'Brien, a polio patient who has yet to leave his lung:

The Man in the Iron Lung

I *scream*
The body electric
this yellow, metal, pulsating cylinder
Whooshing all day, all night
In its repititious, dull mechanical rhythm.
Rudely it inserts itself in the map of my body,
which my midnight mind,
Dream drenched cartographer of terra incognita,
Draws upon the dark parchment of sleep.
I *scream*
In my body electric. (cited in Seavey, Smith & Wagner, 1996)

Although it was frightening, when gripped in the acute phase of illness, many patients perceived the lung as a "savior," as indeed it was. Regina Woods, author of *Tales from Inside the Lung and How I Got Out* wrote, "I was no longer struggling to breathe and the whole thing seemed simply wonderful. So wonderful that I cannot remember a night before, or since, of such sheer comfort. I did not know that these things signaled a worsening of my condition and were viewed by my family with great alarm" (Woods, 1994, p. 5). Getting the patient into the lung, it turned out, was not the problem—it was getting them out.

HOSPITALS AND NURSING, 1929–1955

As is widely documented, the hospital had become the preferred site for care of the ill. Although hospitals had originally been charity-based facilities for long-term care of the chronically ill, by the 1920s they were firmly established as scientific facilities for acute interventions (Howell, 1989; Lynaugh, 1989). Their size and number increased dramatically, and hospitals had already modified their philanthropic ethos with a business sensibility (Rosenberg, 1987; Rosner, 1989). They began attracting middle-class, paying patients. The rise of the third-party payment system in the 1930s continued the trend of hospital utilization, as did other factors, such as the increased use of graduate nurses within the hospital structure (Kalisch & Kalisch, 1995; Melosh, 1982; Reverby, 1985, 1987; Starr, 1982). Medical technology had come to play an important, even central, role before the introduction of the lungs.

X-rays and electrocardiograms (EKGs) allowed doctors to literally "see" inside the human body. Anesthesiology and asepsis encouraged surgical intervention. Diagnostic laboratories enabled doctors to identify and eventually treat specific microbes (Howell, 1989). Concurrent with these innovations was a continued increase in the stature of medicine in the early twentieth century (Louden, 1997; Magner, 1992; Porter, 1997).

In the 1930s, the staffing of hospitals changed from a student nurse labor force to employed graduate nurses (Kalisch & Kalisch, 1995). Paramount among the reasons for this shift was the Great Depression. Patients, still perceiving hospitals as charity institutions and no longer able to afford to pay private-duty nurses in the home, flocked to them; out-of-work private-duty nurses begged for employment and accepted low wages and a roof over their heads. Studies over a number of years supported a graduate rather than student workforce. Additionally, the nursing leaders of the time, many of whom were both nursing educators and hospital administrators, supported this move. In the late 1920s, the American Hospital Association had instituted a voluntary accreditation system; increased emphasis was placed on hospital management, efficiency, and the bottom line. Many nurse leaders saw the alignment of nursing with the increasing scientific strength of medicine—most of it taking place on the stage of the hospital, along with the management of nursing, its personnel, and procedures, in the "scientific" movement toward increased efficiency—as a strategy for advancing their agenda of professionalization for nurses (but that is another story) (Melosh, 1982; Reverby, 1985, 1987).

Although many diploma schools closed in the 1930s and some advancement had been made for university education for nurses, the majority of the nurses of the day were educated in hospital schools of nursing. Many would seek hospital employment after graduation. The pay was low; the hours were long. Eighty-four percent of hospitals offered room, board, and laundry as part of a nurse's wages. Some argue that nursing leaders struck a pact with the devil—yielding to pressure from hospital administrators for lower wages in exchange for control of the hierarchy (some things remain the same), many seeking the leverage of middle-management positions.

In regard to nurses' relations with physicians, in some senses the nurses gained. When nurses were employed by a hospital, doctors lost some of their economic and social control over nurses. The bureaucratic structure of the hospital diffused medical authority and offered a modicum of support for nurses when conflicts arose with physicians.

Hospital nurses occupied strategic positions in the hospital hierarchy; the nurse commanded the domain of her ward. As advances in medical science continued, nursing and medical work became more intertwined. The nurse's close observation of very sick patients became more critical to their very survival, as more life-saving treatments became available. Nowhere was this more true than in the care of the patient in the iron lung.

NURSING CARE: CONSTANT AND RELENTLESS

In a 1938 article titled "The Essential Features of Poliolyelitis," published in the journal *Public Health Nursing*, Dr. T. Campbell Thompson noted, "In no disease, except perhaps pneumonia, is expert nursing care so essential. Rest, complete and prolonged, mental and physical, is by far the most important single factor in aiding the poisoned motor cells in the spinal cord to recover" (Thompson, 1938, p. 145). This sentiment is echoed in numerous sources, by physicians, nurses, and patients. One article notes: "Professor Drinker has stressed more than once the fact that, even if a respirator works perfectly, it will not take the place of nursing care" (Norcross, 1939, p. 1067). Prevention of pneumonia, breakdown of skin areas, and physiologic changes resulting from the patient's severe restriction of movement were all designated as important nursing responsibilities associated with respirator care.

An *American Journal of Nursing* article states: "It is important that the nurse always be present so that the patient may be closely observed" (Harmison, 1935, p. 480). The position of the body must be changed every 2 hours. Leakage of air must be guarded against because the negative pressure is lowered if any air seeps through. "The ordered rate and depth should be kept constantly and recorded frequently" (Harmison, 1935, p. 480).

It was important to guard against pressure sores, especially around the neck, where the fitted rubber collar often chafed. Application of a cotton collar, or "flannelette," or a strip of "soft, chamois skin" between the skin and rubber diaphragm was recommended. Ideally, the rubber should never touch the skin. Washing the neck with cool water and alcohol was recommended as a good preventive measure.

Although the patients could eat, sleep, and talk while in the "tank," they must be taught to swallow only on expiration to prevent strangling. It was also necessary for the nurse to feed the patient. One source recommended gently placing one teaspoonful of liquid into the side of the mouth at a time and monitoring the patient's ability to swallow.

One nurse informant stated:

> The care of the polio respirator patient is a tremendous responsibility. It is physically exhausting in actual physical energy expended to care for the patient, and it is a mental strain trying to imbue him with confidence and a hopeful outlook. It is a great mental strain also watching for signs indicating a change (adverse) in the patient's condition. (Manfreda, 1991, p. 7)

The life of the patient in an iron lung was always in the nurses' hands.

> One of the biggest mental responsibilities is remembering to check on the respirator pressure. Pressure may be lost from the smallest leak occurring around the head opening, a porthole door being left open, incomplete closure of the head and body parts of the respirator, or an unplugged opening, such as the opening designed to admit intravenous tubing. A patient's life could be lost from pressure failure. (Manfreda, 1991, p. 7)

These portholes were those devised by Dr. Wilson and Professor Drinker after the lung's first use in 1928. They allowed access to the patient. One source describes them as follows: "The portholes are constructed in a manner similar to the openings for the head, with rubber diaphragms for the hand to go through so that as much of the vacuum may be preserved as possible" (Harmison, 1935, p. 481). Modifications continued to be made. For example, one article notes that most of the portholes were placed near the upper part of the body, making care of the patient's feet difficult. In this case, the hospital engineer devised a plan where other openings could be made. Specifically, four new ports and windows were added to the end of the machine, which ". . . made our work much easier and more efficient" (Helling, 1941, p. 1323).

Another nurse informant described the work as follows:

> One had to learn to quickly adapt to being able to put equipment into the machine and get it out properly. One had to be able to utilize linens for moving the patient properly. The adaptation of support . . . in the way of rolls of linens and pillows, again for support . . . maintaining proper body alignment was essential, or you ended up with scoliosis, and limbs that were not able to be [used] . . . to recover. (Nurse informant 4; personal communication, July 15, 1999)

NURSING CARE: FEAR AND BRAVERY

It was about the years of the polio epidemic that "... fear hung like heat in the summer air" (Black, 1996, p. 43). This fear was as real for the nurses and doctors who cared for these patients as for the general public— perhaps more so. After all, no one knew how contagious the disease was or how it was transmitted. What precautions should be taken and for how long? We questioned some informants regarding their memories of fear. One answered:

> Yeah, I think everybody did in those days, that was assigned to it. . . . I mean, you had to gown up, wear a mask, you did all this. . . . I think there was a greater fear of contracting polio than AIDS today. . . . Because you knew if you got it you could be crippled for life. . . . During the infectious stage, nurses were afraid. (Nurse informant 3, personal communication, July 8, 1999)

When asked if they ever refused to care for a patient, the informant said she did not really know about that, because, as a student (which she was), she ". . . didn't have much right to refuse." They were told that they needed the isolation experience.

One physician described his experiences as a resident at the University of Minnesota Hospital during the epidemics of 1948 and 1949 in the following terms: "It was like being in combat. You have to be on the ball and ready to go all the time. You were tired, exhausted, and frightened at the same time ". He went on: " We didn't want to get polio ourselves. We were all concerned as heck about it because we'd bring it home . . . you couldn't avoid it. Because you were covered with saliva, you'd bring it with you" (Seavey, Smith, & Wagner, 1996, p. 115).

Nurses were recruited for "polio duty." Their salaries were underwritten jointly by local hospitals and chapters of the National Foundation for Infantile Paralysis, and they received slightly higher rates of pay. However, there was no differential allowed, because ". . . the NFIP had insurance coverage for nurses who contracted polio" (Whitman, 1949, p. 33). This insurance covered medical and hospital expenses, as well as a salary stipend on a decreasing rate over a period of a year. Dr. Joseph Melnick, a scientist at Yale University who was central to the testing and development of the oral polio vaccine, likened the polio epidemics to the AIDS epidemics of today (Seavey, p. 227).

NURSING CARE: WORKING TOGETHER

Teamwork was essential for all phases of the care of lung patients, a requirement that is stressed in all sources. Pictures surveyed in nursing texts, as well as a review of procedures, all portray a team of workers, usually nurses, facilitating the movement of the patient into the lung. Getting organized to "put" the patient in the lung was a rather complex procedure, minimally requiring four people. A variety of equipment had to be assembled and prepared. One text suggests the following procedure for taking the patient out of the respirator, something that took place initially for only short periods of time: "All articles and equipment should be assembled. Two to four nurses should be available to perform the necessary procedure. The doctor should hyperventilate the patient. The stretcher should be withdrawn quickly and the nurses should work together very rapidly and *in unison* to complete the nursing care in the shortest possible time" (Tracey, 1949, p. 568). A great source of anxiety for all concerned was a power outage. Such an event took maximum teamwork. Nurses, doctors, the maintenance man—anyone available—were expected to operate the bellows by hand. As described by one informant: "This is extremely hard to do, the person pumping tiring within a minute or two" (Manfreda, 1991, p. 7). The teamwork in this situation was essential for the patients survival: "The staff on duty (doctors, nurses, orderlies, aides), in short everybody available and able, lined up and in relays we kept the respirators going."

Another nurse recalled that her greatest fear was a power failure. She added, "There was never enough help. Those were the days I recall working twelve plus hours per day. Without a day off for weeks on end" (Nurse informant 1, personal communication, June 30, 1999). Nurses continued to work for low wages, a practice begun in the 1930s and carried into the postwar era. Interestingly, not all nurses seemed excessively concerned about this situation. Victoria Grando argues that women of the postwar period found strengths in achievements within their domestic confines (Grando, 2000, p. 177). One nurse is quoted as saying:

There *may* be some more interesting occupation than nursing . . . but I do not know what it could be. The suspense of watching a patient's physical and psychological reaction to good care is dramatic. Until you see a patient you expected to die walk out of the hospital, you don't know what durable satisfactions are. (Weligoschek, 1950, p. 80)

The concept of teamwork extended to the organization of care on the ward. The polio epidemics provide an early example of patient triage and the practice of grouping very ill patients together to render more effective care. When asked about the number of patients cared for and how they were able to do it, one nurse responded, "We have all eight respirator [patients] in the room if necessary. You see they were rather large, and it made the nursing care much more easy to do. You could stand there and see every patient" (Interview).

Additionally, teamwork operated in the efforts of the National Foundation for Infantile Paralysis, which worked hand in hand with the Red Cross throughout the epidemics. They coordinated efforts to move lungs to where they were needed, to educate health care professionals, such as nurses, in the care of polio patients, and to dispatch corps of workers to the sites of the latest epidemics when needed. This is a story in itself.

NURSING CARE: MASTERING THE MACHINE

The nurses had to learn every aspect of handling the machine (and, hence, the patient in the machine). One nurse described being on duty on a Sunday. There was one machine on standby, and they had to use it. That left one inoperable machine. The nurse called the engineer and said that the machine had to be fixed: "He looked at me and he looked at the machine and he said, 'I've never seen one before.' " She continued, " 'Okay,' I said. I rolled up my sleeves, I put a sheet on the floor and I said, 'Let's take it apart.' And I took it apart, I laid out every nut and bolt that we removed, I found the problem, and put everything back together. And that was a sight to see! Me, crawling around under the machine in a white uniform, a cap on my head. But we did it. And it was operable. (Nurse informant 4, personal communication, July 15, 1999)

The negative pressure of the machine was usually set somewhere between 14 and 18 respirations per minute by turning the regulating wheel by the motor. Most sources note that the attending physicians are responsible for prescribing the proper rate, the negative pressure, and the internal temperature of the apparatus. Sources note that most likely the physician will make the initial adjustment of the machine itself, both of the pressure within the lung, estimated at between 10 and 20 centimeters of water pressure, controlling depth of respirations, and of the respiratory rate. However, sources note that it is the responsibility of the nurse to watch the breathing of the patient and make any necessary adjustments in depth and rate of respirations.

The nurse, as master of the machine, had the important responsibility of adapting it to the individual patient. These nurses had to be attuned to their patients, to their every breath and to any small sign of distress or change in color. They had to be prepared to suction, adjust the tilt of the machine (which could be done to facilitate postural drainage), provide oxygen, or get the physician when a tracheostomy was indicated. The nurse provided the important human link between the patient and machine.

There was a flip side to the mastery of the machine. The machine gave the nurses tremendous control over their patients. The following quotation from patient Regina Woods is but one example of many such quotations found in the patient literature:

> Various ways were tried to get me and those like me out of the lungs that lined the halls like so many yellow caskets, their motionless inhabitants filled with fear and rage. Fear they would not survive the next attempt to help them and rage that they could do nothing to strike back when the keepers went beyond the bounds of human decency. . . . (Woods, 1994, p. 6)

Such sentiments were interspersed with wonderful stories of caregiving and nurturance provided to patients by nurses. Discussions with nurses who had cared for these patients were revealing. One told us of her frustration and difficulty in caring for a young woman in an iron lung, a "chronic"—in other words, beyond the acute, immediately life threatening stage of the disease, but still lung dependent. The nurse recalled that ". . . she wanted to be waited on constantly. And then I had the frustration of not being able to care for my other patients. And being a young nurse, I couldn't comprehend why she was so demanding" (Nurse informant 3, personal communication, July 8, 1999). Reflecting on this situation today, she explained how she did not interpret her behavior as the anxiety that it was but rather that she was a selfish person. The nurse stated, "I wasn't mature enough to understand what she was going through. . . ." This nurse also stated that this situation occurred during her pediatric rotation. "And being at that hospital, supposedly learning my pediatric experience, this being an adult, it was like this isn't fair! I'm being used! . . . and we really felt we were being dumped on! But immaturity was part of our problem too."

Another nurse informant said, "The psychological needs were so vital and yet we didn't attach as much importance to those things in those years as we do today. . . . We weren't as empathic. We weren't as understanding." She spoke of the need for "far better understanding" and concluded with the statement: "We were so harassed with keeping our patients alive and working the hours that we did, and having our own frustrations that we couldn't do more than we were doing, and seeing this never ending constant admission of patients . . ." (Nurse informant 2, personal communication, July 6, 1999).

THE NEED FOR CARING, IDENTIFIED

The psychological side of the care of patients was to change tremendously between 1929 and 1955. During the 1930s, very little attention was paid to the psychosocial side of patient care. Children were separated from parents, and those who became excessively distraught were viewed as being overattached to the mother, according to one source, consistent with the Freudian views that dominated the day. Parents who were excessively anxious were considered "psychologically immature." Nurses were cautioned not to be too sympathetic to the children, that an objective (i.e., professional) attitude was to be maintained at all times. Families were allowed to visit only once a week and for a very brief period, especially during the acute phase of the illness. Children would theoretically make a "better adjustment" to their illness in this way.

One source, from 1937, argued that the hospitalized child should be surrounded by an atmosphere of "neutrality"; having no visitors was thought to be better than having anxious families and friends hovering nearby. According to a 1935 *New England Journal of Medicine* article, for a child who had completely recovered, "the disease seems to have no darker memories than an attack of measles" (Barbour, 1935, p. 565). Another source boldly asserted, "No crippled individual must be left to indulge in his own thoughts" (Kidd, 1943).

By the end of the epidemics, things had begun to change in this arena. By 1947, articles were appearing in the professional literature encouraging the nurse to "Give him the chance to 'get it off his chest' "(Seidenfeld, 1947, p. 369). This enlightened article encouraged nurses to be "open, specific, and above board" with their patients, even the children. Consistently in the literature was the need for the nurse to individualize care to the specific patient and the need to see the whole person.

CONCLUSIONS

By 1928, much of the care of the sick had moved into the hospital set-ting. The hospital had become the stage on which emerging technolo-gies were utilized. And the graduate nurse place of employment was shifting from its base in private-duty nursing, essentially contract work, to employment by the hospital. Thus nurses were most instrumental in the implementation of the radical new technology, the iron lung.

The brave and resourceful nurses who cared for patients in iron lungs in the first half of the twentieth century became technically pro-ficient "masters of the machine" while attempting to hold onto tradi-tional nursing values. The goals of keeping their patients alive and at-tending to multiple physiologic needs, compounded by large numbers of very ill patients during the epidemics, took first priority. The pre-vailing psychological mores of the era did not support sensitivity to a patient's emotional needs. Although psychological approaches were to become more enlightened during the late 1940s and the 1950s, these ideas, though disseminated in professional journals, had not been mainstreamed into nursing curricula. Young nurses and student nurses in particular were not always prepared to meet the overwhelming emo-tional needs of iron lung patients. Students continued to be "used" for service needs, with not enough time and support to provide the high level of care that some of these patients needed.

However, in the main, nurses did a heroic job in meeting the over-whelming nursing care needs of the iron lung patient. It was the re-sponsibility of the nurse to "mold" the technology to the individual pa-tient. The nurses caring for patients in iron lungs had to be attuned to their respiratory needs at all times to keep them alive, which meant being with the patient physically and psychically. Decisions had to be made regarding suctioning, postural drainage, giving oxygen, and the need for emergency tracheostomy, and nurses had to make these minute-to-minute decisions. Nurses positioned the patients every 2 hours and fed them, teaspoonful by teaspoonful if necessary. Nurses had to adjust the gauges on the lung, regulating the depth and rate of the pressure to fit a patient's needs. In a way, they could be said to have "breathed" with the patient. And nurses activated the team nec-essary to "man" the bellows by hand during power outages. Addition-ally, similar to the work of nurses in the early ICUs identified by nurse historian Julie Fairman (1992), "The intense needs of acutely ill pa-tients supported closer relationships between physicians and nurses" (p. 58).

The "constant and relentless" care rendered by nurses in the first half of the twentieth century caring for patients in iron lungs demonstrated technological mastery combined with exquisite sensitivity to the patients' physiological needs. Aspects of this care also cast light on less pleasant aspects of nursing practice—episodes of startling insensitivity, even cruelty. Historian Thomas Olson argues that the "handling, controlling, and managing" abilities of nursing students were what was valued between 1915 and 1937 and that the "language of caring" was absent (Olson, 1987, pp. 68–72; Rinker, 2000, pp. 133–134). This investigation reveals knowledgeable, brave, committed, and creative nurses confronted by overwhelmingly ill patients, frightening and new technology, low pay, and work in hospitals where they were largely powerless. Margaret Sandelowski, for examples, notes, "Specialty nursing practices built around technologies remaining in medical jurisdiction serve primarily the interests of organized medicine and hospitals" (Sandelowski, 1999, p. 61). In essence, the physicians "controlled" the lungs; they set the pressures. These nurses were often students, young, and educated to prioritize physiological needs over psychological ones, often contrary to their own caring instincts.

Historical inquiry into the nature of nursing practice as well as patients' perceptions of this practice has the power to illuminate important knowing. What nursing strengths were demonstrated and what limitations? In incidents of "bad practice," what were the antecedents? What environments can be fostered that support expert and caring nursing? We need to celebrate and highlight the strengths of our practice, the often overlooked contributions of nurses providing "constant and relentless" care, and we need to study episodes of uncaring nursing care, because they constitute equally important sources of knowledge. These understandings can assist current and future nurses in providing competent, yet compassionate and caring, nursing care.

REFERENCES

Barbour, E. H. (1932). Social aspects of poliomyelitis. *New England Journal of Medicine*, 207, 1195–1196.

Barbour, E. H. (1935). Adjustment during the four years of patients handicapped by poliomyelitis. *New England Journal of Medicine*, 213, 563–565.

Barnett, A. (1954). *The iron cradle*. New York: Crowell.

Bates, P., & Pellow, J. (1964). *Horizontal man*. London: Longman.

Beisser, A. (1989). *Flying without wings*. New York: Doubleday.

Benison, S. (1967). *Tom Rivers: Reflections on a life in medicine and science.* Cambridge, MA: Harvard University Press.

Berg, R. (1948). *Polio and its problems.* Philadelphia: Lippincott.

Bigland, F. (1956). *The true book about Sister Kenny.* London: Heinemann.

Billington, R. (Ed.). (1975). *Allan Nevins on history.* New York: Scribner's.

Black, K. (1996). *In the shadow of polio.* Reading, MA: Addison-Wesley.

Bowen, C. D. (1970). *Family portraits.* New York: Scribner's.

Carter, R. (1966). *Breakthrough: The saga of Jonas Salk.* New York: Doubleday.

Cohn, V. (1955). *Four billion dimes.* Minneapolis: Minneapolis Star & Tribune.

Cohn, V. (1975). *Sister Kenny.* Minneapolis: University of Minnesota Press.

Cook, B. W. (1992). *Eleanor Roosevelt: Vol. I, 1884–1933.* New York: Viking Penguin.

Davis, F. (1963). *Passage through crisis.* Indianapolis: Bobbs-Merrill.

De Kruif, P. (1926). *Microbe hutey.* New York: Harcourt Brace.

De Kruif, P. (1962). *The sweeping wind: A memoir.* London: Oxford.

Dowling, H. (1977). *Fighting infection: Conquests of the twentieth century.* Cambridge, MA: Harvard University Press.

Draper, G. (1916). *Acute Poliomyelitis.* New York: GP Putnam.

Draper, G. (1935). *Infantile Paralysis.* New York: Dutton.

Drinker, P., & McKhann, C. (1929). The use of a new apparatus for the prolonged administration of artificial respiration. *Journal of the American Medical Association 92,* 1658–1660.

Dunphy, L. M. (2001). "The steel cocoon: Tales of the nurses and patients of the iron lung, 1929–1955." *Nursing history review, 9,* pp. 3–34.

Fairchild, L. M. (1952). Some psychological factors observed in poliomyelitis patients. *American Journal of Physical Medicine, 31,* 275–281.

Fairman, J. (1992). Watchful vigilance: Nursing care, technology, and the development of intensive care units. *Nursing Research 41,* 56–60.

Farrell, J. G. (1965). *The lung.* London: Scribners.

Fisher, P. J. (1967). *The polio story.* London: Dutton.

Freidel, F. (1954). *Franklin D. Roosevelt: Vol. 2. The ordeal.* Boston: Little, Brown.

Gallagher, H. (1985). *FDR's splendid deception.* New York: Dodd, Mead.

Gould, T. (1995). *A summer plague: Polio and its survivors.* New Haven, CT: Yale University Press.

Grando, V. (2000). A hard day's work: Institutional nursing in the post WWII era. *Nursing History Review 8,* 169–184.

Greteman, T. J. (1944). Nursing care of acute poliomyelitis. *American Journal of Nursing, 44,* 929–933.

Grinell, S. H. (1989, Fall). A post-polio 'Normal's' reconciliation with the ghost of polio past. *Polio Network News.*

Hall, R. (1990). *Through the storm.* St. Cloud, MN: North Star Press.

Harmison, B. (1935). Nursing care of a child in the respirator. *American Journal of Nursing*, 35, 479–481.

Hawkins, L. C., & Lomask, M. (1957). *The man in the iron lung: The story of Frederick B. Smite*. Surrey, England.

Helling, H. (1941). The patient in the respirator. *American Journal of Nursing*, 41, 1322–1324.

Hobson, H. (1978). *Indirect journey: An autobiography*. London: Heinemann.

Howell, J. (1989). Machines and medicine: Technology transforms the American hospital. In D. E. Long & J. Golden, (Eds.), *The American General Hospital* (pp. 109–134). Ithaca: Cornell University Press.

James, B. (1961). *Living forwards*. London: Scribners.

Kalisch, P., & Kalisch, B. (1995). *The history of American nursing*. Philadelphia: Lippincott.

Kidd, D. B. (1943). *The physical treatment of anterior poliomyelitis*. London: Faber & Faber.

Kottke, F. J., & Kubicek, W. G. (1949). The care of the patient with bulbar-respiratory poliomyelitis. *American Journal of Nursing*, 49, 374–378.

Kriegel, L. (1991). *Falling into life: Essays*. San Francisco: North Star Press.

Lash, J. P. (1972). *Eleanor and Franklin*. New York: Simon & Schuster.

Le Comte, E. (1957). *The long road back: The story of my encounter with polio*. Boston: Little, Brown.

Levine, H. J. (1954). *I knew Sister Kenny: The story of a great lady and little people*. Boston: Little, Brown.

Lippman, T., Jr. (1977). *The squire of Warm Springs: FDR in Georgia*. Chicago: Playboy Press.

Louden, I. (1997). *Western medicine*. New York: Oxford University Press.

Lynaugh, J. (1989). From respectable domesticity to medical efficiency: The changing Kansas City hospital, 1875–1920. In D. E. Long & J. Golden, (Eds.), *The American General Hospital* (pp. 21–39). Ithaca: Cornell University Press.

Magner, L. (1992). *A history of medicine*. New York: Marcel Dekker.

Manfreda, E. (1991, Spring). Polio nursing: An abbreviated report to the Wallingford chapter of the American Red Cross on my experience as a polio nurse in Akron, Ohio, August–October, 1952. *American Association for the History of Nursing Bulletin*, 30,6–8.

Marshall, A. (1955). *I can jump puddles*. Sydney, Australia: Haley.

Marshall, P. (1962). *Two lives*. London: Hutchinson.

Marshall, P. (1964). *The raging moon*. London: Hutchinson.

Melosh, B. (1982). *The physician's hand: Work culture and conflict in american nursing*. Philadelphia: Temple University Press.

Mendelson, I., Solomon, P., & Lindemann, E. (1958). Hallucinations of poliomyelitis patients during treatment in a respirator. *Journal of Nervous and Mental Diseases*, 126, 421–428.

Milam, L. W. (1984). *The cripple liberation front marching band blues*. San Diego: Mho & Mho Works.

Morgan, T. (1985). *FDR: A Biography*. New York: Simon Schuster.

Muldar, D. (1998). Clinical observations on acute poliomyelitis. *Annals of the New York Academy of Sciences*, 1–10.

Murphy, Robert F. (1987). *The body silent*. New York: WW. Norton & Company.

Norcross, M. F. (1939). The Drinker respirator. *American Journal of Nursing*, 39, 1063–1068.

Olson, T. (1987). "Laying Claim to Caring: Nursing and the Language of Training, 1915–1937." *Nursing Outlook*, 41(2), 68–72.

Opie, J. (1957). *Over my dead body*. New York: Dutton.

Parisi, C. (1951). The patient in the respirator. *American Journal of Nursing*, 51, 360–363.

Paul, J. R. (1971). *A history of poliomyelitis*. New Haven, CT: Yale University Press.

Plagemann, B. (1949). *My place to stand*. New York.

Porter, R. ((1997). *The greatest benefit to mankind*. New York: HarperCollins.

Prugh, D., & Tagiuri, C. K. (1954). Emotional aspects of the respirator care of patients with poliomyelitis. *Psychosomatic Medicine*, 16, 104–128.

Purdy, K. (1953a, October). . . . The rest of me is alive. *McCall's*, 32–93.

Purdy, K. (1953b, March). What are little boys made of? *Reader's Digest*, 42–44.

Reverby, S. (1985). The search for the hospital yardstick: Nursing and the rationalization of hospital work. In J. W. Leavitt & R. Numbers, (Eds.), *Sickness and health in America* (pp. 206–218). Madison: University of Wisconsin Press.

Reverby, S. (1987). *Ordered to care: The dilemma of American nursing, 1873–1945*. Cambridge, MA: Harvard University Press.

Rinker, S. (2000). To cultivate a feeling of confidence: The nursing of obstetric patients, 1890–1940. *Nursing History Review* 8, 117–142.

Robinson, H. A., Finesinger, J. E., & Bierman, J. S. (1956). Psychiatric considerations in the adjustment of patients with poliomyelitis. *New England Journal of Medicine* 254, 975–980.

Rogers, N. (1992). *Dirt and disease: Polio before FDR*. New Brunswick, NJ: Rutgers University Press.

Roosevelt, A. (1949, July). My life with FDR, Part 3: How polio helped my father. *Woman's Day*.

Roosevelt, E. (1962). *The autobiography of Eleanor Roosevelt*. London: Hutchinson.

Roosevelt, E. & Brough, J. (1974). *An untold story: The Roosevelts of Hyde Park.* New York: Dell.

Rosenberg, C. 1987. *The Care of Strangers.* Philadelphia: University of Pennsylvania Press.

Rosner, D. (1989). Doing well or doing good: The ambivalent focus of hospital administration. In D. E. Long & J. Golden, (Eds.), *The American General Hospital* (pp. 157–169). Ithaca: Cornell University Press.

Sandelowski, M. (1999). Venous envy: The post WWII debate over IV nursing. *Advances in Nursing Science* 22, 52–62.

Seavey, N. G., Smith, J., & Wagner, P. (1996). *A paralyzing fear.* New York: TV Books.

Seidenfeld, M. A. (1947). The psychological considerations in poliomyelitis care. *American Journal of Nursing,* 47, 369–370.

Seidenfeld, M. A. (1948). The psychological sequelae of poliomyelitis in children. *Nervous Child,* 1, 14–28.

Seidenfeld, M. A. (1955). Psychological implications of breathing difficulties in poliomyelitis. *American Journal of Orthopsychiatry,* 25, 788–801.

Smith, J. S. (1990). *Patenting the sun: Polio and the Salk vaccine.* New York: Morrow.

Starr, P. (1982). *The transformation of American medicine.* New York: Basic Books.

Strauss, E. (1979). *In my heart I'm still dancing.* New York: Dutton.

Thompson, C. T., (1938, March). The essential features of poliomyelitis. *Public Health Nursing,* 30, 142–147.

Tracey, M. A. (1949). *Nursing: An Art and Science.* St. Louis, MO: CV Mosby.

Visotsky, H. M., Hamburg, D. A., Goss, M. E., & Lebovits, B. Z. (1961). Coping behavior under extreme stress: Observations of patients with severe poliomyelitis. *Archives of General Psychiatry,* 5, 27–53.

Ward, G. C. (1989). *A first class temperment: The emergence of Franklin Roosevelt.* New York: Harper & Row.

Weligoschek, J. "Personal experiences with polio." *Trained Nurse.* (February, 1950). 68–69, 74.

Whitman, T. "The Polio nurse." A Personal Account. *Trained Nurse,* June, 1948, 33–34.

Wilson, J. L. (1944). The use of the respirator. *Journal of the American Medical Association,* 117 (6), 278–279.

Wilson, J. L. (1968). Memoirs of the development of the respirator. Unpublished memoirs, parts of which are published in Paul, J. (1971). *A history of poliomyelitis* (pp. 324–334). New Haven, CT: Yale University Press.

Woods, R. (1994). *Tales from Inside the Iron Lung and How I got out of it.* Philadelphia: University of Pennsylvania Press.

15

Interpretive Analysis
The Method

Richard MacIntyre

To some extent, all research is necessarily interpretive because all of it is predicated on assumptions and traditions expressed in languages. Some social scientists argue that, despite several positivistic methods grounded in the traditions of rationalism and empiricism, all research is best understood through the interpretive paradigm (Rabinow & Sullivan, 1987; Packer & Addison, 1989). This chapter will not provide an extensive defense of that argument, variants of which can be found in the work of several nurse scholars, including Thompson, Allen, and Rodrigues-Fisher (1992), Munhall and Oiler Boyd (1993), and Benner (1994). In this chapter, interpretive research is approached through the traditions developed in the humanities.

Interpretive analysis that employs critical theory has been used as a "research method" in literature classes for decades. English professors introduce students to theorists such as Marx, Weber, Freud, and Foucault, and students use them to explore, analyze, and interpret the

Editor's note: In this chapter on method, the author makes extensive use of examples from his own research to explicate the processes inherent in the method. This "example" chapter presents a critical interpretive analysis of the social construction of AIDS. This research was published for a lay audience as *Mortal Men: Living with Asymptomatic HIV,* (Rutgers University Press, 1999). Chapter 16 provides a background for the method and other material not covered in the book. The role of critical theory will also be apparent in that chapter.

literature of Shakespeare, Proust, and Joyce. One drawback of this approach is that student papers sometimes demonstrate a better understanding of the theory than of the literature that the theory was supposed to help elucidate. But, in general, the theories provide a framework that helps students discover an organized approach to interpreting literature. Papers using this approach often seem less subjective, more organized, and more socially relevant.

The intersection of literature departments with the social sciences in the last half of the twentieth century is not surprising. Literature is brimming with references to ideas, values, and institutions—both contemporary and historical. But, as universities placed more value and a greater percentage of resources in the sciences, scholarship that seemed more objective became preferable to yet another creative interpretation of Keats. If Freud could be seriously applied to Shakespeare, then psychoanalysis was growing in the way that a science should, and Shakespeare proved his relevance once again.

The danger, of course, is that students are often tempted to superimpose the theory onto the text, like a cookie cutter onto dough. Formed into the shape of the theory, the text can be interpreted. But it often suffers much violence in the process. As lenses, theories can obscure as well as illuminate.

In the hermeneutic (interpretive) tradition, persons are sometimes approached as texts (or dramas). Although thinking about persons as texts is less reductive and more contextual than many other research approaches, the differences between persons and texts are nonetheless marked. Those who learn to read, respond to, and interpret texts learn about themselves and their relations to their worlds. When nurses approach patients' stories as texts, they do so to better understand two complex scenes. One is the scene where sickness or the threat of sickness enters the patient's world. The other scene is where the patient enters the world of health care, the nurse's world.

The early critical theory work in nursing focused on issues of race, gender, and class and challenged researchers in the hermeneutic tradition to identify links between lived patient experiences and the social structures that sustained them (Thompson, 1992). However, if the *primary* goal of researching lived experience is to identify the social structures that sustain positive and negative experiences, one runs the risk of subordinating experience to those structures and losing much of it in the process. This challenge is the same as that faced in English literature departments. The theoretical framework can overshadow the text that it is being used to illuminate. However, to ignore social forces and structures is to artificially disconnect people from their worlds. This is true whether one is interpreting literature or lived experience.

Munhall (1994) notes that the greatest aim of interpretive research is to understand particular meanings "in pursuit of understanding what it means to be human" (p. 32). By "what it means to be human," Munhall is not asking an abstract theoretical or theological question. Rather, the interpretive researcher asks (1) how being is created or transformed through experiences and (2) how social or environmental forces structure human experience. It is not enough to identify oppressive structures in science, technology, and other powerful relations. The human sciences are interested in how we *are* with the structures of science, technology, and relatedness (Munhall, 1994).

Interpretive work can employ critical theory to elucidate the relation between experience and relevant social structures. When the primary goal of research using critical theory is to create social change, the research is used to validate preexisting theoretical or ethical positions. When critical theory is employed within an interpretive framework, the primary goal is not social change, but rather to uncover new or hidden or ignored meanings or practices that bind experience to the social world. Within a critical interpretive framework, the possibilities for social change are enlarged if the experiences of marginalized groups (and the marginalized experiences of dominant groups) are translated so that commonalities and distinctions between the normative and the marginalized can be recognized. A number of thoughtful essays exploring the relation between phenomenology, hermeneutics, and critical theory can be found in books by Thompson, Allen, and Rodrigues-Fisher (1992) and Benner (1994).

Nursing theories and medical frameworks tend to be superimposed on the life-worlds of patients, and the preservation and understanding of their humanity are often lost in the process. This is not just true in health care. Human cultures employ theories and myths to help frame and sustain social worlds. Tony Kushner's (1993) *Angels in America: Part Two, Perestroika* opens with an old Bolskevik delivering an agitated monologue on the centrality of theory:

(With sudden, violent passion) And *Theory*? How are we to proceed without *Theory*? What System of Thought have these Reformers to present to this mad swirling planetary disorganization, to the Inevident Welter of fact, event, phenomenon, calamity? Do they have as we did, a beautiful Theory, as bold, as Grand, as comprehensive a construct? . . . Change? Yes, we must change, only show me the Theory, and I will be at the barricades, show me the book of the next Beautiful Theory, and I promise you these blind eyes will see again, just to read it, to devour that text. Show me the words that will reorder the world, or else keep silent. (pp. 13–14)

Kushner's *Angels in America* brims with theoretical constructs drawn from American religion and politics. These constructs form a powerful backdrop against which the audience watches Prior live with AIDS. At times, theory and experience clash and crash. One can never stand in entirely for the other. In Part One, *Millennium Approaches*, Louis tries to locate himself within the safety of theory, and Prior insists that Louis's theory does not cover his particular situation:

Louis: You can love someone and fail them. You can love someone and not be able to . . .

Prior: You *can*, theoretically, yes. A person can, maybe an editorial "you" can love, Louis, but not you, specifically you, I don't know, I think you are excluded from that general category. . . . A person could theoretically love and maybe many do but we both know now you can't. (Kushner, 1993, pp. 78–79)*

There are certainly many approaches that one might take to doing interpretive critical theory. The one offered here is intended as a guide, not a rulebook.

Articulating a Rationale for a Critical Interpretive Method

Before they embark on any study, it is essential that researchers locate themselves in relation to existing scholarly traditions and the discourse on methodology. The following example illustrates why one might choose and how one might defend the selection of the critical interpretive framework that was used for the dissertation phase of this project.

The contributions of rational empiricism toward human health need not be underestimated to realize that the central concern of any human discipline must be a situated understanding of human persons (Taylor, 1989). Because people live in discrete worlds, rational constructs about the atemporal and context-free nature of human phenomena are often

---

*Used with permission from Tony Kushner.

of little use to the professions charged with caring for people as they are found in the empirical world—that is, individual persons, particular families, and specific communities.

The methods of traditional science cannot effectively guide or direct the scholarly endeavors of the caring professions. The quest for an absolute certainty, the goals of prediction and control, the focus on reliability and validity have all contributed to the objectification of human persons and phenomena. Although prediction and control are appropriate goals in many spheres of science and human life, knowledge gained in pursuit of these goals often benefits those who would profit from managing or manipulating people more than it does the people themselves.

Neither are the goals and methods of traditional science appropriate to guide or direct the scholarly work of the practice disciplines including education, psychology, and management. Human practices *can* be abstracted into theory, and structures for human practices *might* someday be developed. But, when understanding human practices is subordinated to formal structures and theories, the essential, empirical, and lived realities of nursing and other human practices elude us. This leads inevitably to an impoverished discourse of practice. The preoccupation with method over content in both nursing research and curriculum development interferes with developing an understanding of our patients, our practices, and our scholarship. A delimited professional discourse hampers our efforts to articulate and market our services to the public. It also hampers our ability to advocate for that public.

A critical interpretive framework is the better paradigm for nursing for three reasons. First, a larger part of human experiences and the empirical world relevant to nursing can be investigated with critical hermeneutics. A critical hermeneutics can avoid or at least grapple with the dualistic problems of rational/emotional and mind/body. Second, a critical hermeneutics has a better interpretation of positivistic science than positivistic science has of hermeneutics and critical theory. Third, a critical hermeneutics makes use of both rationality and method, whereas positivistic science equates its rational method with truth and tends to deny or ignore the essential hermeneutic nature of its own first principle—radical doubt (Taylor, 1985a).[1]

---

[1] Positivism, the dominant paradigm for modern science, posits that theory can never be proved but only disproved. This is because all theories are based on earlier theories, definitions, assumptions, and observations, none of which can be proved except through reference to earlier "proofs" that are also based on assumptions. Thus, science begins with assumption, or what Hegel called radical doubt.

For purposes of the study presented in Chapter 16 [see MacIntyre (1999) for the full study], persons are understood in the hermeneutical and phenomenological traditions as texts (Taylor, 1985a) or works of art in progress (Habermas, 1971). Texts can be studied for structure or meaning or both, but the propensity in the human and social sciences has been to study texts for structure. Dunlap (1990) identifies content analysis as the major alternative approach to hermeneutics and offers a comprehensive critique of its shortcomings. The main problem with content analysis and other qualitative methodologies popular in the social sciences is a paradigmatic confusion that too often results in neither good science nor heuristic relevance.

In accord with Rorty (1982) and Taylor (1989), the ethnography of the illness experience of Benner and Wrubel (1989), and the interpretive ethnography of Geertz (1972), the study presented in Chapter 16 avoided predetermined methods. In my graduate work, I found only one of several methods texts useful—namely, Van Manen's (1990) *Researching the Lived Experience*. Mostly, Van Manen's book gave me permission to dialogue with my community, develop my own voice, and focus on interpretation instead of procedure.

BURNS'S STANDARDS FOR QUALITATIVE RESEARCH

Evaluative standards are a good place to start when thinking about method and a strategy for approaching any research project. Burns (1989) enumerated five standards for evaluating qualitative research that received wide acceptance in nursing. The first two of these five standards—descriptive vividness and methodological congruence—and several of the attendant threats to those two standards are considered next.

Burns's (1989) first standard, descriptive vividness, is accompanied by nine attendant threats. Five of these threats relate to problems with the written description—lack of essential information, clarity, credibility, depth, and writing skill. Two have to do with observation and include poor observation skills and inadequate length of time in the field. Two have to do with the researcher and include poor self-awareness and "a reluctance to reveal self in written material" (p. 48).

Insider Orientation

This section shows how researchers might explicate their relations to their subject matter and is an example of an "insider" orientation.

I was a member of San Francisco's gay community from 1975 to 1998. This journey has not been wholly academic. It has been deeply personal. From the beginning—which for me was sometime in 1982—people I knew were getting AIDS. Like many of the participants in this research, I did not know all of them well. One was a man who cut my hair for a while. But, as the numbers grew, the epidemic drew closer to my own door. Both my dissertation and the book that followed show a complicated and somewhat incestuous network of interrelations that both constituted the gay community during the decades of the 1970s and 1980s and contributed to the spread of the HIV infection, the subject of this study.

My good friend Micky died in 1983. His picture is still on the table in my living room. My ex-lover, Steve, was sick by 1985, the year in which his ex-lover, Kim, died. My new lover, Martin, and I stayed at Kim's house on the last night to help keep him comfortable. Martin and I tested positive for the virus a few months later, in September of 1985. It came as no real surprise to us. I had been having "safer sex" since late 1982, assuming that AIDS was caused by a virus. If I had avoided it, I did not want to contract it. If I had contracted it, I did not want to infect others or to increase my own exposure. But Martin and I were not surprised to discover that we were both positive.

My ex-lover, Steve, died in 1986. Two weeks before the first anniversary of his death, Martin was diagnosed with AIDS. Martin died in November of 1987. Between Steve's and Martin's deaths, I worked as an on-call nurse for the San Francisco AIDS Hospice and Homecare team.

The year 1988 was a good year. New Year's Eve was particularly memorable—no one really close to me had died that year. In 1989, a very good friend, Howard, died. My best friend, Gabe, went on AZT. My brother Bob married Audrey, a friend and colleague. They had met at Steve's memorial service in 1986. 1990 also was a good year. No one close to me died. Bob and Audrey had a baby girl, Jordanna. In August of 1991, my best friend Gabe died. Thus, it is as an insider that I approach the concerns of the asymptomatic HIV-positive gay community. In 1988, I reentered the doctoral program from which I had been on leave since 1984.

Deciding on a Focus.   When doing critical interpretive work, researchers find it helpful to situate both their personal and their intellectual orientations to their subject matter. This provides a context that others can use to develop rival interpretations from other perspectives.

The academic nursing community at the University of California, San Francisco, helped shape my thinking and focus my interests. A brief synopsis of this academic journey follows. My liberal politics might have led me to intravenous drug users, women, or gay Blacks and Hispanics with HIV. My background as a nurse and my experiences of caring for friends and lovers with acute physical illnesses might have led me to problems associated with advanced AIDS. My long-standing interest in politics and public policy might have prompted research on insurance or employment discrimination, policies of the Food and Drug Administration or the Centers for Disease Control, or cost-effective health care delivery systems.

My interest in alternative/holistic therapies and health practices almost persuaded me to search for the ultimate survival regimen—some elusive combination of Eastern and Western therapies, personal willpower, positive thinking, and spiritual enlightenment. Three things worked against this temptation: the literature on death theory; the "conversion experience" and accompanying "glory theology" (Luther, cited in Schmidt, 1990) that seemed to form a pattern in the survival literature; and the deep ambivalence I felt about the position that survivor stories should occupy in the community. This ambivalence is manifest in the debate between Des Pres (1976) and Bettelheim (1980) on the meaning of surviving the holocaust. Collecting "long-term survivor" stories to help people live longer seemed an admirable goal. But I was not sure that the knowledge in which I was most interested would be embedded in survivor stories rather than in the stories of those who succumbed. I was torn between studying survival and learning how embodied human beings fought, faced, and embraced vulnerability and death. I could not allow survival stories to point to any kind of light, path, salvation, or truth that would in any way denigrate the stories of those who had succumbed. I had too much love invested in some of those other stories.

My dissertation sponsor, Patricia Benner, encouraged me to drop the either-or construction and establish my own ground. "Can't it be what it is like to be a survivor in [a] relationship rather than the 'King of the Mountain' routine?" she asked. That seemed right. Surviving, living, or dying with HIV—the stories are about people coping with information about their health status and experiencing the sicknesses and deaths of their friends and loved ones. The stories that emerged are about how gay men constructed meaning in a community under siege. They do not offer recipes for survival. They are accounts of survival and death, hope and hopelessness, decision and indecision.

Concept Identification and Abandonment.   Well before the preceding questions were addressed in earnest, I was forced to articulate my phenomena of interest in the beginning doctoral course in nursing theory. I had been impressed that, early in the epidemic, theory was more useful than research, simply because we had so little research on which to base our health practices and looked forward to learning more about the relation between developing theories and health practices. As a person with HIV, I was a part of numerous public and private conversations in which people paid attention to what seemed to be working for whom. To bring some coherence to those conversations, I felt I needed a concept. Some of this "felt need" was due to the environmental influences that impinge on doctoral students in nursing. A favorite question among first-year students was, "What is your concept?" To build a theory, one needed concepts (Stevens, 1984).

Rew, Stuppy, and Becker (1988) "upped the *ante*" by asserting that construct validity was the essential link between practice, theory, and research. I was not altogether impressed by this reductive approach to theory or knowledge development. Having not yet been formally introduced to methods of grounded theory, hermeneutics, or phenomenology, I proceeded to identify choosing and coping, as my concepts of interest—much like declaring an undergraduate major that one hopes to change.

I watched as gay men tried to choose what treatment path to follow and, at the same time, I observed other behaviors such as anger, activism, and helping others. These behaviors I lumped together as coping. Choosing had promise as a concept because it fit squarely into the North American Nursing Diagnosis Association (NANDA) taxonomy—something I thought might eventually be developed into nursing theory. This taxonomy listed choosing as one of nine major human response patterns. MacIntyre, Tueller, and Wishon (1988) used the NANDA taxonomy in their nursing care plans for people with HIV infection.

Finally, coping seemed broader than choosing. I wanted a broad concept that would include facing, denying, choosing, reacting, and ignoring HIV disease—not one that would prematurely narrow my focus to something that might not ultimately be important or even interesting. The first nonobsolete definition of coping given by Webster (1972) is maintaining a contest or combat situation, generally on even terms and with success. This definition is particularly interesting in light of Dreuilhe's (1988) extended military metaphor describing his own "fight" with AIDS. But, as this autobiographical account of one man's own war against AIDS demonstrates so vividly, the odds are not even. Success is uncertain. If coping means "overcoming" life-threatening illnesses, then it is an outcome rather than a process, smaller, not larger, than choosing. The research of Lazarus and Folkman (1984) and Benner and Wrubel (1989), however, defines coping as a process rather than an outcome. Fortunately, Patricia Benner guided me away from a concept-driven project.

Beginning Orientation to Structured Fieldwork and Methods.   At the beginning of my second year, I began a two-quarter sequence in field research with Dr. Leonard Schatzman. According to Schatzman (Schatzman & Strauss, 1973), the research problem is typically developed out of a literature review and framed within the relevant theoretical constructs of the discipline. A design is selected that fits the problem and data are subsequently collected and analyzed. However, field researchers make decisions and develop attitudes about a "number of methodological and philosophical issues . . . often long before any particular research project is undertaken" (p. 1). This has certainly been true in my case. A precise "problem statement" never emerged. According to Schatzman (1973),

> Conventional wisdom suggests that a researcher prepare a relatively articulated problem in advance of his inquiry. This implies that he would not, or could not, begin his inquiry without a problem. Yet, the field method process of discovery may lead the researcher to his problem *after* it has led him through much of the substance in his field. Problem statements are not prerequisite to field research; they may emerge at any point in the research process, even toward the very end. (p. 3)

Whereas it is extremely beneficial for researchers using this method to clearly articulate research questions, such articulation is not so much an end as the beginning of interpreting what is of critical importance. Descriptions of my phenomena (which are presented more fully in the section titled Elements of the Study) continued to change. In my field research course, I developed a pilot proposal and began collecting and analyzing data. The questions that guided the initial interviews were:

- What do asymptomatic HIV-positive gay men think about standard and alternative approaches to the management and treatment of HIV infection?
- What does HIV mean to them; what are their concerns about it; how do they see themselves in relation to HIV; how is it affecting

their lives; and finally, what kind of decisions are they making about monitoring and treatment options?

Within a year, this description seemed a bit narrow. In addition to what HIV-positive gay men were thinking, I was also concerned with what they were *experiencing* and how they were feeling. By the end of the project, I discovered how experiences with living with asymptomatic HIV were connected to larger structures including beliefs about health, illness, mortality, and the health care system.

After my first interviews, I had conversations with two participants who indicated that I should (1) ask questions about how people felt about AZT after they decided to take it and (2) ask more focused questions about safer sex. My initial interest was in how HIV-positive people made choices about monitoring and treatment options. While the ultimate focus was broader than coping or choosing, this underlying interest affected the construction of the interview guide. Although I was not sure if safer sex needed to be more specifically addressed, I recognized a need to elicit how treatment choices had affected lives. The interview guide developed before the first three interviews was revised to include these areas and is presented in Table 15–1.

Methodological Congruence

Burns's (1989) second criterion is methodological congruence. In the perspective taken in this study, persons were not viewed as having bodies, but rather as being embodied. Both the body and the mind are knowers, the body experiencing and knowing in a nonreflective manner. This phenomenological view of person as described by Proust (1913/1981), defined by Heidegger (1962), and more recently articulated by Taylor (1985a, 1985b, 1989) and Benner and Wrubel (1989) formed the framework for this study. In this view, persons are partly constituted by their worlds, the meanings that they develop about those worlds, and their self-interpretations. This world is not something to which the self simply reacts. The world is also partly constituted by the self. The world both limits and creates the possibilities that are available to persons. Indeed, our worlds and bodies are the ground of our experience and, hence, the ground for critical interpretive research.

Burns's (1989) criterion on methodological congruence includes four related standards: threats to auditability, ethical rigor, procedural rigor, and rigor in documentation. Although the study is not auditable per se, enough verbatim data are reported to facilitate alternative

TABLE 15–1   INTERVIEW GUIDE

A. General Effect of AIDS Epidemic on Life
   1. Grief/loss issues
   2. Sexual issues
      a. Personal decisions about safer sex
      b. Problems or concerns about following through with those decisions
      c. Ideas and feelings about changes in sexual practices
   3. Spiritual/religious issues
B. Brief Medical History
   1. Dates suspected and confirmed HIV seropositivity
   2. Current frequency of monitoring laboratory work and results
   3. Treatments and lifestyle changes, if any
C. Understandings, attitudes, and beliefs and experience with standard treatments
   1. AZT
   2. T-cells
   3. Other
D. Interests in alternative treatment modalities
   1. Acupuncture
   2. Chinese herbs
   3. Support groups
   4. Other

interpretations. A profound respect for the persons and experiences disclosed, a sensitivity to matters of confidentiality, and a genuine concern for consequences that can result from writing about marginalized communities have, I trust, resulted in ethical rigor. Procedural rigor is a standard imported from science and can best be understood in an interpretative study as reportorial accuracy. Interpretation is not accomplished through procedure, however, no matter how rigorous. Rigor in documentation requires that the author present all the elements of the study:

> phenomenon; purpose; research question; justification of the significance of the phenomenon; identification of assumptions; identification of metatheories; researcher credentials; the context; role of the researcher, ethical implications; sampling and subjects; data-gathering strategies; data analysis strategies; theoretical development; conclusions; implications and suggestions

for further study and practice; and a literature review (Burns, 1989, p. 48)

Several of these elements are addressed in the next section.

Elements of the Study

Phenomenon.   The broad phenomenon under study is gay men living with asymptomatic HIV-infection. Asymptomatic is a relative term that is intentionally not operationally defined. By asymptomatic I mean people who have not had pneumocystis, Kaposi's sarcoma, and other significant opportunistic infections. Some participants had lymphadenopathy, hairy leukoplakia, thrush, or fatigue.

Some members of the academic community argue that the term "asymptomatic" ought not be used, because it implies the absence of psychosocial problems or, worse, denigrates the significance of psychosocial problems. I have two responses. First, the term asymptomatic has meaning in the lay population and ought not be discarded because of turf wars within the "priesthood" of health care professionals. Second, abandoning the term "asymptomatic" is an insidious form of medicalization as the "priesthood" seeks to bring ever larger parts of the population under its purview. I am willing to drop the term if and when the HIV/AIDS community drops it, but I believe there are significant qualitative distinctions between living with clinical AIDS and living with nonclinical HIV disease. The term *preclinical* perpetuates the hopelessness discourse about HIV. *Nonclinical* may be an appropriate substitute.

Purpose.   The purpose of this study is to increase understanding of gay men's lived experience with HIV infection through an exploration of meanings, associated informal models of explanation, and patterns of coping that these men developed in response to monitoring, treatment options, and the threat of AIDS. In addition, there are personal purposes and meanings for my doing this study.

When I die, I assume that some holy committee will ask me to give an account of myself. The demographic summary of my earthly incarnation will likely read: gay man, nurse, teacher, graduate student; lived in San Francisco during the AIDS epidemic. In addition to satisfying the tenure requirements of my employer, my motivation for doing this research is to satisfy the "committee" on the other side. The purpose of this research was to become increasingly aware of and sensitive to my brothers' and my own humanness; to come to a better understanding of what my brothers and I were experiencing; to more effectively care for myself and my brothers.

Kierkegaard (1846/1962) would insist that an understanding of persons is *experienced*. Understanding goes beyond probability statements, populations, abstractions, and universals. Understanding goes beyond the reflective appreciation and vicarious experience (Kierkegaard, 1843/1971) that comes from reading an ethnography of a strange culture—for example, beyond the sexual revolution. Understandings must go beyond matters of justice (Kierkegaard, 1843/1987)—for example, beyond AIDS activism. Understanding goes beyond coming to terms with mortality (Kierkegaard, 1855/1967)—for example beyond good deaths and the "all we need is love" movement. Understanding aspires to embrace an emerging faith (Kierkegaard, 1848/1985) in what it is to be a person—mind and body, mortal and immortal, sick and healthy, hopeful and resigned. The purpose is primarily moral and only secondarily useful; more about faith than works. Luther (1520/1988) wrote:

> Though you were nothing but good works from the soles of your feet to the crown of your head, you would still not . . . [read: fulfill the requirements of a modern secular humanist] since God [humans] cannot be worshiped [served] unless you ascribe to him [them] the glory of truthfulness and all goodness which is due him [them]. This cannot be done by works but only by the faith of the heart. (p. 16)

Utilitarian research, like Luther's works, is meaningless without a commitment to an understanding of humankind. The "glory of truthfulness and all goodness" of human beings is what Kierkegaard and every other moral philosopher is seeking.

This project is both similar and dissimilar to Krieger's (1983) research in a midwestern lesbian community. Like Krieger, I am using the research as a source of insight "both about others and about myself" (p. 321). I agree wholeheartedly with her position on self-disclosure:

> In social science, I think, we must acknowledge the personal far more than we do. We need to find new ways to explore it. We need to link our statements about those we study with statements about ourselves, for in reality neither stands alone. (p. 321)

Krieger (1983) focused on identity and belonging and found the lesbians in her study somewhat lacking in both respects. Krieger's work developed out of a prior interest in identity and belonging. However, I was not engaged in this research to "find a way out of a problem" (Krieger, 1985, p. 321). Furthermore, I did not "hide" my voice, merge it with the others, or merge other voices with my own.

Lines of Inquiry. Five lines of inquiry were developed after the first year of collecting and writing beginning interpretations of the transcripts. None of them appeared in the interview guide, because they did not relate to how people in my community were talking about HIV. These lines of inquiry provided a focus for analysis.

* What self-understandings and experiences increase or decrease a person's willingness to consider various treatment options?
* Are treatment and monitoring decisions congruent with the HIV-infected person's self-understandings and experiences?
* How does the medical establishment's approval or disapproval of various treatment options influence a person's choices and self-understandings?
* How do family and community mores and expectations about asymptomatic HIV infection influence a person's choices and self-understandings?
* What are the interpretations, informal explanatory models, and meanings associated with T-cell counts, percentages, and ratios?

A caveat or confession may be in order here. I did not post these questions on the wall of my study for continued guidance in writing analyses or interpretations. I think that the process of writing and rewriting questions and lines of inquiry helped me focus on what I thought was important. But any more conscious focus on "questions" would have interfered with my ability to respond to the voices in the texts. Munhall (1994) emphasized the importance of acknowledging our unknowing. I interpret this unknowing to include an awareness that our research questions might not get at the heart of what is important. This leads to openness. Munhall states that knowing "that you do not understand someone who stands before you, and who perhaps does not fit into some preexisting paradigm or theory is critical to the evolution of understanding meaning for others" (p. 63).

Justification of Significance of Problem. The significance of HIV infection in those lives of gay men living with asymptomatic HIV infection before the advent of the new protease inhibitors is profound and needs no further "justification" whatsoever. However, in deference to convention, the following professional context is offered. The research agenda developed by the National Centers for Nursing Research established seven priorities. Several of the topics listed under these priorities pertain to asymptomatic HIV-positive gay men, including:

- Identification of cofactors among high-risk groups which are correlated with increased risk of (a) becoming infected with the AIDS virus and (b) developing AIDS . . .
- Survey of patient preferences with regard to delivery of care options during various stages of illness . . .
- Effect of HIV infection among asymptomatic individuals on sexual behavior with homosexual partners . . .
- Psychological and social impact of HIV-positive status on healthy individuals . . .
- Impact of counseling programs on practices of HIV-positive individuals (National Institutes of Health, 1987, as cited in Larson, 1988, pp. 61–62).

Of these priorities, the "psychological and social impact of HIV-positive status on healthy individuals" was most pertinent to this study.

In 1993, The National Institute of Allergy and Infectious Diseases released new guidelines for antiviral therapy in HIV disease. These guidelines, also reported in the June 17, 1993, issue of the *New York Times* concur with one of the central assumptions in this study:

No average patient exists. Some patients will do better, and others, worse, than what clinical studies would predict. The HIV epidemic has forced clinicians to recognize the limitations of medical technology and reminded us that the finest expression of medical practice still lies in the optimal blend of current science and the "art" of patient care. (Sande, 1993)

Organizations such as the AIDS Foundation in San Francisco have used focus groups to help develop advertising campaigns designed to help people overcome their reluctance to get tested and to seek medical help. Before 1996, medical help included T-cell monitoring and, if indicated, drug treatment. After 1996, "viral load" testing and improved drug treatments became available. But, to date, there is little or no empirical evidence to help patients and physicians determine the best time for instituting antiviral therapy.

The premise behind such public health advertising campaigns is that it is better for people to overcome their fears and denial and to seek treatment. However, the literature does not indicate that fear and denial are the major problems confronting people who are not fully complying with standard medical recommendations. Even if these problems are major, the story is incomplete. To help patients overcome fear and denial, fear and denial must be understood in relation to the patient's personal meanings and lived experiences.

Identification of Assumptions. My own orientation to and beliefs about HIV, T-cell monitoring, viral-load testing, death, survival, AZT, and aggressive antiretroviral treatment are disclosed throughout the extensive monologues and dialogues between myself and the participants. These are not presented in Chapter 16 but are more than evident in *Mortal Men* and other publications (MacIntyre & Holzemer, 1997; MacIntyre, Tueller, & Wishon, 1998, MacIntyre, 1999; Freeman & MacIntyre, 1999).

Identification of Metatheories. Instead of "metatheories," this project began with the identification, articulation, and defense of epistemological positions summarized earlier in this chapter. No formal "theoretical framework" directed the study. The frameworks that guided this study were the assumptions about knowledge development and the experiences of the researcher with the phenomena. The five lines of inquiry heretofore listed developed out of my experience with HIV/AIDS and my initial positions on epistemological and ontological issues. These experiences and positions are reflected in both the interview guide and my statements and questions within the interviews themselves.

Theoretical frameworks often reduce qualitative research findings to the obvious, tell us little more about the theory, and serve only to fulfill the demands of a "sacred cow." In this study, no predetermined theoretical framework guided data collection, and critical theory was used only sparingly to assist with interpretation. The theories discussed in *Mortal Men* and in Chapter 16 are included both to disclose the perspective and orientation of the researcher and to assist with the interpretive work.

Role of Researcher. I decided to do this research primarily to pay greater attention to the ongoing informal discourse between gay men with asymptomatic HIV infection. My role was to articulate that discourse for the community in order that it might proceed more formally and be taken more seriously and that it might evolve, develop, and contribute to our emerging understandings of ourselves and our worlds. Like everyone else, I am both a participant in and an observer of that discourse.

Ethical Implications.   The issues raised in this research are inherently ethical and moral in nature—disclosure, self-care, and self-understandings. Two ethical principles, autonomy and beneficence, provide a critical reflective stance for the analysis and interpretation of participants' stories and reflections about interactions with health care providers. However, in keeping with an interpretive phenomenological approach, every effort is made to present meanings using the terms and voices of the participants. Confidentiality is always a difficult matter when doing research in one's own community. A risk of participation in this type of research may be a loss of privacy. Procedures to protect the confidentiality of participants included changing names and, occasionally, occupations and cities. Race is rarely disclosed for the same reasons.

Sampling and Subjects.   The research participants were HIV-positive, asymptomatic, gay men, ages 21 to 46. Seventeen participants were interviewed at length. A masters student conducted three of the interviews. A convenience sample of participants who had previously identified themselves as HIV-positive to the investigator was used. Whereas some participants were monitoring blood work, taking AZT, or enrolled in other studies, they were otherwise free agents and not under medical supervision for symptoms. In the preceding several years, people I knew had expressed interest in participating in such a study.

I decided to interview people who were part of my own community network, rather than people who visited a specific AIDS clinic or support group, for several reasons. First, people who are associated with a particular clinic or support group are connected by virtue of a medical problem or psychosocial concern. They are not necessarily a community or representative of a community. In choosing myself as a kind of central point in the sample (all respondents are minimally "connected" by virtue of an acquaintance with me—many are also friends with one another), I have selected a natural community. Because I am a member of that community and made every effort to create an egalitarian space for dialogue, I was privy to a high level of candor and openness. My own story is clearly evident throughout the interviews that I conducted. At one point in an interview, the roles were completely reversed.

Most study participants were white (one Black, one Hispanic), college educated, HIV-positive, gay men living in San Francisco or New York. The following occupations were included: telephone man, student, freelance writer, nurse, physician, travel agent, insurance broker, executive vice president in a large securities firm, major shareholder/owner of a successful family business, advertising executive, cook, freelance computer specialist, architect, special education teacher, and artist. None of the participants had significant symptoms at interview. Approximately 20 additional people are referred to in my field notes in the same age and socioeconomic range. Most of the respondents reported using recreational drugs.

The theoretical sampling categories used in this study included people who (1) were not monitoring their T-cells; (2) were participating in alternative treatments; (3) were pursuing aggressive (and occasionally experimental) treatment through standard medical practice; (4) had just started taking AZT; (5) had only been recently tested; (6) believed strongly in denial; (7) seemed especially fearful; and (8) were long-term seropositives. For those who were monitoring T-cells, counts ranged from 200 to 1200.

I had great aspirations after reading the first transcripts, feeling that there was enough data for ten dissertations. I decided to bring together an interdisciplinary group of graduate students interested in HIV and phenomenological approaches to research. We had a few meetings that I summarized in my diary. My idea was to have several of us doing interviews, transcribing and analyzing the data, and critiquing one another's work. Instead of looking at between 20 and 30 interviews, we could look at 120 or so. Unfortunately, there were too many problems for us to overcome, including dissimilar theoretical backgrounds and different approaches to the interview, different notions of what constituted scientific research, and different positions on the nature and purpose of the health care disciplines.

Data-Gathering Strategies. A 1- or 2-hour open-ended interview based on the interview guide was conducted in a participant's home or other place of his choosing. Interviews were taped after verbal permission was given for doing so. Brief field notes were taken, which included notes on conversations with and observations of people in the community, newspaper clippings, and notes on public speeches. Interviews were transcribed verbatim.

Like Munhall (1994), I am uncomfortable with the term *interview*. What I wanted to get was each participant's story. I usually opened with a question such as "When did you first hear about HIV?" That gave the participant permission to start his story wherever he pleased. I used the interview guide to make sure that I had covered all of my issues, but often they were addressed spontaneously. In general, I tried to err on the side of being too conversational rather than feigning a privileged position or voice. I was, after all, HIV positive my-self. One of the reasons for doing this research was that the conversa-tions that I was having with other HIV-positive people on the street and in cafes were far more interesting than most of the research that I was reading. I wanted to spend much more time coming to terms with those conversations. My strategy was therefore to tape conversations with some of the same people with whom I had been discussing HIV for years.

Data-Analysis Strategies.   Interpretive work includes a search both for exemplars and for paradigm cases in the data and thematic analy-sis (Benner, 1985). Exemplars are stories or vignettes that serve as a "strong instance of a particularly meaningful transaction, intention or capacity" (Benner, 1985, p. 10). In the same vein, paradigm cases reveal particularly strong patterns of meaning. Paradigm cases may be evi-dent to researchers before they clearly understand what their mean-ings are. Four paradigm cases were selected from the data and pre-sented in the dissertation stage of the study, and exemplars from field notes and other interviews were used in the analysis chapters. How-ever, it is not always necessary to identify paradigm cases and exem-plars at the outset of analysis. Sometimes it is best to focus on the in-terpretation and analysis of one transcript at a time. What is of central importance will emerge during this process.

Step One: Editing and Analysis. The first specific scheme used in this study was to translate or shape the transcripts into stories. That process entailed a good deal of editing, reorganizing, and interpreting the interview transcripts. (The original transcripts were, of course, pre-served.) I started with the story that I thought would be easiest for me to tell—the one that I thought I had best "heard" and understood. This entailed helping the reader see who was speaking, not just in medical terms but in relation to me and to his community. Sometimes sections of the transcript were "cut and pasted" to improve the flow and con-sistency of the story.

I used a basic word-processing program and found it helpful to high-light the entire transcript, indent the left and right margins and choose a new style that I called "quote." This reminded me of the indented quotations I had used in school papers and I realized that writing the research project was not entirely different from writing other papers. I used the "normal," nonindented style for my initial interpretations and analysis. I put notes to myself and questions for my editors, fellow stu-dents, and committee members in italics. That way I had everything pertinent to the project in one place—the "interview data," my emerging analysis, and the questions that I wanted to raise with others.

This process takes a long time and is the most important part of the analysis. Sometimes I would reorganize sections of the dialogue only to discover that I had interrupted the flow too much. This was often because a secondary issue was embedded in the primary issue that I was trying to isolate for story-telling purposes. Another decision that had to be made over and over again was where to interject my analysis into the dialogue. I discovered that "it all depended." There were instances where it seemed appropriate to let the dialogue run for five or more pages. At other times, it seemed necessary to comment on every line. These decisions should be based solely on what is the clearest way to communicate the story and interpretation to the reader—not on some notion of what is right or wrong.

The editing process is a learning experience for the new researcher. At first, editing is done very conservatively to preserve the participant's voices. Throughout the process, the researcher learns that an effective interpretation requires that a good story told around a campfire or over a cup of coffee must undergo much editing if it is to be just as well told in written form. The translation from the tape-recorded story to the transcript to the written text requires an enormous number of crucial decisions about organization. Although it is perfectly normal for a story that is told verbally to loop back on itself and to jump from place to place, most readers expect stories to proceed in a more organized format.

Some researchers have decided that it is best not to rearrange transcripts but to lightly edit them for readability and deposit them more or less in their entirety into a chapter with an analysis at the end. They argue that the sequence in which a story is told has significance. My own position is that, when sequence has significance, it should be pointed out and discussed by the interpretive researcher.

After transcripts of interviews are produced, the critical interpretive researcher has two major tasks. The first is a translation (through editing and reorganization) of an oral story into a written one where significant meanings, ambiguities, and contexts are illuminated. The second is to provide insightful interpretations of lived experience within a social framework. To that end, it is necessary to remember that listeners and readers have very different expectations and needs.

According to Van Manen (1990), writing is a measure of our analytic thoughtfulness. Writing helps us see meanings and lived experiences, focuses our understandings, and is the vehicle through which we can illuminate these understandings for others. Critical interpretive research is primarily a form of writing, rather than the final stage in the research process. Reading and writing promote and sustain the conversations that we as nurses have about our patients, the discourse about nursing practice, and the discourse about HIV in affected communities. Writing, rereading, and rewriting increase the precision and quality of interpretive work.

Step Two: Preparing an Index. After a transcript was shaped into a coherent story with interpretive analysis, it would often be more than 100 pages long. To help me find whatever I might be looking for and to outline the content areas that I had covered, I constructed a 3- to 4-page index of themes or content areas for each transcript. Do not do this before you have finished several drafts of the story and interpretation or you will just have to do it again when the page numbers change. Wait until you are satisfied that you have both told the story and provided a good interpretation. The index provides a ready organized reference to themes and content areas within each story while allowing the researcher to organize and tell each story in its own terms. In other words, it is not necessary to superimpose a singular format onto the stories, but being able to abstract common themes and content areas into an index facilitates comparative analysis. Do not try to be completely consistent with index categories at first. You can always reorganize the index later. Feel free to include short modifying phrases under categories such as Recreational Drugs: theories about; celebration of; struggles with. These phrases will help identify which aspects of a given topic were covered in a particular interview and which were left out.

Step Three: The Grand Index. After all transcripts had been converted into edited and organized stories and indexes had been created, a "grand index" of themes and categories was created to facilitate better access to the content and themes in each story. Preparing the "grand index" required rereading various parts of the edited transcripts. The question, "Is this section sufficiently like the others that I have grouped under this heading?" will present itself several times and requires that the sections be reread to determine if a new heading is needed. These index headings are not as formal or central to the analysis as are the codes, dimensions, constructs, or themes used in many qualitative projects. However, the process of constructing an index is a useful step in the interpretive process.

Step Four: More Interpretation. In the dissertation phase of this project, I presented four of the edited, reorganized, and interpreted transcripts in a long chapter of paradigm cases. This chapter was followed by two more interpretive chapters. In the first chapter, I compared the belief structures and social positions of those who believed strongly in Western medicine with membership in a state church. Established Western medicine also has its heretics who interpret and critique health practices with other frameworks from the social sciences or holism. There were several participants whose beliefs were clearly within the realm of medical heresy. Other men in this study articulated health beliefs that, in a religious context, would be considered agnostic (those who did not believe in Western or alternative medicine) or ecumenical (those who wanted to do it all). The final interpretive chapter outlined several ways of understanding CD4 counts within the framework of (1) a state church, (2) heresy, (3) agnosticism, and (4) ecumenicism.

The process of moving from the dissertation to the book took several more years of analysis and writing. In that phase, I deemphasized the connections that I had made between individual beliefs about health and standard approaches to religion. This was done to avoid what might look like categorizing the participants. In the book, I wrote an introduction outlining my concerns with HIV/AIDS research followed by a chapter that documented my own story. I then served as a narrator to tell 10 additional stories in a sequence that showed how my own understanding unfolded. The first story in the dissertation became the last story in the book. Relations between experiences and social structures were analyzed and discussed, but the experiences of each participant were kept in the foreground. In this phase, I removed many of the questions and comments that I made in the course of the interview to preserve the voice of the participant. This sometimes required adding a phrase or two to what the participant actually said for context.

Theoretical Development.   Critical and interpretive theory differs from conceptions of theory aimed at explanation, prediction, and control of human phenomena. Critical and hermeneutic theory provide a perspective or an interpretation aimed at understanding some phenomenon (Jorgensen, 1989). This study did not result in a new interpretative or critical theory. Not all interpretive or ethnographic research results in theory, but all should nonetheless facilitate greater understanding and insight. Future interpretive work with this data may lead to more refined and focused interpretations that might in turn lead to a more integrated articulation of meanings, concerns, and self-understandings. Future critical work with this data (or that of another study) might lead to a more refined account of health beliefs. But neither interpretative theory nor critical commentary is the ultimate goal of this work; understanding is.

Validity Issues

To address content validity, data was gathered from several sources including the formal interview, field notes on conversations between participants and the investigator, and, in at least two instances, the participants' own writing. Interviews were conducted over a 3-year period and most of the participants were available to the investigator throughout that time. There were multiple stages of interpretation. Interpretations were presented to selected study participants, HIV support-group members, and other asymptomatic, HIV-positive gay men for their feedback. My interpretations have tended to resonate with the lived experiences of people in the community.

Reliability and validity are nonetheless inappropriate terms for interpretative research. Interpretative research is either full of errors or biases that might have been reasonably prevented or it is not. Like investigative journalism, interpretative research is either good or bad, interesting or boring, insightful or superficial. It is not so important that interpretative research be "right." Research that produces alternative interpretations from the participating communities, whether lay, professional, or academic, has done its job. What is important is that interpretative research in the human sciences sustain an ongoing dialogue. Arguments about the validity of methods are irrelevant. In fact, these arguments miss the point entirely, because interpretative research does not make ultimate, ahistorical, or absolute truth claims. This does not mean that interpretive work embraces relativism. Interpretative studies seek to articulate a "best account" and must compete with rival interpretations. If a meaningful discourse is to be sustained in the human sciences, it will have to be more about content than about method. Rival interpretations help sustain such a discourse.

Limitations of Methods

While collecting data, I often felt like a novice investigative journalist. Much cultural knowledge is structured through investigative journalism. One major distinction between investigative journalism and interpretive research is that researchers are often under fewer time constraints than are journalists. While writing textual interpretation, I felt as if I had returned to my days as an undergraduate. I was never given a method for interpreting texts. My undergraduate experience as an English major and my undergraduate teaching experience in the great books were both shaped by faculty decisions to discourage students from reading criticism and to develop their own critical abilities. One liability inherent in this study and any other is the researcher's own limited experience and perspective. I had neither the field experience of an investigative journalist, the reading or writing ability of a professor of literature, the cultural expertise of an anthropologist, nor the training of a philosopher. Although gay, I had not been an avid reader of gay writers and have only recently come to appreciate their importance. Nurses are nonetheless experienced readers of live human texts, and it is from my perspective as a nurse that this work proceeded. The result was neither journalism nor literature, but a novice's first effort that was presented as a doctoral dissertation and then as a book.

Burns's remaining three standards are analytical preciseness, theoretical connectedness, and heuristic relevance. These standards relate to the stories and interpretations and are not specifically evaluated here. The full text (MacIntyre, 1999) contains substantial analysis and material from interviews so that the reader can evaluate whether the stories and interpretations are precise enough. Because the purpose of this study has nothing to do with confirming or disproving theory, Burns's standard on theoretical connectedness was replaced by thematic connectedness. Judgments about the standard on heuristic relevance also must be left to the reader. I struggled to make this study relevant to both the gay and the professional nursing communities. Chapter 16 focuses on a critical interpretive review of the literature that does not appear in the book.

Chapter 16 is also an example of how critical theory can be used to frame social context. Other examples of this approach can be found in the critical review of research in alternative medicine and HIV (MacIntyre, Holzemer, & Philipek, 1997; MacIntyre & Holzemer 1997; Freeman & MacIntyre, 1999) and in the historical overview of HIV/AIDS (MacIntyre, 1999).

REFERENCES

Benner, P. (1985). Quality of life: A Phenomenological perspective on explanation, prediction, and understanding. *Advances in Nursing Science, 8*(1), 1–14.

Benner, P., & Wrubel, J. (1989). *The primacy of caring: Stress and coping in health and illness.* New York: Addison-Wesley.

Benner, P. (Ed.). (1994). *Interpretive phenomenology: Embodiment, caring, and ethics in health and illness.* Thousand Oaks, CA: Sage.

Bettelheim, B. (1980). *Surviving and other essays.* New York: Vintage Books.

Bourdieu, P. (1990). *The logic of practice* (Richard Nice, Trans.). Stanford, CA: Stanford University Press.

Burns, N. (1989). Standards for qualitative research. *Nursing Science Quarterly,* 2(1), 44–52.

Des Pres, T. (1976). *The survivor: An anatomy of life in the death camps.* New York: Oxford University Press.

Dreuilhe, E. (1988). Mortal embrace: Living with AIDS (L. Coverdale, Trans.). New York: Hill and Wang. (Original work published 1987)

Dunlap, M. J. (1990). *Shaping nursing knowledge: An interpretative analysis of curriculum documents from NSW, Australia.* Unpublished doctoral dissertation, University of California, San Francisco.

Freeman, E. M., & MacIntyre, R. C. (1999). Evaluating alternative medicine and HIV disease. *Nursing Clinics of North America, 34,* 147–162.

Geertz, C. (1987). Deep play: Notes on the Balinese cockfight. In P. Rabinow & W. M. Sullivan (Eds.), *Interpretive social science: A second look* (pp. 195–240). Berkeley: University of California Press. (Original work published 1972)

Habermas, J. (1971). *Knowledge and human interests* (J. Shapiro, Trans.). Boston: Beacon Press. (Original work published 1968)

Heidegger, M. (1962). *Being and time* (7th ed.). (J. Macquarrie & E. Robinson, Trans.). New York: Harper & Row.

Jorgensen, D. L. (1989). *Participant observation: A methodology for human studies.* London: Sage.

Kierkegaard, S. (1843/1971). *Either/or* (Vol. I). (D. Swenson & L. Swenson, Trans.). Princeton, NJ: Princeton University Press.

Kierkegaard, S. (1843/1987). *Either/or* (Vol. II). (H. Hong & E. Hong, Trans.). Princeton, NJ: Princeton University Press.

Kierkegaard, S. (1846/1962). *The present age* (A. Dru, Trans.). New York: Harper & Row.

Kierkegaard, S. (1848/1985). *Fear and trembling* (A. Hannay, Trans.). New York: Penguin.

Kierkegaard, S. (1855/1967). Training in Christianity (W. Lowrie, Trans.). Princeton, NJ: Princeton University Press.

Krieger, S. (1983). *The mirror dance: Identity in a women's community.* Philadelphia: Temple University Press.

Krieger, S. (1985). Beyond "subjectivity": The use of the self in social science. *Qualitative Sociology,* 8(4), 309–324.

Kushner, T. (1993). *Angels in America, part one: Millennium approaches.* New York: Theatre Communications Group.

Kushner, T. (1994). *Angels in America, part two: Perestroika.* New York: Theatre Communications Group.

Larson, E. L. (1988). Nursing research and AIDS. *Nursing Research*, 37, 60–62.

Lazarus, R. S., & Folkman, S. (1984). *Stress, appraisal, and coping*. New York: Springer.

Luther, M. (1520/1988). *A treatise on Christian liberty* (W. A. Lambert, Trans.). Philadelphia: Fortress Press.

MacIntyre, R. C., & Holzemer, W. L. (1997). Complementary and alternative medicine in HIV/AIDS, part II: A literature review. *Journal of the Association of Nurses in AIDS Care*, 8(2), 25–38.

MacIntyre, R. (1999). *Mortal men: Living with asymptomatic* HIV. New Brunswick, NJ: Rutgers University Press.

MacIntyre, R. C.,Tueller, B., & Wishon, S. L. (1988). Nursing care plans for people with HIV infection. In G. Gee & T. A. Moran (Eds.), AIDS: *Concepts in nursing practice* (pp. 215–258). Baltimore: Williams & Wilkins.

MacIntyre, R. C., Holzemer, W. L., & Philipek, M. (1997). Complementary and alternative medicine in HIV/AIDS, part I: Issues and context. *Journal of the Association of Nurses in AIDS Care*, 8(1), 23–31.

Munhall, P. (1994). *Revisioning phenomenology: Nursing and health science research*. New York: National League for Nursing Press.

Munhall, P., & Oiler Boyd, C. (1993). *Nursing research: A qualitative perspective*. Sudbury, MA: Jones and Bartlett.

Packer, M. J., & Addison, R. B. (Eds.). (1989). *Entering the circle: Hermeneutic investigation in psychology*. Albany: SUNY Press.

Proust, M. (1981). *Remembrance of things past* (T. Kilmartin & S. Moncrieff, Trans.). New York: Random House. (Original work published 1913–1927)

Rabinow, P., & Sullivan, W. M. (Eds.). (1987). T*he interpretive turn: A second look* (2nd ed.). Berkeley: University of California Press.

Rew, L., Stuppy, D., & Becker, H. (1988). Construct validity in instrument development: A vital link between nursing practice, research, and theory. *Advances in Nursing Science*, 10(4), 10–22.

Rorty, R. (1982). *Consequences of pragmatism*. Minneapolis: University of Minnesota Press.

Sande, M. A. (1993, June 25). HIV therapy guidelines issued. *News from* NIAID. National Institute of Allergies and Infectious Diseases.

Sarter, B. (1988). T*he stream of becoming: A study of Martha Rogers' theory*. New York: National League for Nursing Press.

Schatzman, L., & Strauss, A. L. (1973). *Field research: Strategies for a natural sociology*. Englewood Cliffs, NJ: Prentice-Hall.

Schmidt, S. A. (1990, March). The suffer's experience: A journey through illness. *Second Opinion* 13, 91–108.

Stevens, B. J. (1984). *Nursing theory: Analysis, application, evaluation* (2nd ed.). Boston: Little, Brown.

Taylor, C. (1985a). *Human agency and language: Philosophical papers* (Vol. 1). Cambridge, England: Cambridge University Press.

Taylor, C. (1985b). *Philosophy and the human sciences: Philosophical papers* (Vol. 2). Cambridge, England: Cambridge University Press.

Taylor, C. (1989). *Sources of the self.* Cambridge, MA: Harvard University Press.

Thompson, J. L. (1992). Identity politics, essentialism, and constructions of "home" in nursing. In J. L. Thompson, D. G. Allen, & L. Rodrigues-Fisher (Eds.), *Critique, resistance, and action: Working papers in the politics of nursing.* New York: National League of Nursing Press.

Thompson, J. L., Allen, D. G., & Rodrigues-Fisher, L. (Eds.). (1992). *Critique, resistance, and action: Working papers in the politics of nursing.* New York: National League of Nursing Press.

Van Manen, M. (1990). *Researching lived experience: Human science for an action sensitive pedagogy.* New York: SUNY Press.

Webster (1972). *Webster's new collegiate dictionary* (7th ed.). Springfield, MA: Merriam.

Religion as Metaphor
Interpretive Analysis

Richard MacIntyre

LITERATURE REVIEW

Critical theory can be used to analyze and interpret literature reviews and the social contexts relevant to research studies. A critical literature review helps researchers identify and clarify values and assumptions that bear on the project at hand. Rather than trying to "bracket" these values and assumptions as suggested by some phenomenological methodologists (Crotty, 1996), researchers in the interpretive tradition should try to clearly articulate them (Allen, 1992). The clear identification of values and assumptions allows readers to situate the researcher's position within the relevant histories and social discourses. It also facilitates dialogue and rival interpretations.

This chapter uses critical theory to present an interpretive analysis of the early social response to HIV and AIDS, the general focus of the research project. Critical theory was used as an approach to frame and interpret analytically the social text produced in response to HIV and AIDS.

Ideologies of Health and Illness

Sociologists, anthropologists, and other thinkers have been describing similarities between religion and the modern institutions of science for more than 100 years. Even cartoons and the television series *Star Wars* refer to science as the religion of the twentieth century. This comparison is nowhere more apparent than in the medical sciences. Goethe feared that the world was turning into one giant medical institution, and Reiff believed that hospitals were replacing churches and parliaments as the archetypal institution of Western culture (cited in Zola, 1984).

During the Middle Ages and the Renaissance, behaviors and attitudes that fell outside of socially sanctioned norms were viewed as sins. As society developed a more secular orientation, these same aberrant behaviors and attitudes were reconstructed as crimes. In the scientific era, many behaviors and attitudes found to be more than 2.5 standard deviations from the mean were reconstructed as sicknesses. Fox (1984) described the evolution of sins to crimes and of crimes to sicknesses. She also noted a concomitant shift in the institutions charged with controlling deviance from churches to courts to medical institutions.

Several scholars have discussed problems with this evolution, including the increasing "medicalization" of nonnormative behaviors (deviance) and life in general. Advocates for medical science purport that it has a more objective, less dogmatic approach to human problems. Critics assert that medical science is no less dogmatic in its pronouncements on the causes and treatments of human problems than are religious authorities and has contributed to a more objectified and dehumanized understanding of life. Indeed, the most outstanding dissenters in medical science are often regarded as heretics, from Thomas Sazz to Peter Duesberg.

Although science has largely replaced religion as the dominant framework for understanding life, suffering, and death, almost every culture—including our own—has symbolically located health and illness within the domains of the sacred and the profane (Zerubavel, cited in Wolf, 1993). To understand the meanings that asymptomatic HIV might hold for a group of gay men, HIV and AIDS must be located within the dominant culture's constellation of health and illness. In turn, health and illness must be situated within the domains of the sacred and the profane so that the contexts in which health beliefs and healing practices are sanctioned or dismissed can be examined. One of the central "findings" of this project was that the range of beliefs and practices associated with health, illness, and treatment was very similar to the range of ideologies on religion—member of dominant or state religion, heretic, agnostic, ecumenicist. These similarities were discussed in depth in the dissertation phase of the project and presented again in a less categorical manner in a text intended for lay audiences (MacIntyre, 1999).

The Social Response to AIDS

The remainder of this chapter argues that the early social response to AIDS was an acute manifestation of cultural death anxiety. The concepts of contagion, moral panic, stigma, taboo, and cultural death anxiety can help facilitate our understanding of the social construction of AIDS.

Contagion.   For Sontag (1988), *plague* was the dominant metaphor for AIDS. Sontag defined plague as the highest standard for collective calamity, evil, or scourge. But AIDS did not come to signify a *collective calamity* for the nation as a whole as long as it was confined to gay men and intravenous drug users. Rather, the collective calamity began when hemophiliacs became infected with the disease and the safety of the nation's blood supply was questioned. AIDS continued as a "collective" national problem because heterosexual men could be exposed to HIV through prostitutes and because children could be exposed to HIV in utero or through an infected mother's milk. Inherent in this distinction is the concept of contamination of innocents by the guilty.

Public hysteria about contamination from AIDS continued to be rampant despite medical evidence showing that AIDS was not casually transmitted. As late as fall, 1985, "a *New York Times*/CBS poll found that 47 percent of Americans believed that AIDS could be transmitted via a shared drinking glass. . . ." (cited in Brandt, 1987, p. 192). In 1999, a directive by the government ministries in the Socialist Republic of Vietnam barred HIV-positive people from providing direct services in hotel rooms, from providing food or care to children in creches or kindergartens, and from work in hair cutting, hair drying, and hair washing. The reasons for these directives could not have been to protect the public from HIV-positive people. There is no scientific basis for it. The reasons must be located elsewhere.

Scholars outside of medicine use terms such as plague, pollution, contamination, moral panic, and stigma to describe the social meanings of AIDS (Brandt, 1987; Watney, 1987; Sontag, 1988). The contagion metaphor has been applied to homosexuality in general. Watney's (1987) description of attitudes toward homosexuality in England helps explain how 47 percent of the most modern, scientifically oriented society in the twentieth century could imagine that AIDS could be transmitted by drinking glasses. He quotes from a 1961 text on sex education:

> The greatest danger in homosexuality lies in the introduction of normal people to it. An act which will produce nothing but disgust in a normal individual may quite easily become more

acceptable, until the time arrives when the normal person by full acceptance of the abnormal act becomes a pervert too. (p. 23)

Somehow, a sexual expression that is "disgusting" becomes appealing when a "contagious" predator seduces an innocent victim. Such a perception derives from the heterosexual "nature" paradigm for sexuality: males are naturally predatory and females are just as naturally preyed upon (Watney, 1987). Part of homophobia thus comes from projecting the predatory nature of heterosexual men onto gay men who are then fantasized as being so powerful and potent that innocent heterosexual men might be seduced. The victims are thus "feminized" or functionally castrated by these powerful seducers (Watney, 1987). The other part of homophobia derives from our misogynist attitudes toward men who seem to be like women. Men who are "feminized" are at once feared (could this happen to me?) and loathed (for having allowed it to happen). If homosexuality is contagious, it is easy to understand why people might believe that AIDS could be acquired from drinking glasses—even in a "scientific" society.

Moral Panic.   Moral panics arise when events or groups emerge to threaten social interests and identities. Which group emerges to fulfill this definition tends to be shaped by the media, whose role is to communicate norms and boundaries. Moral panics both construct and reinforce a public identity or self (Watney, 1987). In America and Western Europe the public self is created through a continual repetition of images and symbols designed to reinforce a white, heterosexual identity. Moral panics bring the public's deepest interests into sharp contrast with its deepest fears. They consequently define the public self by clearly differentiating it from an unhealthy "other"—from what it is not.

Stigma and Taboo.   The public, or collective, identity is circumscribed by boundaries that protect it from contamination by the lives and habits of others. Fears, stigmas, and taboos help construct those boundaries that separate self from not-self. The concepts of stigma and taboo refer to both the sacred and the profane and can help shed light on the social construction of both AIDS and homophobia.

The term *stigma* derives from *stigmata*, defined by Webster (1972) as "bodily marks or pains resembling the wounds of the crucified Christ and sometimes accompanying religious ecstasy" (p. 861). The stigmata are at once sacred, representing the suffering of Christ, and profane, representing a violation of Christ's body. To receive the stigmata is to be blessed by God; to be stigmatized is to be cursed by a culture. To be blessed by God is clearly preferable to being cursed by one's culture, but Goffman (1986) focuses on the latter and identifies three kinds of stigma that refer to our biopsychosocial natures.

The first type of stigma has to do with an abomination of the body (bio); the second with individual character defects (psycho); the third with a fear of the "other" based on race, religion, or nationality (social). Each of these types of stigma can lead us to a more comprehensive understanding of the moral panic surrounding AIDS and the "core of being" that panic disturbs. Although the connotations associated with stigma are largely negative, the word suggests that stigmatized peoples suffer public evils much as Christ did. Jesus was put to death in part because he refused to submit to religious authorities, and these authorities feared that his power would threaten theirs. Stigmatized people are threatening because they are feared.

Taboos have their origin in a fear of how mysterious or demonic powers might be manifested in a community. But taboos differ from religious or moral prohibitions. Religious and moral prohibitions result from a system of thought that gives justification or reasons for their necessity. For example, religious prohibitions against homosexuality in particular and sexuality in general can be understood through a concept of nature (i.e., what is natural, what nature intended), a need for procreation, or a need for social-political order and control. Taboo restrictions lack any type of justification primarily because the feared power is both unknown and unbounded. Taboo serves to protect people from an overwhelming sense of fear and dread by isolating and ritualizing relations with people, objects, and events that possess extraordinary mystery. In 1913, Freud enumerated several objectives of the taboo that include (1) securing people against the wrath of the gods; (2) protecting important persons (chiefs and priests); (3) safeguarding the weak from the power of these important persons; (4) protecting people against corpses; (5) guarding the chief acts of life (birth, initiation, marriage, sexual functions) against interference (Freud, 1918).

Sexual behavior in general, and gay sexual behavior in particular, has always been associated with powerful mysterious or demonic powers and subject to strict taboos. Because gay sexual behavior does not result in procreation, it is frequently seen as a violation of the sacred, heterosexual, life-affirming "nature model." Furthermore, AIDS linked gay sexual behavior directly to death just when the link between sexual behavior and death was receding from the collective memory of the dominant culture. Successful repression includes forgetting the wish to forget, the act of forgetting, and the antecedent condition making forgetting possible—in this case, antibiotics. But taboos against male homosexuality also function to protect men from themselves, from feminization, from their own misogyny. Men were not to be preyed upon sexually. Just as in psychoanalytic theory in which a child fears punishment from the parent whom he wants to replace, so predatory male behavior engenders fears of being preyed upon. Gay men are fantasized to be the devils capable of meting out that punishment—devils inspiring fear and dread.

Thus the fear that AIDS engenders in the public is associated both with powerful cultural taboos and with all three types of stigma identified by Goffman (1986): stigmas of body, character, and otherness. All three of these types of stigma have to do with deep-seated fears, and these fears are at the root of the moral panic engendered by AIDS. Punishment or death often follows stigmatization, reinforcing the strength of a culture's taboos and the "moral" purpose behind its stigmatization. Those who adopt the public persona of the dominant culture can take comfort in imagining that adhering to cultural taboos will provide protection from mysterious forces such as death.

Cultural Death Anxiety and the Origin of Fear and Dread.   The concepts of contagion, moral panic, stigma, and taboo refer to beliefs and behaviors that are deeply routed in culture. The remainder of this chapter will argue that these beliefs and behaviors are formed in response to the fear associated with unresolved anxieties about death.

Freud's last work, An *Outline of Psycho-analysis*, published in 1940 after his death, postulated two basic instincts from which all human activity is derived:

> After long hesitancies and vacillations we have decided to assume the existence of only two basic instincts, Eros and *the destructive* instinct. . . . The aim of the first of these basic instincts is to establish ever greater unities and to preserve them thus—in short, to bind together; the aim of the second is, on the contrary, to undo connections and so to destroy things. In the case of the destructive instinct we may suppose that its final aim is to lead what is living into an inorganic state. For this reason we also call it the *death instinct*. (Freud, 1949, p. 1)

The majority of Freud's work concerned the function of Eros and libidinal energy. Freud did not even develop a concept analogous to libido for the death instinct, but he did state that some part of the death instinct remains within us (like libidinal energy) until it at last succeeds in killing us. Freud concluded that individuals die from their internal conflicts and that our species dies of its unsuccessful struggle against the external world. Thus Freud posited an individual self that contains the seed of its own destruction.

Brown (1985) pointed out that an essential conflict between the self and the culture results when our only hope for health lies in our ability to translate the instinct to die into an instinct to kill. He rejected Freud's dualistic ontology and postulated that it is anxiety about death—not the death instinct—that is problematic. For Brown, the conscious fear and repression of death is found only at the human level. If this is not an absolute distinction between human beings and the animals, it is certainly qualitatively significant. People store up their dead, build immortal cultures, and make history—all in an attempt to escape from death. But, for Brown, death anxiety is the same as life's anxiety and to escape death is to escape our individuation:

> At the simplest organic level, any particular animal or plant has uniqueness and individuality because it lives its own life and no other—that is to say, because it dies. (p. 104)

Brown is saying that the "death instinct" helps us separate into unique individual beings, just as Eros helps us unite with others and feel connected to the universe. The death instinct (mortality) gives people their independence and individuality. Thus, the fear of death becomes the fear of separation and individuality.

Brown's contribution helps explain the phenomenon of moral panic. If persons fear separation and individuation, then socially constructed public identities can help reduce that fear. The media fulfill this function by regularly presenting images of the ideal identity (white, heterosexual families) and by periodically publishing stories that portray the nonideal, or nonconformed (nonwhites, gays, single people) as a threat. The fear of individuation can also be seen in our willingness to submit to control of all kinds, including the control and regulation of sexual behavior.

Becker (1973) posited a slightly different dualistic problem for human beings—the relation between the self and the body.

> The person is both a self and a body, and from the beginning there is the confusion about where "he" really "is"—in the symbolic inner self or in the physical body. Each phenomenological realm is different. The inner self represents the freedom of

thought, imagination and the infinite reach of symbolism. The body represents determinism and boundness (pp. 41–42).

Kierkegaard set up the problem in a similar manner (Kierkegaard, 1983). Persons are a synthesis of the body (the finite) and the mind, or self (the infinite). Both the body and the self present problems. If the self is not adequately anchored in the body, schizophrenia, the sickness of infinitude, results. If anchored too securely, depression, the sickness of finitude, results. Becker (1973) thinks that the finite body is a problem for the infinite mind or "self." Unlike the animals, humankind is not primarily driven by instincts and alive in the moment. The inner symbolic self is all too aware that it is tiny, powerless, and perhaps even meaningless in relation to the vastness of the universe that it perceives. Becker concluded that the very idea of such a self-conscious animal is both ludicrous and monstrous because it means knowing that "one is food for worms" (p. 87).

The self needs to defend itself from its creatureliness and accomplishes that in part by building a "character." This character helps let one "pretend and feel that he is somebody, that the world is manageable, that there is a reason for one's life, a ready justification for one's action" (Becker, 1973, p. 87). In the 1970s, gay men and women developed new identities and new possibilities for character. Previously, this development had been difficult for many homosexuals because heterosexuality is such a major component of the public identity. The construction of an identity was a major theme in the stories of the gay men in this study.

> *Gabe:* In the late '70s and early '80s gay men operated upon a certain set of assumptions. Like any community, most of our assumptions were not articulated, but nevertheless loomed so large that perhaps they now need to be articulated. One of those assumptions was that sex was healthy, literally and metaphorically. Another was that sex did not need to be monitored. Any kind of attempt to monitor or regulate it was viewed as a residue of Victorian repression or puritanical impulses. . . .
>
> For some good reasons, our culture followed a very conservative impulse, one that clearly favored stability. As a result, there were very few outlets in the late-twentieth century for a middle-class person such as myself to explore the unknown, the exotic. Sex provided that outlet for my generation, especially for gay men. You could just plunge into the unknown, the exotic, and emerge differently, into new

senses of the self. The self was something to be created and reinvented. You went to the baths with a self that could be constructed, manipulated, altered, modified, right there on the spot. All of a sudden AIDS came along, and I don't mean to be crude, but it was no longer as adventuresome and no longer as fun. So that impulse, that arena of play, that arena of the dissolution of the self was lost to me for many, many years. And I mourn losing that sense of adventure as well as the deaths of my friends.

Eric: There was a sense of community that was glued together through sex, which I think was fine. There was just a sheer enjoyment of sex. Sex became a folk art, and people were busy practicing. It's like we were employing homophobic tendencies to break down our homophobic selves—to break down the man in us, to create a new gay individual, on a personal level and on a community level. Sex does have a masochistic aspect that is completely valid and unavoidable, though I think it reached a threshold that ultimately produced ill health.

Kirk: I used to be a major party animal, and I used to be able to really carry on in college. When I first came out, I could be ridiculous. I used to think that some sort of death wish was behind some of my behavior. . . . [But] I wouldn't trade a night in the bathhouse for anything! And I feel compassion for these guys who are twenty and are coming out, and they never get to spend a night in a bathhouse and fuck around with eight people in one night. I mean, that's letting your libido go crazy. That's letting your fantasy run wild. It was great to have that experience. . . . [But] the physical act of sex is not the most important part of relationships. The most important part of relationships is the bonds that you form, the emotional, the spiritual, the intellectual bonds that you form.

When AIDS hit, some gay men decided that it was more important to preserve these relatively new identities, character roles, and cultural possibilities than it was to fight AIDS directly. But others, including Eric, noted that the hypersexuality associated with the new gay identity was as obligatory as it was emancipating.

Richard: How do you account for still getting fucked without condoms after having decided that the behavior was linked to AIDS?

Eric: It just goes to show how obligatory sex was at the time, how absolutely essential it was to have sex. There is still a strong forceful imperative to have sex. Back then it was truly oppressive.

Another participant, Ron, talked about how the company that he kept greatly affected his behavior.

Ron: I actually know a lot of people who were not into anal sex. I had a roommate who always felt like he was an outsider because he didn't like anal sex. He always had to make excuses. Safe sex was the greatest thing for him because he didn't have to make excuses anymore. There were certainly times when I had anal sex when I didn't want to. I just felt, well, okay, if they want to do it, let's do it and get it over with. . . .

I don't really do drugs on my own, but if I'm around certain friends, I do them. . . . I [also] have a few friends that I used to do drugs with. . . . They don't want to do drugs anymore, but I would do drugs with them if they wanted to. I like being around them, so if they wanted to go for long walks and knit sweaters, I'd probably want to do that with them. If they wanted to do drugs and have wild sex, I'd do that too. I just like being with them. I'm sort of a follower that way, so if they're not doing drugs, I'm not doing drugs. Even drinking is the same. If my friend orders a Calistoga and I was going to have a beer, I'll just order a Calistoga. I'm sort of a copycat person. Not with everybody, just with certain people. So my act has sort of been cleaned up for me.

Character, whether the traditional heterosexual one or the newly created gay hypersexual character of the 1970s and 1980s, lets one live automatically and uncritically (if not unconsciously) in one of the programmed character roles in the culture. Some of our social constructed character is necessary. The Eros instinct drives us to unification with others. But Kierkegaard described the despair or sickness that can result when the self gives itself over to the character roles available in the culture:

But whereas one kind of despair plunges wildly into the infinite and loses itself, another kind of despair seems to permit itself to be tricked out of its self by "the others." Surrounded by hordes of men, absorbed in all sorts of secular matters, more and more shrewd about the ways of the world—such a person forgets himself, forgets his name divinely understood, does not dare to believe in himself, finds it too hazardous to be himself and far easier and safer to be like the others, to become a copy, a number, a mass man. (Kierkegaard, 1983, pp. 33–34)

This is the normal man for Kierkegaard: his individuation lost, his self merged with and protected by the more powerful public identity.

According to Brown and Becker, the primary repression in society is not seeking pleasure through sexual activity but the consciousness of death. Becker removes the pathological connotations associated with Freud's death instinct and Brown's death anxiety and gives us two positive instincts: the need to merge and to achieve unity and transcendence; and the need for individuation, separation, and freedom. Becker reverses Freud's and Brown's description of the instincts. He contends that the individualized self, or ego, is a product of Eros rather than the result of human mortality. And rather than equating the death instinct with separation, freedom, and individuation, Becker sees it as the expression of a need to merge, unite, and identify with a larger power or force. Thus Thanatos becomes agape love; Eros, self-love. Wilber (1986) expanded on these revisions with a psychoanthropological analysis of the evolution of human consciousness. His work, drawing heavily from Freud (1949), Brown (1985), and Becker (1973), asserts that the evolution of human consciousness has some parallels with early human development. His conception of Eros and Thanatos is similar to Becker's. Early humans, like the newborn infant, did not distinguish between subject and object, between their mothers' bodies and their own; between the world and themselves. Wilber cites the Eden paradise myths as evidence for a time of unconscious embeddedness with nature. Like Brown and Becker, Wilber ties our individuation to a consciousness of death. As our self-consciousness merged, as our Eros instinct asserted its individuality, so our consciousness of death and our need to repress it also came into being.

Regardless of which name (Eros or Thanatos) is applied to the instinct for unification and transcendence and which is applied to the instinct for individuation and freedom, humankind's first attempts to come to terms with death anxiety are found in taboos (Wilber, 1986). Totemic cultures formed and people were able to "merge or unite" with a larger power, even if it was only the larger power of the totemic clan. Religious sacrifice offered one way to appease the unknown force that demanded our deaths. Taboos marked the boundaries between life and death; us and them. War offered another possibility. If we and our gods could overcome them and their gods, the cultural immortality project also was strengthened. Sexual taboos offered still another way of controlling mortal and fickle bodies that could sicken and die. Whether the body is conceived of as an offensive, mortal shell (the Greek view) or as a temple for spirit (the Christian view), the mortal body has been both objectified and divided from the self.

The Perversion of Eros and Thanatos

Returning to Goffman's (1986) definition of stigma, we can clearly see why the public reaction to AIDS is so hostile. Since the time of the early Greeks and Romans, we have posited our inner spiritual selves as having been in conflict with our mortal, evil bodies (Bullough & Bullough, 1977). Kierkegaard calls it a conflict between finitude and infinitude; Becker and Brown, between the need for unity and individuation; Freud, between life and death instincts. Health is the result of having both together, repressing neither. But as each of the foregoing theorists point out, this task is very difficult: individuals and societies alternate between repressing, perverting, or misdirecting both instincts.

The instinct toward unity and connection helps protect the self through identification with something larger, stronger. The aim of this instinct is transcendence—not, as Freud would have it, the death of the physical body. The vastness of the universe becomes less frightening and overwhelming if one can somehow identify with and rest in it. When the instinct toward unity achieves a transcendent identity or consciousness, there is no conflict with the opposite instinct toward individuation. A transcendent consciousness or perspective can appreciate both unity and differentiation simultaneously. A transcendent perspective can bring a measure of understanding to the seeming conflict between life and death.

Often, people lose themselves in the process, give themselves over to slavish tyrants, adopt the character roles of the culture, worship false and lesser gods. This perverse identification with the public, rather than a sacred identification with God, the universe, or the transcendent self, accentuates our fear and loathing of finite, individuated bodies— of individual self-expression, of sexual freedom. Without a meaningful relation with a powerful God who could protect it from evil, the public self sees devils and demons everywhere. The public self is fearful that differentiation will fragment its precarious identity, and so it creates taboos—sexual and otherwise.

Gay men violate the taboos and threaten the public's fragile, worldly identity. Those who by necessity would individuate themselves from socially constructed norms, who would violate the taboos on sexual expression, must be killed or banished for the public self's defense. Denied communion with and meaningful participation in public life, gay people hold the stigma of a culture that both fears and loathes its own embodied mortality. Thus it is the threatened public self that resists rational AIDS policies. Policies that could save lives through appropriate sexual and drug education would undermine the public's fragile identity and empower its favorite scapegoats.

The efforts to recriminalize homosexuality in America and other countries are about maintaining our false god, our public self. Watney (1987) reports that for the first time in British history, a bill was introduced that would criminalize lesbianism, in addition to male homosexuality. This bill is proposed in the name of protecting the public from AIDS. But, because lesbians are at lower risk for AIDS than is any other segment of the population, something else is obviously going on. The first fear of this largely heterosexual male legislative body was of homosexual men, and it derived from a projected fear of their own predatory behaviors. The move to outlaw lesbians seems to be about losing prey. But the greater fear is for maintaining the socially constructed self that works to reduce our death anxiety.

Identification with the public self seeks to satisfy both instincts, unity and individuation. But, just as the public self fails to provide for transcendence, so does it fail to give a real identity. The media-sustained public self needs an "other" if it is to meet its second ontological need, individuation. The "normal" public self has no individuated identity apart from an "other," apart from being defined by who it is not. This "other" is found in the form of other races, religions, economic classes, and sexualities through which the leveled and normalized public self can feel differentiated. The stigmatized "other" is readily available to the public self through the moral panic over AIDS in the form of gay men, intravenous drug users, ethnic minorities, and prostitutes. Without a truly individuated identity, the normalized self resorts to fantasies of omnipotence resulting in serious misperceptions about individual character and patterns of individual behavior. Brandt (1987) notes:

> Behavior is not always subject to rational control. . . . The underlying assumption about behavior, and one deeply ingrained in our culture, is that it is entirely voluntary. According to this logic, once appropriately informed about risks, individuals "should" modify their behaviors. Moreover, we know too little about how

to assist individuals who seek to make, and maintain, difficult behavioral alterations. (p. 191)

The assumption that character and behavior result from an expression of individual will derives from an inflated sense of a separate self. The notion of an entirely separate self, created by the will alone, results in an unwillingness to engage in the collective actions that are necessary if collective public health problems are to be overcome. It explains the reluctance of the Reagan and Bush administrations to spend monies appropriated for AIDS. Why should public funds be spent on a disease that could be largely avoided if only separate selves exerted individual wills in conformance with public standards of morality? If developing AIDS can be perceived as a failure of individual will and character (and it generally is), then all three of Goffman's (1986) stigmas converge on the person with AIDS. He is an "other"—someone unlike and foreign to the public self. He has violated social taboos concerning the body through homosexual acts or drug use. And he is deficient in the strength of individual character that the public self fantasizes itself to possess.

The stigmatization of AIDS can be understood as a perversion of the dual ontology of humankind. When our innate need for unification is translated into a fear of death, a public self replaces the transcendent self. When our innate need for individuation is translated into fantasies of omnipotence, tyrants dispensing judgment and death replace heroes dispensing salvation and life.

Social policy is frequently designed to maintain and protect the social identity, rather than to save money and lives. For example, we have been more inclined to fund widespread HIV testing than to fund AIDS treatment and prevention programs. Like the Biblical separation of the sheep from the goats at the Last Judgment, HIV testing separates the saved from the damned, ensuring eternal life for the socially constructed public identity (sometimes the majority) and eternal death for the "other." Nothing resolves our own deep-seated fears about death better than the sacrifice of an "other."

FORECASTS OF DOOM

This section includes a chapter excerpted from *Mortal Men: Living with Asymptomatic HIV* (MacIntyre, 1999). As with most of the chapters, it begins with a segment that both paints a picture of the time and culture and reveals some personal experiences that shaped my emerging point of view. The chapter on Matthew is included as an example of a member of the state church—someone who believes strongly in Western medicine. Although Matthew does not blindly follow his physician's advice, he demonstrates a clear belief in pharmaceutical intervention. Other chapters in *Mortal Men* tell the stories of men whose health beliefs could be characterized as ecumenical, agnostic, or heretic. However, Matthew's story is important for many other reasons, including the fact that he was the person in our extended circle of friends who had been documented as HIV positive for the longest length of time—since 1979.

Introduction

There was only one reason for a San Francisco homosexual to be on Fourth Street in the middle of the day. Sandwiched between a gas station and a cheap motel, the clap clinic was a venerated San Francisco institution. The first few minutes were always the most awkward. It wasn't standing before the massive desk or facing the dozen or more subaltern officials and clerks who moved behind it. Most of these were occupied with incomprehensible duties, and only one or two attended to the line. No, it was standing with your back to the one or two hundred patients in the seats behind you. These were the people you might know— or might want to know.

To show I was neither intimidated nor repentant, I always wore Levi's and a black leather jacket, but not a trashy shirt. And yet it was all quite awkward. How do you cruise at the clap clinic? And how do you not cruise when you're in a room full of gay men who have nothing else to do? That, together with the fact that the whole flock was "grounded," made the whole thing weird and depressing.

As numbers were called, we watched each other get up and walk to one of the tiny cubicles that lined the room. Between each call, we retook our seats with the rest of the mostly male group. I couldn't tell you what percentage might have been straight, because I saw only the gay men. There weren't many prostitutes, though, of either sex. They had long ago learned how to avoid such trouble or else got their care from the privates.

The first call was to an office on the right wall. The social worker had your record—an eight-and-a-half by five-and-a-half-inch card with room for about thirty visits. When that filled up, the social worker stapled on a second. I knew a couple of guys who had three. The second call was usually to the physician. Their offices were in a hallway to the left of the main desk in the front. The third call was to the nurse who administered injections or gave pills, depending on the protocol. Her quarters were on the left wall, in the rear of the room. Even if you got shots, you usually had to take some pills as well. The water fountain was in the middle of the wall on the left. Some guys faced it straight on and bent their butts to the crowd. Others favored a forty-five-degree approach, while the more timid tried to keep their bodies parallel with the wall. The whole ordeal could take up to two hours.

One February day in 1978 a social worker at the clap clinic asked if I would be interested in participating in a hepatitis study. They were looking for people who had never had hepatitis B. When I initially came down with hepatitis in 1976, they had told me it was hepatitis A, so I volunteered. They drew some blood, tested it for hepatitis B, and after three weeks or so told me that I had indeed been infected with hepatitis B and was therefore ineligible for the study. Nine years later, in 1987, they telephoned me again. They'd saved some of my blood from that 1978 test and wanted permission to test it for HIV. They also wanted some fresh blood. I readily agreed and made an appointment to sign forms and give another sample. When I went for the results, I already knew I was positive. That had been confirmed in 1985 when Duckus and I had taken the test. But I hadn't ever had my T cells checked, so that was the only source of concern.

I knew the T-cell counts of only three other people. Duckus, who had been diagnosed with pneumocystis, had a count of 30. Two friends from the gym who seemed very healthy had counts around 450 and 700. I knew we would eventually have population statistics that would tell us what was normal, but "normal" might vary widely from person to person. I knew it would be easier to decide what my own future T-cell counts would mean if I could compare them against both population parameters and my own past history. So even though the professionals were saying, "They didn't mean anything," I wanted the number for historical purposes. In situations new to medicine "not meaning anything" is always code for "We have not yet determined what this means."

This new research project wasn't housed in the same building as the old clap clinic, but a lot of the faces were the same. My appointment was with a friend from the gym. "I've got good news and bad news," he said. "Which do you want to know first?"

"The bad," I responded, without the slightest hesitation.

"Well, the bad you already know, so it's not really news for you. Your blood was positive for HIV."

Despite the fact that he knew that I knew, he nonetheless delivered the "bad news" with one of those open expressions that gives permission for a reaction, that even seems to hope for one. I had none. I'd been living with this for quite some time. Steve had been dead almost two years now. Duckus had already come down with pneumocystis. Now this guy whom I knew from the gym, with whom I'd had several conversations about being positive, was "giving me news." Maybe it's because he was sitting behind a desk. I guess they had a training session or something. Whatever.

"So what's the good news?"

"You were HIV negative in 1978."

"Why is that good news?" I asked. "I was hoping I was positive in 1978. That would mean I had survived this thing for nine years already, at the least."

"Because our research shows that the only thing that correlates with survival is time since infection."

"What! That's impossible. What sort of factors are you looking at? How are you collecting the data?"

"We're looking at everything. We have an incredibly sophisticated design that looks at all aspects of sexuality, drug use, psychological testing, demographic factors. We have a top team of public health professionals, epidemiologists, survey researchers, biostatisticians. I know it is not very hopeful, but that is what the research is showing. To date, the only thing that correlates with survival is the length of time since becoming infected. So it is very good that you weren't infected in 1978. It isn't uncommon for people to live with this thing for five years, and of course research continues to look for treatments."

"So what are my T cells—good or bad?"

"Well, your T cells are 714, which is high, but that really doesn't mean anything. I can't emphasize this too strongly. T-cell levels have not yet been correlated with survival. We don't know what T cells mean. Some people are living a long time with very low T cells, and some people are getting sick with relatively high T-cell counts. Not even drug use has been correlated with survival time. The sad thing is, the only thing that correlates with survival is time since getting infected."

"Yeah, right. I know they don't mean anything yet. But they will someday. What kind of qualitative data are you collecting?"

"For those who were positive in 1978/80 we're asking a lot of questions, especially about sex and drug use."

"And what about those who were negative in the early stages? Are you asking them the same questions?"

"Unfortunately, there isn't enough funding to do everything we'd like to do."

I suspected that increased funding wasn't the problem. I suspected that the entrenched methods and procedures of the public health establishment were the problem.

"The reason nothing correlates with survival," I answered "is that you're probably not asking the right people the right questions. It's pretty presumptuous, don't you think, to say nothing correlates with survival just because you haven't found anything yet?"

"Well, of course, as we get more data, things might change. All of us hope something will correlate with survival. Hope is very important, but science is important, too. This is an incredibly well designed study."

"Have you written down that I tested positive in September 1985, or is this research going to show my HIV-positive test date as 1987?"

"I'll write it down if you like, but the statistics will be run on the 1987 test date. This is very rigorous scientific research, and the grant requires that we gather verifiable data. I'm sure you know when you were first tested, but as you know, many people are not reliable historians."

"My concern is that your results are not going to be reliable either. Yet you'll convince the public it's the gospel truth because you've done such good science. If you don't ask people when they tested positive, you won't ever be able to go back and run your statistics again—once for your verifiable stuff and once for what people in the community are saying—even if you do get more funding."

He indulged my harangue about this type of epidemiological work for a while, and I left the office depressed. Maybe nothing but time since infection would correlate with survival. That was really disappointing. It meant that the virus was stronger than everyone, that the virus would catch up with everyone. Survival itself lessened one's chance for survival. I didn't really know what data they were collecting or how they were analyzing it, but I was deeply suspicious. Just because science had not discovered anything that affected disease progression (other than time since infection) did not mean genetic or psychosocial correlation's did not exist. However, the pronouncements of researchers were made with such conviction that even skeptics such as myself were sometimes tempted to abandon their hope.

A few months later I was having breakfast with Gabe and reading the *Chronicle*.

"Jesus!" I screamed across the breakfast table. "Who do these jerks think they are? Are they just idiots or what?"

"The bit about the average survival time?" Gabe asked calmly.

"You already read it?"

"Before you got up."

"What in God's name do they mean by average? Where do they manage to find averages? They won't be able to find the mean until the last one of us drops dead. Any average calculated before that is going to be short. Any projection that they tweak from the data so far is only going to represent the ones who died first. This is just crap. Probably hundreds of thousands of dollars' worth of crap."

"Are they assuming that the group of us with HIV are distributed over some sort of bell curve?" Gabe asked, trying both to soothe my nerves and engage my rational processes.

"Probably. But that is a guess out of nowhere. The assumptions behind these statistical projections are never discussed. The survival curve for people with HIV could take a dozen different shapes, but the ones who will live the longest are clearly not comparable to those who will die first. And the people who were infected early may well not be comparable to the people who were infected five years later. And neither group may be comparable to those who are being infected today. Supposedly this virus is mutating, but even if it isn't, those who got infected in 1979 probably include a greater proportion of people with weaker immune responses to this virus. All they know is the average length of time it took for the first 30 percent to drop dead. They don't know how long it's going to take for the next 30 percent to die. They sure don't know how long it's going to take the last 30 percent to die. And by that time people will have eaten so many pharmaceuticals that they'll never be able to calculate an average survival time that means anything at all."

Later I discovered the assumptions behind their statistical methods weren't discussed in the scientific journals that published the studies either. Perhaps that was because the audience reading scientific journals already knew the theoretical assumptions behind each statistical method, so it would be redundant. Perhaps lay journalists covering medical news simply needed to be educated. But I suspected that the problem wasn't confined to journalists. Most of the American researchers in the social and medical sciences I'd met were either unable or unwilling to discuss the philosophical assumptions on which their methods were based. The doubt that used to be a hallmark of good scientific thinking had been preempted by a devotion to instruments of measurement and profitable products.

As time went on, this became less and less surprising to me. For nearly four decades now sociologists have been describing how the modern medical industry has assumed much of the authority and responsibility that used to adhere to the church. Today medical science charges dissenters such as Robert Root-Bernstein (1993), Joseph Sonnabend (1992), and Peter Duesberg (1996) with heresy. Today medical science is the nearly indisputable arbiter of truths concerning all matters related to health and illness.

Interview with Matthew

I met Matthew and his lover, Robert, at the gym in the late 1970s. To my mind, they were the epitome of a successful open gay relationship. (They had been together for 15 years when Robert died.) Both were extremely bright and very handsome. Popular, promiscuous, and successful, Robert was a brilliant economist whom I both loved and admired, and Matthew reminded me of my lover, Steve.

I interviewed Matthew because he had been HIV positive since 1978, his status having been documented because of his participation in the San Francisco hepatitis study. Thus, he was the longest documented survivor of HIV whom I knew. My closest friends and I had often theorized about what kind person might survive HIV infection. Because Matthew was our living example of a survivor, he had became a kind of lay case study and a reason to hope. I was of course interested in life style and medical decisions, but what I found was a story of love, irreplaceable loss, and a reluctance to be perceived as any sort of model survivor. As soon as I turned on the tape recorder, Matthew took over.

Matthew: I'm better off answering specific questions than rambling on about my story.

Richard: Okay. When did you first—

Matthew: Is the tape on?

Richard: Yeah.

Matthew: Oh. Let me fix my hair.

Richard: When did you first hear about AIDS?

I continued, trying to take a bit of control.

Matthew: I don't know. I think I've lost my sense of time. I had a friend over last night for dinner, and he mentioned his lover had died five-and-a-half years ago. I would have sworn it was around three years ago. If I'd thought about it, I could have figured it out by going back from when Robert got sick in 1986. It was before that. So I seem to have lost my time line. My guess is that I started hearing about it probably seven or eight years ago.

Richard: Which would make it 1982 or 1983.

Matthew: In that general time frame. I knew relatively early because one of the first cases in the city was a friend of mine. I remember when they were diagnosing one or two cases a week, and I thought that was a lot. So it was fairly early.

Richard: When did you take the HIV test? Was it before Robert was diagnosed?

Matthew: No. At that point we both felt that there was no reason to take the test because you couldn't do anything about it. It just would have upset us. The city had already contacted me to say that they had blood samples of mine from 1978 and blood samples from Robert from 1979. So we knew that those were sitting there. We had a long history at the clinic and were just waiting for a reason to take the HIV test. About a month after Robert was diagnosed with KS [Kaposi's sarcoma],[1] we left for Europe for two months. When we came back, I had the test.

Richard: What was it like to get the test results? Was it hard?

Matthew: It was very difficult because there's always a chance that you're negative, even though you assume you're positive. One reason you don't get tested is that you think there's a chance that you're negative. I had a friend whose lover had died of AIDS, yet he tested negative. But my reaction to being positive wasn't as bad as it could have been. If I had gone in and been told I was positive, I think it would have felt like the earth was moving and the floor was falling out from under me. But I was basically told, "You're positive, and you've been positive since 1978." So I was already positive for quite a number of years.

Richard: What did that mean to you? How did you interpret that?

Matthew: I interpreted that as a good sign. At that point they didn't really know what the incubation period was, but they were talking about two to three years. I was well beyond that, so I figured it was a good sign. I would have been more concerned if I hadn't been positive in 1978. I felt better having all those years under me. As it turns out, I don't feel better about it now, because they've just changed the incubation period to eleven years.

Richard: Eleven and a half—they change it every year.

Matthew: Yeah. They keep raising it. I thought that I was past the incubation period, but it's just not happening that way. I'm at twelve-and-a-half years now.

Matthew was not the only person who was disappointed by the news that the average length of time from infection to AIDS was increasing. When he got tested in 1986, being HIV positive since 1978 seemed to mean that he had a high chance of being in the group that might "survive." In 1990, when this interview was conducted, the expanded aver-

---

[1] Early in the epidemic, Kaposi's sarcoma was one of the leading causes of AIDS death among gay men. That this cancer has been rare to nonexistent among people with AIDS who are not gay has led some to question of whether other factors besides HIV, such as Kaposi's sarcoma, may be contributing to some AIDS.

age time from infection to AIDS (from about 5 years to 11 years) meant that he was only 1 year beyond the average. What should have been interpreted as good news for HIV-positive people became bad news for those who had always striven to be as far "above" the norm as possible, whether in regard to grades, sports competitions, or salaries. With HIV, death had defined the norm from the beginning. Even after the virus failed to kill all of its victims in the monolithic fashion that the experts expected, even when the predicted "average" survival time increased from 5 to 11-plus years, death still defined the norm. To beat death, we had to somehow beat the average, and the average time had grown so long that it was impossible to beat.

To Matthew, this annual change said the same thing that it did to several men in my community: "This is your year to die. We thought it was last year, but we were wrong. It's this year." Whether from AIDS researchers' inflated sense of self-importance or from the media's uncritical faith in their utterances, a measure of cruelty emanated from those reports that affected even those of us who doubted them from the beginning. Several men in this study were angry about those projections, not so much because they were so far from the truth, but because they were swallowed whole by the mainstream press. If the press moved just a few of its political pundits to the biomedical beat, the modicum of doubt, skepticism, and alternative thinking kept alive in our political discourse might produce a revolution in America's thinking about sickness and health. In fact, academic thinking is way behind what people are practicing. One-third of Americans already use alternative medical practitioners (Eisenberg et al., 1993).

Richard: So you've been positive since 1978. You found out in 1986. When did you start measuring T cells?

Matthew: In 1986. As long as I was positive, I wanted to know what was going on, so I started measuring T cells. They've always been in the same range, between 500 and 600. There was one test that was way higher than that, and I just assumed that it was a fluke, not an accurate test.

Richard: Have you done anything in terms of lifestyle changes or anything as a result of being positive or having 500 or 600 T cells?

Matthew: It's not that I have 500 or 600 T cells. I think I would have made the same changes if they were 700 or 800. I started taking acyclovir four years ago because I thought that

AIDS was eventually going to be associated with herpes.[2] I'd never had it, so I figured, Why bother getting herpes? My doctor said it wasn't harmful, and I felt like I was doing something, so I've been taking acyclovir since 1986. I've tried various things. I took that muck you put in the blender, AL-721. I did that for about a year. I've tried various things. I still do acyclovir, and I started AZT two months ago.

Richard: Tell me about the acyclovir first. How much do you take?

Matthew: It varies. At different times I've been on different amounts, from as many as ten a day to as few as three a day. At the moment I'm on six a day. I'm taking six AZTs, so I thought six would keep it simple.

Richard: Does your physician have any recommendation on how much acyclovir you should take? Has he given you any sort of range?

Matthew: His recommendation is none. He really doesn't think it makes much difference if I take three or four or five or six. He was more comfortable with six than ten, but he lets me participate. I figure it's my decision since it's my body.

Richard: So you took acyclovir to prevent herpes. Why did you take AL-721?

Matthew: Well, the initial reports on AL-721 looked promising. It was totally nontoxic, and I figured, Why not do it as long as there are no side effects, other than being inconvenient? Things come out and you hear great things about them, and then you hear nothing else about them ever again, and you figure, well, they must not have found anything. I didn't see anything negative about it—except that it didn't do anything. But I never saw anything positive about it again.

I read a report that said people taking it had fewer night sweats and less thrush, but that it didn't change T cells and had no effect on the immune system. I stopped taking it, too, even though I thought the conclusion of the study that debunked it was crap. Egg lecithin doesn't kill

---

[2]Several people in my community sought to avoid sunburn, poison oak, and herpes outbreaks because, in the gay press, these conditions had been associated with increased viral replication.

thrush by itself. It has to affect the immune system. They're all looking for a cure, and AL-721 wasn't a cure. I think we all stopped taking it at about the same time.

Richard: What about going on AZT? How did you decide to do that?

Matthew: My decision about that was from the research coming out. They only get T cells within a range, so there's no real difference between 525 and 475. My doctor seemed to think that, when you get below 500, you should start AZT. They have an attitude of "when, not if." It's like they're waiting. It's sort of creeping up on you. I figure as long as it's going to be eventual—and they keep telling me it's eventual, that it's going to happen, that they're going to drop another 25 or another 10 or whatever—I might as well just start it now.

Richard: What were your physician's arguments?

Matthew: For not taking the AZT? There's no research done above 500, no statistics to show that it does anything. The only studies were in the 200 to 500 level. Granted, it was significant, but the sample was so small that he didn't consider it relevant. But I disagree. I know a number of people who are taking AZT and have had dramatic increases in their T cells, which I find strange.

Richard: Is it like the acyclovir? You just feel like you should be doing something?

Matthew: Well, it's not just feeling that I should be doing something. I have this horrible feeling that at some point we'll find out that this is what you should have been doing all along, and now it's too late. You should have been doing this two years ago or whatever. I guess I figure I should do something. AZT is all that's out there at the moment that's approved, and it seems to be relatively nontoxic or relatively safe. I had a friend who was just killed by ddI—from pancreatic failure.[3] I don't have those worries about AZT. Since I've started taking it, I had my blood work done again this week, and my red and white cells are fine. The doctor said that my white cells were up and so were my red cells.

---

[3]DdI was the second antiviral drug approved for HIV.

Richard: So you're obviously not getting anemic from it. You said you've been on it for two months?

Matthew: Yeah.

Richard: Have you had any side effects?

Matthew: I get tired in the middle of the afternoon, and I seem to urinate at night. I have to get up to go to the bathroom three or four times.

Richard: What do you do when you're tired in the middle of the afternoon?

Matthew: Lie down usually.

Richard: Do you sleep?

Matthew: Not usually. Sometimes a little bit. If I sleep, it's like fifteen minutes or something. One day when I was in Florida in a shopping mall with my mother, I had to sit down because otherwise I was going to keel over. I've gotten that tired a couple of times.

Richard: When you say you felt like you were going to keel over, what do you mean?

Matthew: I felt like I was just going to fall asleep. I was that tired.

Richard: Did you feel a little light-headed?

Matthew (laughing): No more than usual.

I just felt tired—and heavy—like my body had to go down. The other side effect is that I seem to have not a great deal of interest in sex, which is highly unusual for me. I'll have a date over, and instead of having sex, we'll watch TV and I'll fall asleep. Or the other night the guy I've been dating was out of town. About 10:30 I was going to go down to Folsom Street to party at the 890 (a sex club), but I thought I'd rather go to sleep. Sounded like more fun. So I went to sleep.

Richard: Are there any other things you feel like you're not doing because you're HIV positive?

Matthew: I don't think so. I pretty much do what I want. I look at other people, and they have all kinds of other difficulties. I don't have any financial problems. I'm able to busy myself, to buy houses, and to do what I want. I don't worry about getting sick most of the time, but I don't want to put myself in a situation where I'm in the middle of something and then get sick. If I weren't worried about getting sick, I would have built a new house instead of buying a new house. I'd like an estate on eighty or one hundred acres, with a caretaker's house and a guest house to get people out from under my nose when they're there. I would have built a relatively simple house—by my standards, which I guess wouldn't be all that simple. But I couldn't see being in the middle of construction and then getting sick.

Richard: Have you made any changes with drugs or alcohol?

Matthew: My drug use was always less significant than people thought it was. I didn't really do that many drugs. Robert liked poppers. I didn't give up grass and I won't. I don't do it that often, and it's not a big deal.

Matthew took care of himself by doing what he wanted to when he wanted to. When he got tired, he napped; he stopped. His immediate feeling or state of mind was far more important than meeting some preestablished expectations, his own or those of others. Even when he planned a date or a trip to a sex club, if his attitude or energy changed, he went with it.

Matthew was also a man who thought things through for himself. He generally accepted the medical establishment's appraisal of the situation: "They have an attitude of when, not if," and he decided to begin using pharmaceuticals early. His explanation for taking acyclovir and AZT before his physician recommended it had nothing to do with needing hope, power, or control. Matthew understood himself as having power and control already. Rather his attitude was expressed in very pragmatic terms: "I figure as long as it's going to be eventual— they keep telling me it's eventual . . . I might as well just start it now." Although Matthew organized much of his story around the loss of his lover, Robert, he did not tell it in terms of having to make changes or give things up.

Matthew: Once Robert was diagnosed and we got over the initial shock, things didn't change much. The major change was that Robert wasn't going to work anymore. He went on disability and was home all the time. After three or four months had gone by and he seemed fine and nothing happened, AIDS just became something to live with. For at least a year I really didn't think in terms of Robert's getting any sicker or about anything further than the moment. You never know. Some people just go on. Then about two years after he was diagnosed, we noticed some changes in his health.

Richard: So for two years you tried hard to just kind of deny it?

Matthew: I don't think we were denying it. The previous idea was that you get AIDS and you died. People all around us were dying, and that was a constant reminder. But the new idea developing was that you have AIDS and you live with it. After being diagnosed, AIDS was our life. But then life went on. Then when Robert got sick, AIDS became our life again.

Richard: What has sex been like since AIDS or since Robert was diagnosed?

Matthew: At first we stopped having sex with other people. We had been fairly promiscuous. I remember when I went to something or other and they asked me what I missed the most about sex in the old days, and my answer was, 'Being called a slut and taking it as a compliment.' We didn't know many people with AIDS at first. Then we called someone up to have sex with, and the person had been diagnosed two days earlier. At that point we both stopped having sex with other people.

Another change was rubbers. We hadn't been using rubbers with each other. We figured we'd been having sex for ten years together without rubbers and if we'd exposed each other, we'd exposed each other and that's the way it is. After Robert was diagnosed, one of the doctors said that repeated exposure may not be good, so we started using rubbers with each other. Robert liked them less than I do. Then about a year after he was diagnosed, I started having sex with other people again, and I just assumed everybody was positive. That was my attitude. It was always very, very safe. It slacks up a little sometimes, but I think it's still within safe-sex guidelines, from beating off to intercourse. But intercourse is always with rubbers, and I don't believe in coming in a rubber. I think there's too much potential to tear.

I realize that on the spectrum of things, everybody's idea of 'safe' is different, and some people would say that I'm being very safe, and others would say I'm not being safe enough. My guess is that, if I were negative, I would probably have a different set of guidelines. I'm not comfortable going out with people who think they are negative. I figure they may be negative, they may not be negative, but I don't want anyone to feel that I'm responsible for making them positive. So I prefer going out with someone who's positive.

Richard: You mentioned also that about a year after Robert was diagnosed, you started having sex with other people. What was that about? How did that work for the two of you?

Matthew: It just sort of happened. It was no big deal. Robert wasn't much interested in sex, and I still was. Robert became interested in sex only with certain people, and he was interested in doing things that I wasn't into. He had a couple of little sex friends, and most of my sex was like at the 1808 Club, you know, beating off and stuff.

AIDS can bring people together or pull them apart. After a while Robert just developed other interests. He had his spiritual people and his crystals and things that I did not share an interest in. It didn't create friction to have different interests. It just created a separation. My feeling is that whatever one believes, if it helps them, then that's good. But some of the stuff with psychics got to be a bit much for me. We went to this thing in Palo Alto where there was another voice going through the body and stuff. I figured they were profiteering off a lot of us, and I got annoyed with it. It's one thing to have Lazarus, but it's another thing to have Lazarus stores.[4] Robert would tell me that Lazarus wasn't the one profiteering; it was the channel. You'd think that Lazarus would speak to the channel and tell them not to profiteer. Robert could certainly afford it, but I had friends who had limited resources and were spending their money on this.

But people explore until they find what fits. Robert went into each thing with gusto and picked up pieces of each thing that worked for him. Some things worked better than others, and he stuck with them. He took what he could from things that didn't really work and just combined them into his little patchwork of whatever was going to help. I had interest in some things and doubts about others. Some of it seemed totally ridiculous. It was difficult at times for me to not share that with him, which was not being very supportive, but I could only go so far with some of it.

---

[4]Lazarus was a popular disembodied spirit channeled by a clairvoyant. Lazarus gave people advice on health and other matters. Lazarus tapes and books were for sale in many urban gay neighborhoods. San Francisco's Castro district even had a Lazarus store.

Matthew: I almost felt like I lost Robert about six months before he died. There was suddenly this wedge between us that wasn't there before. I felt I was there as a caretaker. There was an emotional change maybe four or five months before he died, but I was aware of it before his final illness. I withdrew a little bit. There's probably still something that hasn't come out. I don't know. I had very little in the way of tears after he died. I was just sort of numb for a while. I think a lot of it was just pushed out of my mind.

I still have Robert in the box upstairs. I haven't opened it, and I'm reluctant to part with it. I was going to take some of his ashes to Italy and some to the country, but I figured, well, I don't want to have him all over different places. How would he get back together again? I find it strange that I'm keeping the box of ashes there. I used to keep it out on the bathroom counter, but yesterday I put it away, under the counter. I was straightening up, and I figured it had been there for two months. When I was in the other house, I didn't want it in the closet because it was dark. I find it all a little peculiar.

Richard: I haven't scattered Duckus's ashes. If I ever do, it will be in one place.

Matthew: Why?

Richard: I think that that's what he would want. Yet he never told me exactly what to do with them.

Matthew: Robert didn't care. He was quite specific that he didn't care what happened to them. I thought I might take a cup of it and dump it in the river in Florence—or someplace—but who knows.

Richard: I don't know where to put Duckus because I don't know where I'm going to put me. Do you ever think about that?

Matthew: No, because I haven't decided what will happen to me. I don't know that I want to be cremated. I may want to go into the family plot. On the other hand, being underground sounds so unappealing. But I don't want to be burned either.

Richard: Being underground goes on and on and on. At least the burning is fast.

(laughing): It's all quite weird.

Matthew: I'll tell you what bothers me, and it's way off. I can't believe that they've not come up with a term for a deceased

lover. You'd think with all the creative minds—the the-
atrical, verbal, spiritual minds—that there'd be some sort
of term. When I talk about Robert, I don't want to call him
my former lover. I feel funny referring to him as my deceased lover. I really don't know how to refer to him when
I talk about him, and I've talked to other people who have
lost their lovers, and they all feel the same way. There's
no word for it. Wouldn't you imagine that someone would
come up with that?

Richard: What does the heterosexual community use? Do they
have such words? They don't. I don't think they do.

Matthew: But you're referred to as a widow or a widower. There's not
even a word for that for us. It's not really correct to be considered a widower. I just don't feel comfortable with that.
We need something that's not masculine/feminine, something "nondenominational." How do you refer to Duckus?

Richard: As my lover. Then I have to explain that he's gone. It's
weird. It's always awkward.

Matthew: It's awkward for the other person because then you have
to explain that they've died. It's socially awkward, and it's
emotionally awkward, which I think is more important.

Richard: What's dating been like since Robert died?

Matthew: I think another relationship is improbable. I think I'll date
people. Once I thought about whether I'd like to live with
someone I was dating, but then I thought, no. By the time
you hit forty, you have your home, your friends, and your
own way of doing things. Then suddenly there's someone
new. In the old days you did things together. You bought
a house, you furnished an apartment together, you made
friends together. I have all that stuff now, and the last
thing I'd want is someone moving in here who didn't have
my taste. I know, bad taste is really just taste that isn't my
taste. If their taste is too good, it's bad to me. The right
amount of funk, the right amount of this. I'm looking for
me. So I think that seems improbable.

Richard: That you'll find somebody like you?

Matthew: It's not really me because I wouldn't go out with me, but
someone who has interests that are similar enough, taste
that is overlapping enough, all that type of stuff. I think
that seems improbable. The people that I go out with
seem to be less sophisticated than I would like. That's an

elitist attitude, but you spend twenty years looking at art, going to the ballet and the opera, analyzing films, whatever, or just looking at things with a certain analytical eye. Then you meet someone who's very nice, and they've spent that time in the discos. It's just a difference in experience and what you see when you're with someone. I could go with Robert to some little town in the middle of nowhere, and we'd find things that were absolutely awe-inspiring. We could sit and look at the stonework in a wall for an hour—just a bunch of rocks piled up three hundred years ago—and see something in it and appreciate it. How do you find that again? Someone else might say, "Gee that's a nice wall."

Matthew: When we'd take trips, we wouldn't want to just be everywhere at once, so we'd try to get a focus. We'd focus fairly arbitrarily. One year we decided that what we were interested in were floor patterns. We were in various cathedrals in Italy, and everybody was looking at the stained glass windows, and we're photographing the floors. It's hard to do this with other people.

Richard: You mentioned a support group. Have you ever felt a need to get involved in a group that dealt with grief issues, especially in terms of Robert?

Matthew: Well, in my Friday group we devoted a meeting to my grief. That's the thing to do. But I haven't gone to one of their grief groups. I think my grief is something private, and I don't think it would help me to sit with a bunch of strangers and talk about my grief. In order to understand my grief, you'd have to know me and you'd have to know Robert.

There were a number of issues that created a sense of loss for Matthew before Robert died. They had a long history of supporting each other's divergent interests, but Robert's diagnosis brought these differences into stark relief. There was a wedge between them that hadn't been there before. Part of that wedge was certainly due to changing sexual and spiritual interests, but part of it was due to the simple fact of Robert's getting sicker. Matthew tried to support Robert's new directions, but that attempt came from his new role as a caregiver, not out of the long-term relationship they had enjoyed together.

Matthew was well aware that AIDS brought some people closer and pushed others apart, but a "big picture" awareness did not end his story. Matthew did not need information or processes. He knew what was going on inside himself. Matthew's grief was private. This is something health professionals and academicians must take seriously. The movement to capture the most fundamental aspects of our humanity in concepts, precise definitions, and universal social interventions often does more for academic careers than it does to relieve human suffering or develop better understandings of the human condition. Talking about grief is not the same as grieving. Sharing stories of deep personal loss with a therapeutic community of strangers is a modern invention that does not work for everyone. Although professional strangers are certainly necessary in modern times, they are no substitute for a community where life is celebrated and death is shared. Even when mourning is shared, the most profound grief is both private and universal, but rarely social.

Matthew also saw his long-term asymptomatic status as something personal and refused to help me develop a theoretical understanding of surviving HIV.

> *Richard:* I'd like to share some of my own impressions about how you are dealing with all of this, to see what you think of them. I know that a newspaper would say that you're average—that you've lived the average amount of time since being HIV positive. Of course, as you keep living longer, they keep upping the average. But never mind what the statisticians are saying about the future. You're the longest surviving HIV-positive person we know about. So I'm pretending that I'm an anthropologist going to those places where people live to be 110 and asking them what the secret of their longevity is.
>
> *Matthew:* I don't like that. A couple of years ago someone said, 'You're the kind of person who gives us hope because we see that you've been positive all these years and you seem to be fine.' It's a responsibility I'm not real thrilled about. I have the feeling that if I get sick, it's going to wreck all these people. I figure it would be enough for me to be sick without worrying about how everyone else might react. I could imagine people coming over and not being sure if they were concerned about me or about themselves.
>
> *Richard:* I can understand that, but right now you have managed for a long time with this, and our community needs to paint profiles of survivors. Whether you get sick or not, at

this point you're still in the survival mode. Gabe and I were talking about survival last week. You're not the only one, but we used you and a couple of other people to generate some initial thoughts about what it might take to survive this thing. I think you are an interesting model for survival because you're one of those people that combines a lot of opposites. You care about other people but are totally self-obsessed. You are as anxious as anyone, but you know about what help is available. You look at it all and don't really believe in any of it. Skeptical, yet engaged. It's almost a kind of healthy neurosis that's not about denial or acceptance or belief. You seem to be walking this very fine line. It's not about repressing a huge amount of feelings; it's not about giving vent to all the feelings. You're this odd combination of responses to—

Matthew: Then how come I can't get a good date?

Matthew neither confirmed nor denied the interpretive analysis that Gabe and I had constructed to explain why someone might survive with HIV. Matthew was not interested in our theories of survival and changed the subject with one of his typical wisecracks. And, whereas Matthew's story revolved around the loss of Robert, it cannot be adequately framed or interpreted with psychosocial concepts such as grief, social support, hope, or fear. To know Matthew's loss, you had to know Matthew, and what emerged most clearly from his story was an incredibly strong sense of self.

But Matthew's story was not simply a collection of idiosyncratic concerns. Losing people before they died or deciding what to do with a loved one's ashes reflects wider cultural concerns that become increasingly relevant as lesbians and gay men establish new identities, families, communities, and traditions. Matthew was extremely interested in community and participated in programs that lent support to people with AIDS. He never blamed the dominant culture for failing to develop effective treatments or for denying us a language in which to express our love and our grief. He was a part of that dominant culture and simply asked why the smarter members of our community had not already invented the language that we needed.

Likewise, decision-making theory does not help us understand Matthew's choice about early intervention with AZT. Matthew was certainly aware of a possible downside to taking AZT too early, but his decision was not framed as a rational cost-benefit analysis. Rather, he expressed it in terms of the mistake he did not want to make—waiting too long before taking advantage of something that would have helped. Nor was his story primarily about hopes or fears. For instance, Matthew seemed less overtly fearful than Nathan, but also less overtly hopeful. As much as possible, Matthew even avoided casting the lifestyle changes that he made in the 1980s in terms of HIV. Instead, matters such as reducing recreational drug use were presented as outcomes of his own personal development, his own changing desires.

Despite the fact that the numbers keep pushing him closer to the norm, Matthew remains one of our longest-known survivors, having tested positive in 1978. Twenty years later, in 1998, Matthew still has not developed AIDS. Perhaps it is good that he rejected the poster-boy role. The new research protocols do not count him as a long-term survivor anyway. He does not meet the new criteria for a "long-term nonprogressor." Almost none of us does. We do not have enough T cells.

REFERENCES

Allen, D. J. (1992). Introduction. In J. L. Thompson, D. G. Allen, & L. Rodrigues-Fisher (Eds.), *Critique, resistance, and action: Working papers in the politics of nursing*. New York: National League of Nursing Press.

Becker, E. (1973). *The denial of death*. New York: Free Press.

Brandt, A. (1987). *No magic bullet: A social history of venereal disease in the United States since 1880*. New York: Oxford University Press.

Brown, N. O. (1985). *Life against death: The psychoanalytical meaning of history* (2nd ed.). Middletown, CT: Wesleyan University Press.

Bullough, V., & Bullough, B. (1977). *Sin, sickness and sanity: A history of sexual attitudes*. New York: New American Library.

Crotty, M. (1996). *Phenomenology and nursing research*. Melbourne: Churchill Livingston.

Duesberg, P. (1996). *Inventing the AIDS virus*. Washington, DC: Regnery.

Eisenberg, D. M., Kessler, R. C., Foster, C., Norlock, F. E., Calkins, D. R., & Delbanco, T. L. (1993). Unconventional medicine in the United States: Prevalence, costs, and patterns of use. *New England Journal of Medicine*, 328(4) 246–252.

Fox, R. (1984). The medicalization and demedicalization of American society. In P. R. Lee, C. L. Estes & N. B. Ramsay (Eds.), *The Nation's Health* (2nd ed.) (pp. 145–159). San Francisco: Boyd and Fraser.

Freud, S. (1918). *Totem and taboo*. (A. Brill, Trans.). New York: Vintage. (Original work published 1913)

Freud, S. (1949). *An outline of psycho-analysis* (J. Strachey, Trans.). New York: Norton. (Original work published 1940)

Goffman, E. (1986). *Stigma: Notes on the management of spoiled identity* (2nd ed.). Englewood Cliffs, NJ: Touchstone.

Kierkegaard, S. (1983). *The sickness unto death* (H. Hong & E. Hong, Trans.). Princeton, NJ: Princeton University Press. (Original work published 1849)

MacIntyre, R. (1999). *Mortal men: Living with asymptomatic HIV.* New Brunswick, NJ: Rutgers University Press.

Root-Bernstein, R. (1993). *Rethinking AIDS: The tragic cost of premature consensus.* New York: Free Press.

Sonnebend, J. (1992, December). In D. Hopkins, Dr. Joseph Sonnabend. *Interview Magazine.* pp. 24–125, 142–143.

Sontag, S. (1988). *AIDS and its metaphors.* New York: Farrar, Straus & Giroux.

Watney, S. (1987). *Policing desire: Pornography, AIDS and the media.* Minneapolis: University of Minnesota Press.

Webster (1972). *Webster's new collegiate dictionary* (7th ed.). Springfield, MA: Merriam.

Wilber, K. (1986). *Up from Eden: A transpersonal view of human evolution.* Boston: Shambhala.

Wolf, Z. R. (1993). Nursing rituals: Doing ethnography. In P. L. Munhall and C. O. Boyd (Eds.), *Nursing research: A qualitative perspective.* New York: National League of Nursing Press.

Zerubavel, E. (1979). *Patterns of time in hospital life.* Chicago: University of Chicago Press.

Zola, I. (1984). Healthism and disabling medicalization. In P. R. Lee, C. L. Estes, & N. B. Ramsay (Eds.), *The Nation's Health* (2nd ed.) (pp. 160–169). San Francisco: Boyd and Fraser.

17

Action Research
The Method

Carolyn L. Brown

Health care practitioners love what works. They seek positive *outcomes* from their practices, whether direct patient care, administration, or education. The common denominator binding practice-oriented disciplines together is interest in results created from actions taken within the practice arena. Practitioners see a problem or issue, create a plan to resolve it, enact the plan, and use a "fly by the seat of our pants" approach based on expediency to determine the success of the outcome. If we meet the needs of the moment, put out today's fire, we are pleased with the outcome. Today, institutional administrators tell us that, if we meet the bottom line, contribute to the profit margin, get patients up and out the door quickly without their returning to the emergency room within a few days, have students who graduate without undue cost, we have done a good job. But, when the novice asks us, "How do you know you did a good job? How did you know what to do? Did you use a theory to guide your plan?" and myriad other questions, we have no answers. We essentially fly by the seat of our pants and keep few records other than that we have succeeded in the short run. We learned about research in our research classes (probably why you are reading this chapter now), theory in theory classes, and how to do what we do in our practice-oriented classes, with the little that we know of evaluation left to the research classes.

In an interview for Joel Kurtzman (1998), Chris Argyris spoke of the need to get to knowledge for action. Argyris has a long history of blending the practical need for action in the practice with the academic disciplines. He stated, "Let me also say at the outset that I'm interested in action, and not simply knowledge for the purpose of understanding and explaining. I'd love that, but it has to be knowledge for understanding, explaining, in order to act" (p. 1). Argyris talked about Model I behavior; behavior resulting in actions based on unquestioned acceptance of assumptions guiding everyday practice. With Model I behavior, the practitioner acts according to theory that does not encourage inquiry into or testing of the theory in use. Model I guides "seat of the pants" actions, doing what feels right intuitively and with little or no reflection on process or outcome. In contrast, Argyris pointed out, "With Model II, you encourage illustration, you encourage inquiry, you encourage testing" (Argyris in Kurtzman, 1998, p. 6), thus providing the foundations for action research. Those engaged in practice should find the notion of action research, reflective inquiry leading to informed action to improve practice, particularly attractive. In nursing, Holter and Schwartz-Barcott (1993) described the usefulness of action research to nursing practice.

ACTION RESEARCH DEFINED

What *is* action research? Definitions vary widely. In search of an answer to this simple yet very complex question, I came upon a book titled *Action Research as a Living Practice* (Carson & Sumara, 1997). As a title and as an approach to inquiry, I find this notion particularly attractive. It originated in the Department of Secondary Education at the University of Alberta, a place known to be friendly to qualitative work and home to the Institute for Qualitative Methods. Carson and Sumara ask a foundational question, "What are the relationships among forms of *educational* action research, written reports of action research, and the lived experiences of action researchers?" (Carson & Sumara, 1997, p. xii). The reader may easily substitute any discipline for *education* because action research is in no way limited to education. Action research, according to these authors, "is a lived practice that requires that the researcher not only investigate the subject at hand but, as well, provide some account of the way in which the investigation both shapes and is shaped by the investigator" (p. xii). In health care, such an approach calls us to be accountable for our practices, our outcomes, our ethical responsibilities within economic constraints, and our processes. Action research provides a way to live practice as a part of the overall living of our lives; it brings together the whole of that experience. Action research provides a way to be accountable for the how, what, and why of practice; a way to *enact* meaningful practice.

HISTORY OF ACTION RESEARCH

In the twentieth century, inquirers diverged from principles established in the Enlightenment period—a period bringing humankind out of the Dark Ages into the Age of Reason and the birth of science as presented to current students for the first time in kindergarten curricula and reinforced all the way through formal education. Peter Reason (1998) proposed a dialectic of thought in regard to this important period in the history of the world.

> [This more] . . . orthodox scientific world view . . . represents a liberating step for human society in releasing itself from the bonds of superstition and Scholasticism. From another perspective, it is a movement to narrow our view of our world and to monopolize knowing in the hands of an elite few, and is fueled by patriarchy, alienation, and materialism; it is the product of a society committed to the domination of nature and of other peoples . . . (Reason, 1998, p. 261)

Such ideas are antithetical to action research, a type of inquiry founded in ideas of participation and usefulness. Disciplines focused on knowledge for use, where action research provides a useful approach, include education, social work, nursing, organizational development, and business, among others.

Over time, action research has come to be associated with varied degrees of participation by persons undertaking the research rather than with traditional researchers who come to the research setting with preconceived ideas of what should be studied and how. In traditional research, the plan for the research comes from the top down, meaning that the researcher plans the research, controls for as many variables as possible, and imposes the plan on the subjects, who, in the best designs, are compliant. They agree to be acted upon to inform the research, thus contributing to knowledge. Extant theory often gives rise to a hypothesis, the researcher's best guess about outcomes of the research. In contrast, the focus of action research is everyday practice. It is useful and is usually based on full participation for all who take part in the research process. Its purpose is to create and evaluate change that works for all research participants. The research is not created from the top down, but rather employs the talents and knowledge of participants to create practical actions based on reflective practice, yielding outcomes relevant to that practice. No one is acted upon but rather participants act *with* researchers.

Historically, Kurt Lewin, a social psychologist, is given credit for creating the grounding for action research (Greenwood & Levin, 1998). His work, starting in the United States (he fled Germany's repressive Nazi regime) in the 1940s, gave rise to a simple model of change. This model was created by Lewin to envision action to achieve a goal: unfreeze, change, refreeze. In fact, this grounding for action research was so simple that it caught on with practical-minded clinicians and managers who wanted visible results now, results demonstrating effectiveness of programs or clinical interventions. Lewin's model lends itself to action research in that participants in the research from practice and the academy come together as equals in a process to craft research from inception to evaluation. The aim is to create some sort of change of benefit to all parties.

The Tavistock group, also an early founder of action research, formed in Great Britain after World War II and continues to occupy a central role in action research as a way to humanize work settings through psychoanalytic and psychological principles. In 1947, the Tavistock Institute, stressing social science in action, formed as an independent nonprofit group to "combine research in the social sciences with professional practice" (Tavistock Institute, 1999). A spinoff of the early work of this institute moved the world of work from the Tayloristic machinelike view of workers as cogs in a factory assembly line to seeing them as contributing, thinking, feeling human beings. Those trying to improve industrial work, through varied action foci, moved industry toward more democratic models with emphasis on participation (Greenwood & Levin, 1998). The work of the Tavistock Institute continues today through independent, interdisciplinary action approaches to organizational change and evaluation in "new and experimental programs, particulary in health, education and community development" (Tavistock Institute, 1999).

Chris Argyris, in concert with Donald Schön (Anderson, 1999), formed a bridge from the historical to the present through conceptualizing the idea of "action science," a way of conceptualizing action research still important today. Argyris has worked in this area since the 1970s with a particular interest in *organizational* change (Argyris, 1993). Schön's work contained a more psychological twist, with strong emphasis on reflective practice. Both advocated for positive change in varied practice settings. In *Action Science*, Argyris, Putnam, and McClain Smith (1985) spoke about intervention in a current situation such that the situation improves. Intervention, in this context, may be equated with change or action. In a recent interview (Argyris interviewed by Kurtzman, 1998, p. 1), Argyris explained his passion for action in relation to knowledge when he emphasized that knowledge must be useful. Central to Argyris's work is the notion of "theory in use" and espoused theory in relation to actions of individuals. People "espouse certain theories to explain what the world is about. But what really influences their actions are their theories in use. These are designs that tell people how to behave" (Argyris interviewed by Kurtzman, 1998, p. 1). As a result of using either espoused theory or theory in use, two types of learning take place:

> Single-loop learning refers to a situation where people or organizations alter their behavior but do nothing to change the behavioral strategies that gave rise to the problematic situation initially. . . . By contrast, double-loop learning results from responding to a problem by stepping back and examining alternative larger frames into which the problem can be put. The immediate problem is understood to be the product of a context that itself must be altered. (Greenwood & Levin, 1998, p. 190)

Greenwood and Levin, in their discussion of Argyris's work, linked models of action to the two types of learning. They described Model I as being related to "unilateral control over others. Few people espouse Model I, but many people practice it" (Greenwood & Levin, 1998, p. 192). The result is behavior aimed to please rather than to deal openly with real problems. Model I actions create images, not solutions. Model II theories of action, they stated, result in relations with slight or no defensive base, greater risk taking, and freedom to choose. In the collectives of individuals in organizations, "The result is the creation of a *community of inquiry* in which issues and conflicts can be opened up and in which both single- and double-loop learning occurs" (Greenwood & Levin, 1998, p. 192).

Argyris's work in action science relies heavily on the notion of intervention. I find myself asking whether all action aimed to create a more positive outcome needs to be an intervention. Intervention disrupts, occurs between events, often is imposed by others, and interferes with the status quo. Must all change in action research come from planned disruptions? But questions such as these flow from each person's philosophy, or even the Zeitgeist, and lead to the question of who participates in action research? Who, when, why, and whether to intervene rest in the nature of the expectations of the participants in the action research project. All of this leads again to the notion of participation in the action research process. Readers who think of engaging in research or inquiry leading to action and hope for positive results may imagine themselves at the center of the process. Action research may be seen as a way to achieve the hoped-for results and to get people to listen, all the while tracking process and contributing to the body of knowledge about the project. Participation as central to action research is briefly discussed next.

CONTEMPORARY ACTION RESEARCH

People often associate research with experts. Experts are the ones who know enough about the organization or practice of whatever discipline to ask the right questions or make the right hypotheses. Practitioners often feel intimidated by the lofty knowledge of the researcher. The persons at the bottom of the hierarchy, as it is often imaged, defer to the researcher, who frequently comes from academia, a place not unlike a magic kingdom where riches surely dwell and a strange foreign-sounding language provides the medium for communication. These persons—patients, students, residents, the ordinary person hoping to benefit from knowledge—see themselves as *subjects*, not as a part of this important-sounding research process.

Peter Reason discussed three conceptualizations of participative inquiry in his chapter in *Strategies of Qualitative Inquiry* (Denzin & Lincoln, 1998). Each of these approaches used action research as its foundation. In this chapter, Reason (1998) discussed cooperative inquiry, participatory action research, and action science or action inquiry. Reason discussed his own philosophy regarding participative research structures when he said,

> Let me be clear that my personal and professional commitment is to contribute to the emergence of this more participative worldview; that I write this chapter as an advocate of the methods presented rather than as an outside reviewer. I have devoted the past 15 years of my professional life to the development and application of co-operative inquiry in which the emphasis is on working with groups as co-researchers. . . . It seems

to me to be urgent for the planet and for all its creatures that we discover ways of living in more collaborative relation with each other and with the wider ecology. I see these participative approaches to inquiry and the worldview they foster as part of this quest. (Reason, 1998, p. 262)

John Heron's (1996) model is one of cooperative inquiry, whereas Ernest Stringer (1996) and Davydd Greenwood with Morten Levin (1998) provide guidelines for action research without participation as a central focus. Reason (1998) highlights the feminist blend of ideas of action research with empowerment of people, a central thesis of Glittenberg's work with action research presented in this book (see Chapter 18). Ideas surrounding how varied actors participate in the process of inquiry are important to action research, and they surface repeatedly in the different approaches. In this section, the work of researchers from varied disciplines is presented. The next section presents a synthesis of models of action research for the beginning researcher/practitioner—a guide. Last, a brief description of action research within nursing in a health care organization is presented and critiqued.

Cooperative Inquiry: John Heron (1996)

Heron (1996), in his introduction, provides what he calls a brief history of cooperative inquiry. Key to the notion of cooperative inquiry is the idea that "Each person is co-subject in the experience phases and co-researcher in the reflection phases" (p. 1). Although Heron's cooperative inquiry shares some of its history with action research grounded in the work of Kurt Lewin (1952), much of the foundation for cooperative inquiry rests in the idea that "It is a vision of persons in reciprocal relation using the full range of their sensibilities to inquire together into any aspect of the human condition with which the transparent body-mind can engage" (Heron, 1996, p. 1). Heron bases his work on the phenomenological tradition, believing that the researcher can produce valid inferences only when honoring full participation of all actors in an inquiry process. One cannot perform an experiment on another as object while engaging in cooperative inquiry. Coequal partnerships form the essential core for cooperative inquiry and differentiate it from other forms of action inquiry. In cooperative inquiry, the researcher does not stand apart from the process of the inquiry in any way and does not drop into the research setting with his or her own environment or self being immune to change. The whole—including the context of the researchers' homes and work settings and the assumptions undergirding academia and the research itself—becomes of concern as the questions, processes, and outcomes of the research process flow from genuinely coequal generation of inquiry. Heron sees action research as a necessary part of the cooperative inquiry process, coming into play "in the action phase of a co-operative inquiry, when each person is busy implementing some action-plan decided on in the prior reflection phase. The skills of action inquiry are thus a fundamental component of co-operative inquiry, but they also reach far beyond it" (pp. 8–9).

Action Research for Practitioners: Ernest T. Stringer (1996)

Stringer (1996) provides a model for community-based action research, an approach linking "processes of inquiry to the lives of people as they come to grips with the problems and stresses that beset them in their day-to-day lives" (p. xv). Community-based action research provides a useful approach to inquiry for *practitioners* from all disciplines: "teachers, health workers, social workers, community workers, administrators, and other human service workers . . ." (p. xvii) with practitioners placed in the role of *research facilitator.* Stringer sees the role of the practitioner as providing "leadership and direction to other participants or stakeholders in the research process" (p. xvii). Practitioners may also ask outside consultants to join them in leading the research process should their knowledge gaps or job demands invite such a collaborative approach.

Stringer (1996) sees research as a simple process, one used by all of us every day. It entails a problem, an inquiry process, and an explanation allowing for understanding the problem, culminating in *"actions* that attempt to resolve the problem being investigated" (p. 5). He sees the process as a continuance of processes that we use to solve day-to-day problems. For example, in nursing, such simple questions as who needs to take part in patients' care, how care should be prioritized, what to include in care, and so forth, constitute everyday problems requiring solutions that include action.

Anthropology and other social science disciplines form the root of action research. Glittenberg's work (see Chapter 18) speaks to doing ethnography that, in essence, turned into action research. As stated earlier in the present chapter, action research is related to efforts to improve the situation for participants. Community-based action research as used by Stringer (1996) fits this definition. It is social in nature, "always enacted through an explicit set of social values" (p. 9) through processes that are democratic, equitable, liberating, and life enhancing. "As they collectively investigate their own situation, stakeholders build a consensual vision of their life-world [resulting not only in] . . . a collective vision but also in a sense of community" (p. 10). Given the contemporary focus of nursing on community-based education and programs, Stringer's approach seems particularly well suited to solving problems that arise owing to changes in both educational and care delivery programs.

The essence of action research, for Stringer (1996), rests in the following statement and highlights the difference between action research and traditional research approaches: "You know . . . the difference with your work is that you expect something to *actually happen* as a result of your activities" (p. 11). In collaboration, practitioners and others create a way to take "systematic action to resolve specific problems" (p. 15). The approach is simple, once all inquirers have agreed to the basic philosophical principles undergirding the approach. It consists of *looking* at the situation to gather information about it and fully describe it; *thinking* about the situation to roll it about in the mind, forming tentative hypotheses about why and how the situation exists as it is (hypothesizing and generating theory); and *acting* through processes of planning, implementing, and evaluating. Stringer cautions practitioners to avoid thinking of these processes as linear. One does not simply look-think-act and then you are done. The processes take place in a spiral-like format, all taking place simultaneously, yet moving the whole of the activity to a higher point in the spiral. For example, while one is carrying out a part of the process, one is gathering information, all the while reflecting on the information gathered and thus informing the next action phase of the project. All of these processes (looking, thinking, acting) are inherent—in fact, are second nature—in the actions of any practice discipline. Perhaps formal evaluation is the least used in practice, because most practitioners take the informal view that if everyone is happy, the change is visible, and we have met the bottom-line expectations of the higher ups, the less-reflective "fly by the seat of the pants" approach was successful. The patient got well, the child learned, the organization made money.

Practitioners take a more formal evaluative stance when things do not go as planned or when some of the stakeholders are not happy. Then more evaluation processes are sought to preclude the recurrence of the error.

Like the other action researchers presented in this chapter, Stringer (1996) believes that "Community-based action research seeks to change the social and personal dynamics of the research situation so that it is noncompetitive and nonexploitative and enhances the lives of all those who participate" (p. 19). Rather than adversarial in their approach, those engaged in community-based action research act consensually *with* other stakeholders, rather than having the central intent of confronting and eradicating oppression. The primary mode of action of this type of research is to link people together, even those who may be in conflict, in order to find mutually acceptable and beneficial solutions to problems.

> Its intent is not only to "get the job done," but to ensure the well-being of everyone involved. This notion runs contrary to many of the imperatives enshrined in bureaucratic practices that make up much of our public life. We have come to accept the impersonal, mechanistic, and allegedly objective procedures common to many health, education, and welfare services and business corporations as a necessary evil. We endure hierarchical and authoritarian modes of organization and control despite the sense of frustration, powerlessness, and stress frequently felt by both practitioners and the client groups they serve. (Stringer, 1996, p. 19)

Most practitioners hope to empower those they serve, as well as to enhance their well being. In order for practice disciplines to be effective, the will of the people served in planning for change must take center stage. Thus, research that fully acknowledges the personal worth of individuals, families and communities, and extends maximum choice potential for the same, stands a much better chance of success. Stringer's approach mirrors Lincoln and Guba's (1989) in *Fourth Generation Evaluation* through emphasis on full participation in the research process, equity for all participants, and co-participant roles for all involved in the research process. Authoritarianism and superiority of the knowledgeable researcher are ruled out. While the research proceeds, community is built. Thus, the researcher and/or practitioner do not enter the research situation with any particular set of expectations other than to take direction from the developing community and initially, to address the situation posed by the community and deemed to be in need of solution.

Participatory Action Research:
William Foote Whyte (1991)

Whyte (1991), as editor of *Participatory Action Research*, highlighted three branches of thought influencing the development and practice of participatory action research (PAR). He clearly situates PAR in social research approaches, participation in decision making for all levels of organizational personnel, and "sociotechnical systems thinking regarding organizational behavior" (p. 7). He divides his work into two parts—PAR in industry and PAR in agriculture—with examples of PAR presented from work done in different nations of the world. Whyte and others decry the hegemony of the well-entrenched positivist approach to scientific research. The work of Whyte (1991) lays the groundwork for the later work of Greenwood and Levin (1998) on action research. Whyte, Greenwood, and Lazes (1991) defined PAR:

> [S]ome of the people in the organization or community under study participate actively with the professional researcher throughout the research process from the initial design to the final presentation of results and discussion of their action implications. (p. 20)

PAR is applied research, with all participants in active engagement with the research process. Perhaps one of the most important contributions of Whyte, Greenwood, and Lazes (1991) is the notion that PAR is clearly interdisciplinary. Each discipline contributes its own unique perspective, adding richness and relevance to the outcome. They also noted that PAR, like other qualitative approaches, is informed by "continuous learning" through constant inclusion of data from all participants as information to be used to correct the research process. All participants become more acutely aware of the problems, examine the incoming information, have an active role in the research process, and warrant the practical usefulness of emerging theory, which is subject to on-the-spot testing through the PAR process. Also growing out of Whyte's (1991) work on PAR is Elden and Levin's (1991) model for cogenerative learning (p. 130). This model was called a model for PAR Scandinavia Style: The Co-generative Way; it clearly depicts the roles of insiders and outsiders, an idea that I adapted in a simple model for those who wish to begin a PAR project (Figure 17–1).

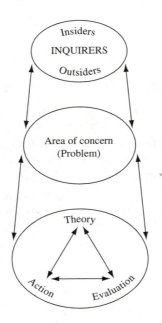

Figure 17–1   Action research cycle.

A GUIDE FOR ACTION RESEARCH

The action research cycle presented here is both simple and complex. It is a meld of the thinking of many in the field and is presented in a "cookbook" fashion. Bear in mind, the process is not linear, step-by-step, as it will appear on presentation. What is required varies according to the setting, the actors, and the desired outcomes. As in any good recipe, the mix requires fine tuning, with varying amounts and preparation of each ingredient. At first, the cook will follow the recipe exactly as it is written. Experience provides the wisdom to make the fine changes necessary for the mix to turn out extremely well. An experienced action researcher (cook) knows, almost intuitively, what needs to happen at each step in the process. Mistakes will occur. Such mistakes may require that the researcher start over or the mistake may simply be folded into the end product. Process and outcome vary.

Starting Out
All action research, like most qualitative work, begins with noticing something. In action research, we usually notice something that needs

some change, some action to bring about the desired change. Often, when we first notice that something needs to change, what needs to be changed and how to change it eludes us. We experience a sensation or thought that something is not right the way it is. Sometimes, as in Glittenberg's work (Chapter 18), knowing happens dramatically. A whole community arises in anger at the event of a young man's death; factory or hospital workers go out on strike to protest the erosion of wages and benefits or the diminishing to the danger point of resources for giving adequate care; a nation reverberates to the threat of impending war or to children killing children in public schools. Or, less dramatically, a nurse notices that patients released from the hospital shortly after admission return with symptoms dramatically worse or with an iatrogenic infection; an administrator notices that the hospital is losing good nurses and cannot so easily replace them from the shrinking pool of available experienced personnel; nurses are leaving the profession and faculty in a school of nursing notices dramatic decreases in enrollment. Both the dramatic and the mundane examples create a sense of unease, a knowing that something must be done. Noticing creates a call to action. Very often, what occurs next is problem solving, with action taken. The process stops there. Little is learned from the situation other than how to solve the next problem. Students continue to learn the same old theories that do not work, because the theories are not informed by practice, by actions that work and that have been incorporated into the body of a discipline's knowledge base. Action research corrects that problem by contributing useful theory to knowledge.

So, after noticing, those who notice make a commitment to do something; something likely to make a difference for more than the current problem—action with a long-range objective, not just putting out the fires of the emergency and being satisfied with the short-haul success in the present.

Very often those who first notice a problem of concern are those "in the trenches," those responsible for producing effective efficient services or products. Also, very often these people are not proficient researchers. They may not even know the most current information available about the area of concern. When struggling from day to day, practitioners barely have time to look up the latest drug, the latest treatment, or the latest teaching approach. Who has time for the latest management technique, the best way to empower people, the best way to contribute to knowledge so that the huge bank of information in the ranks of practice is not lost?

Deciding Who Takes Part

The next step is to decide who needs to be invited to work on the area of concern. I should take a moment to state that, just as often as not, the ones who notice may be clinicians/researchers from outside the system or recipients of services who bring the area of concern to the attention of the local clinicians. No matter who does the noticing, for action research to ensue, the information must be taken to the next step: deciding whom to tell, whom to bring into the circle of potential actors for the project.

In Figure 17–1, the arrows between the inquirers and the area of concern are double headed. They represent the interaction between who is part of the action research cycle and the area of concern. This is so in the following way. Who we are, our professional "set," provides a particular lens through which to view and interpret a situation. Thus who we are determines, in part, what we see as an area of concern. However, the particular area of concern, once noticed, demands the participation of certain persons, often called stakeholders. Who needs to be a part of the process? The problem calls for action, a solution. An early decision is whether those who notice the area of concern then help to determine whether the solving of the problem will move the process to action research or whether that decision rests with others. If a longer-term solution is sought, very often someone outside the situation is sought to assist and very likely this person will come from a university setting where knowledge for the future in the form of theory, with this theory based in research, is highly valued. The "insiders" often ask these folk to join the effort because they recognize that they have limited time to research the area of concern and a lack of advanced, up-to-the-minute knowledge about how to undertake research to generate the most credible (valid) results. At this point, resources also are at issue. *Who will pay for the costs of the project?* Are the potential benefits great enough to warrant the expenditure of resources? In the Glittenberg example, external grants paid for the project. In regard to an organizational concern, if the payoff is deemed adequate, the organization will pay for the project. How this decision is made will have a lot to do with who takes part in the project.

Who needs to be part of the process also includes deciding what one thinks about *empowerment and the sharing of power*, and about *participation and inclusion*. These two areas intertwine, meaning that what one believes about empowerment and the sharing of power influences how and which actors are included in the process. The more genuine sharing there is at all phases of the research cycle, the more participants are empowered and the more they will contribute. The "up" side to full empowerment and participation comes when actors can truly say, "We did it!" Full empowerment and participation mean that, the more the actors share in responsibility for both the process and the outcome of the action research endeavor, the more they own it. The "down" side of full empowerment and participation for all actors means that the researcher relinquishes full control over the process and outcome. The researcher and all other participants become coequal partners and must truly believe that each participant in the cycle contributes material of importance. One must relinquish the Orwellian stance in *Animal Farm*: the pigs are more equal. All participants have equal value.

In taking on the values of full participation and empowerment, all parties must recognize that the process of coming to agreement about all decisions takes much more time than does a more traditional top-down leadership approach. In this day of moving quickly and economically, the action research process may not be the most efficient solution for the short term. However, when all have a stake in the validity of the project, the potential for success grows. Insider and outsider roles blur. When the project is truly a "we" endeavor, no participant can later point fingers and say, " 'They' didn't know what we are really like, so 'they' made a mistake in recommending a particular action." So, all share equally in the success or failure (or some outcome in between) of the endeavor. No one takes the major credit for the project; nor can anyone blame someone else for difficulties or failures.

How to gain full participation and empowerment includes many different strategies. An initial group meeting of participants starts the project off on the right foot. Here the group may talk about beliefs undergirding the project, making explicit the underlying philosophies of the participants. Determining stakeholders (those who have a stake in the outcome of the project or will be affected by its process) is imperative at this early stage, as is how to achieve full participation. How stakeholders can best take part also may be determined through these initial meetings.

The Action Research Triangle of Knowledge

In Figure 17–1, double-headed arrows extend between the area of concern and the processes of creating theory, determining actions, and evaluating. Double-headed arrows also link the *triangle of theory–action–evaluation*. The double-headed arrows in the model speak to the interactiveness of the process. All actions happen simultaneously, not in a step-by-step format. Theory is formulated by each person and by the group as it grapples with the nature of the area of concern and who needs to be included. This is the first level of theory, a theory in use, according to Argyris (1993; Anderson, 1999). It is less formal than traditional ideas of theory. Theory here provides a loose map of the territory, rather than a rigidly determined map of verisimilitude. Theory in use helps the inquirers to know what to notice, how to interpret it, whom to ask to join the endeavor, what actions will be taken, how to interpret and evaluate the processes and outcomes, leading to new theory in use. The cycle is complete and repeats itself, continuously moving to the next level. Thus, the cycle repeats in a spiral fashion rather than a circular fashion, which denotes closure. In the action research cycle, closure occurs only when participants agree that the cycle is complete.

The process for action research can be seen in Glittenberg's example in Chapter 18. Her description of trying to build a snowman while studying snow in the middle of an avalanche speaks volumes about the action research cycle. Approaches to action research take form through the process of doing the research itself. As the process unfolds, the aims of the research become clearer, albeit at all times modifiable. Nothing is concrete. Thus, the process of living in the situation while that same situation continues applies to the full triangle of knowledge—theory–action–evaluation. Action research is in constant motion, constant action if you will. It takes its approaches from an ongoing evaluation process leading to theory leading to actions. Thus, when Glittenberg says that participants in one project stated, in regard to a very far reaching program to eradicate health hazards, "There are no flies," the project achieved the outcomes that it sought. Disease-bearing flies and their filthy habitats have disappeared. The contribution to scholarship comes through theoretical descriptions communicated to others who would aim for similar ends. Testing theory comes through applications of the material published, not in the way of verisimilitude but in the way of providing a lens through which to see and evaluate. The lenses are tested for usefulness.

The reader will notice the lack of a linear lockstep approach to how each part of the process takes place. There is no other way to present "how to" other than to say that the process of the action research project dictates the next steps in the process. All steps are going on simultaneously and feed one another. To engage in action research, all participants must have faith in the process, in one another, and in the approach itself.

An Experience with a "Failed" Action Research Project

In the early 1990s, an academic nurse researcher worked with a community hospital group on a participatory action research project. At first, her role in the project was unclear in that the basis of her entry into the facility was her knowledge of empowerment and organization, not her knowledge and expertise as a researcher. She had been asked to assist on specific organizational matters related to the department. Several problem areas were discussed and agreed to by the chief nursing officer and the researcher. In the early stages, the researcher agreed to lead the group in a strategic planning session for the nursing department, an approach that helped the department take its direction from its members. Because the researcher could see the merit of doing the project as research and because she had been heavily influenced by work on empowerment and by William Foote Whyte's book titled *Participatory Action Research*, after the first strategic planning session, she began to talk with the chief nursing officer about the merits of beginning to define their work as PAR. The nurse executive agreed, and they began to work according to Elden and Levin's Co-generative Learning Model (1991). In this model, insiders and outsiders defined a project together, which is what had, in fact, already been done through many discussions and through the departmental strategic planning session.

The direction sought was a greater voice in decisions for the nurses. As the project unfolded, more and more action began to occur in the direction of creating a shared governance model to allow staff nurses and nurse managers to have more active and real participation in the decisions affecting them and their patients. The nurses were energized and felt good about what they were creating. Unfortunately, the rest of the people in the hospital became more and more uneasy. The hospital had always been patriarchal, albeit benevolent. In fact, before the present leader, the CEO was dubbed "father," and the then director of nursing was "mother." Very little in the institution ever changed. In fact, at one time, the entryway to the hospital, designed with beautiful cut stone work, was seen as symbolic of the unchanging nature of the hospital and its unyielding stances regarding nursing and any other changes.

Outside the small community where the hospital was situated, massive change was taking place in the health care sector, changes that would ultimately affect this hospital. Managed care was being adopted at breakneck speed, and the government was tightening regulation and spending while increasing scrutiny of billing practices. Hospitals had little room for discretionary decision making in how they allocated responsibility for expenses incurred in the treatment of patients. Small, stand alone hospitals were being gobbled up to form larger profit-driven corporations. As did many threatened institutions, instead of becoming more and more flexible to allow rapid response to change, the hospital tightened its structures more and more. Fear began to grow. A scapegoat was sought and found in the person of the nurse executive who was blamed for much of the unrest. She was offered an opportunity to resign and, in typical corporate practice, escorted off the property. A few weeks later, the researcher met with the acting nurse executive (a person without academic credentials beyond a diploma from a 3-year nursing school and no education in administration), who told her that the project had been placed on hold. That was the end of it. The project went no farther.

What happened? For one, the nursing department tried to act without fully acknowledging stakeholders in the rest of the hospital and the community, the political environment. Much of what project participants were trying to do was right and in keeping with the principles of action research. However, ignoring the political environment was a fatal flaw. In addition, creating a genuine participatory process for the project in an otherwise benevolent autocracy was a mistake. Full and genuine participation was not congruent with the rest of the system and resulted in anxiety. The executive who commissioned the work was out of synchronization with the rest of the institution and with the nursing department, one that a few short months before had been led by a director of nursing with no higher education. Although members of the rest of the administration paid lip service to wanting a better prepared nurse executive who would help move the department into step with contemporary practices, they did not fully understand what they sought. For many reasons, a project based in principles of empowerment could not succeed in that institution at that time.

Engaging in an action research project is always a complex and unpredictable process. From its inception, it fits into the qualitative, naturalistic paradigm where the context is highly interwoven and situational. Little or nothing is controllable. The process contains the nucleus of the project's aims. So, in many ways, though the project did not come to a clean and neat conclusion, it was not a failure. Those who participated learned much about themselves, their workplace, what is necessary to create democratic decision making in an organization, who needs to take part when a change is made, and how to survive when the outcome is not the desired outcome.

REFERENCES

Anderson, L. (1999). *Action research papers*: Argyris and Schön's theory on congruence and learning. Available: http://www.scu.edu.su/schools/sawd/arr/argyris.html.

Argyris, C. (1993). *Knowledge for action*: A guide to overcoming barriers to organizational change. San Francisco, CA: Jossey-Bass.

Argyris, C., Putnam, R., & McClain Smith, D. (1985). Action science: concepts, methods, and skills for research and intervention. San Francisco, CA: Jossey-Bass.

Carson, T. R., & Sumara, D. J. (1997). *Action research as a living practice*. New York: Peter Lang.

Denzin, N. K., & Lincoln, Y. S. (Eds.). (1998). *Strategies of qualitative inquiry*. Thousand Oaks, CA: Sage.

Elden, M., & Levin, M. (1991). Co-generative learning: Bringing participation into action research. In W. F. Whyte (Ed.), *Participatory action research* (pp. 127–142). Thousand Oaks, CA: Sage.

Glittenberg, J. (2001). Action research: Building a snowman while you study snow in the middle of an avalanche. In P. Munhall (Ed.), Nursing research: A qualitative perspective (pp. 523–533). Boston: Jones and Bartlett.

Greenwood, D. J., & Levin, M. (1998). *Introduction to action research*: Social research for social change. Thousand Oaks, CA: Sage.

Heron, J. (1996). *Co-operative inquiry*: Reserach into the human condition. Thousand Oaks, CA: Sage.

Holter, I. M., & Schwartz-Barcott, D. (1993). Action research: What is it? How has it been used and how can it be used in nursing? *Journal of Advanced Nursing*, 18(2), 298–304.

Kurtzman, J. (1998). *An interview with Chris Argyris*. Available: http://www.strategy-business.com/thoughtleaders/98109.

Lincoln, Y. S., & Guba, E. G. (1985). *Naturalistice inquiry*. Beverly Hills, CA: Sage.

Orwell, G. W. (1946). *Animal farm*. New York: Harcourct Brace Jovanovich.

Reason, P. (1988). *Human inquiry in action*: Developments in new paradigm research. Newbury Park, CA: Sage.

Reason, P. (1998). Three approaches to participative inquiry. In N. K. Denzin & Y. S. Lincoln (Eds.), Strategies of qualitative inquiry (pp. 261–291). Thousand Oaks, CA: Sage.

Stringer, E. T. (1996). Action research: A handbook for practitioners. Thousand Oaks, CA: Sage.

The Tavistock institute: Social science in action. (1999). Available: http://www.tavinstitute.org.

Whyte, W. F. (1991). Participatory action research. Thousand Oaks, CA: Sage.

Whyte, W. F., Greenwood, D. J., & Lazes, P. (1991). Participatory action research: Through practice to science in social research. In W. F. Whyte (Ed.), Participatory action research (pp. 19–55). Thousand Oaks, CA: Sage.

18

Building A Snowman While You Study Snow in the Middle of an Avalanche

Jody Glittenberg

"They've killed me, Momma," cried Oscar as he lay dying, another victim of a stray bullet from a gang-related drive-by shooting. Moments earlier he and his three older sisters had been opening his presents, celebrating his eleventh birthday, October 6, 1996. It was a beautiful evening, so the family had gone to enjoy soft drinks on the front porch when suddenly two cars filled with rival gang members came barreling down the street, rapid gun fire spurting in all directions—one bullet struck Oscar, and he died moments later in the arms of his hysterical mother. Sorrow and outrage grew in the small Mexican American town, long held hostage by the ever-increasing street violence; it was incensed—losing one of its most promising youngsters. Local news media began to unfold the story of Oscar, a model student in a barrio of poverty-stricken, recent immigrants. Media pounded on the facts that gang-related violence was not the only form of civil disorder in this small town where prostitutes and drug dealers openly conducted their trade and local residents never left their homes after dark, fearful for their lives. The townspeople and leaders were dismayed and in conflict about what could be done to change this destructive path. In the street, Oscar's parents and sisters, I, and thousands of others marched to protest this growing violence, shouting, "Enough!" "Enough!" We, the protesting people, tried to bring the community into a collective action toward changing the path of continued slaughter of innocent people. Oscar became the symbolic martyr for the town, as churches filled with concerned citizens from all walks of life and emotional issues were debated hotly. Several federal grants were received to improve the community police force and for some youth programs. Tougher laws were passed to round up hardened criminals and get them behind bars.

I had been doing ethnographic research in their town since I first arrived at the University of Arizona, in 1992, because I saw a community at risk. I had a group of minority high-school students do a Project GENESIS (General Ethnography and Needs Evaluations in a System) in the town in 1995, as a way to seek preliminary data to obtain funding through the National Institute on Drug Abuse (NIDA). I was to do an ethnographic study of alcohol- and drug-related violence by living with the people in this distraught town. The study, funded for 3 years, began in 1997. The research team consisted of Dr. Charles Anderson, a legal anthropologist, Richard Corona, a research specialist with years of drug rehabilitation counseling experience, and Mary Lou Chacon, an administrative assistant, a single mother with a teenaged daughter. We were all into the fray, partnering with the people in the poor barrio, becoming part of the solution. In this chapter, I will describe the process of initiating action research, the dilemmas faced, and the ethical concerns in doing such research.

ETHNOGRAPHIC RESEARCH: STUDYING SNOW IN THE MIDDLE OF AN AVALANCHE

The action research that I do is ethnographic. Michael Agar once described ethnographic research as "studying snow in the middle of an avalanche" (1999, personal comment). Action research goes a step beyond merely studying the snow; action research, to me, is like *building* a snowman (i.e., snow person) *while* you study snow in the middle of an avalanche. There is *action* in action research, not just on your part as a researcher, but also on the part of all the *people* being studied. You are not just studying action—you *are* the action. You, all, must become part of the "snow"—in the middle—as you partner with those wanting to understand their problem better and to find solutions to eliminate the problem. Action research demands a fire in the belly, a courageous heart, a brain with the capacity for multidimensional, multitask participation, a level of insatiable energy, and a constant vigilance toward ethical choices—it takes all five elements to carry the project from beginning to end.

HOW I LEARNED ACTION RESEARCH: ETHNOGRAPHY WITH EMPOWERMENT

I learned action research through practice by combining my knowledge of ethnography (learned as an anthropologist) with knowledge about empowerment (learned as a nurse working beside a dedicated medical missionary in Guatemala—Doc Behrhorst). My knowledge about doing ethnographies came from my doctoral studies in anthropology when I did my dissertation field research in two Guatemalan highland villages (1973–1975), comparing the cultural contexts in which family reproduction took place (Glittenberg, 1976, 1994). This study period was followed by another 5 years of doing ethnographic studies in 4 squatter settlements and 21 villages and towns in the highlands and lowlands of Guatemala in a National Science Foundation funded project studying how a developing country copes and recovers from a devastating natural disaster (Glittenberg, 1985). Owing to the political terrorism in Guatemala, I returned to the United States in 1982 and began teaching at the School of Nursing, University of Colorado. Here I was inspired to teach graduate students a different way of doing community health assessments. Rather than the usual top-down way of assessing the effectiveness of health professional studies, I sent the students forth to *live with the people* to learn from the people how they viewed health. Through field work, the students found that the people were not a simple set of vital statistics. Nor did the people see the health department as the only holy temple of health; rather, students found that the people used all types of alternative healing. The people also conceptualized the community in different categories (e.g., "old timers," "new comers," "red neckers," "dirt baggers," etc.) instead of the health department's categories of ages 1–5 years, 5–15 years, and so forth, and by sex. The people organized and held in their minds an *emic*, or insider's, view of their community. Students found that a sociocultural history of each community existed in the minds of the people; this collective knowledge (some real, some mythical) gave the people a powerful way of dealing with problems.

The students collected a vast amount of data by living with the people and by studying historical documents and published facts. Through focus groups and key informant interviews, they reached an even closer understanding of the whole culture—the way in which the prescribed roles and statuses of each group operated on a day-to-day basis. Data about these cultural rules and norms were collected and organized into the *etic* (outsiders') categories of social institutions such as family, religion, education, economics, power/politics, and health. The organized categories, when put all together, formed a community profile of each town or system. This profile was presented to the townspeople at a public hearing.

Collecting data for ethnographies and constructing the profile are like the Sherlock Holmes technique of using a magnifying glass to examine bits and pieces of evidence and then putting them all together to solve a mystery. The bits and pieces of the mystery are found in cultural symbols, such as verbal and nonverbal language, and in the symbolic interaction of these bits and pieces. When all these data are combined, a pattern emerges that is unique for each group or system; for instance, the ethos, or cultural pattern, of one community is different from that of another—for example, Athens and Spartus in Ancient Greece were quite distinct even though they were close in proximity. Another example is a department store such as Nieman Marcus compared with a Wal-Mart.

Systems are organized for a purpose—for survival—through multiple processes of adaptation and adjustment. When challenged, a system survives through adaptive processes; a system is ever changing, dynamic. This ongoing, dynamic process is a major challenge for anyone doing ethnographic research—because the snow does not stay the same or in one place; it keeps moving on, much as the elements that make up a system shift, move, appear, and disappear.

I named this new model of community assessment Project GENESIS for General Ethnography and Needs EvaluationS In a System; the acronym describes not only the process but also the process as a new beginning (Glittenberg, 1983). GENESIS is a model still used in teaching graduate students at the University of Colorado and has been adopted by several other universities in the United States, Australia, Israel, and the Philippines. It has been used with various groupings of people (e.g., a hospital, an apartment house, a high school, a university, a barrio, an island, and perhaps others). GENESIS can be used in simple or complex systems.

Two aspects of the Project GENESIS model are common to ethnography and to action research: the *partnership through invitation* and the *evaluation process*. Partnership through invitation occurs before any research is begun. An invitation from the leaders of a group of people requests study. When the invitation is accepted (by the research team), it is done as a partnership with a commitment from the people being studied that they will participate in the data collection, the interpretation of the findings, and the plan of action toward a solution. I, as the principal investigator, have always initiated an invitation, as an educative process. For instance, the first town in which a Project GENESIS was done was a ski resort; vital statistics revealed that this town had the highest suicide rate in the state. I presented these figures to the mayor of the town, and asked, "Would you like help in understanding why this problem exists and ways in which it might be changed?" The answer was affirmative, so I then proceeded, with his assistance, to set up a community meeting to which all the leading citizens were invited (e.g., business people, clergy, educators, health care providers, police and legal representatives, elected officials, and others). From that first community meeting, the plans for the action research were discussed, and the townspeople made commitments to participate.

One "agency," or organization, volunteered to coordinate the research process and to arrange for homes, hotels, and so forth, in which the students could stay for 2 or 3 days. The coordinating group also made appointments for key informant interviews with the identified leaders. These informant interviews were the first-level designated interviews. These leaders then suggested names of other informed people, by using a snowball technique to spread interviews out to the rest of the town or organization until the categories were "saturated" (i.e., information obtained was redundant). The usual number of completed interviews in a group/town is about 100. The field notes were discussed each night in a team meeting, and the leaders within each of the social institutions (religion, economics, education, family, law/politics) evaluated what further data were needed. A series of secondary data were collected before, during, and after the fieldwork was done, such as historical documents, newspaper articles, and photographs. Subsequent to the intense fieldwork, the students and faculty returned to the university for continued interpretation of the data and development of a community profile and a case study report. After the profile and report appeared complete, a presentation date was set (usually within a few weeks) with the townspeople. Students and faculty returned to the town and presented their findings for further input from the community partners, and together they developed a plan of action.

I have found no better way of teaching students the importance of ethical, thorough, systematic data collection—in sum, to be credible, trustworthy, and accountable researchers—than to have them prepare the report and then present it orally to the townspeople. In addition to the public hearing, a written report was given to each participant; this report was part of an action plan. It was not a report meant to catch dust on some bureaucrat's shelf, because it belonged to the *people*. It was meant to be a working document, changing every year. The total cost to the University of Colorado School of Nursing was approximately $2,000 for each Project GENESIS, which included transportation costs and printing of the reports. The community itself contributed in-kind expenses feeding the students and providing an office in which to work.

Another important aspect of action research is an understanding of empowerment. There are a number of examples of empowerment programs—community development projects—such as community conscientiousness building of the Catholic church in Latin America, credited to Freire in the 1970s. My own understanding of empowerment came from working with medical missionary Carroll Behrhorst (Doc, mentioned earlier), a physician from Winfield, Kansas, who went to Guatemala in 1960 with his family of six children to cure disease. However, instead of putting on Band-Aids as a *missionary*, Doc found himself as a *man with a mission* dedicated to reversing the poverty and subsequent ill health and early death among the Mayan Indians of highland Guatemala (Barton, 1970; Glittenberg, 1974, 1994; Lueke, 1993). His program, the Behrhorst Development Program recognized by the World Health Organization as a model of primary health care, took shape through empowerment as Mayan Indians learned to read and write in Spanish and then later in their native language, became educated as teachers, nurses, physicians, and business people; collectively shared their individual incomes through cooperatives; and finally found the power of their voices and votes in the election of representatives to the Congress in the Republic of Guatemala. Doc Behrhorst deeply respected the Mayan cultural beliefs and practices. His life was based on principles of social justice, in accord with a Chinese motto written on a plaque above his simple desk in Chimaltenango, Guatemala: Go to the people, live with the people, love them, learn from them, so that when you leave they will say, "We did it ourselves!" Doc died from a heart attack in his beloved Guatemalan home, May, 1990, after living long enough to see his goal of having a *Mayan* physician become director of the Program and the Indian hospital and clinics. Doc's work was done. His work lives on (Glittenberg, 1990).

EVALUATION: HOW IS IT MEASURED?

Evaluation of the work, like the whole process of action research, is not a simple endeavor. The process of action research maintains rigorous standards that parallel those of quantitative investigations, but with one major difference—the *people are partners in the evaluation*. Evaluation of the adequacy, the completeness, and the credibility begins on the first day of contact *with* the people and it ends the last day *with* the people when both the community or group's partners and the research team say, "It is complete—this is our community." Answers to "What have we learned?" may vary, but they should be consistent, cohesive, and point to practical solutions with the use of local resources and an ongoing process of action and research. "What are we learning?" evaluates process, whereas "What have we learned?" evaluates outcomes.

An Example: There Are No Flies

As an example of evaluation in action research, consider my work with the World Health Organization in the Philippines. I visited a primary health center and talked with leaders of a group of 10,000 very poor people living in a neighborhood without running water or a sewer system. This group of people had partnered with health care providers in the project, and the group was pleased with the progress being made in their action research study. I asked the president of the neighborhood committee, "What changes have you seen since this program started?" He looked around carefully, eyeing the shacks, the railroad tracks that went through the neighborhood, and the hundreds of children running playfully around, and said, "There are no flies!" That simple statement stood as a powerful evaluation of what had happened in the partnership formed for controlling waste disposal for 10,000, for bringing in potable water, and for general cleaning of the footpaths and sanitation. The statement gave an emic—insider's view—of cultural values as well as a reality measure of the "possible." It gave me a measure of *empowerment*, for the people themselves were controlling their destinies and their health, and they knew it.

Evaluation is not just of the product, because in action research the *process* is more empowering. If researchers come into a community and "do" the research—a top-down method—they usually consult very few of the people living there. Perhaps they speak to a sample sufficient to meet a donor's requirements or those of a publication. They may publish a slick report that may be sent to certain people in the community, but it is not a part of the process of change and action, and too often the report has little effect on the situation at hand.

Evaluation took a different form in the first Project GENESIS by empowering both students and townspeople to see their roles as participants in solutions. Too often students have little investment in the collective learning of their cohorts of students; nor do they see the value of their talents being used for the betterment of humankind. We are a nation of rugged individuals—we tend to say, "I did it myself!" But, within the action research model is an acknowledgment—a knowing that we are not alone, we did not learn it "by ourselves," but rather our intellects and our talents are shared, given away, and enriched by other intellects and talents, the Others. In GENESIS, becoming a scholar, a scientist, or a nursing leader is not done as a single person, but rather "becoming" is a process potentiated by our colleagues, our mentors, and our students/partners. In action research, shared responsibility means that it is a "we" project and a "we" process. Sometimes the process has less participation from one side or the other, but the ideal action research is one of balance, harmony, and commitment. Ethically, action research is done with the people and, ethically, they own the solution. At times, I have questioned this ownership when I felt that another solution perhaps was preferable, but, in my experience, the people-based solution is the right one, and I have learned to honor that ownership.

PROGRESS IN THE MEXICAN AMERICAN TOWN

The NIDA-sponsored research dealing with violence in a Mexican American town described at the beginning of this chapter is now moving into its third year of funding; we are currently conducting a household survey and are finding that most of the people are plain, good, hard-working poor people. Reaching the point of doing this survey consisted of multiple steps. I shall describe them briefly.

The Beginning: 1997

In the two years of waiting for an approved funding source, the original research team had dissipated. Attrition was expected. It is what happens in life while one is waiting for reviews. Two team members had moved away and one had another grant, so I started to develop another team from scratch. Fortunately, I had worked with Dr. Anderson on another small study and was deeply impressed by his abilities and his ethics. I was lucky to be able to hire him full time as a program coordinator but quickly promoted him to a research associate professor and coinvestigator. We next hired a research specialist who had worked in a previous study with Dr. Anderson, Roberto Corona, an extraordinarily talented, intuitive man with Yaqui and Mexican heritage. Mary Lou Chacon was my third blessing as a perceptive, motivated young single mother who had lived in the barrio as a young woman. She knew many people living there. We hired her as our secretary and soon promoted her to administrative assistant. Our team then was complete. Balance of talents in action research is critical, as is trust in one another. In this team, we had both qualities, and we truly enjoyed working together.

To be closer to the people, we rented an apartment, through HUD housing, right in the middle of some very violent activities. Through developing a plan of action, we committed to many activities aimed to enrich the lives of our neighbors: health clinics, classes for building social skills, beautification of the grounds, lectures on health-related subjects, cleaning up the area, helping undocumented people deal with becoming citizens, classes on parenting, and "safe sex" classes; these activities represent "building a snow man while you're studying snow in the middle of an avalanche." We held an open house during our first days in the apartment and were not surprised when only children came. We had to build trust—that took time. When Mary Lou, her teenaged daughter, and her grandnephew moved into the apartment, this was the answer, because Mary Lou was one of them—a good neighbor and an extraordinary person with many talents. Not only was she trusted, but she organized three large parties for the children and helped teach the women how to contact donors for food and toys. A Halloween party was a great success and was followed by a Christmas party to which more than 1000 children came. Next was a successful Easter egg hunt. The real empowerment has come through the coffees held by Mary Lou each week in the apartment, where timid, often illiterate women have begun to share their fears and their dreams.

We have many other examples of partnering with the people. Some have been successful, whereas others have not. We organized a community advisory board to help evaluate our progress and to critique our study. The members asked that we not make public the study, because they were afraid that it would label the community as being "derelict, crime filled, and lazy." We have honored that wish. The title of our program, Community Empowerment Partnership Project, known as CEPP, was accepted.

The Second and Third Year to Date

At the beginning of the second year, we moved into a second office in the community—a simple storefront office across the street from one of the most violent bars in town. Community health students use this space as their office for work in the community. The office is headquarters for our household survey and will be a place for our continuing key informant interviews. From our front window, we witness drug dealing and prostitutes looking for tricks. We also see the positive changes being made within the whole town.

Weed and Seed, a federally funded program to provide block grants for the purpose of weeding out the bad, e.g., crack houses and seeding in the good, e.g., establishing safe havens for street kids, was initiated at the beginning of the second year of study. From this grant, many positive changes are visible to the eye. A domestic-violence program has shown definite signs of changing from domestic violence being an accepted occurrence to a zero tolerance policy.

Will the changes be permanent? The people wish for a safer town without the drug dealers, prostitutes, and gangs. We found a glimmer of hope while living in the HUD apartment and have seen more social services being offered; sidewalks are adorned with art works, and alleys have been cleaned. Slum lords are out and crack houses are being torn down. To date, there have been no more drive-by shootings—no more Oscars lost to gang violence. We wish to go forward in a more focused action research effort, looking specifically at the culture of drugs and narrowing the scope toward rehabilitating addicts and prostitutes. There are resilient people living among us, and through action research we are providing bridges for their strengths to become more explicit and visible. When we leave, we hope they will say, "We did it ourselves!"

REFERENCES

Agar, M. (1999). Workshop on ethnography. First International Conference on Qualitative Research Methods. University of Alberta, Edmonton, Canada, January 11, 1999.

Barton, E. (1970). *Physician to the Mayas: The story of Dr. Carroll Behrhorst*. Philadelphia: Fortress Press.

Fetterman, D. M. (1996). Empowerment evaluations: An introduction to theory and practice. In D. Fetterman, S. Kaftarian, & A. Wandersman, (Eds.), *Empowerment evaluation: Knowledge and tools for self-assessment and accountability* (pp. 3–49). Thousand Oaks, CA: Sage.

Glittenberg, J. (1974). Adapting health care to a cultural setting. *American Journal of Nursing*, 12, 2218–2221.

Glittenberg, J. (1976). *A comparative study of fertility in two highland Guatemalan towns: A Latino and an Indian town*. Unpublished dissertation. University of Colorado, Boulder.

Glittenberg, J. (1983). Project GENESIS: A community assessment model. In P. Morley (Ed.), *Transcultural nursing theory in teaching, research, and practice*. Salt Lake City: University of Utah, College of Nursing Press.

Glittenberg, J. (1985). Social upheaval and recovery in Guatemala city after the 1976 earthquake. In J. Laube (Ed.), *Perspectives on disaster recovery*. Norwalk, CT: Appleton-Century-Crofts.

Glittenberg, J. (1988). The Behrhorst program: A model of primary health care. *Journal of Professional Nursing*, 6, 400–459.

Glittenberg, J. (1990). Doc Behrhorst: His work is done . . . his work goes on. *Journal of Professional Nursing*, 10, 408.

Glittenberg, J. (1994). *To the mountain and back*. Prospect Heights, IL: Waveland Press.

Glittenberg, J. (1998). The power of literacy. In D. Masson (Ed.), *Policy and politics for nurses* (3rd ed. pp. 633–636). New York: Saunders.

Luecke, R. (1993). A New Dawn in Guatemala: Toward a worldwide health vision. Prospect Heights, IL: Waveland Press.

Part III

Other Considerations in Qualitative Research

The following chapters address a variety of questions and concerns, frequently expressed not only by students of nursing science, but also by faculty, consultants and reviewers of qualitative research. In Chapter 19 is a discussion of ethical considerations in qualitative research and closely related to insuring those ethical dimensions; a discussion on institutional review boards is the subject for Chapter 20. Chapter 21 is a new chapter on interview strategies and analysis by Janice Morse. Carolyn Oiler Boyd describes the issues and the possibilities about combining qualitative and quantitative methods in Chapter 22.

Chapter 23, by Julie Evertz, discusses the evaluation and critiquing of qualitative research. Chapter 24 helps the researcher with suggestions for qualitative research proposal and reports. Chapter 25 is another new chapter and is on the sources for qualitative researchers to be found on the Internet by Maureen Duffy. The content in Part III does not intend to provide the *only* answers to these questions and concerns, and the reader is encouraged to study the references for additional perspectives. For example, the question of combination of methods is a subject that has provoked heated discussions, so if the reader is to be truly informed about the critiques, additional reading is necessary.

Indeed, the journey of learning about qualitative research methods, if started with this text, is just the first part. Perhaps along the reader's journey, a qualitative researcher will be born and this volume will represent his or her gestation.

19

Ethical Considerations
in Qualitative Research*

Patricia L. Munhall

As members of the scientific community, nurse researchers have become adept at identifying and applying criteria for evaluating the various aspects of quantitative research. We may have even surpassed our colleagues in other disciplines in the level of rigor applied when evaluating the design, method, and protection of human subjects of a study.

With regard to the protection of human subjects, I like to think that rigor is founded on a profound reverence for human beings and their experiences. As nurse researchers, we have become increasingly sophisticated in our qualitative research endeavors and have begun to identify distinct considerations and criteria for viewing the ethical dimensions of qualitative research.

Naturalistic, direct involvement and participation with people necessitates acknowledging the subjective nature and activity of the researcher as the main "tool" of research. Qualitatively oriented nurse researchers prize this direct involvement yet, contextually, are faced with the canonization of objectivity detachment of prevailing convention. In contrast, qualitative nurse researchers face the "nitty gritty," the

*Reprinted with permission of Western Journal of Nursing Research, 10(2), 150–162, 1988.

serendipitous, the passions, the complexity of subjectivity, and at-
tachment to people and their vicissitudes.

The purpose of this chapter is to provide one of the stepping stones
needed to differentiate criteria that are essential and appropriate for
qualitative research methods in nursing. This discussion will focus on
selected ethical considerations with the following themes interwoven
throughout: ethical means and ends, collaborators as means, conflict
methodology, models of fieldwork, and process consent. Potential for
role conflict within the investigator is discussed from the perspective
of the therapeutic imperative and the research imperative.

UNDERLYING ASSUMPTIONS AND DILEMMAS

In the tradition of qualitative research methods, I would like to state,
or bracket, here my own beliefs and values and their implications for
ethical considerations when doing qualitative nursing research:

1. The therapeutic imperative of nursing (advocacy) takes
   precedence over the research imperative (advancing
   knowledge) if conflict develops.
2. Nursing reflects a deontological ethical system (people are not
   to be treated as means). However, if individuals consent to be
   part of our research, they have, in essence, joined the research
   enterprise. Instead of being called subjects or objects, they are
   now collaborators (Punch, 1986).
3. Informed consent is a static, past-tense concept. Qualitative
   research is an ongoing, dynamic, changing process. Because of
   unforeseeable events and consequences, a past-tense consent
   is not appropriate. We need to facilitate negotiation and
   renegotiation to protect our collaborators' human rights.
   Therefore, a verblike consent seems necessary and the concept
   of process consenting reflects the ongoing dynamic nature of
   qualitative research.

ETHICAL MEANS AND ENDS

Bellah (1981) sets our stage for ethical dialogue with the premise that
all inquiry has normative commitments. Arguing that all social inquiry

is linked to ethical reflection, he uses the expression "moral sciences" interchangeably with "social sciences." He states: "Social science must consider ends as well as means as objects of rational reflection" (p. 2).

Laudan (1977) also focuses on the consequence side of science when he states: "Science is essentially a problem-solving activity" (p. 66). Wilson and Fitzpatrick (1984) state that the purpose of nursing science is "to render reality intelligible as it relates to human health and development" (p. 41).

The question to be asked from an ethical perspective then is: Toward what goal and for what end? For our purposes here, let us suggest that, for the most part, nurse researchers are very much interested in "problem solving" or "problem preventing" research and that our motives are to produce an end that is in some way considered "good." In this way, research assumes a normative commitment, something that "ought" to be. The most apparent example of this commitment is that many of our research endeavors focus on facilitating "health." The search for a means to produce a desired health outcome requires critical ethical reflection.

Other aims that we have in addition or in conjunction to the attainment of health are assisting people to reach their potential, to self-actualize, and to reach their maximum well-being. Actually, many of these ends are equivalent to or similes of the concept of health.

Acknowledgment that our aims have normative commitments is critical because we then move on to ways (means) of achieving our decided good. In essence, our aims become prescriptive. An example may serve to illustrate this point.

Ethical Aims

One of our normative commitments is to help individuals achieve their maximum potential. In this pursuit, we do a qualitative study of a group of "underachievers" who are not attaining full intellectual potential or physical health potential. The ethical questions that arise include whether the ethical aim is to assist those subjects whom we study or future generations. What do the underachievers whom we study have to gain from our studying them? Further, is it a given that our mission is to help people reach their maximum potential if unrequested?

Although our society has accepted and promoted some goods, we need to reflect upon them. Some may actually be in opposition to others. For example, a "steady state" or some form of "equilibrium" may indeed *be in opposition* to an achievement ethic. In qualitative research, knowledge of our collaborators' aims and normative commitments is an intrinsic component of the research process. We need to reflect on our own and, perhaps more importantly, their normative commitments.

Ethical Means

In *The Prince*, Machiavelli proclaimed his aim of a free, independent Italy, free from outside governance as an end that was readily proclaimed as good. However, his means to that end illustrated moral vacuity. Machiavelli believed that corruption is natural to man. However, by generalizing a behavior to *all* "men," he justified his means in order to obtain an end. Human experimentation is based on the "ends justifying the means" principle.

Changing people's behaviors, often an aim in the helping professions, contrasts sharply with understanding different behaviors and accepting and supporting those differences. Perhaps not all people need or want to reach their maximum potential. Some philosophers, such as Kant, believe human beings have a moral obligation to reach their maximum potential. The question then becomes, Do nurses have a moral obligation to help others attain a moral obligation? This is an example of an ethical consideration that needs in-depth exploration by nurse researchers.

Aims Versus Means

Ethical consideration in qualitative research (and quantitative as well, though it is not spelled out) entails knowing explicitly and implicitly what our ethical means and aims are. Entering and participating with our collaborators seems a precious experience that calls upon us to reflect, know, and bracket what our ethical means and ends are. A negotiated view requires such reflection.

Perhaps the most critical ethical obligation that qualitative nurse researchers have is to describe the experiences of others in the most faithful way possible. This ethical obligation is to describe and report in the most authentic manner possible the experience that unfolds even if contrary to your aims. Perhaps it might appear wonderful not to strive to maximum achievement of your potential! Not having to achieve a level of significance to accomplish your aim may be the highest degree of freedom possible when doing research.

THERAPEUTIC VERSUS RESEARCH IMPERATIVE

Ethics is a tangled web of principles where one can usually see the position of the opposition as having some legitimacy. That is why ethical dilemmas are thorny, at best. In the instance of the therapeutic imperative and the research imperative, the ethical systems of deontology and utilitarianism potentially conflict. The nurse who is doing research needs to acknowledge what her therapeutic imperative is. Is it deontological, where the individual is not a means to an end but an end as such? Is it advocacy for human beings? Is it based on justice, beneficence, and respect for patients' rights? The researcher also needs to reflect on the research imperative. Is it utilitarian, where people are used as means to further knowledge? Is the researcher imposing possibly uncomfortable conditions on her participants? Is the researcher working under a utilitarian posture where the ends may justify the means? In qualitative research, some conflicts that present dilemmas for researchers are as follows:

Means	*Ends*
Entry	Departure
Confidence	Disappointment
Elation	Despondency
Commitment	Perceived betrayal
Friendship	Desertion

From a utilitarian perspective, those results listed at the right may seem unavoidable in fieldwork. From the deontological perspective, they are ethically problematic.

Role conflict evolves from behavioral expectations that may differ in the nurse's therapeutic imperative from those in the researcher's imperative. Given the potential for harm in fieldwork, consideration must be given to these dilemmas so as to minimize them or prevent them from occurring. Communication is an essential process, as is a team or joint approach to research. Perhaps even the term *participant-observer* could be abandoned, simply titling all those taking part as *participants* or, as already mentioned, *collaborators*. It may be helpful to understand, from a human perspective, that, if there is to be a departure, that all who take part are prepared and that the researcher, too, often does feel sad. In essence, there is a real "joining" of feelings and understandings.

IS BEING A COLLABORATOR A MEANS TO AN END?

Suppose a nurse-anthropologist-researcher asked you to participate in her study titled, "Contemporary Women's Hassles: An Exploratory Study," and she asked whether she could visit you in your home at various times when you were available to "sort of" observe and interview you. In addition, she asks, Would it be all right to visit you in your office? Rock (1979) states: "No sociologist I know would himself agree to become a subject of observational research" (p. 261).

Well, what is at stake here? When I think of this, very much is at stake, and we need to walk in our collaborators' shoes. Sure, there are hassles for the contemporary woman, but having this researcher come into my home seems not only another hassle, but perhaps a crisis! One needs to be concerned about the usual ethical considerations of fieldwork: privacy, confidentiality, achieving accurate portrayal, and inclusion and exclusion of information. In this instance, however, as in many others, the psychological burden and threat that an outsider might pose need serious consideration. Regardless of all of our efforts to act in the collaborators' best interest, some invasion, as it were, occurs to the person or people involved. The end that we hope to accomplish may be laudable, but we are cajoling ourselves, I think, if we are not aware that there is some inconvenience or discomfort in the process of being observed. The unknown consequences of the observation, it seems, could contribute to a pervasive state of anxiety for the participants, whether consciously or unconsciously. Rather than the casual "Within 2 to 3 weeks the person or persons seemed comfortable with my presence" or "I was virtually unnoticed after 2 or 3 weeks," we need, as advocates, to attend to other possibilities that occur with observations. We can ask ourselves, "Would we be comfortable until the results were in?" Empathizing with and attending to the process of being an observee must be ongoing on the researcher's part. We may feel blended into a culture, but that does not mean that the observees are experientially where we are.

As already mentioned, nursing seems to espouse the deontological principle that human beings are to be treated as ends and not means. In contrast with that system is utilitarianism, which argues that the ends justify the means. From that perspective, one can use another person for the good of others and to advance further knowledge. Technically, the research enterprise turns people into means and, though one could argue that this occurs far less with qualitative research, the potential still remains. We have come to some peace with this issue through the process of informed consent, where, in effect, the individual joins the research enterprise. Joining the effort accords individuals the opportunities of contributing to society, of being of service and perhaps advancing a cause of their own. We may not have thought of informed consent from that perspective, but ethically it helps to resolve the means–end dilemma and makes the term collaborator much more accurate.

INFORMED CONSENT IN QUALITATIVE RESEARCH

Fieldwork that is existential and authentic requires the negotiation of trust between the researcher and the participants. Entering into fields in the various roles of participant-observer is a privilege. We are "allowed" into someone else's world with its customs, practices, and events, which we promise to describe faithfully and without bias. While we are negotiating entry into this world, we invite the participants to become part of the research enterprise and validate that agreement with an informed consent.

Informed consent has been defined as:

> knowing consent of an individual or his legally authorized representative, so situated as to be able to exercise free power of choice without undue inducement or any element of force, fraud, deceit, duress, or other forms of constraint or coercion. (Annas, Glantz, & Katz, 1977, p. 291)

Typically, informed consents include the title, purpose, and explanation of the research and the procedures to be followed. Risks and benefits are to be clearly spelled out. A statement that the participant has had an opportunity to ask questions and that the participant is free to withdraw at any time also is included (Field & Morse, 1985). This model of informed consent evolved out of experimental research; some of it is applicable to qualitative research, but to resolve some of the aforementioned dilemmas more seems needed.

PROCESS CONSENT

Because qualitative research is conducted in an ever-changing field, informed consent should be an ongoing process. Over time, consent needs to be renegotiated as unexpected events or consequences arise. I may, in a weak moment, sign a consent for our previously mentioned researcher to observe me in my home, but without the full realization of what the consequences might be. To be ethical in this situation, the researcher needs to assess the effects of involvement in the field and continually acquire new permissions. Maybe children will react negatively to an outsider in their home, and perhaps the contemporary woman will find that keeping some semblance of cleanliness of her home on a daily basis is just the hassle that will take her over the edge.

Common sense plays a large part in renegotiating informed consent. If our focus should change, we need to ask participants for permission to change the first agreement. This is important from the perspective of sensitivity to our collaborators as well. They may wonder why you "lost" interest in a particular part of the field and chose something that you obviously have found "special." Continually informing and asking permission establishes the needed trust to go further in an ethical manner.

Secrets

Another area that needs ethical consideration in fieldwork is confidentiality of the exchanges between the researcher and the participants. Both informed and process consent should carefully delineate the data to be included in the study. Role conflict can be generated when the participant wants to tell you a secret or an off-the-record remark. The "nurse" listens to this, and in fact, knows that a bond has been established that is valuable. However, the "nurse researcher" and participants will probably be better off if the researcher gently reminds the participant of the purpose of the study and that all communication is supposed to be part of the study (Field & Morse, 1985). If it is possible, as may be the case in a health care facility, the participant can be referred to an appropriate person with any information not relevant to the study. The idea here is to discourage participants from telling secrets unless these secrets can be part of the study. This, of course, needs to be done with the utmost care, because secrets are treasures, *but, more importantly, imply promises to keep them.* Most often these problems can be discussed quite openly with collaborators.

Witnessing unethical or illegal conduct can pose another ethical dilemma. If we are nurses and, as such, the clients' advocates, we cannot place the research imperative above the therapeutic imperative. Some (Estroff & Churchill, 1984) suggest that clear procedures be established prior to the start of the study that spell out the channels the researcher will go through if unethical or illegal practices are witnessed. Researchers are morally obliged from the therapeutic imperative to report such violations. The ethical dilemma of whistle-blowing helps us to understand this particular problem.

Findings and Publication

Anonymity of subjects individually or as a group is often a requisite of qualitative research. However, sometimes individuals and cultures allow themselves to be identified. An understanding about anonymity is part of the informed and process consent. What is often not mentioned or planned for is publication and dissemination of findings. With all research, what the researcher intends to do with the findings needs to be a part of the consent. A longitudinal view from point of entry to publication needs to be agreed upon with the collaborators. Being observed can be quite different from reading a description of yourself or of your culture or from hearing from someone who has such information. To prevent misunderstandings, all taking part need to agree on the various stages and activities of the entire project. What will happen to the descriptions? Will they be presented at a conference? Will they be published, and where, and for what purpose? All collaborators need to agree to dissemination of findings, from an ethical perspective of deontology, because they are part of the entire project. Because we may not foresee the consequences of publication, it is wise in this litigious society to protect not only our collaborators but also ourselves.

CONFLICT METHODOLOGY

Conflict methodology in fieldwork is built on the interactionist and ethnomethodological perspective, adding the belief that ordinary social life is characterized by deceit and impression management (Douglas, 1979). Opponents of this method maintain that the researcher is justified in using similar techniques, because it is the explicit purpose of research to expose the powerful and that deception is "legitimate" (Punch, 1986, p. 32).

The argument is based on an end that may in itself be highly moral (recall Machiavelli); yet the means are acknowledgedly unethical, but within the conflict methodological view, justified. There are ethical arguments advanced for conflict methodology, but, if civilization hangs on to the Kantian principle, certainly this is a most dangerous practice.

The counterargument to justifying deceit is nicely summed up by Warwick (1982):

Social scientists have not only a right but an obligation to study controversial and politically sensitive subjects . . . but this obligation does not carry with it the right to deceive, exploit or manipulate people. My concern with backlash centers primarily on the alienation of ordinary individuals by research methods which leave them feeling that they have been cheated, deceived, or used. (p. 55)

In nursing research, deception, exploitation, or manipulation of people would be ethically antithetical to all that we philosophically stand for professionally. Our concept of client advocacy precludes the use of conflict methodology. In addition, we need to be alert to *nuances* in our research that could cause individuals to feel "cheated, deceived, or used." I have often heard collaborators comment that they were supposed to receive a copy of the research report but never did. Thus they feel cheated. In some of our methods and consents, the collaborators actually see the report or description before finalization for their response and agreement to the portrayal. This may also assist in validation and an accurate portrayal. From an ethical perspective, we need to determine which models of fieldwork seem consistent with our belief system.

MODELS OF FIELDWORK

The extent to which invasion into a social setting is ethical is often a matter of common sense. The researcher needs to be aware of what is not being told, as well as what is being said. The extent to which the research is a covert or overt operation also is open to ethical evaluation. Here, again, the ethical aim needs to be clear. There is a fine line between doing anthropological research and an "investigation" in the journalistic or "FBI" sense.

Punch (1986) conceives of three models of fieldwork and relates them to ethical features of trust and deceit:

1. The *hypothetical "problemless"* project: For instance, a graduate student gains entry into a commune, shares daily life, is accepted, departs to write a description, and allows the culture under study to read and validate what has been written. There is no high trauma, drama, or problems and, as Punch (1986) points out, this type of study is like the classical ethnography when the investigator could be sure that the Ashanti and Nuer would not be scouring the anthropological journals with their lawyers for negative references to tribal life. Today, I am not sure that we can even say that!

2. The *"knotty"* project: The institution erects barriers against outsiders and gaining access becomes difficult. An example might be a state mental institution where those associated with certain practices fear publication in the interest of preserving the institution's and their own reputation.

3. The *"ripping and running"* project: There is deliberate concealment, which, in addition to being ethically indefensible, is illegal. This model depends on an unrevealed person posing as a member of the group. This practice has the connotations of spying and undercover investigating and certainly violates civil liberties.

Many of us doing fieldwork like to believe that, as moral agents, we may come to identify problems and abuses within cultures or institutions. Because of that ethical aim, we may be tempted to justify unethical means, such as bending the truth, to gain entry in order to obtain an accurate portrayal. Such practices again constitute conflict methodology and have serious consequences for collaborators and researchers in the field.

The second and third models of fieldwork hold the potential for moral, social, and political change. However, in the long run, using these two models will have the effect of "closed doors" in the field due to loss of trust, credibility, and confidence in nurse researchers. The last model of fieldwork violates the very foundation of our nursing practice. Whistle-blowing again is the topic that needs to be addressed and certainly is not limited to practices witnessed by researchers. For instance, in any type of health care facility where unethical practices exist, the moral obligation of reporting such practices belongs to all involved. However, as was mentioned under process consent, preplanning for such events, should they occur, is one way of ensuring that your course of action is known and has been agreed on prior to the commencement of the study.

SUMMARY REMARKS

There is much more to be discussed within the topic of ethical consideration of qualitative research. There is much still to be discussed about qualitative research methods in nursing. So these remarks are not concluding but contribute to the dialogue centered on the developing interest in these methods. One facet is clear: one cannot transpose criteria for quantitative research and apply them to qualitative research.

The static, past tense of informed consent does not adequately protect human subjects in qualitative studies. For that matter, it may not always do so for quantitative methods.

The most glaring difference, however, springs from the dynamic, process-oriented qualities of qualitative research. Qualitative research could be thought of as a verb, a process, with the ethical components constantly being scrutinized. "Process consenting" might be a way to remind ourselves of the ongoing nature of discussing with our collaborators the means and the aims of our study.

In addition, our therapeutic imperative and research imperative need to be as clear as possible. From an ethical perspective, the therapeutic imperative provides the research imperative, so that efforts to avoid any difficulties or disadvantages to the collaborator need our constant vigilance if the research is to proceed ethically.

Because we, as nurses, have the ethical theme of deontology threaded throughout our philosophies, I think we are humanistically ahead of many other disciplines in considering the ethics of our research enterprise. Our egos are not split. We are patient-client advocates, where trust, compassion, and empathy encompass all our nursing endeavors, including research.

REFERENCES

Aamodt, A. (1983). Problems in doing nursing research: Developing criteria for evaluating qualitative research. *Western Journal of Nursing Research, 5,* 398–402.

Annas, D. J., Glantz, L. H., & Katz, B. J. (1977). *Informed consent to human experimentation: The subject's dilemma.* Boston: Ballinger.

Bellah, R. (1981). The ethical aims of social inquiry. *Teachers College Record,* 83(1), 1–18.

Douglas, J. D. (1979). Living morality versus bureaucratic fist. In C. B. Klockars & F. W. O'Connor (Eds.), *Deviance and decency.* Beverly Hills, CA: Sage.

Estroff, S. E., & Churchill, L. R. (1984). Comment (Ethical dilemmas). *Anthropology Newsletter*, 25(7).

Field, P., & Morse, J. (1985). *Nursing research: The application of qualitative approaches*. Rockville, MD: Aspen.

Laudan, L. (1977). *Progress and its problems: Towards a theory of scientific growth*. Berkeley: University of California Press.

Punch, M. (1986). *The politics and ethics of fieldwork*. Beverly Hills, CA: Sage.

Rock, P. (1979). *The making of symbolic interactionism*. London: Macmillan.

Sandelowski, M. (1986). The problem of rigor in qualitative research. *Advances in Nursing Research*, 8, 27–37.

Warwick, D. P. (1982). Tearsome trade: Means and ends in social research. In M. Bulmer (Ed.), *Social research ethics*. London: Macmillan.

Wilson, L., & Fitzpatrick, J. (1984). Dialectic thinking as a means of understanding systems in development: Relevance to Roger's principles. *Advances in Nursing Service*, 6(2), 41.

ADDITIONAL REFERENCES

Amason, J. P. (1990). Cultural critique and cultural presuppositions: Hermeneutics and critical theory. Philosophy and Social Criticism 15 (1), 125–150.

Aamodt, A. (1983). Problems in doing nursing research: Developing criteria for evaluating qualitative research. *Western Journal of Nursing Research*, 5, 398–402.

Denzin, N., & Lincoln, Y. (1994). *Handbook of qualitative research*. Thousand Oaks, CA: Sage.

Erlandson, D. A., Harris, E., Skipper, B. L., & Allen, S. D. (1993). *Doing naturalistic inquiry: A guide to methods*. Newbury Park, CA: Sage.

Lincoln, Y., & Guba, E. (1985). *Naturalistic Inquiry*. Beverly Hills, CA: Sage.

Schutz, S. (1994). Exploring the benefits of a subjective approach in qualitative nursing research. *Journal of Advanced Nursing*. 20 (3) 412–7.

Watson, J. (1990). Caring Knowledge and Informed Moral Passion. Advances in Nursing Science 13. Sept.: 15–24.

Watson, J. (1995). Postmodernism and knowledge development in nursing. *Nursing Science Quarterly*, 8 (2) 60–4.

Wilde, V. (1992). Controversial hypothesis on the relationship between researcher and informant in qualitative research. *Journal of Advanced Nursing*, 17, 234–242.

Van-Amburg, R. (1997). A Copernican revolution in clinical ethics: engagement versus disengagement. *American Journal of Occupational Therapy*. Mar.: 51 (3) 186–90.

20

Institutional Review of
Qualitative Research Proposals
A Task of No Small Consequence*

Patricia L. Munhall

PLACING THE TASK IN CONTEXT

A colleague of mine sent her research proposal to a large university hospital where the sample for her study was to be derived. She followed the format precisely and was somewhat surprised when she was asked to appear before the institutional review board (IRB) of the hospital. When she arrived, she was astonished to find 26 members of the board present. They discussed the project with her for 2 hours and engaged in what appeared to be an internal struggle over the design and conceptual framework of the study before granting her permission to conduct the study.

My colleague's study was a traditional quantitative research project. Ironically, the study was not to be conducted within the institution itself; rather, the nurse-researcher wanted to do a follow-up mailing to all patients who had had hip-replacement surgery. My purpose in this chapter is to place the review of qualitative research proposals in a perspective from which this context can be understood. According to

*Reprinted with permission from Sage Publications; *Qualitative Nursing Research*: A Contemporary Dialogue, J. Morse (Ed.), 1989, 1991, pp. 258–271.

Noble (1985), IRBs often pose problems for researchers, *regardless* of the research method: "A frequent solution . . . is to engage in minimally clinical projects, such as research involving healthy, intelligent, middle-class clients . . ." (p. 293).

Using this solution, many researchers have looked for subjects outside institutions, which is one alternative. However, because many nurse-researchers are committed to research within institutions, the aim of this chapter will be to facilitate the IRB process, specifically with qualitative research proposals.

The Setting

In this chapter, the presentation of qualitative research methods to IRBs in institutional settings will be addressed. Similarities of IRB requirements for qualitative and quantitative research designs will be discussed. Departures and additions specific to qualitative research methods will be analyzed, with emphasis on the educational aspect of research proposals. The idea of process consent also will be examined, and the appearance of qualitative researchers before IRBs with research proposals will be discussed.

Institutional review boards are the conscience of an institution. They are deeply concerned with human rights and human dignity. The principles of patient autonomy and rights of privacy, confidentiality, anonymity, self-determination, and safety are critical components of the philosophical statements of IRBs.

The most important aspect of any research proposal is the education of our colleagues about qualitative methods and the assurance that we have the same concerns for the dignity and rights of our human subjects. A psychological principle pervades this need for education because most people are generally invested in the status quo, that is, the familiar. Individual members of IRBs are, for the most part, accustomed to the traditional quantitative research design and thus feel a certain amount of confidence when reviewing these proposals. Qualitative research designs within the traditional medical science setting present problems for these IRB members and raise questions simply because the reviewers are unfamiliar with the more unstructured qualitative research methods. This leaves the qualitative nurse-researcher with a task of no small consequence.

The Challenges

Qualitative research in institutional settings presents different challenges from those of more traditional research methods. The three main challenges in receiving permission to conduct qualitative research in institutions are:

1. The IRB's unfamiliarity with the methods, language, and legitimacy of qualitative research;
2. The structural–functionalist perspective that pervades most institutions; and
3. The conscious or unconscious perception of the similarity of qualitative research methods to investigative-type journalism.

Although these challenges are interrelated, each one will be addressed separately.

Unfamiliarity with Qualitative Research Methods

Most IRBs (and, in fact, most grant review panels) have members who are unfamiliar with the aims and outcomes of qualitative research. At present, many IRBs are developing guidelines and are uncertain about the role that the boards play in their institutions. Their task is complex—so complex that a request for the release of names to do a follow-up mailing to former patients (as previously described) resulted in a major meeting of the IRB. The receipt of a proposal with a method called "phenomenology" also may result in an invitation to provide further information.

Phenomenological studies aim at understanding a phenomenon by studying the essences of a life experience with thoughtful attention, and they search for what it means to be human in the attempt to discover plausible insight. Many members of IRBs are not familiar with such language in a research proposal. They will ask, "What is phenomenology?" or "What is grounded theory?" Although these questions do not spell disaster for proposed qualitative research projects, they do complicate matters because these important questions are asked from the structural–functional perspective of institutions.

The Structural–Functional Approach of Institutions

The structural–functional perspective is often viewed as the sacrosanct way of organizing a bureaucratic institution. Roles are prescribed, functions are distributed, behavior and outcomes are predictable, and all should go well according to fixed rules and procedures. The values in our health care institutions seem removed from or, at best, unrelated to qualitative research aims. For the most part, within our health care institutions, pragmatic goals prevail. There should be an action, an intervention, and a concrete observable task with a measurable outcome.

Pragmatism in research is narrowly perceived—for example, the idea of testing something to solve some problem. The idea that understanding preceding experience or any lived experience has pragmatic value is not self-evident from the highly structured functional perspective. From this perspective, the search for "meaning" appears irrelevant. It is this search for meaning that creates confusion in some minds about the difference between qualitative research and investigative journalism.

Similarity of Qualitative Methods to Investigative Journalism

All research methods are essentially investigations, but perhaps they are more threatening to individuals when unstructured interviews and the possibility of a participant observation technique are part of the research design. Quantitative research designs are by nature more specific, the variables are already known, and the researcher searches for relations between variables. On the other hand, discovery, the finding out about something otherwise not fully understood, is often the aim of qualitative research designs.

Within institutions, such studies may be perceived as threatening. Interviewing patients may cause staff to worry about negative information that the patient may give—for example, complaints, reporting incidents, and so forth. If there is to be observation, who does not experience some anxiety about the idea of being observed? Fear, then, is an important feeling to consider, and one that cannot be summarily dismissed: What if you do "discover" some "negative" findings that do not reflect well on the institution or staff?

These challenges must be addressed in any proposal presented to an institutional review board. The strategies for meeting these challenges include education and translation, the establishment of compatible values, and the generation of trust.

MEETING THE CHALLENGES

Education and Translation

Becoming sympathetic to the concerns and psychological dynamics of the members of institutional review boards is the best place to start. In many cases, qualitative research proposals may not be understood by these people, may be contrary to the way that they think, and may be threatening to them. In addressing these challenges, one should realize that the normal human response to change is resistance. Many qualitative nurse-researchers in institutions have reported that "resistance" was the only response to their research proposals and that they have had to change their proposals or move out of the institution. Although this situation is unfortunate, it can be prevented if qualitative nurse-researchers will educate their colleagues who sit on IRBs about the nature and philosophy of qualitative methods.

Most board members are thoroughly familiar with the methods associated with the Western mind-set of objectivity, control, prediction, and so forth. No one needs to explain ex post facto correlation, experimental design, or statistical test, but phenomenology, grounded theory, ethnography, or whatever qualitative research method is going to be used must be explained. Not only must it be explained, but it must be presented in language that can be understood by people familiar with deductive, pragmatic, numerical ideologies.

There is a need to explain in concrete terms the primacy of perception, embodiment, and the philosophical concepts. All these ideas should be clearly stated in language that the reader will understand. For example, in submitting a proposal for a qualitative research project that will examine the needs of patients who have had a mastectomy so that appropriate nursing interventions can be developed, language such as "the lived experience" of having a mastectomy, consciousness, and essences may be used but need to be explained. Is this a capitulation, a compromising of our principles? On the contrary, it is the recognition that it can take years to understand these concepts and that, in a proposal, there is a limited amount of time and space for explanation. So, instead of a capitulation, it is actually a pragmatic action for a pragmatic setting. If the institution uses a structural–functionalist approach, it is unrealistic to think that this perspective will not also be reflected in the process of an IRB review.

Compatible Values

In structural–functional bureaucracies, the reality is that the search for meaning, the apprehension of essential relations among essences, the thematic analysis of cultures, the perception of another's world, and the discovery of core variables are at odds with the predominant problem-task orientation. Helping patients find meaning does not rank high among institutional objectives. So this objective must be stated in the proposal in pragmatic terms—such as, this study will result in improved nursing care or act as the basis for developing nursing intervention. The qualitative method must also appear structured, even if the design allows for fluidity and some flexibility. As far as possible, research aims should be compatible with the aims of the institution. The members of the IRB must not think that they are making an exception by accepting a qualitative research proposal, because it appears different from their value orientation. It is best, from any point of view, to *demonstrate the convergence of values* between the institution and the qualitative study by stating how the study's *quest for discovery is laying the groundwork for nursing intervention.*

Generating Trust

Developing trust and alleviating fear or anxiety or both within the institution is critical to a successful qualitative research proposal, and it is also one of the more awkward challenges. This awkwardness arises from the perplexing situation in which the staff worry about the researcher having access to potentially damaging information or observing poor nursing care. They wonder what the researcher is going to do with possible "negative" findings.

The difficulty can be dealt with by pointing out that quantitative researchers in institutions may witness and be part of the same environmental activities as qualitative researchers and that the staff themselves are probably aware of whatever problems exist. Ideally, ethics committees or quality assurance programs address these problems, yet there is always the possibility that qualitative research may uncover some problems, and consequently, the staff may feel threatened.

The first step in dealing with this problem is to include a category for "unexpected findings" in the proposal and to carefully spell out what channels the nurse-researcher will use to share such findings. If the members of the IRB understand that *the discovery of findings that indicate problems is important* so that they can then be solved, members and staff might be more assured. Again, education is important for achieving this perceptual shift. Traditionally, IRBs are familiar with research that attempts to *solve problems.* The value of research that may *identify problems* so that they, too, may be addressed needs to be stressed, and stressed, and stressed. Indeed, it is critical to identify the right problem *before* testing solutions.

Sometimes this is difficult to do, such as when patients complain during interviews about poor nursing care. A good qualitative researcher looks at the larger context (before reporting such a result, ethics demands that the lens of the study must be widened) and finds that there is inadequate staffing. Although the administration may not be happy with that finding, the nurses on the unit will be glad to have such an important need substantiated. At other times, the problem is thornier. Perhaps the poor nursing care is the result of an incompetent nurse. Although the nurse-researcher cannot be the only one to know of this, he or she is ethically obligated to report such a finding through the channels that are established prior to starting the project (see the example in Field & Morse, 1985, pp. 48–49). Although this is essentially "whistle blowing," with its attendant consequences, sometimes good, sometimes bad, this action embodies the belief that "the therapeutic imperative of nursing (advocacy) takes precedence over the research imperative (advancing knowledge) if conflict develops" (Chapter 19 herein).

These problems have fewer ramifications for researchers not researching in their home institutions, and, if possible, it may be wise not to conduct research in one's home institution. Additionally IRBs have members who wish to protect their institutions or their own reputations or both. This difficult problem should be addressed in qualitative research proposals in positive, helpful terms and fully discussed with staff. They, too, need to be fully informed about the research project.

Similarities Between Qualitative and Quantitative Proposals

There are many similar areas in qualitative and quantitative proposals that are of concern to institutional review boards. More than likely, the same form will be used for both types of methods, and the researcher will be asked to address the following areas:

1. Objective of study
2. Research methodology
3. Characteristics of group(s)
4. Special groups (children of compromised adults)
5. Type of content
6. Confidentiality of data
7. Possible risk
8. Nonbeneficial research

Although there may be other variables, ensuring that individual rights and human dignity are protected needs to be demonstrated and documented. Often, institutional review boards have more elaborate requests than those listed here, and qualitative research proposals are often evaluated on the basis of adherence to traditional scientific method. Scientific legitimacy, then, is being evaluated rather than human subjects' protection. This may not be a problem 10 years from now, but, today, proposals come back from IRBs with questions that indicate reluctance to approve the proposal because the board does not understand the method and its concomitant language. As previously suggested, educating members of IRBs about the scientific legitimacy of qualitative studies is an additional task for qualitative nurse-researchers. What follows are some distinguishing characteristics of qualitative research that need to be addressed in IRB proposals.

Departure and Additions for Qualitative Research Proposals

A brief overview of the aim and purpose of qualitative research methodology may precede the proposal or, perhaps, be the introductory paragraph, depending on the institution. This overview does not have to be a highly sophisticated discourse about worldviews and paradigms, with quotations from Husserl, Erasmus, or Speigelberg; rather, a simple paragraph explaining how qualitative research methodology seeks to discover new knowledge, uses narrative descriptions in the findings, includes interviews with individual participants, and so forth, is all that is necessary. Stating that these aspects of the methodology can be used to build on one another may be important. Nurse-researchers often get into difficulty by discussing intersubjectively, going "to the things themselves," living the question, and so on. Understandable language is critical.

Objective of the Study.   As previously discussed, the objective of the study should be ultimately stated in pragmatic language. Often the aim of qualitative research is stated in existential terms. Remember the setting and take the existential purpose one step farther by showing how the study might, for example, (a) improve staff performance or (b) assist the patient in recovery.

This approach is appropriate because it is the qualitative research baseline that enables quantitative researchers to develop hypotheses for nursing intervention, staff performance, and assisting patients in their recovery. Stress the importance of the study in pragmatic terms.

Research Method.   Perhaps the most important part of the proposal, the research method offers the best opportunity for educating members of IRBs. Introduce the method, the rationale for choosing the method, and the outcome of this method. Take the reader through a step-by-step narrative in language that is familiar. This may mean taking the proposal that was written for nursing colleagues of a similar bent and translating it for persons who may be puzzled by the use of the word "phenomenon." For example, instead of saying "lived experience," just say "experience." In fact, someone once asked me what other kind of experience there is! Perhaps replacing the phrase "ontological commitment" with "it is my belief that" also will be helpful.

Although it may be human to want to impress one's colleagues with a high level of abstraction, it will probably be counterproductive. In any case, it seems paradoxical when qualitative research is actually very interested in the concrete. No one wants to feel inadequate, and it seems unwise to send out proposals loaded with unfamiliar language. Again, to achieve IRB approval, *members must be able to read* qualitative research proposals *without a dictionary*!

So qualitative researchers need to be clear and emphatic about their research methods. They need to teach about the method and its pragmatic usefulness to nursing sciences in language that will not distract the readers but keep them focused on the substance.

Consequence.   There is a debate in the literature about whether informed consent is necessary when observations and discourse take place in the course of a nurse's routine work (Noble, 1985; Oberst, 1985). Interviews have often been exempt from formal informed consent procedures if individual verbal consent is given. However, I fear we will be on a slippery slope if too many of these exceptions to the written consent process are allowed. Common sense needs to prevail.

Within institutions, qualitative researchers need to anticipate a request for informed consent. If more than one interview or observation is going to take place, the idea of a process consent seems to exemplify a negotiated view of not only the "phenomenon" but also the study itself (Chapter 19). All consents need to take into consideration the capacity of the person consenting, full disclosure of the research activity, and the freedom to voluntarily enter and withdraw. An inclusive consent can be found in Field and Morse (1985).

A proposal for process consent is suggested because an informed consent represents a past-tense concept. Qualitative research is often an ongoing, dynamic, changing process. A process consent offers an opportunity to actualize a negotiated view and to change arrangements if necessary. A process consent encourages mutual participation and, perhaps, mutual affirmation for the participants and the researcher.

A process consent for qualitative nursing research should be developed with the research participants' input, ideas, and suggestions and reviewed at specific times if necessary. This approach is appropriate if the researcher is going to be doing observations or participant observations over a period of time. In addition to the informed consent, a process consent should address some of the processes listed in Table 20–1.

It is probably wise to have information about self-disclosed secrets in the process consent. It should be stated that all data obtained will be part of the study. In other words, secrets should be discouraged if they cannot be included in the study. It is best to explain to the participants that some secrets pose a dilemma for researchers who are also concerned about the patient's well-being. The question of secrets and patients' confidentiality needs to be planned, and ethical dilemmas need to be considered before the proposal is written (see Chapter 19).

TABLE 20–1   PROCESS CONSENT

Researcher and participant as collaborators come to agree on:

  how you will enter the field

  how often, for how long

  how you will leave the field

  how you will prepare to leave

  how you will share the information

  how you will keep the information anonymous and confidential

  how you will assure an accurate portrayal

  what you will do if focus changes

  what you will do with "unanticipated findings"

  what you will do with secrets and confidential material

  what you will do with inclusion and exclusion of information

  where the findings are to go

Comments by participant

Comments by researcher

Dates reviewed and changes made

Signatures

Note: Each study would require a specific process consent, depending on the substance of the study. This process consent is in addition to the usual components of informed consent.

Confidentiality and Anonymity.   The same guarantee of confidentiality of data and anonymity of participants that quantitative researchers give must be made a general principle of qualitative research. This is a *general* principle because some institutions allow their identities to be known, especially if the study is going to reflect positively on them. In addition, some participants enjoy being identified in certain kinds of interviews or studies. However, the general principle is to maintain confidentiality and anonymity.

In qualitative research, can we promise confidentiality when we include precise quotations from the transcripts in our publications? The answer is "no," but we can provide anonymity by protecting the identity of the participant. Consequently, individuals and institutions will want assurances that only the researcher(s) will have access to the data and that there will be no identifying evidence, such as names on cassettes, names on computer printouts, and so forth. They will also want information about how and where the data will be stored.

In this section of the proposal, it might be helpful to identify the lines of communication that have been established for reporting findings. Information concerning the plans for disseminating the findings (i.e., publication, presentation, and who will receive final reports) should be included and mutually agreed on.

Possible Risks.   Qualitative research is considered noninvasive, but, in a sense, that is a limited perception of the word. Although it is true that qualitative researchers do not physically alter the participants with interventions, there are invasions of their space and psyches. Although such invasion is often therapeutic, it can pose possible risks if certain precautions are not taken.

It is well substantiated that talking has therapeutic benefits. Patients in institutions, or staff for that matter, often find relief just "getting it out of their systems" or "off their chests." Nursing intervention often provides opportunities for patients to ventilate their feelings, and interviews provide such opportunities. Attention is usually viewed as a positive experience, and being important enough to study can be viewed positively. That someone's experience is worth studying can have a validating effect.

Are there risks in qualitative research? One reviewer from an IRB asked about "triggering" an emotional response within an informant. This possibility cannot be lightly dismissed if the experiences under study are highly charged. Because of their training, nurse-researchers are usually able to intervene appropriately and make good assessments about how a patient is responding. It may be normal if a patient becomes upset in the course of an interview, and the nurse-researcher must be supportive and manage the interview with good clinical judgment. Arrangements also should be made with the patient's primary caretaker to support the patient after leaving the field. Aamodt (1986) writes:

> In the Human Subject Consent Forms we had said there were no psychological or social risks. Because communication in response to client feelings is an expected nursing intervention, to ignore such a need could be classified as irresponsible. We planned that interviewers would not be the primary caretaker of the child, and when the situation demanded it, the child and parent were referred to the primary caretaker. (p. 167)

An inaccurate portrayal of participants or situations can cause harm. A statement of how you intend to ensure the accurate description of participants and situations should be included in this section of the proposal. Validation by the participants is respectful and necessary for authentic representation. The harm/benefit question is succinctly placed in context by Morse (1988) when she states:

> Are the risks to the participant any greater than the everyday risk from confiding in a friend? And the "friend" in this context is a registered nurse who is accustomed to handling confidential information, counseling the dying and the distressed, observing and listening. Yet, suddenly, because the information is obtained under the auspices of "research" (rather than practice), the activities of the nurse may be considered by the IRB as potentially harmful. We must learn to trust our colleagues. (p. 214)

Nonbeneficial Research

This section of the proposal addresses research that is devoid of therapeutic purpose for the participant. Again, the opportunity to verbalize and be appreciated for sharing often does have therapeutic effects. This section should not be problematic, particularly in light of what has been previously discussed.

Presenting to the IRB

When presenting to an IRB panel, anticipate as many questions as possible. Consider the presentation a wonderful opportunity to discuss your study. However, educating IRB members about your research methods and translating them into clear, concrete, pragmatic terms should also be done in the verbal presentation. Know who the board members are and avoid answering questions in a philosophical or existential style. If there is a member of the clergy on the board, he or she might understand your answer, but the lawyer, the physician, the two laypeople, the banker, and the accountant might not, so keep your discussion clear and precise. Remember, the intentions of the IRB are the same as yours: to protect the patient.

In summary, writing clearly (especially philosophical translation), suggesting compatible values between the institution's goals and the research goals, developing trust, and establishing clear lines of communication are important areas to consider when submitting a qualitative research proposal to an institutional review board.

REFERENCES

Aamodt, A. (1986). Discovering the child's view of alopecia: Doing ethnography. In P. Munhall & C. Oiler (Eds.), *Nursing research*: A *qualitative perspective* (pp. 163–171). Norwalk, CT: Appleton-Century-Crofts.

Field, P., & Morse, J. (1985). *Nursing research*: *The application of qualitative approaches*. London: Croom Helm.

Morse, J. (1988). Commentaries on special issue. *Western Journal of Nursing Research*, 10(2), 213–216.

Munhall, P. (1988). Ethical considerations in qualitative research. *Western Journal of Nursing Research*, 10(2), 150–162.

Munhall, P., & Oiler, C. (1986). *Nursing research*: A *qualitative perspective*. Norwalk, CT: Appleton-Century-Crofts.

Noble, M. (1985). Written informed consent: Closing the door to clinical research. *Nursing Outlook*, 33(6), 292–293.

Oberst, M. (1985). Another look at informed consent. *Nursing Outlook*, 33(6), 294–295.

ADDITIONAL REFERENCES

Burns, R. (1989). Standards for qualitative research. *Nursing Science Quarterly*, 2, 44–52.

Denzin, N., & Lincoln, Y. (1994). *Handbook of qualitative research*. Thousand Oaks, CA: Sage.

Erlandson, D. A., Harris, E., Skipper, B. L., & Allen, S. D. (1993). *Doing naturalistic inquiry*: A *guide to methods*. Newbury Park, CA: Sage.

21

Types of Talk
Modes of Responses and Data-Led Analytic Strategies

Janice M. Morse

Analysis of interview data has by and large focused on the substantive content. That is, when using content analysis, the researcher has coded the transcripts by *subject content*, placing all data relating to similar topics in the same category. Thus, analysis has been driven primarily *by actual events and transitions between these events* rather than by the researcher also looking for—and analyzing—other, less explicit substance that lies beneath the obvious. This chapter is a plea for an additional level of analysis; that is, one that incorporates the interesting and important aspects of the interview *form* in the analysis.

A concrete approach to analysis tends to keep the research descriptive. The research loses a great deal of meaning, perhaps even losing the primary essence of the interview. Furthermore, when I explain to students that the most significant and powerful qualitative research is interpretative, they counter that they "do not know how to interpret" or "do not know how to increase the abstraction of the analysis from the interview itself." Thus, the aim of this chapter is to bring some of these

Acknowledgments: An earlier version of this chapter was presented at the AQR Conference, July, 1999, in Melbourne, Australia. I thank Mary Haight, M.A., for her contribution. The research was supported by AHFMR Health Scholar Award and MRC (Canada) Senior Scientist Award.

techniques to the fore, to make the less-obvious voices in the interview transcript audible, and to discuss alternative levels and types of analysis that are possible.

CHARACTERISTICS OF UNSTRUCTURED, INTERACTIVE INTERVIEWS

Unstructured, interactive interviews are used when the researcher has little information on a topic and, therefore, assumes the stance of a receptive, nonjudgmental listener or learner.[1] The researcher asks a minimal number of questions, perhaps only one "grand tour" question (Spradley, 1979). The participants are given space to "tell their stories" at their own pace, starting wherever they wish to start and proceeding with minimal interruption. The researcher is an active listener who tracks each story as it is told and stacks questions about alternative pathways to be asked at a later time. Questions that the researcher may ask are done without interrupting the flow of the narrative or are asked at the end of the interview or in subsequent interviews.

The content of unstructured, interactive interviews varies: An interview may consist of a description of ongoing events (in which case, the interview would be conducted at various points in the experience) or it may follow the completion of the event, with the participant being asked to relate "the whole story." Participants define the parameters of the events themselves; so, as the researcher increases the number of participants in the study, there is some variation not only in the experience of the event, but also in the parameters, focus (including those of the self or others are presented), levels of generality, and perspectives. Rather than adding confusion, these differences add the neces-

---

[1]Some reviewers for the journal *Qualitative Health Research* have challenged the notion of an "unstructured" interview, suggesting that if "unstructured" interviews were possible, then the information obtained would have no focus. Indeed, that is not the case. Consider the context of the interview: Participants know that they have been invited to participate in the study because of some experience they have had and they have received a full description of the research project in the process of giving their consents. Therefore, by the time a researcher reaches the point of asking the first question, the participant knows what experiences to relate. For instance, in my study of dying, the first 'question' was simply a statement by the interviewer, "Whenever you are ready. . . ."

sary richness required for saturation.[2] The goal of the analysis of unstructured interactive interviews is to produce rich descriptions that will enable comprehension, synthesis, an increase in the level of abstraction, and theory development.[3]

In this chapter, I refer to the *form*, or the *structure*, of the interview as the course of the story line, level of intensity of the interview, and the interview focus and scope; that is, all the structural features of the interview that are not directly related to the topic being discussed. It includes the degree of description, the emotional tone, and the degree to which the participant was a "good informant," that is, the ability to be reflective, talk, and share experiences.

The Course of the Story Line

The story line is how a participant chooses to relate the story. Unstructured, interactive interviews begin tentatively, with the participant first providing some context so that the story will make sense. As the participant begins to tell the main story, the intensity and the emotional depth of the story increase. Occasionally there will be "critical junctures" in the story line, with the participant choosing to follow one of two paths and continue the interview into another segment or story, whereas the other path is left unexplored. The interviewer must remember critical junctures so that, at the end of the interview, the researcher can take the participant back to those points and ask about alternative story lines:

> You told me that when you received news about the positive biopsy you resisted your husband's pleas to seek alternative therapy and to follow the physician's recommendations. Can you tell me about that time and the alternative therapy?

Note that the emotional depth of the account is reached after the participant "settles" into the story. The participant becomes internalized, lost in the telling, losing eye contact with the interviewer and apparently looking off into the distance. As emotional depth is reached, the participant's eyes may tear, and the participant may cry, but, by the end of the story, the participant regains emotional stability, as

---

[2]Unstructured, interactive interviews are not usually "one shot" data-collection events. The investigator may return to seek additional information—in particular, to seek information on the applicability of information obtained from other sources for this case.

[3]For a complete description of this analysis process, see Morse (1994).

evidenced by the tone of voice. The interview invariably concludes with lighthearted and irrelevant gossip and social talk. Norris (1989), in her study of mothers providing consent for their adolescent daughters' abortions, notes that, although these stories were exceedingly emotional, by the end of the interview the tone was one of lighthearted talk. In this way, the interview process itself is cathartic, providing a therapeutic release for the participant.

The Timing of the Interview

Consideration must be given by the investigator to when the interviews are best conducted. Interviews may be conducted immediately after the event, during the event, with several interviews being conducted over time in order to complete the event, or sometime after the event, with the participant chronologically reconstructing the events. Sometimes "event sampling" may be used, with interviews conducted with people who are at various stages in the process.

The timing of the interview is important because it affects the nature and quality of the information obtained. Some argue that the interviews should be conducted soon after the event to prevent "forgetting," but my experience has shown that the timing of these interviews depends on the research question and the data required. For example, if the researcher's question addresses interaction or decision making, either the interviews should be conducted as soon as possible after the interaction or the decision was made or the interaction should be recorded directly and the methods of conversational analysis used. If, however, the research question pertains to relationships or to the outcomes of the decision, then interviews are best timed after the event. For instance, when I began my own research on trauma patients, I incorrectly believed that the interviews should be conducted as soon as the condition of these patients permitted; that is, after the discharge from the intensive care unit (ICU). These interviews were terrible. Patient after patient gave a recitation of events in monotonic manner, and these accounts were devoid of emotion and contained no experiential information. When we changed our strategy and conducted these interviews 6 months later, when people were discharged from the rehabilitation hospital, the interviews were all that we had expected—rich and descriptive. We know now that several factors account for the change in the quality of these interviews. When patients were interviewed just out of the ICU, they were enduring, focused on the present and suppressing emotion (see Morse & Carter, 1996). They had not had time to "make sense" of their injuries or time to evaluate the effect that these injuries would have on their lives. Further, I have argued elsewhere that the assumptions underlying qualitative interviews is violated when we interview those who are newly sick: the assumptions are that the informants are experts, yet those newly ill or injured are in a bewildered state, not expert at all (Morse, 2000).

On the other hand, patients who were discharged from the rehabilitation hospital had time to reflect on the consequences of their injuries. Furthermore, their recall of events was enhanced: flashbacks had filled in memory lapses, and some had sought information from ICU staff and emergency medical technicians (EMTs) about "what they did" and "what happened." They were now in a stage of *suffering* (rather than enduring) and able to reflect on the consequences of their injuries. Finally, although these participants had had an opportunity to report what had happened throughout the course of the hospitalization to therapists and others, several reported that the unstructured interview situation gave them an opportunity to tell their stories for the first time "all at once" and therefore provided them with an opportunity to "put it all together." First-time stories are usually better than those that have become rote with telling.

Interview Threads and Themes

When recalling past events, participants tend *not* to tell their stories as a comprehensive whole from start to finish. Rather, they compartmentalize their stories by linking related events, telling the story of one set of common events and then returning to the beginning to report on another thread or set of related events. These threads may or may not become analytic themes in the completed study.

For example, in our studies of enduring and suffering, participants are given the option of structuring their stories as they choose. Our initial question is simply, "Tell me . . ." Invariably participants begin by giving us a comprehensive overview of the illness. Next they report on what we call the "medical story"—a chronology of the illness from diagnosis to the present, including treatments, surgery, and their interactions with physicians. We then hear about their responses, what they *thought* and how they acted and responded during the illness; and, finally, we hear the peripheral story, about their families' responses, the effect on their jobs, and so forth. We call these various strands *parallel stories* because they may need to be reconstructed or mapped to obtain a comprehensive overview.

But all participants do not present data in the same form. Others may use events, reporting on their experiences by attaching illness events to major changes in their lives: the marriage of their children, a husband's retirement, the birth of their grandchildren, a major vacation, and so forth. Still others may center their stories on changes in levels of disability, places of residence, and so forth. The important point is to identify the structure of the interview threads and themes and to use these points analytically because they are significant to the participants. In particular, if the illness trajectory is important in the analysis (as with grounded theory), recognizing the points that participants use to anchor their stories is helpful when analytically moving from the general to the specific and developing a generalized story across all participants. To identify common events, it may be necessary to map and to reconstruct events or responses on the same time line so that the researcher may synthesize the experiences.

The Form of the Interview and Coding Patterns

Coding is simply the identification and labeling of pieces of data. However, the process of coding includes decisions about what is and what is not relevant to the research question, degrees of significance, and which pieces of data are related and are to be placed together in the same category. At its lowest level, coding for content analysis collects and labels groupings of data from one or more interviews collected from one or more participants. When data are interpreted, the process of interpretation lifts data to a level of abstraction apart from the original data. And, according to the method used, coding patterns vary. For instance, with grounded theory, segments of the interview are considered apart from others, according to the stages and phases of the process. Data forming the core variable, however, are derived from a theme running through the entire interview.

Less discussed are what I call *shadowed data*. In the process of the interview, the participant may speak for her- or himself and for others like, or not like, her- or himself. In doing so, the participant is sorting the world for the analyst. Participants also do this by defining parameters, reporting the frequency of occurrence, sorting the commonplace from the exceptional (thus defining norms), and reporting on best and worst cases (thus defining extremes). *In this way, awareness of the structure of the interview while the interview is taking place, and certainly during analysis, enhances understanding and facilitates analysis.*

Moving the Interview Between Levels of Theory

We interview because we, as researchers, do not know what our participants think. But our participants are not generally naïve, unsophisticated, or stupid. They come to the interview with a certain amount of knowledge. Working beyond description—for instance, exploring concepts such as health—results in one learning what participants have been carefully taught. This is why studies exploring *health* give us regurgitated knowledge about vitamins and the importance of exercise, sleep, and eating right rather than the kind of information that we need to know, whatever that may be. Interviews are not a *test* of knowledge. I learned this the hard way. Once, when exploring health in an inner city, an elderly lady said, in response to the question "What, to you, is health?"

> Well, my dear, if I knew you were going to ask that, I would have looked it up in the dictionary.

Perhaps many of these health studies are using the wrong methods and should actually be quantitative surveys. Researchers must always be aware of whether they are working inductively or deductively and identify the level of their data.

Explore transcripts for threads of theoretical perspectives and identify them. Just as analysis is not atheoretical, the words of our participants are also not atheoretical. At the moment, we are conducting a study of enduring to die, and, when interviewing nurses about their patients, we learn that a surprising number of nurses are using Kubler-Ross's (1969) stages of dying to describe patient states. If we wanted to know about Kubler-Ross's theory, then we would read her work rather than interview; if we wanted to know about how Kubler-Ross's theory was and still is used and if that was our research question, then maybe these interviews would be helpful. But our research asked about patients and their responses to dying, and those interviews that were couched in a Kubler-Ross framework and provided a glimpse of reality through that particular theoretical lens were not used in our analysis.

Similarly, the participants may themselves have political or religious or other type of agendas and use the interview as an opportunity to further these agendas. So what do you do with this information? Note that the decision to discard or to use this information depends on the research question.

Moving the Interview Between Levels of Data

How does the researcher move the interview between levels of abstraction? We do so by *identifying parameters* of the interview; that is, by noting the scope of the participant's references, using levels of generality and specificity in the interview text.

The Self/Multiple Occurrences.   In an interview, parameters are defined by the participant first stating a generalization, usually by reporting on experiences of multiple instances of past events from one's own experience and then giving a specific example (Figure 21–1). The nature of the example must be noted because sometimes the example will be an exception.

Sometimes, when a common alternative exists, it may be countered with another specific example. Noting the frequency of occurrence in the text aids in recognizing patterns:

> *I:* How do you manage the doctors? Can you tell me that?
>
> *S:* We talk a lot. I ask them a lot of questions, and I try to state my needs as clearly as possible, although I play the passive patient and I just go along with whatever they say. When they told me today that I should stay in another week, they wanted to keep me in another week, because it's in my best interest, I didn't make a fuss, although it would have been easy to just say I want to go home today, and I think it's my right to choose that, but it would just hurt me in the end, I suppose.

Notice how the interview "funnels" from the general to the specific—in this case, from the *self* to *multiple or repeated occurrences*:

> *S:* We talk a lot. I ask them a lot of questions, and I try to state my needs as clearly as possible, although sometimes (*Generalized: common exception alternative*) I play the passive patient and I just go along with whatever they say. (*Specific example*) When they told me today that I should stay in another week, they wanted to keep me in another week, because it's in my best interest, I didn't make a fuss, although it would have been easy to just say I want to go home today, and I think it's my right to choose that, but it would just hurt me in the end, I suppose.

Uncovering.   One interview strategy used to aid in the funneling of interviews I call *uncovering*. First, a generalized question is asked to elicit

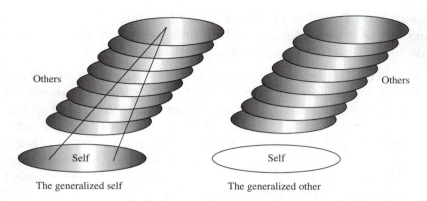

Others

Others

Self

Self

The generalized self

The generalized other

Figure 21–1 Perspective of the generalized self and the generalized other.

a generalized response, which is then brought to specifics by asking for the example:

Generalized question

I: Now when people come to visit you, how do they act toward you as a sick person?

Generalized response

S: They've been really good actually. A few of them passed out when they seen the pins in my legs.
I: They fainted right on the floor?
S: Two did, I think.
I: And then?
S: Well they kind of came to.

Bringing it to specifics

I: Tell me. . . .
S: Well, the first one was a friend of mine that works in the hospital here. I was still in the x-ray room, and she works in x-ray. I been telling the x-ray technicians that I knew her and she came in, so they told her that there was someone there that she knew, so she poked her head in, and there I was laying or sitting there. She came over and talked to me and started getting like turning colors and wobbling and she fell over.

Generalized Question to "Worst Case" Example.   The scope or parameters of a topic may be elicited by moving from the generalized case to the best- or the worst-case example:

> *I:* Do you have any memories of some very unpleasant situations?
> *S:* Yup. Yeah, there was one incident. It was just after I had moved into Edmonton and, by then, things had, the colitis had become what I call just a minor inconvenience for the most part I thought. But there was one day: I lived in a suburb of Ottawa, so I used to take the bus to work. It was about a 40-minute trip. This one day I was back in Ottawa on business. But we hadn't moved, so I was staying at home. Got on the bus and was fine but got within about 10 minutes of the office and the cramps got really severe, really bad. Literally walking up to the building feeling so bad that I thought I was going to have to. . . .

The Generalized Self/Generalized Other.   Important features of the participant's world may be understood by examining the text to determine the ways in which the participant sorts classes of people. We have, for instance, the *generalized self*, which entails identifying with a class of people with similar experiences. For instance, a participant with a spinal cord injury may use "we" to refer to all people with spinal cord injuries or, more broadly, all those in wheelchairs:

> At first, *you* don't want to go back in the world; *you* don't want to face people. *You* don't want to go to malls; *you* don't want to go to restaurants, but—at first I found it really, really hard. Especially in the wheelchair. Everybody, it doesn't matter, *you're* at everybody's mercy.

The linguistic indices are important. I argue that the patients use of *you, your,* and *you're* (*the generalized self*) is an attempt to normalize incomprehensible changes to the self.

There are those who are not like the participant, the *objectified other*—those like *that.* The *generalized other* refers to a group of people who behave in a particular way or who have characteristics that are *not* shared by the participant. Now, let us look at some data to see how these indices can be used analytically:

> A little kid came up and asked me, "What happened?"—you know, "Where's your hand?" . . . And, you can't say, "Look, kid, beat it," you know . . . 'cos they're innocent—they don't under-

stand what is going on. I just told him, "Well," I said, "I really—
I had a bad accident, and I, uh—lost my hand." And he says
"Well, were you awake when you lost it?" And I said, "No, no, I—
I was asleep. The—the doctor took it off, you know." And he was
just dumbfounded. He couldn't—couldn't see how you could
lose your hand. It's just something you didn't lose, you know,
like—he thought—I'd lost it. It just happened to . . . fall off.

Notice that the first "you know" is an example of the *generalized self*. The
next "*they're*" and "*they*" are examples of the *generalized other*: "cos *they're*
innocent" and "*they* don't understand."

Now in our transcripts we have some confusion. Some patients used
what we will label the *generalized self* in referring to themselves and their
injured bodies. They spoke about themselves and their own body
parts as "you," "your," and "you're." Often, the use of the generalized
self was a genuine generalization, in which the participants spoke
about experiences common to everyone. Now we can use this ambiguity to move the analytic strategy one step farther and explore the indices of the generalized self or the generalized other in relation to the
self; that is, as signals of embodiment and disembodiment.

We identified four types of signals used to refer to the *self* (i.e.,
the embodied self, the disembodied self, the embodied other,
and the generalized self) and three types of references to *others*
(i.e., the embodied other, the objectified other, and the generalized other). Next, by using different types and levels of interview
data, we can move beyond description to interpretation and to
theory development.

TABLE 1   LINGUISTIC SIGNALS OF EMBODIMENT/DISEMBODIMENT
             USE FOR SELF AND OTHERS

FOCUS	SIGNAL	MEANING
Self	I, my, me, mine,	Embodied self
	It, the, this	Disembodied self
	We, us, our	Embodied other
	You, you're, your	Generalized self
Others	My [doctor], our [diabetes]	Embodied other
	The [doctor]	Objectified other
	They	Generalized other

An Example: The Disembodied Self

Transcripts from patients who were burned were fascinating when we explored for signals of disembodiment (Morse & Mitcham, 1998). A lineman who suffered electrical burns and multiple amputations spoke about his experience as follows:

> Both *hands and wrists* were burnt, which were the . . . entry sites. And . . . *both feet* were burnt . . . *the right side* being the worst . . . . *Right side* of *both hands and feet* because I had—*my right hand was up high.* So naturally it entered *the right* the most . . . whatever was left over came down and went into *the left* . . . *it* still sustained some damage. . . . *The right hand* had to be removed. . . . And *the right leg* was burnt quite badly and the whole outside of *the leg* was burnt down to *the bone*—you could see *bones and sinews* in there, and *the very bottom*—it also exited—not on *the bottom of the foot* but . . . *the bottom of the leg,* like right at the side of *the foot* was really burnt bad, too.

By developing conjectures to explain this use of pronouns and testing these conjectures in data sets from patients who had experienced different intensities of pain and different relations with their bodies, we were able to demonstrate that linguistic indices of disembodiment were a strategy used to control agonizing pain by psychologically detaching the body part. As we followed the interviews over time, we were able to discern the points in the rehabilitation process where participants "took their bodies back" and again incorporated them into their body images.

The Embodied Other

There is much work to be done in exploring the function of the embodied other. For example, although the use of the inclusive "we" is common in the doctor–patient relation ("How are *we* today?"), Roberts (1999) notes that the function of this use of the pronoun has not been seriously explored.

Exploration of the use of pronouns in interviews can be a source of new insights into our participants' lives. For instance, in a recent article by Tappen, Williams, and Touhy (1999), self-descriptions of elderly people with middle- or late-stage Alzheimer's were used to determine their sense of self. The use of first-person pronouns was an indicator to determine the persistence of the sense of self.

Summary

To summarize the strategies presented here, analyze the type of talk in the interview rather than the topics being discussed. This analytic use of form can both enrich and expand analysis, linking it and developing it theoretically. The strategies are:

1. Trace the course of the interview to highlight the story line and to identify transitions and the function of the examples. Examine the transcript for level of generality because this enhances the scope of the study and reduces sampling.
2. Identify the threads and themes of each interview to determine if the story line is comprehensive or in parallel form. Mapping the interview threads and themes facilitates the merging of stories and the development of a generalized story.
3. Map the emotional intensity of the interview. Rote interviews are less rich than interviews that contain the story told for the first time—that is, when a participant is putting his or her story together for the first time. If the story is too hard to tell, it will have gaps and omissions.
4. Identify the level of sophistication or level of education of the participant. Does the interview consist of regurgitated book learning? Reveal a desire to please? Is there a theoretical overlay in the data? Or has the participant a political or religious agenda? It is important to remember that decisions to incorporate or to discard these data depend on the research questions asked. If you decide to discard the data, do not erase it; simply put it aside in case you realize later in the study that it was more significant than previously thought.
5. Seek and identify the linguistic features in other interviews, seek contextual explanation, and seek theoretical rationale. Look for the unexpected use of pronouns in references to self and to the other. Check occurrences in the participant's and others' interviews. Seek contextual explanation and theoretical rationale.

In this chapter, I have tried to demonstrate a different perspective for conducting textual analysis, which, if used, will move the analysis beyond a content/category sort. Original insights into transcripts or new questions and theoretical insights may be developed by analyzing the use of pronouns, exploring the form of the interview, and looking beyond the immediate topical content. Qualitative research, in the discovery mode, is an important tool for getting into participants' worlds and gleaning new and significant insights.

REFERENCES

Kubler-Ross, E. (1969). *On death and dying.* New York: Macmillan.

Morse, J. M. (1994). "Emerging from the data": Cognitive processes of analysis in qualitative inquiry. In J. Morse (Ed.), *Critical issues in qualitative research* (pp. 23–43). Menlo Park: CA: Sage.

Morse, J. M. (2000). Researching illness and injury: Methodological considerations. *Qualitative Health Research,* 10(3), 538–546.

Morse, J. M., & Carter, B. (1996). The essence of enduring and the expression of suffering: The reformulation of self. *Scholarly Inquiry for Nursing Practice,* 10(1), 43–60.

Morse, J. M., & Mitcham, C. (1998). The experience of agonizing pain and signals of disembodiment. *Journal of Psychosomatic Research,* 44, 667–680.

Norris, J. (1989). Mothers' involvement in their adolescent daughters' abortions. In J. M Morse & J. L. Johnson (Eds.), *The illness experience: Dimensions of suffering* (pp. 201–236). Newbury Park, CA: Sage.

Roberts, F. D. (1999). *Talking about treatment: Recommendations for breast cancer adjuvant therapy.* New York: Oxford University Press.

Spradley, J. (1979). *The ethnographic interview.* New York: Holt, Rinehart and Winston.

Tappen, R. M., Williams, C., & Touhy, T. (1999). The persistence of self in advanced Alzheimer's disease. *Image: Journal of Nursing Scholarship,* 31(2), 121–125.

22

Combining Qualitative and Quantitative Approaches

Carolyn Oiler Boyd

Combining research methods in a study, or research triangulation, is an issue in the nursing discipline as it has been for many years in psychology and sociology, and it is one of the manifestations of the division between the qualitative and quantitative traditions in research. Fielding and Fielding (1986, p. 10) noted that this issue, in psychology, is apparent in the tension between clinical and experimental methods; in sociology, it is apparent in the separation between fieldwork and statistical work. Further, they traced the differences in points of view to the hypothetic-deductive approach in quantitative research and the analytic-inductive approach in qualitative research. A third point of view posits the advisability of using both approaches to arrive at a superior research product; it is this view that draws protests from some camps and that will serve as the primary focus of this chapter.

Knafl and Breitmayer (1989) reported that, originally, the term "research triangulation" was "a technical term used in surveying and navigation to describe a technique whereby two known or visible points are used to plot the location of a third point" (p. 210). They explained that it first appeared in the social sciences in the 1950s as a metaphor to refer to the use of multiple methods to measure a single construct. The earliest references to triangulation in the research methodology literature, then, were concerned with enhancing the validity of quantitative findings through confirmation, or convergence, of findings from two or more instruments and/or data-collection procedures and techniques. Today, amid controversy, research triangulation is a term that refers broadly to the research practice of combining methods within a single tradition (quantitative or qualitative) or across those traditions. The overriding purposes of triangulation are to increase the reliability and validity of a study or to increase the comprehensiveness of a study, including those studies that are carried out in phases over a protracted period of time, or both.

In this chapter, the purposes of triangulation, types of triangulation, and applications in nursing studies are discussed, serving, in part, to enable the reader to engage in or to observe the controversy with a clear sense of the broad and particular meanings of triangulation and how it has been, and could be, used in nursing research. The controversy over combining qualitative and quantitative approaches in a single study is presented with an effort to transcend a simplistic view of the differences between the qualitative and quantitative traditions in research in the arguments either for or against this practice.

PURPOSES OF TRIANGULATION

As already stated, there are two overriding purposes for combining methods in research. The first is to increase the reliability and validity of a study, otherwise known as convergence or confirmation. In essentially quantitative studies, when there is measurement of discrete variables, the researcher may perceive a need to provide confirmation of findings from measurement. This confirmation could be accomplished by triangulating in another measure of the same variables. Qualitative strategies such as interviews might be conceived as such a measure, just as the addition of another instrument is so conceived. For the quantitative researcher, all the traditional rules of quantitative research continue to apply, and the integrity of the research remains essentially quantitative. Findings from this other measure or measures would be expected to converge with, or confirm, those obtained through initial or primary measurement if that instrument is reliable and valid. Convergence might be the purpose of administering a scale measuring a construct of caregiver burden in an essentially qualitative study as well. However, one sees fewer examples of this in the literature. It is becoming increasingly common nevertheless—a function perhaps of qualitative researchers needing to document in statistical form that their qualitative findings are valid from the positivist point of view. This problem with the concept of truth in research continues to vex qualitative researchers despite excellent explanations of how reliability and validity are interpreted and protected in qualitative approaches.

The second primary purpose of triangulation is to increase the comprehensiveness of a study. The idea here is that one method provides at best a partial picture of a complex phenomenon with many perspectives or aspects that need to be understood. Two or more methods are thus selected within one or the other of the research traditions or across those traditions. Some common ways to express this purpose are:

- *To provide qualitatively derived richness or detail in description or explanation of a phenomenon or both.* In quantitative inquiry, this purpose is usually viewed as complementary to the quantitative findings. In a qualitative inquiry, it is generally at the heart of the research and is often expressed in the research design through the inclusion of multiple methods selected from within the qualitative tradition.

- *To achieve a more complete understanding of the phenomenon under study, especially when the phenomenon has multiple aspects or perspectives to consider.* For the quantitative researcher, the option that meets the purpose of comprehensiveness might be conceived in two types of measurement such as the use of a broadly designed survey of adult women in a selected geographical area to ascertain usage patterns of mammography services and of a more detailed questionnaire administered to a random sample to obtain detail concerning such questions as how subjects determine a need for such services. Or researchers might regard some aspects of the phenomenon under study as measurable and others as needing to be explored qualitatively, leading to triangulation across research traditions. Such triangulation might, for example, include solicitation of data from nurses about caring as an aim and activity, from nursing management about their views, from patients about being cared for, and from nonparticipant observers of the interpersonal exchange in nursing care delivery. Or, comprehensiveness might be considered temporally and data might be generated at multiple points in time, producing multiple perspectives on, for example, the experiences of a child during and after the divorce of his or her parents.

- *To compensate for the weakness of one method via the strengths of the other; that is, to maximize validity of a quantitative study or to achieve a holistic understanding in a qualitative study.* In a quantitative study of loneliness in institutionalized elderly, for example, the measurement process may be recognized as posing a threat to validity. Qualitative method might be triangulated into such a study by collecting observational data descriptive of the manifestations of loneliness, and thereby the threat is counteracted. In a qualitative study of the same phenomenon, the addition of a measure of loneliness administered to elderly residents might be included in the study's design to compensate for possible reactivity to the research process.

It bears mentioning that, in triangulated studies, there is often a relative emphasis on their being essentially quantitative or qualitative. Methodological options are viewed by some as a menu of data-generation strategies or techniques and are used accordingly, with a sense of full freedom to select strategies that best serve identified purposes. There may, however, be important differences in the application of those strategies and in the gestalt of the design and analysis, based on the researcher's allegiance to one research tradition over the other.

Both purposes of triangulation—to enhance reliability and validity and to increase comprehensiveness—are accommodated by routine features of many qualitative inquiries. The incorporation of multiple data sources provides a check on the reliability of researcher-as-instrument and increases the credibility of findings. The conduct of an inquiry over a protracted period of time and the validation of findings with informants or the inclusion of judges in analysis of data accomplish this as well. In this sense, most qualitative studies are triangulated by nature. The issue, then, is clearly concerned with triangulation across qualitative and quantitative methods. In this narrower sense of the meaning of triangulation, the purposes heretofore discussed emerge from and relate to the quantitative paradigm in nursing research. Researchers who choose this approach in their studies thus reveal a positive regard for the coexistence of both research traditions if not an explicit allegiance to the quantitative paradigm.

TYPES OF TRIANGULATION

Four types of triangulation are distinguished in the literature: theoretical, data, investigator, and methodological triangulation (Denzin, 1978). Each type will be explained briefly, with an emphasis on methodological triangulation, which serves to focus the argument about combining qualitative and quantitative methods.

Theoretical Triangulation

Theoretical triangulation is the use of several different frames of reference in the analysis of data. This type of triangulation is commonplace in qualitative research when data have been analyzed in the discussion of findings and how they relate to the existing theory, research findings, and clinical practices. However, theoretical triangulation usually refers to the effort to test two or more theories with the same database by using each theory, in turn, to analyze the data. For example, in her study of women's responses to battering, Campbell (1989) compared two theoretical models—grief and learned helplessness—for their relative explanatory applicability for these responses.

Data Triangulation

Data triangulation refers to the use of a variety of sampling strategies or multiple data sources. It, too, is characteristic of qualitative studies, particularly those using grounded-theory and ethnographic approaches (and, properly, those adhering to phenomenological criteria). It is geared toward enhancing the internal validity of findings. Informant guardedness, for example, would be revealed in the prolonged period of fieldwork in which one "samples" that informant repeatedly. Researcher bias, as another example, is less likely to be maintained in the avalanche of data that contradicts him or her. In quantitative studies, this type of triangulation is seen when researchers use different measures of the same variable—for example, different measures of pain. It also refers to such strategies as data collection from the same subjects over time and sampling from more than one group and more than one situation. For example, measuring professional values of graduating seniors, recent graduates, and RN students might aim at revealing the effect of the curriculum on socialization into the profession.

Investigator Triangulation

Investigator triangulation refers to the use of multiple observers in a single study, as seen in studies conducted by research teams. This type of triangulation usually introduces theoretical triangulation by virtue of the various theoretical perspectives introduced by the team members. It also serves as a check on researcher bias and thereby contributes to internal validity in a qualitative study.

Methodological Triangulation

Methodological triangulation is simply the use of multiple methods in a single study, and as such this type of triangulation is the focus of attention in the controversy over combining qualitative and quantitative approaches. There are two subtypes of methodological triangulation: within method and between or across method triangulation. Within method triangulation is illustrated when one method, such as survey, is selected and several different data-collection strategies are used within that method, as, for example, the use of several measures of social support. This subtype is employed for the purpose of establishing convergent validity of confirmation of findings on one measure by the findings on the other. The second subtype, between or across method triangulation, is an approach that combines qualitative and quantitative approaches. It serves the purpose of establishing convergent validity as in the within method subtype or the purpose of disclosing paradox and contradiction in the findings.

APPLICATIONS

Comprehensiveness in a quantitative study can be achieved through the use of case study to illustrate the full meaning of quantitative findings. Qualitative data obtained from interview are not uncommonly used to clarify and amplify responses to questionnaires and scales. Alternatively, in qualitative studies, responses to questionnaires or scales can be used to give direction to the fieldwork, giving the researcher some beginning orientation to people's concerns or their beliefs, for example.

To achieve convergence, researchers may validate empirical constructs through interview or observational data. They may verify quantitative findings with qualitative findings or vice versa. In either case, the findings from one type of data generation are compared and contrasted with those from another type of data generation. If findings converge, they point in the same direction, to the same conclusions. In some cases, there may be "leftover" findings that require explanation. They do not fit in with the bulk of findings, but they do not contradict them either. Flaws may be located in the instrumentation or in data-collection procedures or in statistical analysis procedures; that is, there may be a failure in comprehensiveness. The deviant findings in such a case may give direction to future instrument development, for example. In other cases, the qualitative and quantitative findings may "fight" each other, offering up contradiction. Again, the researcher may search for flaws in the study. Finding none, he or she might turn again to the purpose of comprehensiveness as a possible explanation for contradiction. In qualitative research in particular, contradiction may simply point to a need for expansion in concepts so that the range of human variety is adequately accounted for in the data. Here, the quantitative researcher's concerns with means and medians are at odds philosophically with the qualitative researcher's concerns with the range of human possibilities. The odd case, the one that does not fit in with the others, is critical to disclosing those possibilities. The search for possible ways to be human in any given context is of particular interest to the phenomenological researcher and is of general interest for all qualitative researchers. Nonetheless, the tension between the particular and the universal exists not only between the quantitative and the qualitative orientations; it also exists within the qualitative tradition. The purpose of comprehensiveness is for some qualitative researchers interpreted to mean that a research interest in coping or in using the health care delivery system, for example, is necessarily concerned with an accounting for the variety believed to exist.

Two studies using multiple triangulation, and recently reported in the literature, will be reviewed to illustrate ways in which triangulation might be used. The first is an essentially qualitative study, according to the authors' designation; the second is an essentially quantitative study.

Knafl and Breitmayer (1989) reported on their use of multiple triangulation to achieve comprehensiveness in a qualitative study in process of how families define and manage a child's chronic illness. In Table 22–1, the authors' framework for evaluating the comprehensiveness of their study is indicated by listing each type of triangulation and the approach and purpose/goal for that type.

For investigator triangulation, four team members were assembled who had a general interest in how families respond to a member's chronic illness. The team members were diverse, however, in regard to their particular expertise with parents, children, or siblings; knowledge of differing aspects of the relevant literature; theoretical backgrounds; and research training. This diversity produced in the research team a complementarity that contributed to the purpose of comprehensiveness in the research.

Data triangulation was used across the three dimensions of person, time, and situation by collecting data from: (1) chronically ill children, their parents, and their siblings (person); (2) families in which a child

TABLE 22–1 FRAMEWORK FOR EVALUATING THE COMPLETENESS OF A QUALITATIVE STUDY BY USING MULTIPLE TRIANGULATION

TYPE OF TRIANGULATION	APPROACH	PURPOSE/GOAL
Investigator	Four member team	Substantive, theoretical, and methodological diversity.
Data Source	Person Time Situation	Represent individual perspectives over time and across a variety of situations. Theoretical sample.
Method	Intensive interviews Child Behavior Checklist (CBCL) Family Environment Scale (FES) Harter Perception Profile(HPP)	Identify individual definitions and management behaviors. Explore outcomes of definitions and behaviors.
Unit of Analysis Theory	Individual Family Development Application	Conceptualize individual and family unit response. Conceptualize family management style. Interpret individual and family unit response patterns.

Source: From "Triangulation in Qualitative Research: Issues of Conceptual Clarity and Purpose" by K. Knafl and B. Breitmayer, 1989. In *Qualitative Nursing Research: A Contemporary Dialogue* (pp. 213–214), edited by J. Morse. Newbury Park, CA: Sage Publishers, Inc. Reprinted by permission.

had been recently diagnosed and families in which a child had been diagnosed for some time (situation); and (3) two data-collection sessions, spaced 12 months apart (time). Two levels of data analysis, the individual and the family unit, were featured in this study to emphasize the person dimension of the data triangulation. Methodological triangulation was used through combining qualitative and quantitative data-generation strategies: structured instruments, observations, and intensive interviews. Theoretical triangulation in this theory-generating (in contrast with theory-testing) study was to be used in two ways: first, existing theories were to be used to interpret the data and, second, at the conclusion of the research process, findings were to be discussed in relation to other theories of family response to chronic illness (Knafl & Breitmayer, 1989, pp. 214–218).

TABLE 22–2   Multiple Triangulation: Application in a Study of the Relation Between Disaster-Related Stress and Health Outcomes

Type of Triangulation	Approach Features
Data	Study groups: 1. Bereaved group without property loss 2. Bereaved group with property loss 3. Permanent property loss 4. Vacation-home loss 5. No disaster loss Instruments randomly arranged, mailed at 1 year and 3 years post-disaster Follow-up interviews with subsample from each study group
Investigator	Multiple investigators
Theoretical	Tests of magnitude-of-loss hypothesis and two rival hypotheses: self-efficacy and social support
Methodological	Multiple statistical techniques Analysis of structured interview data

Source: Murphy (1989).

All four types of triangulation were also illustrated in Murphy's (1989) report of a study that aimed to assess the relations between disaster-related stress and mental and physical health outcomes after the Mount St. Helens volcanic eruption in 1980. Both purposes of convergence and comprehensiveness were served by triangulation in this study. The mediating effects of self-efficacy and social support on the stress–health relation were examined, and the effects of mass media coverage on recovery were explored. Table 22–2 summarizes the main features of multiple triangulation in this study.

Data triangulation entailed collecting data from five mutually exclusive types of study participants as listed in Table 22–2. Study instruments, arranged in three random orders, were mailed 1 year and 3 years post-disaster. This approach enabled the researchers to compare data across the study groups and longitudinally, from 1 year to 3 years post-disaster. Follow-up interviews were conducted with subsamples from each of the five study groups to obtain in-depth information regarding perceived disaster stress, coping strategies used,

588 Nursing Research: A Qualitative Perspective

and perceived recovery. Investigator triangulation was achieved through the participation of multiple researchers in this 8-year research project and included multiple interviewers and initial and secondary analyses of data. Data analysis included the use of various theoretical and methodological approaches by the research team members. Theoretical triangulation was used to test the major hypothesis that the effects of loss are proportional to their magnitude, as well as two rival hypotheses of the mediating effects of stress on health, social support and self-efficacy. In methodological triangulation, multiple statistical techniques were used to demonstrate the independence of linked pairs of bereaved participants and to test the magnitude-of-loss hypothesis, and interview data were analyzed to identify stressors and mediators of stressors.

THE CONTROVERSY, WITH AUTHOR COMMENTARY

Curious about how we tend to talk past one another and finding nursing's progress toward better understandings of opposing views slow at best, I will present two polarized points of view about research triangulation, with special attention to how they do and do not speak to each other. For the reader who strives to arrive at a personal judgment concerning the wisdom or the legitimacy of combining qualitative and quantitative research approaches, this discussion of opposing views may help to clarify what is at stake as well as the differences and difficulties in these arguments.

Moccia's (1988) argument against combining research approaches is selected to represent this stance because it is such a cogent explication and because it serves to complement the careful grounding for qualitative research laid out in Chapters 1 through 3. Gortner's (1990) argument for a philosophy of nursing science that clearly consigns qualitative researchers to an ancillary role in the discipline is also selected for two reasons. First, it, too, is a cogent explication of a view that dismisses qualitative research as a misdirected, otherwise worthy, endeavor. Second, few articles have appeared in the preceding decade that pointedly, and publicly, articulated the concerns and criticisms of many nurse researchers and students of nursing research. The arguments of each of these scholars will be described, accompanied by the author's commentary. It is hoped that the commentary will be successful in extending the necessary ongoing dialogue in this controversy.

Moccia (1988) argued against "appeasement and compromise" in decisions concerning whether and when to use qualitative or quantitative methods or a combination of the two. She cited four problems in the compromise approach:

1. The reality of limited resources of time, energy, and expertise in any given study or for any given researcher;
2. The flawed assumption that nursing research questions are atheoretical, lending themselves to a variety of methodological options;
3. A denial of the significance of the influence of philosophies of science in research and theory development; and
4. The avoidance of commentary on the political function of research traditions (p. 2).

In arguing for a reframing of the debate about methods in nursing research, Moccia offered the clarification that we are faced with a very fundamental choice about what nursing is to become: the choice of methods is really about the choice of continuing to develop knowledge that is aimed at prediction and the control of people and their problems or the choice of aligning ourselves with methods that serve recipients of nursing care, methods that assist people with understanding their experiences. But this equates research with practice: every situation presents a research project, and, surely, Moccia is not arguing that qualitative research findings do not constitute knowledge that can somehow be used to assist others outside of the situation that produced the findings.

Qualitative research produces a certain *kind* of knowledge. It produces knowledge of the range of possibilities, given shared historicity, which does offer a degree of predictability in health care situations. Qualitative research also contributes to what is understood about the nature of being human. It serves to relate us to one another, opening up a new sense of community with others, which, in turn, is linked to behaving more humanely with one another. Qualitative research thus has a sensitizing effect in the nurse–patient relation that has valuable, "good" outcomes for people in nursing.

Nursing necessarily uses many knowledges to practice holistically, in recognition that multiple perspectives constitute truth. It has chosen to strive for holism in its orientation, its intending, toward the practice world. Because truth is a matrix of perspectives, because being scientific in the positivist tradition is one of those perspectives, and because a view of the person as object yields a perspective as nearly true as any other, nurses need to synthesize multiple perspectives to accomplish their practice aims. If nursing scholars fail to interpret the relevance of research findings to practice in terms of a synthesis that admits multiple perspectives, it is not likely that practice will achieve an art–science coherence, a holistic orientation, or a distinctive character that renders nursing with an identity in the health care field.

As Moccia indicated, the question of combining research approaches pivots on the consequences of choice for nursing morally, ideologically, and politically. The kinds of questions posed as research questions, the kinds of data admitted as research data, and the processes used to generate the data all contribute to the definition of nursing and ultimately to practice activities themselves. But nursing does use other sciences, which confuses the issue. If one accepts the notion that there is (or could be) a unique body of knowledge in nursing or a unique application of knowledge, this is to say that nursing has boundaries and a perspective that distinguish it from other disciplines. For some qualitative researchers, the qualitative approach focuses our attention on certain kinds of phenomena from a particular perspective that is congruent with nursing intentions but is also clearly contrary to the positivist tradition in research. The relevance of qualitative methods for them has more to do with defining and creating nursing than with the methods per se. As Moccia (1988) stated,

> The research activity contributes to the emergence of a world or reality that was not there before the research. Through such research the knowledge created is logically characterized by the same attributes that identify human phenomena, e.g., the rational and the emotional, the objective and the subjective, and the passionate and the controlled. Logically, then, such characteristics also describe the science created through such an approach to research. (p. 3)

The idea of creating knowledge rather than discovering it is a unique feature of at least some interpretations of qualitative research. Through interview, for example, the researchers' reflections on and presentations of their experiences in language form create certain meanings that might not otherwise appear for them. Still, as research that produces knowledge, qualitative research must be understood as just one possible mode of awareness. Although it strives to give voice to human experiences, it is just one perspective on those experiences. Qualitative research cannot claim to have an exclusive corner on truth. Qualitative research findings are holistic only in the sense of meaning and coherence within the perspective of research partici-pants. They are not holistic in the sense of disclosing all possible per-spectives; nor is this generally the aim of qualitative studies. This dis-tinction from the sense of the term "holistic" when used to describe nursing care is important.

In Moccia's view, the methods debate concerns a distinction "among research activities that serve nurses and nursing, those that serve pa-tients and the public's health, and those that serve both" (1988, p. 6). She argued against the effort to predict and control on the bases of both the resistance of holistic human phenomena to prediction and control and the interest of nurses in their patients as autonomous, self-determining subjects rather than objects. Yet, to recall the kinds of knowledge that qualitative research produces, knowledge of some of the possibilities and even of probabilities does not have to be applied so as to cut off other possibilities, choice, and uniqueness. It seems to go without saying that nurses need to be able to predict (in a general way) such human experiences as pain and suffering, grieving, birthing, and so on, in order to anticipate and deliver needed care. This does not mean, for example, that a nurse can or should be able to predict precisely how John Doe will respond, but nurses do need to predict that he is likely to have pain, that his cultural history and identification may influence his response in certain ways, or that the meaning of his diagnosis to him is likely to be influenced by sociocultural meanings in certain ways. Being human does mean something; we do share a com-mon world of objects; we share multiple capacities, a common stock of everyday knowledge, and a common range of human possibilities within the contexts of the various worlds in which we find ourselves. This commonality includes those perspectives, among others, that are particularly focused in medical science and health care technology. In fact, because of our continually changing contexts, the work of qualita-tive research is never finished.

To be in health care situations with patients and to contribute meaningfully to those situations, nurses continue to need access to the multiple perspectives that constitute holistic assessment and in-tervention. If nursing is to claim the patient's experiencing as its unique focus, this claim will be furthered by such access. Why do qual-itative research if not to disclose shared humanness and human pos-sibility? We cannot, should not, close off our scientific mode of aware-ness. But, we should not adhere strictly to it if nursing's ambition to be expert in human experiencing of health and health care situations is to be realized.

Qualitative methods are designed to get inside the skin of the actors in these situations. However, as Gadow (1977) explained, both the lived body and the object body need to be understood to practice nursing. She stated:

> The history of professionalism in nursing suggests that nursing has focused exclusively upon the lived body and the object body in turn. . . . Nursing can now surpass both of these extremes: the nurse, as advocate of the patient's wholeness, is committed to advocacy of neither the shattered lived body nor the duly imposed object body. Nursing can, in short, make possible for the patient an enrichment of the lived body by the object body, and an enlivening of the object body by the lived body. The nurse can assist the patient to recover the objectified body at a new level at which it is neither mute immediacy nor pure otherness, but an otherness-made-mine, a lived objectiveness. . . . The nurse assists me, the patient, to live my objectness as my own, instead of allowing it to remain alien. That unity which I achieve is more fully expressive of my totality than even the lived body was. (pp. 24–25)

In this way, nurses are in a position to offer assistance to patients with a truly humanistic science, not merely with well-honed counseling skills but also with substantive knowledge about human health experiences.

Gortner (1990) acknowledged the significance of nursing values and nursing philosophy in traditional ways; that is, she cited the guidance of values in nursing activities, including scientific enterprises, and suggested:

> What well may be foundational in humanistic philosophy (concern for person and meaning) can remain as philosophy; it need not be translated into scientific strategies . . . and used to the exclusion of other options. Further, the practice of science and the scientific method, the search for explanations, regularities, and predictions about the human state should not be viewed as being incompatible with professional beliefs about practice and societal and personal worth. (p. 102)

She went on to cite the foundational nature of humanistic philosophy in Scandinavian nursing research as evidence of the potential for an intimate link between nursing philosophy and nursing research, noting that the "renewed interest in humanism and history has infused us with an appreciation for and sensitivity to the human condition, in the links between objective measures of reality and personal subjective ones" (1990, p. 103). What Gortner accomplished with this statement was reinforcement of an essentially dichotomous split between our humanism and our science—one that was reaffirmed in Gortner's proposal for a nursing science philosophy. In this proposal, she established that human understanding, arising from interpretations of phenomena from the patient's perspective, is a basic premise in nursing science, but then went on to reaffirm the positivist tradition with its emphasis on measurement, causal inference, and knowledge that allows for prescriptions for practice (pp. 103–105).

Despite the respect accorded to qualitative methods as an aid to the linkage between philosophy and research, they are not included in nursing science, which Gortner defined as public knowledge, meaning, in turn, intersubjective consensus among scholars. In so doing, Gortner neglected to attend to strategic points about the irreconcilability of the philosophical frameworks that support two research traditions in a variety of disciplines and to attend to the claims of intersubjectivity as an essential feature in the qualitative paradigm. However, she credited the idea of grounding quantitative research formally and practically in a body of knowledge generated through qualitative research, which was a promising overture of compromise in its most positive sense. Recognizing qualitative research as truly foundational to quantitative efforts in the field would be doubtlessly facilitated by a comprehensive inclusion of the former in nursing science. To do so requires, as Moccia stated, redefinition of science and the profession. To arrive at this redefinition, there must be continuing attention, specifically, to the nature of reality, truth, and human experience. Although not all nursing scholars may be inclined to ponder such philosophical questions, their importance is brought into relief by the neglected discussion of these premises by those who either oppose qualitative methods altogether or who regard them as merely a collection of techniques that may be applied to quantitative purposes.

Gortner's essay represented the kind of appeasement and compromise position that Moccia criticized. On the surface, considerable appreciation was expressed for qualitative researchers whose interest resides in "human understanding," which, for Gortner, was a worthy endeavor in nursing philosophy but distinct from scientific activities. The problem in this stance is the failure to include qualitative research as part of legitimate science, which will prevent adequacy in the body of knowledge that nursing produces. The idea that values and meanings determine our research behavior as well as our practice behavior is not recognized as a tangible and practical feature of qualitative research activity. Values are dismissed as if they had no practical consequences for public knowledge, as if there really were an absolute truth awaiting discovery. Gortner's essay is seductive in its appeal to a desire for orderliness in the discipline, with clear separation of nursing science from other nursing activities despite a weakly described linkage among them. The reaffirmation of the positivist tradition in the point of view represented by Gortner's proposal is perhaps an expression of the preference to continue in the mainstream of scientific endeavors in health care and a reluctance to confront the fact of choices before us.

To wait out the death of the debate is to refuse choice. It is not enough to say that values and philosophy are nice and, of course, there is interaction between nursing philosophy and nursing research. Consciousness has been raised, and, increasingly, researchers are recognizing that their use of research techniques has consequences for research participants and for the evolution of nursing practice in health care. When viewed as merely a collection of techniques, qualitative research methods can be easily triangulated in studies, as illustrated by the applications described earlier in this chapter. Goodwin and Goodwin (1984), for example, lay out this view directly: "The qualitative-quantitative distinction is primarily one of methods of data collection, analysis, and interpretation" (p. 378). Inattentiveness to the philosophical framework for qualitative research, or rejection of it, allows this.

An alternative basis for triangulated research can be located in an understanding of nursing phenomena from a practice perspective such as that explicated by Gadow (1977). The kinds of questions about these phenomena—in fact, the very emergence of phenomena as nursing phenomena—should be grounded in nursing philosophy if that philosophy really means something about nursing or for nursing. Clarity in identity and purpose will go far in guiding researchers in what they attend to, how they proceed with attending to it, and their use of the information produced by the research effort. Phenomenologically, what is argued is a need to establish a phenomenological baseline for our concepts, our theories, and our subsequent science. Other disciplines and other schools of thought within the nursing discipline might refer to this baseline to do science in the positivist tradition, and such science, in turn, will continue to become a part of our worlds, transforming human experience and creating new possibilities. In this sense, the work of establishing a phenomenological base-line is continuous. We have witnessed, for example, modification in theories of grieving as more is learned about how people live through grieving. We have come to understand that the timetable for grieving varies considerably; that the meaning of loss is open to a range of possibilities; that living through loss is highly contextual, highly embodied, highly enmeshed in a range of possible perspectives; and clearly intersubjective.

Duffy (1987) provided a discussion of benefits of triangulation that focuses the potentially complementary and supplementary relation of qualitative and quantitative methods (p. 132). From a view of differences between these two approaches as differences in not only techniques but also perspectives, she suggested that each perspective has limitations, and thus the overriding purpose of triangulation is to counterbalance the weakness of one perspective with the strength of the other. When one's attention is drawn to the world of nursing practice, various practical concerns surface, notably the need of nurses for concepts and theories to guide practice in the hectically paced world of health care. There has been unquestionably insufficient knowledge for them to use to size up situations quickly; to recognize who among their patients needs and chooses to explore and to determine their experiences; to know not only how to guide, but where; to know when and how to apply information in health-producing ways; to determine coherence in health care situations that are intimidatingly complicated with multiple participants and multiple perspectives. Nurses cannot be expected to approach each patient care situation without such knowledge; that is to say, without such generalizations about possibilities and probabilities. We do need science, and science is concerned not only with regularities, but also with possibilities.

There is an appeal to the idea that nursing would define itself as being, by choice, concerned with particular aspects of truth that are addressed by the qualitative research paradigm. As noted in Chapters 1 through 3, this kind of explicit acknowledgment of the discipline's interest and concern needs to avoid the trap of discounting the presence and import of the positivist perspective in the world. This perspective along with others are "real," are a part of the world to which nurses and patients belong, and thus cannot be discounted in the chosen perspective of human experiencing of the world. Consensus about a nursing perspective, however, does not seem to be imminent.

Practically speaking, then, nursing research is likely to continue to house two schools of thought. (Parenthetically, there is a third school of thought, but one hears little about it in the literature these days; that is, little from positivists who see no merit or authenticity in the arguments of the qualitative paradigm.) The first school adheres carefully to the qualitative paradigm, inclusive of its particular view of the nature of being human and of reality, the nature of nursing practice, and the kind of knowledge that serves the intentions of such a nursing worldview. Researchers who subscribe to this worldview will not triangulate their studies, in part because the introduction of measurement in their relation with participants would alter the nature of that relation and interfere with the data-generating dialogue of mutual benefit to researcher and researched. But, they would not deny the positivist worldview that is such a prominent part of health care situations.

The second school of thought concerns itself less with worldviews, accepts positivist premises as practical at the least, and makes use of qualitative research strategies as needed or desired to broaden understanding of those phenomena selected for research attention. Studies that flow from this way of regarding methodological options might be essentially qualitative or quantitative and might reflect the researcher's selective commitment to one or the other research paradigms. Unfortunately, this second school of thought, as currently practiced in research, does not recognize what is intended in the use of qualitative research to produce a phenomenological baseline; that is, the juxtaposition of quantitative research in a secondary role.

As Gortner and others who promote triangulation have pointed out, the interests and concerns of qualitative researchers are not irrelevant to quantitative researchers. There can be productive dialogue between the two. Neither school of thought necessarily need block the other; multiple paradigms within a single discipline are characteristic of our world anyway. We can live with blatant conflicts in ways of thinking about the discipline and might profit from them. In the meantime, researchers who locate a rationale in the purposes of triangulation explicated in the literature should be welcomed to the discipline's exploration of research methodologies. Appeasement and compromise are among our possibilities, as is the purist approach to qualitative research.

REFERENCES

Barbour, R. S. (1998). Mixing qualitative methods: quality assurance or qualitative quagmire? *Qualitative Health Research*, 8, 352–361.

Campbell, J. (1989). A test of two explanatory models of women's responses to battering. *Nursing Research*, 38(1), 18–24.

Copnell, B. (1998). Synthesis in nursing knowledge: An analysis of two approaches. *Journal of Advanced Nursing*, 27, 870–874.

Denzin, N. (1978). *The research act: A theoretical introduction to sociological methods* (2nd ed.) New York: McGraw-Hill.

Duffy, M. (1987). Methodological triangulation: A vehicle for merging quantitative and qualitative research methods. *Image: The Journal of Nursing Scholarship*, 19(3), 130–133.

Fielding, N., & Fielding, J. (1986). *Linking data*. Beverly Hills, CA: Sage.

Gadow, S. (1977). Existential advocacy: Philosophical foundation of nursing. Presented to Four State Consortium on Nursing and the Humanities, Phase I Conference, Nursing the humanities: A public dialogue, Farmington, CT.

Goodwin, L., & Goodwin, H. (1984). Qualitative vs. quantitative research or qualitative and quantitative research? *Nursing Research*, 33(6), 378–380.

Gortner, S. (1990). Nursing values and science: Toward a science philosophy. *Image: The Journal of Nursing Scholarship*, 22(2), 101–105.

Knafl, K., & Breitmayer, B. (1991). Triangulation in qualitative research: Issues of conceptual clarity and purpose. In J. Morse (Ed.), *Qualitative nursing research: A contemporary dialogue* (pp. 209–220). Newbury Park, CA: Sage.

Moccia, P. (1988). A critique of compromise: Beyond the methods debate. *Advances in Nursing Science*, 10(4), 1–9.

Morgan, D. L. (1998). Practical strategies for combining qualitative and quantitative methods: Applications to health research. *Qualitative Health Research*, 8(3), 362–376.

Murphy, S. (1989). Multiple triangulation: Applications in a program of nursing research. *Nursing Research*, 38(5), 294–297.

Shih, F. (1998). Triangulation in nursing research: Issues of conceptual clarity and purpose. *Journal of Advanced Nursing*, 28, 631–641.

ADDITIONAL REFERENCES

Allen, D. (1985). Nursing research and social control: Alternative models of science that emphasize understanding and emancipation. *Image: The Journal of Nursing Scholarship*, 17(2), 58–64.

Barbour, R. S. (1999). The case for combining qualitative and quantitative approaches in health services research. *Journal of Health Services and Research Policy*, 4(1), 39–43.

Beck, C. T. (1997). Developing a research program qualitative and quantitative methods. Nursing Outlook, 45(6), 265–269.

Coyle, J., & Williams, B. (2000). An exploration of the epistemological intricacies of using qualitative data to develop a quantitative measure of user views of health care. Journal of Advanced Nursing, 31, 1235–1243.

Foster, R. L. (1997). Addressing epistemologic and practicing issues in multimethod research: A procedure for conceptual triangulation. Advances in Nursing Science, 20(2), 1–12.

Glaser, B., & Strauss, A. (1966). The purpose and credibility of qualitative research. Nursing Research, 15, 56–61.

Guba, E. (1990). The paradigm dialog. Newbury Park, CA: Sage.

Guba, E., & Lincoln, Y. (1981). Effective evaluation. San Francisco, CA: Jossey-Bass.

Jick, T. (1983). Mixing qualitative and quantitative methods: Triangulation in action. In M. van Marten (Ed.), Qualitative methodology (pp. 135–148). Beverly Hills, CA: Sage.

Lather, P. (1986). Research as praxis. Harvard Educational Review, 56, 257–277.

Mitchell, E. (1986). Multiple triangulation: A methodology for nursing science. Advances in Nursing Science, 8(4), 18–26.

Milburn, K., Fraser, E., Secker, J., & Pavis, S. (1995). Combining methods in health promotion research: Some considerations about appropriate use. Health Education Journal, 54, 347–356.

Munhall, P. (1986). Methodological issues in nursing research: Beyond a wax apple. Advances in Nursing Science, 8(3), 1–5.

Oakley, D., Yu, M., Zhang, Y., Zhu, X., Chen, W., & Yao, L. (1999). Combining qualitative with quantitative approaches to study contraceptive pill use. Journal of Women's Health, 8(2), 249–257.

Patterson, B. L. (1994). A framework to identify reactivity in qualitative research. Western Journal of Nursing Research, 16, 301–316.

Powers, B. (1987). Taking sides: A response to Goodwin and Goodwin. Nursing Research, 36(2), 122–126.

Schultz, P. (1987). Toward holistic inquiry in nursing: A proposal for synthesis of patterns and methods. Scholarly Inquiry for Nursing Practice, 1(2), 135–146.

Smith, J. (1983). Quantitative versus qualitative research: An attempt to clarify the issue. Educational Researcher, 12(3), 6–13.

Tinkle, M., & Beaton, J. (1983). Toward a new view of science: Implications for nursing research. Advances in Nursing Science, 5(2), 27–36.

23

Evaluating Qualitative Research

Julie Evertz

*I want to beg you, as much as I can,
to be patient toward all that is unsolved
in your heart and to try to love the questions
themselves like locked rooms and like books
that are written in a very foreign tongue.
Do not seek the answers, which cannot
be given you because you would not be able
to live them.
And the point is to live everything.
Live the questions now.
Perhaps you will then gradually,
without noticing it, live along
some distant day into the answer.*
—Rainer Maria Rilke

The evaluation of qualitative research has generated much discussion and debate. I believe that it has done so owing largely in part to the complexities inherent in the various qualitative research approaches. However, regardless of the approach utilized, all qualitative research refers to human science. It is in that distinction alone where much of the debate and controversies exist. I believe that it is also in the context of human science where the evaluation of qualitative research should remain. This chapter considers the epistemology of the two major research paradigms and the role of epistemology within each, revisits past frameworks for evaluating qualitative research, presents current guidelines suggested for the general evaluation of qualitative research, considers the distinctions in evaluating different qualitative approaches, presents general guidelines and challenges in understanding the grant review process, compare the roles of critique and evaluation, and includes a brief discussion of the role of philosophical themes in evaluating qualitative research.

THE POWER OF EPISTEMOLOGY IN EVALUATION

The epistemological differences that prevail in quantitative and qualitative research must be well understood and respected to even discuss evaluation and what that means to either paradigm.

First, the quantitative approach to research has historically been considered the "received view" of the twentieth century that defined "science and research." That statement holds tremendous power. The power lies in wondering what was not or could have been "received." Briefly, some of the basic tenets of quantitative research are:

- Prediction and control
- Valuing of a homogeneous group
- Static reality, which can be held constant
- Logical positivism, specifically, the search for one universal truth
- Social world as given—which implies that humans are reactive
- An independent physical reality
- Reductionism, generalizability, and statistical analysis are valued
- Objectivity and distance are aims
- Measurable, deductive reasoning
- Manipulation
- Linear causality and categorization
- Operationalism
- Laws and quantification

Although there have been changes in how qualitative research is being received, largely owing to greater exposure by those dedicated to human science research, qualitative research has often been referred to as the "nonreceived" view in many traditional scientific circles. The term "nonreceived" speaks volumes to the degree of respect and value that historically has been given to qualitative research, specifically in the grant review processes. Some of the tenets of qualitative research are:

- Humans act upon and create meaning from experiences
- Human beings are active and integrated
- Reality is dynamic, choice laden, and autonomous
- There are multiple unique realities or "truths"
- Social world is created
- Process oriented or an open system
- Subjectivity and individual interpretation is valued
- Characterized by inductive reasoning
- Meanings are context dependent
- Uncertainty is embraced
- Humanism guides the approaches
- Holism described as looking at the whole and not parts
- Heterogeneous groups
- Changes in consciousness and advocacy
- Relativism

Both paradigms are important and appropriate in nursing research. The choice of approach depends upon the research question(s) or phenomenon of interest. In the process of evaluating qualitative research, perhaps the greatest challenge lies in the researcher(s) and all those in the scientific community evaluating a specific study assuring that they have expert knowledge of what they are evaluating, knowing their limitations when they lack knowledge relevant to the qualitative research approach used, and, perhaps most important, admitting their lack of knowledge and then taking the appropriate ethical stance.

FRAMEWORKS REVISITED

A great body of literature addresses quality issues and standards in qualitative research. Much of this literature is directed at providing researchers with guidelines for enhancing the overall quality of their work (Sandelowski, 1986; Guba & Lincoln, 1981; Lincoln & Guba, 1985; Guba, 1990; Denzin & Lincoln, 1994).

In addition to ensuring quality in design, conduct, and reporting of their studies, qualitative researchers recognize the need to clarify evaluative guidelines as appropriate to their specific approaches so that the findings of their research are preserved with the utmost ethical authenticity to the participants and the aim(s) of the study. This may also result in less doubt or lack of understanding for those who judge their efforts.

Concerns about the use of appropriate criteria for evaluating qualitative research are not new. As early as 1966, Glaser and Strauss questioned "the applicability of the canons of quantitative research as criteria for judging the credibility of qualitative research and analysis" (p. 56). They argued in favor of using criteria "based on generic elements of qualitative methods for collecting, analyzing, and presenting data" (p. 56). Since then, other qualitative nursing researchers have developed and presented frameworks for judging the merit of qualitative investigations (Aamodt, 1983; Burns, 1989; Cobb & Hagemaster, 1987; Morse, 1991, 1997; Parse, Coyne, and Smith, 1985). Although these frameworks vary to some degree, in accord with the philosophical underpinnings of the researcher, common beliefs exist. There is agreement that qualitative studies should be evaluated on the basis of their significance, defined as contribution, relevance, importance, and transferability.

Relevant to the importance of context in evaluating qualitative inquiry, Aamodt (1983) discussed the importance of conveying context in which the verbal and behavioral actions of interest take place. Cobb and Hagemaster (1987) addressed the importance of understanding the investigator's role in the research setting. Burns (1989) noted the responsibility of the investigator to present a full description of the actual process of doing the research.

Finally, Cobb and Hagemaster (1987) and Burns (1989) identified the importance of evaluating the clarity and specificity of the analytical activities that lead to or are intended to lead to the study results. They stressed the need to indicate the processes and decisions that underlie the final organization and presentation of the research material. Burns (1989) specifically cited methodological congruence and theoretical connectedness as important evaluative criteria. Methodological congruence requires the reviewer to assess both the underlying assumptions and the specific qualitative approach that guide the research. It includes rigor in documentation, procedure, ethics, and accessability. Documentation of the rigor of a study refers to specifying both the philosophical and the methodological underpinnings of the study. Procedural rigor refers to the ability of the investigator to demonstrate the accuracy and representativeness of the material. Ethical rigor directs the researcher to demonstrate that the participants' rights were protected during the research, and accessability addresses the documentation of the process by which the results of the study emerged from the research material. The standard of theoretical connectedness requires that the theoretical assumptions developed from the study be clearly expressed, logically consistent, tightly reflective of the research material, and compatible with the knowledge base of nursing (Burns, 1989).

These past frameworks vary in purpose and level of specificity. They provided the reviewer with choices available at that time. Each of the frameworks contributed to setting reasonable expectations and standards for reviewers of qualitative research to follow. The selection of which to use depended on the purpose of review and the reviewer's preference.

BREAKING THE FRAME: GENERAL EVALUATION GUIDELINES

Each qualitative methodological tradition has distinct principles by which it may be judged as theoretically, epistemologically, and technically sound. However, many qualitative researchers have synthesized sets of general ideas that are, for the most part, widely accepted across the spectrum of the various qualitative approaches. They are guidelines meant to assist the researchers and reviewers in the evaluation process. They are not mandates by any means; nor do they presume any universal knowledge or criteria to be used (Morse, 1997).

All qualitative research is expected to demonstrate epistemological integrity, ranging specifically from a defensible line of reasoning from the assumptions made about the nature of knowledge to the methodological rules by which decisions about the research process are explicated. The research process must reveal a research question that is consistent with the epistemological standpoint, an interpretation of data sources, and interpretive strategies that follow logically from the question (Koch, 1995; Simmons, 1995; Morse, 1997).

Qualitative studies should demonstrate representative credibility in that the theoretical claims that they espouse are consistent with the manner in which the phenomenon being studied is sampled. For example, in phenomenology, shared elements within an experience would not be expected or proposed at all. In a grounded-theory study that reflects the basic social processes of a dominant cultural group, inferences that the processes are universal across cultures would not be accepted or appropriate. Findings based on a prolonged engagement with the phenomenon are more likely to be held as credible than are those derived from superficial involvement (Erlandson, Harris, Skipper, & Allen, 1993; Morse, 1997).

Reports of qualitative research are expected to reveal an analytic logic that makes clear the reasoning of the researcher from proposal stage to the interpretation and knowledge claims made on the basis of what was discovered in the research. Sandelowski, Davis, and Harris (1989) recognized that good qualitative research has an inherently emergent nature. The adequacy of the decision-making process must be accessible. There should exist an explicit reasoning path that another researcher could presumably follow. Additionally, ethnographic principles of thick description and the phenomenological tradition of saturation demand that we craft research reports that explicate our interpretive claims in verbatim accounts from our data (Morse, 1997).

Finally, qualitative studies should reveal an interpretive authority. Although all knowledge is recognized to be perspectival, there needs to be an assurance that a researcher's interpretations are trustworthy and that they fairly illustrate or reveal some "truth" outside the researcher's own biases, assumptions, experiences, or belief system. There needs to be some sense of confidence about which claims represent individual subjective truths. The researcher's intentions in revealing knowledge about a particular phenomenon must be evident. (Janesick, 1994; Patterson, 1994).

EVALUATING QUALITATIVE RESEARCH WITHIN DISTINCTIVE APPROACHES

Although the general guidelines presented are useful for evaluating qualitative studies, they do not take into account important differences that exist among and within the specific qualitative methods. Each of these methods has its own guidelines concerning aims, evidence, inference, and verification. We must recognize the importance of these distinctions and the resulting confusion that can surround the evaluation of qualitative research.

Qualitative research emphasizes the importance of presenting a rich, contextual understanding of the subject matter under investigation. Different approaches are taken owing to different underlying purposes, procedures, and forms of presentation. Grounded theorists focus on the identification and conceptualization of basic social processes that attempt to explain human behavior. Phenomenologists aim to understand, to the extent possible, the lived experiences of human beings. Researchers using these approaches use different interview strategies and data-analysis techniques. Additionally, there are often differences within a specific qualitative approach. The researcher and reviewers need to take that into account. Ethnographers working from different cultural theories and phenomenologists embracing different philosophical traditions will address different kinds of research questions and will use different data-collection and analysis methods. In addition to being knowledgeable of the general guidelines for evaluating qualitative research that exist to date, as well as the epistemological differences in the research paradigms themselves, the reviewers also need to be aware of differences that cross qualitative approaches and to take these differences into account when reviewing a manuscript or proposal (Munhall and Boyd, 1993).

CHALLENGES IN GRANT REVIEWS

Guidelines for evaluating qualitative research grant proposals exist but are controversial. There are helpful publications that focus on grant writing, most specifically federal grant writing. Federal grant writing criteria can be easily accessed through the Internet at the National Institutes of Health's Website and specifically at the National Institutes of Nursing Research's link.

Qualitative researchers are concerned about whether appropriate criteria are used to evaluate qualitative research grant proposals. This is particularly true in the nonfederal arena, where variances in criteria for evaluation within and among individual organizations persist. There are some common "guidelines" frequently used as important criteria for inclusion in grant review. Table 23–1 summarizes general grant review guidelines:

The reality is that methods for qualitative analysis are less understood than are those of quantitative analysis procedures. Therefore a clear description of a plan for data organization, collection, processing, analysis, and attention to sample as appropriate is needed (Morse, 1997).

The qualifications of the investigator(s) and the research team as well as letters of support, appropriateness of consultants, and each investigator's record of research and professional experience are all significant to a successful grant approval. Having knowledgeable, appropriate, and qualified reviewers is undoubtably important (Morse, 1991).

TABLE 23–1 Common Guidelines for Grant Review

- The degree of scientific contribution of the research.
- The research is likely to yield new information.
- The topic to be studied is significant.
- The parts of the proposal go together in a coherent and consistent manner.
- Literature reviews lead logically to the specific aims, showing what is known and how the study will expand this particular knowledge.
- Importance of the knowledge to the nursing profession.
- The appropriateness of the context of the theory on which the research is based relative to the chosen approach; if no theory is used as a context, the reason for its omission must be justified.
- The method proposed should be sound for the research proposed.
- The method will achieve the aims specified.
- Congruence of purpose, aims, and design must be apparent.
- Stated research question(s) must be consistent with the stated aims.
- Clear description of the proposed research methods.
- Description of preliminary work, pilot projects, and previously related research is helpful.

Regarding nonfederal grant writing, review guidelines are inconsistent and vary tremendously. Researchers would be well served to contact the particular organization from which the grant is being requested to ask appropriate questions relative to evaluation and review specific to the researcher's chosen method before submission of a proposal.

CRITIQUE VERSUS EVALUATION

The idea of critique extends beyond the realm of evaluation. Critique calls for qualitative researchers to account for the ways in which their study findings affect disciplinary and interdisciplinary knowledge. In the health sciences, most qualitative research appears to aim toward knowledge that can potentially or actually influence health care practice. Morse (1997) suggested five elements of critique by which researchers judge their qualitative studies.

First, a criterion by which all health care research should be judged is its moral defensibility. Convincing claims need to exist concerning why we need the knowledge collected from research participants and the purpose of that knowledge once obtained. This element reaches beyond traditional ethics about the protection of human subjects. It stretches into an understanding of how knowledge is used in our society. Further, we must account for the possible uses of our research findings before we know what they include. The findings must demonstrate a potential benefit for the health care of those we serve. This is imperative before we can defend the possible placement of any marginalized group at the risk of social censure or antipathy as a result of knowledge collected through our research or because of the way in which that knowledge is made visible to others whose purposes and power may not coexist with a humanitarian health care agenda (Morse, 1997).

A second criterion proposed by Morse (1997) was that of disciplinary relevance. Accordingly, she suggested that critique includes the issue of whether knowledge obtained is appropriate to the development of the disciplinary science—in this instance, nursing science. What is "accepted" in one discipline is not necessarily so in all health care disciplines. Therefore, and perhaps unfortunately, researchers need to be able to explain the relationships between their research and the disciplinary knowledge that they want to advance before the profession will accept otherwise competent research.

The third criterion proposed by Morse (1997) is one in which the problems inherent in the practical sciences, where conditions of truth and opinion are blurred, are reflected. Morse calls this a pragmatic obligation. This criterion describes the inherent strain within practice realities, in which respect for the uniqueness of individual experience lends itself to an idealist epistemology at the same time that the moral mandate of a practice discipline demands usable general knowledge. Therefore researchers are obliged to consider their findings "as if" they might be applied in practice. No idea should be purely understood as theoretical; nor can qualitative researchers suggest findings with the assurance that no one will put them into practice before they are stamped as "scientifically proved" (Morse, 1997).

A fourth criterion explicated by Morse (1997) is the contextual awareness revealed by the qualitative researcher. The epistemological claims on which qualitative research approaches are based solidly find knowledge within the societies that construct their knowledge. Simply, knowledge is socially constructed and grounded in knowledge. Qualitative researchers have an obligation to recognize that their own perspectives are inevitably bounded by their historical contexts and their disciplinary perspectives. Although elements of our social historical context that are apparent to us can be accessed, explained, and, to some degree, bracketed, we must assume that we are as strongly influenced by other invisible assumptions. Further, owing to the fact that many of our basic assumptions are social constructions, they are likely to be common to others in the field and even to those whom we aim to study. Qualitative researchers need to present their findings as contextual, recognizing that many supposed accepted realities cannot withstand any test of "time" particularly when time is viewed through a philosophical lens.

Lastly, critique of qualitative research requires a respect for ambiguity, the word *validity* and the shared reality explained in philosophy as probable truth. There is no set of standards by which we measure our procedures and findings that can fully account for the idea of truth or for representativeness within the living world; nor can they assure confidence that research findings are absolutely valid, because there are no absolutes. We can accept that there is value in some kinds of knowledge as "probable truth." We must also accept that certain forms of knowledge claims, that superficially seem to meet our best truth criteria, may be proved untrue (Morse, 1997).

Perhaps what might be most helpful is that we reconstruct our reason for doing research as an effort to create meaning, to construct constantly changing images from which our most intensely human, fallible, and temporal views of the world can be altered, challenged, rejected, or assured.

Critique of qualitative research reaches beyond superficial guidelines of evaluation. Critique implores us as qualitative researches to reflect deeply about our reasons for selecting certain questions, about how the knowledge obtained through our research furthers certain kinds of meaning, about how we clearly demonstrate epistemological links within our research through the findings, and finally, about the possible implications of acts based on our researcher, participant (Morse, 1997).

Table 23–2 summarizes the distinctions between evaluation and critique criteria suggested for use with qualitative studies. I have added visibility and voice as a part of the evaluation process, criteria distinct from those of Morse (1997). Although much can be said about both in great detail, visibility refers to the ability of the researcher(s), participant(s), readers, and reviewers of qualitative research to "see" the experience(s) as one with themselves, not just merely "inside" but as the "other(s)." Voice refers to the ability of the researcher, participant(s), readers, and reviewers to "hear" the sounds, whether in words or sounds of emotion, of experience(s), which explicates meaning absent of reductionism of any

TABLE 23–2 CRITERIA FOR EVALUATION AND CRITIQUE OF QUALITATIVE RESEARCH

EVALUATION	CRITIQUE
Epistemological integrity	Moral defensibility
Representative credibility	Disciplinary relevance
Analytic logic	Pragmatic obligation
Interpretive authority	Contextual awareness
Visibility and voice	Probably truth

kind. Both visibility and voice are forms of intense closeness, which I believe is the ultimate goal in qualitative research if we are to attempt to claim any understanding of phenomena. Much about visibility and voice was written by Merleau-Ponty (1968, 1988). Both concepts are addressed in detail within his ontology. Qualitative researchers who aim toward greater understanding must aim toward greater closeness.

PHILOSOPHICAL THEMES IN EVALUATION

Regardless of the qualitative approaches used or the differences that may exist within those approaches themselves, to remain focused on the general philosophical themes that transcend all qualitative approaches throughout the research process from research proposal to a written manuscript may be a means of ensuring that the tenets of qualitative research are intricately woven throughout the research study. Focusing on the general philosophical themes can be a means by which we evaluate and critique these studies while adhering to the philosophical underpinnings of the various approaches. Three major philosophical themes in qualitative evaluation are summarized in Table 23–3.

Experienced qualitative researchers must seek out roles as reviewers for journals and funding agencies. Once such researchers are in these positions, changes can be introduced to allow for a greater understanding of and respect for differences among and within the qualitative perspectives. Reviewers will have an opportunity to decide whether sufficient specific knowledge exists to conduct specific reviews. A grounded theorist, for example, may or may not be able to fairly evaluate phenomenological research. Being clear about what we can and cannot review is important. Whatever evaluative research guidelines are developed in the future, room needs to exist

---

TABLE 23–3   Major Philosophical Themes in Evaluation

- To exist is to be conscious of something in the world.
- Human realities are interactive and transactional with the world.
- Reality and truth depend on the fundamental relation of human existence in a concrete world of others, objects, events, circumstances, and situations.
- We are tied to the world in a perspective created by being bodily situated in the world in a particular way.
- Human realities are always subjective in nature.
- Perception is the original awareness of the appearance of phenomena in experience.

Source: Van Manen (1990).

TABLE 23–4   Major Assumptions of Human Science

- Human science relies on a perspective from the inside.
- The supreme category of the human sciences is meaning.
- The task of inquiry in human sciences comprises interpretation and understanding.

---

for creativity in research—for new and innovative methods. These methods, though ethically sound, should be given visibility and respect. If our ultimate goal is to create useful ways to advance the science, art, and practice of nursing, then all efforts should be made to shorten distance where distance exists and to allow difference an equal voice. As we guide changes in qualitative evaluation, I believe that, while we develop research questions and guide our approach to understanding, it is also important to keep in mind the major assumptions about human science. These assumptions should be inherent in all qualitative research. The three significant assumptions of human science are listed in Table 23–4.

Excellence in qualitative inquiry and scholarship is unquestionably important. Until greater understanding exists regarding the qualitative paradigm in general, qualitative researchers and their studies are destined to endure endless scrutiny. Perhaps it is our challenge as qualitative researchers to ensure that the study of human science always be deeply connected to human beings, to remember that theoretical concepts can be only theoretically correct. They cannot capture the richness and uniqueness of human experience; nor can sterile labels be assigned to the experiences of individual people, societies, or groups. At best, this would be distance. At worst, it would be a betrayal of our humanity.

REFERENCES

Aamodt, A. (1983). Problems in doing nursing research: Developing criteria for evaluating qualitative research. *Western Journal of Nursing Research, 5,* 398–402.

Burns, R. (1989). Standards for qualitative research. *Nursing Science Quarterly,* 2, 44–52.

Cobb, A., & Hagemaster, J. (1987). Ten criteria for evaluating qualitative research proposals. *Journal of Nursing Education,* 26, 138–143.

Denzin, N., & Lincoln, Y. (1994). *Handbook of qualitative research.* Thousand Oaks, CA: Sage.

Erlandson, D. A., Harris, E., Skipper, B. L., & Allen, S. D. (1993). *Doing naturalistic inquiry: A guide to methods.* Newbury Park, CA: Sage.

Glaser, B., & Strauss, A. (1966). The purpose and credibility of qualitative research. *Nursing Research,* 15, 56–61.

Guba, E. (1990). *The paradigm dialog.* Newbury Park, CA: Sage.

Guba, E., & Lincoln, Y. (1981). *Effective evaluation.* San Francisco, CA: Jossey-Bass.

Janesick, V. J. (1994). The dance of qualitative research design: Metaphor, methodology, and meaning. In N. K. Denzin & Y. S. Lincoln (Eds.), *Handbook of qualitative research* (pp. 209–219). Thousand Oaks, CA: Sage.

Koch, T. (1995). Interpretive approaches in nursing research: The influence of Husserl and Heidegger. *Journal of Advanced Nursing,* 21, 827–836.

Lincoln, Y., & Guba, E. (1985). *Naturalistic inquiry.* Beverly Hills, CA: Sage.

Merleau-Ponty, M. (1968). *The visible and the invisible.* (A. Lingis, Trans.). Evanston, IL: Northwestern University Press.

Merleau-Ponty, M. (1988). *Merleau-Ponty's ontology* (2nd ed., M. C. Dillon, Ed.). Evanston, IL: Northwestern University Press.

Morse, J. (1991). On the evaluation of qualitative proposals. *Qualitative Health Research,* 1, 147–151.

Morse, J. (1997). *Completing a qualitative project.* Thousand Oaks, CA: Sage.

Munhall, P., & Boyd, C. (1993). *Nursing research.* New York: National League of Nursing.

Parse, R., Coyne, A., & Smith, M. (1985). *Nursing research: Qualitative methods.* Bowie, MD: Brady.

Patterson, B. L. (1994). A framework to identify reactivity in qualitative research. *Western Journal of Nursing Research,* 16, 301–316.

Rilke, M. R. (1977). *Possibility of being.* (J. B. Leishman, Trans.). New York: New Directions.

Sandelowski, M. (1986). The problem of rigor in qualitative research. *Advances in Nursing Research, 8,* 27–37.

Sandelowski, M., Davis, D., & Harris, B. (1989). Artful design: Writing the proposal for research in the naturalistic paradigm. *Research in Nursing and Health, 12,* 77–84.

Simmons, S. (1995). From paradigm to method in interpretive action research. *Journal of Advanced Nursing, 21,* 837–844.

Van Manen, M. (1990). *Researching lived experience.* Ontario, Canada: SUNY Press.

24

Qualitative Research Proposals and Reports

Carolyn Oiler Boyd and Patricia L. Munhall

Lofland and Lofland (1984) emphasized that a qualitative research project begins with the investigator's personal concerns and entails determining what he or she cares about independently of social science. Personal concerns are thus primary and may or may not coincide with those judged to be of significance in a given discipline. These authors stated:

> "Starting where you are" provides the necessary meaningful linkages between the personal and the emotional, on the one hand, and the stringent intellectual operations to come, on the other hand. Without a foundation in personal sentiment all the rest easily becomes so much ritualistic, hollow cant. (p. 10)

Although personal interest and investment are not unique features of qualitative research, attention to personal concerns and use of that involvement are uniquely important in the qualitative research tradition. This aspect stands in marked contrast to the common practice of delineating a research agenda based on priorities set by funding agencies or some other sanctioning authority. The influence of conventional sanctions on research poses a dilemma for researchers who depend on external approval of their work, and it may be managed at times by casting the proposal in terms that will convince readers of the significance of the proposed research for science. In this chapter, the problem of sanctions is addressed along with other influences on not only what we study, but how. An effort is made to accommodate the legitimate concerns of qualitative researchers who seek approval from funding agencies and from dissertation committees that are relatively unfamiliar with the qualitative paradigm or that interpret and judge qualitative proposals with a positivist orientation. At the same time, however, we intend to protect the nexus of qualitative research philosophy with its methodology and thereby preserve the congruency of substance and form in qualitative research.

In Marshall and Rossman's text titled *Designing Qualitative Research* (1989), the bent toward a positivist interpretation of qualitative research is revealed in an emphasis on a thorough review of the literature and formulation of guiding hypotheses. Although these authors repeatedly stress the importance of flexibility in design to accommodate the unknown and what may emerge in the conduct of the inquiry, their position appears to be one of compromise with the requirements of the positivist paradigm. Qualitative research from such a position is characterized more by its strategies and techniques (that is, by the generation of word data with an effort to maintain the sociocultural context of people's verbal expressions) than by its philosophical premises and broader implications. Nevertheless, this chapter will offer some of the same advice as that given by Marshall and Rossman because, regardless of one's philosophical orientation, when a proposal must be approved by the guardians of the dominant paradigm in our world, the positivist frame must be addressed. We suggest therefore, that qualitative proposals provide readers with:

1. Education about and description of the method from its aim to its outcome. Such detail also enhances confirmability by leaving a decision trail.
2. Justification for using the method through a logically developed explanation of why the researcher has chosen to use it.
3. Translation of language unique to the method in terms that are likely to be understood by readers.

In time, with greater acceptance of qualitative research on its own terms, compromises and translations may no longer be necessary except for those who practice qualitative research as a hybrid model in the positivist tradition.

GETTING STARTED

On some level, most researchers settle on a research topic because of some personal reason. Even for the opportunistic researcher with an eye on funding priorities, personal interest is usually aroused with ties to the researcher as person. For the qualitative researcher, personal interest is a strategic tool in the research project; it provides the energy and the motivation to persevere with the challenges and tedium inherent in any scholarly work. More importantly, however, personal interest can position the researcher to attend to the phenomenon under study in a certain way; it establishes figure and ground for the research endeavor in what can be highly personalized ways that make the research a passion, a preoccupation, an intimate companion. All of these aspects are enabling for the qualitative researcher, making it possible for him or her to be in a state of what Schutz (1970) referred to as wide-awakeness (pp. 68–69). The personal sentiment of which Lofland and Lofland wrote is more than an idle curiosity, more than a mere research interest or agenda. It merges with aspects of one's life that encompass the professional but go beyond it. As a colleague remarked, "I find that I am increasingly interested in geriatrics as I grow closer to being elderly myself." Similarly, some of the authors of this text have had occasion to share notes on the menopausal experience as we search for meaning in this time of our lives. And, as required in phenomenological research, Lauterbach has acknowledged her personal investment in meanings associated with the loss of a pregnancy in her research presentation in Chapter 6. Rather than being biases to confess and then to eliminate, such personal investment in the research topic can be exploited to enhance the research process. The first step in developing a proposal is thus to identify a phenomenon about which one has a vested interest. This step is private and largely invisible. There are, no doubt, multiple instances, if not an established convention, of glossing over this consideration in deference to more practical issues in proposal development.

If the researcher is a "purist," he or she has taken up a position philosophically that establishes a particular way of regarding the nature of being human and of reality and truth, usually in connection with a way of regarding the nature of nursing. For such a qualitative researcher, all questions and problems in the domain (nursing) will be qualitative questions, circumventing the need to dwell on whether to use a qualitative approach in the research at hand. This point bears some elaboration. As a point of departure, the qualitative researcher acknowledges the following premises for his or her work, although these premises may be stated in various ways:

1. Human realities are constituted in human involvement with a world of people, objects, events, and circumstances.
2. Multiple points of view may be taken up in this intending toward a world. The facts of the world alone do not equate with human realities.
3. Reality is constituted in a complex interaction of one's historicity, which includes the common stock of knowledge passed on through the culture in which one resides and a chosen perspective in the world.
4. Although an objective world may be the focus of attention in research, human reality is chosen for attention in nursing research, thus necessitating attention to the complex context in which those realities emerge for human beings.

Thus, to understand people is to comprehend them in their contexts, mindful of the concrete world in which they are enmeshed and attentive to the variety of ways in which it is possible for them to be in that world. The qualitative paradigm thus determines the kind of question posed for research; all questions are qualitative in nature.

On the other hand, for the researcher who reconciles the qualitative and quantitative paradigms, these premises may or may not be considered important or addressed. Because the philosophy and ideology of the qualitative paradigm are not consciously and explicitly adopted as a point of departure, the research idea does not alone determine how the research will be carried through. Rather, a more conventional approach is adopted in which a research question/problem is posed and, after its significance to the domain has been ascertained, a decision-making process is used to determine whether qualitative methods are best suited to the question/problem. Regardless of whether a philosophy drives the question, the adoption of a qualitative design must be defended, and discussion of the heretofore listed premises can serve later in proposal development to achieve this defense.

One can start from the perspective of the qualitative paradigm or be led to it by the nature of the phenomenon under study and the state-of-the-art knowledge about it. At the very least, however, getting started requires reflection on one's own position in the world. In a discussion of getting started in phenomenological inquiry, Van Manen (1990) wrote of orienting to the phenomenon:

It is important, therefore, for the researcher to focus carefully on the question of what possible human experience is to be made topical for phenomenological investigation. . . . This starting point of phenomenological research is largely a matter of identifying what it is that deeply interests you. . . . [T]o orient oneself to a phenomenon always implies a particular interest, station or vantage point in life. (p. 40)

For nurse researchers, this advice means that we orient to life as nurse or perhaps as nurse educator or nurse administrator. It is primarily this orientation that should characterize the selection of a phenomenon for study if the study is to qualify as a *nursing* study. Parenthetically, what it means to orient to life as nurse is itself an interesting question that, despite a long history of contemplation, still eludes us as a discipline. This question is further confounded by the orientation of some nurse researchers as nurse researchers or as social scientists rather than as nurses as such. There are yet other orientations to life; for example, as a mother or middle-aged woman or as a person with a chronic illness or as an artist, any of which may also enter into a nurse researcher's selection of a research focus. These latter orientations have the potential to enhance the intensity and passion with which one begins a study as well as the data to which one has access during the study. It is also true that such involvement through one's given orientations presents challenges to the researcher in managing preconceived conceptualizations during the study—the price of gaining the high ground of insight.

FORMULATING THE RESEARCH QUESTION

Qualitative research questions are characterized by their focus on what is often cited as "lived experience." They are also characteristically stated broadly through language that allows for the flexibility required in the research process while communicating a starting position of openness about the phenomenon under study. If a position of humility is not warranted by the state of the art concerning the phenomenon, research is not indicated. Both features figure prominently in the process of formulating the research question.

As in all research proposals, the question undergoes revision as the proposal is developed and decisions about the study plan are made, however tentative this plan may be. For a qualitative study, the question is born by focusing one's attention on a selected interest. Some qualitative researchers specify the utility of selecting an interest about which one knows little, at least in a formal way, in order to augment the researcher's openness in the conduct of the inquiry. Others, quite naturally, orient to interests that have been central to their careers in nursing. Still others select interests that have been piqued by personal experience that is tied to their professional lives. A psychiatric nurse, for example, might become interested in how people live through infertility and infertility technology if she has herself been diagnosed as infertile.

All qualitative research questions are psychosocial in nature in the sense that they are concerned with living through various health-related circumstances. The focus is on awarenesses, meanings, and the various ways in which these awarenesses and meanings are given expression as well as their consequences for health and the quality of people's lives. In the earlier example, the researcher's lack of professional knowledge about infertility could be used to advantage in that she would be less likely to be encumbered by ready-made, scientific conceptualizations that might obscure her fresh vision of the human experience to be studied. Like the substance of fiction, the selected interest carries with it an angst of some sort that will figure into defending the significance of the study. This angst may be a matter of discontent with measurement of variables, sensibilities about patient experience, or adequacy of nursing interventions in certain situations. The angst, however, regardless of its source, provides fuel for the research endeavor.

The overriding consideration in formulating qualitative research questions, as well as in refining them as the proposal is shaped, is whether they focus on some aspect of human experience *in its context*. Context refers to "the world" in which people live out their lives, the world in which human meanings are constituted. Each qualitative method brings a particular orientation to the research question, but all concern themselves broadly with the task of understanding something about the human condition and why and how it comes to be that way. All recognize that human choices, manipulations, interpretations, and "sense making" figure prominently in the way things are.

The selection of a research focus establishes that phenomenon as important. In so many aspects of women's lives, the phenomenon may profit from being carefully attended to and the research question may focus on providing a rich description of it. A qualitative researcher who cites increased sensitivity to the phenomenon as an aim or purpose of the study is suggesting that this phenomenon is an important one for us to pay attention to and to understand. In so doing, a statement is made about the boundaries and mission of the discipline, and there is an implicit intention to alter the discipline's sensibilities about the objects of its concerns as well as the adopted perspectives on those objects. In other cases, the aim is to go beyond description of what it is to description that sheds light on how and why it is. The point of understanding the how and why of any given human condition is, for nursing, threefold:

1. Such understandings enter into the sense making of which we are capable, and they influence our actions in patients' health circumstances.
2. They constitute impetus and rationale for our actions.
3. When qualitative research is conducted in tandem with quantitative studies, such understanding contributes to the identification of relevant variables, conceptualizations of such variables, and possible relations among variables.

The particular focus of qualitative studies, then, is on human experiencing in the contexts in which such experiencing is studied. The constantly changing landscape of our contexts as well as the variety of contexts in which human behavior can be observed provide an infinite call for qualitative research activity. Presumably, the nursing discipline's concern with health and with doing something constructive about people's health provides the overriding context for all nursing research endeavors regardless of various views on how direct the connection of the research with nursing practice should be. Beyond this overriding context, the qualitative researcher specifies that he or she is interested in the various ways in which people construct their ideas about health matters and how these ideas are played out in their lives, given the worlds to which they are tied. The research question may isolate any of these aspects of this interest and, for example, specify an inquiry into what people perceive in a given situation or how they interpret the meaning of that situation or what can be discerned about the connection between their meanings and their actions in the situation. Some qualitative research questions indicate the intention to investigate the entire domain of the qualitative interest for a select group or for a select situation. These distinctions in the scope of the research question have numerous implications for the type of qualitative research approach best suited to the study and the attending decisions concerning research design or method.

In all cases, the emphasis in qualitative research is on the perspective wielded by those who are in the situation. Research results, then, contribute to insights about why and how human conditions come to be. Such insights are explanatory, dispelling the idea that qualitative research produces description alone. Research that produces description of human perspective itself, if a rich description, simultaneously produces insight about why that perspective is chosen and how it figures into the way things are. The power of description needs to be reconceptualized to better acknowledge its role in a much needed revision of the explanation of phases and processes in theory development.

SIGNIFICANCE OF THE STUDY

It goes without saying that any research study must be important for the development of knowledge in the discipline or for social science generally. Passable theories may become outdated as the contexts in which people live out their lives change (inevitable in health care because of the ongoing changes in health care technology and delivery). Theories may be revealed as biased or as relevant to only a percentage of those to whom they are applied or, in some other way, inadequate as a framework for nursing practice. The phenomena with which they are concerned may be recognized as being infinitely more complex than their accounts of reality, particularly when they have been developed in the absence of adequate attention to lived experiences or with exclusive attention to objective reality in a conception of reality as dualistic. Any of these judgments concerning the adequacy of formal knowledge in the discipline might serve to defend the significance of a qualitative research study.

Significance of a study, then, arises from a judgment that what we know collectively as a discipline is not enough and is grounded in a sufficient review of the literature to document that the proposed study will contribute to knowledge in some way. Perhaps one of the most common pitfalls in developing a proposal is benighted ambition, a well-meaning intention to fill in a knowledge gap completely. Not only is this intention impractical within a single research project, but it is also impossible from the point of view that knowledge changes and must be created anew forever.

The review of the literature to establish the significance of a study varies from the review in quantitative research in this critical respect: what is already known is recognized as partial and tentative and possesses the quality of data rather than a conceptual framework that guides, leads, and filters the researcher's observations and analyses. For the researcher who is studying a phenomenon within the parameters of a specialty in which he or she has taken part in the course of his or her career, the literature review serves a second important purpose that is unique to qualitative research; that is, acknowledging what is already known enables the researcher to bracket this knowledge so that fresh insights may emerge in the course of the study. Particular attention to conventional or customary ways of understanding the phenomenon under study is needed, rather than a comprehensive review that accounts for every point of view. A regard for what is already known as data rather than as fixed reference points also serves this purpose when presented critically by raising questions about this knowledge. These questions will also serve in the refinement of the research question and may be introduced as guiding questions for the research, thus satisfying some researchers' need for more detailed structure in the research question.

SELECTION OF A QUALITATIVE RESEARCH APPROACH

One of the most common questions of doctoral students who have studied the qualitative paradigm concerns which of the many methodologies reported in the literature should be selected to study a given research question. The research question itself is often silent on the matter, an outcome of the precision of the paradigm in directing researchers to the types of questions that are qualitative in nature or, perhaps, the power of the paradigm to generate universally (in that paradigm) relevant questions. Selection of a specific approach, then, becomes a function of other considerations. Any of the following considerations might apply:

1. Those orientations identified in the phase of "getting started" constitute a conceptual orientation that is subsumed within the qualitative research paradigm. If one is particularly interested in intrapsychic processes, for example, phenomenology or case study methods would be compatible and lend direction to design decisions. Alternatively, an orientation toward interpersonal processes might lead one to grounded theory, and an interest in the cultural contexts of human behavior might lead one to ethnography or historical research.
2. Contemplation of the options in qualitative methodology might lead the researcher to select one over others because of its anchor in a disciplinary perspective that is believed to have potential in the investigation of nursing phenomena.

Hutchinson, for example (see Chapter 7), although learned in the various qualitative methodologies, preferred the grounded-theory approach and its anchor in the sociological theory of symbolic interactionism. Each qualitative method carries with it a grounding in the works of particular philosophers and theorists, any one of which might hold particular appeal to a researcher.

3. At times, the researcher may be quite committed to a particular way of stating his or her research question, which in turn points to one method over the others. The following research questions are all concerned generally with families and chronic health problems. The way in which each is stated, however, illustrates the implications for selection of method.

   a. What are the challenges for these families and how do they address them? (grounded theory)
   b. What is the culture of human relationships in a cystic fibrosis clinic? (ethnography)
   c. What are the meanings of health for these families? (phenomenology)
   d. How does Family X perceive and manage health care and day-to-day living? (case study)
   e. What is our sociocultural-political legacy in concepts, values, and attitudes about chronic health problems? (historical research)

   A research question that asks broadly, "What is the lived experience of families in which there are members with chronic health problems?" does not provide sufficient direction in the selection of qualitative method or in the many decisions that must be made about design; without the support of subquestions, it is simply too broad to be useful beyond the "getting started" stage.

4. Some research questions that fail to give a clue to the most useful or appropriate method or both are compounded by the researcher's lack of commitment to any particular perspective offered by the various methods. In this case (and as sometimes practiced by researchers), the method may be synthesized from the particulars of the options. Although there are legitimate questions about this practice, it may represent researchers' interest in developing creative applications of borrowed methods within the discipline of nursing. Such creative and experimental work in methodology is laudable, particularly when it consists of more than a simple cut-and-paste approach.

5. Lastly, a researcher may simply wish to learn a selected method well and will use that method to refine the research question as well as to direct the plan for the research.

In our experience, dissertation committees are usually most comfortable with the selection of a design from the literature and faithful adherence to the methods included in that design. Although it is common practice in published qualitative research reports to cite the use of a particular method for data analysis—for example, Colaizzi's method of data analysis (1978) or the constant comparative method from grounded theory—it is not unusual to find little else in the report that identifies it, for example, as phenomenological or as grounded theory. Rather, such studies are generically qualitative; using the constant comparative method does make a study grounded theory, for example. There are models for us in the education literature for such an eclectic approach to qualitative research design. However, readers should be aware of what may be thin ice in this approach in nursing. We believe that nursing will profit from experimentation with qualitative methods and that social scientists who have developed qualitative designs are no more legitimate sources for designs than methodologists who have emerged or who may emerge in our own discipline. There is, however, a lingering malignant doubt about ideas in nursing that cannot be traced directly and clearly to other disciplines.

To summarize, refinement of the research question is accomplished in tandem with selection of the qualitative approach. It should reflect the particular orientation or perspective that the selected qualitative approach lends to the study. When an eclectic approach is to be used, the researcher will need to explain how his or her choices in the design reflect his or her nursing perspective (or other orientations). In keeping with the idea of researcher-as-instrument in qualitative research, careful attention to the researcher's orientations and perspectives in an explicit way is expected throughout the research process. In the proposal phase, identifying and explicating those orientations and perspectives are part of bracketing (in phenomenological terms) or controlling and monitoring researcher bias (in positivist terms).

INTRODUCTION TO THE STUDY

The first section of the qualitative proposal is usually titled "Introduction" and includes the research question, the aim of the study, the researcher's explanation of its significance for nursing, and the identification of the qualitative approach that will be used to conduct the inquiry. As explicated in the preceding sections of this chapter, the way in which these components of the introduction are communicated and explained is critical for a positive review of the proposal.

The overall purpose of the introduction is to orient the reader to the phenomenon under study and to the general design of the study. It demonstrates how the aim of the study has implications and relevance for nursing, and clearly focuses on the substance of the study. What the researcher needs to convey is his or her perceived justification for studying the selected phenomenon.

Because of the openness of qualitative research to fresh insights, in general, the language used to state the research question will contain phrases such as:

* What is it like to [be in this circumstance]?
* What is [this phenomenon]?
* What is going on [in this situation]?
* What is the meaning of [this experience]?

Identification of a context in which the phenomenon occurs provides further definition of the research question and may be discussed narratively rather than through precision in the research question as such.

The aim of the study should be stated explicitly and related to the strengths of qualitative methodology. Most qualitative studies aim to enhance conceptualization through description of lived experiences that have eluded many of our theories. From this point of view, discovery is an apt way to refer to the aim of such studies. Many nurse researchers take the position, especially in phenomenology, that qualitative research does not necessarily lead to theory development. This position could reflect the interpretation of what is theory. Some researchers maintain that phenomenological narratives can be developed into descriptive theory, whereas others maintain that most qualitative methods' nongeneralizability do not warrant a theory (see Chapter 5). A brief overview of the particular qualitative method selected for the study should be included and should flow logically from the presentation of the research question.

EVOLUTION OF THE STUDY

In this section, the researcher places the study in the context from which it has originated. In a description of the evolution of the study, the researcher again provides a rationale for the study and supports this rationale within the historical context—that which the researcher knows historically—and situates the study in a period of time. Furthermore, the researcher includes the experiential context—that which is in the researcher's own experience. This context needs to be clearly elaborated and includes the researcher's involvement in the experience—the meaning and interpretation of what the researcher is thinking about from the realm of person, thus the personal.

THE RESEARCH DESIGN

Proposal readers frequently need to be educated about the selected qualitative approach or design; for this reason, we suggest that the selected design be presented and explained in a separate section. Some repetition of information is inevitable in this approach, but we have found that it is useful to readers unfamiliar with the various qualitative designs available to the qualitative researcher.

Design includes the philosophical/theoretical premises for research within that design as well as the kinds of questions that can be addressed and a host of particulars concerning methods for answering those questions. In grounded theory, for example, symbolic interactionism is a critical framework for research and thus must be understood and used in the research. In phenomenology, several interpretations of method are reported in the literature; each has implications for the design of studies, from formulation of the question to the substance and form of the research product. To make the researcher's decisions sensible and plans comprehensible, the selected design must be presented and explained in considerable detail. Because integrating this presentation and explanation into other sections of the proposal is not usually satisfactory for the reader, we suggest that it be addressed in a clearly identified, separate section (preceding the section titled "Research Method") in which many of the particulars of the design are applied in the study. The following guidelines emphasize the importance of definition, translation, description, explanation, documentation, and illustration in this section of the proposal:

1. Reiterate the philosophical/theoretical premises of the design.
2. Use primary sources to document the description of the design. In a grounded-theory study, for example, Glaser and Strauss's (1967) work is indispensable.

3. Translate or paraphrase language that has meanings unique to the design. The expression "lived experience," for example, is particularly puzzling to many.
4. Reiterate the rationale for selecting the design, emphasizing how it will help to answer the research question and why this is important to the nursing discipline. For example, if the identification of basic social-psychological processes common to people in the same circumstances will contribute to the development of nursing interventions in their common social-psychological problem, this fact should be highlighted. Citations of studies that used the design can be especially effective in substantiating the claims that are made.
5. Describe the design's methods for generating and analyzing data. Examples from other studies may be useful in clarifying steps of analysis in particular.
6. Predictable questions about reliability and validity should be addressed through a description of the design's provisions for rigor. Kirk and Miller (1986) provided a handy reference on reliability and validity in qualitative research by reframing and responding to the questions in terms appropriate to the qualitative paradigm. Evertz, in Chapter 23 of this book, addresses the use of those terms and presents alternative perspectives for evaluation.

THE RESEARCH METHOD

The research method—that is, the plan to collect and analyze data that will answer the research question—is one element of the design. In qualitative proposals, method is tentative to allow for ongoing decision making through interaction with research participants and discovery of the unforeseen. Some of the same methodological questions addressed in quantitative proposals are equally germane to qualitative proposals. The relevance of each question varies with the research question and the overall nature of the method.

In this section of the proposal, it is helpful to repeat the aim of the study and to relate the methodological particulars to that aim. The language of the design can be used freely, having been defined and explained in the preceding section, and the researcher can now focus on how the design will be carried out within the specific parameters of his or her study.

Sample, Setting, Unit of Analysis (What Will the Sources of Data Be?)

A research question may delineate the fact that research participants' perceptions are the source of data, and the method will reflect this by describing methods to solicit those perceptions. Often, the source is participants' responses to the researcher's questioning through interview. If the occasion for the interview is directly tied to the research project, it is possible and desirable to indicate how the interview will be initiated and sustained. In this case, an interview guide is purposeful and should be included in the proposal. This holds true also for the broad, open question such as "What is it like for you to take care of your mother in her old age?" that constitutes the only prompt from the researcher. More often, however, qualitative interviews are conducted in a conversational manner, and an interview guide merely indicates, rather than prescribes, how the researcher will direct attention to the research question in that conversation. Like social conversations, the course of the qualitative interview cannot be predicted with any precision; nor would such prediction be desirable.

A recurring question concerning sources of data is the matter of sample size. As in quantitative research, the answer is ambiguous—that is, "It depends." In studies that use a single source of data such as a one-time interview or a written response to the research question, one would expect to see larger numbers of participants included in the design. In studies that use repeated interviews that extend over long periods of time, fewer participants might be acceptable. One of the considerations in this decision concerns the amount of data that is likely to be produced by the selected data-generating method, particularly in the context of the overall time frame for the research project. When multiple methods of data generation are included in the study, the "sample" would include not only people who have agreed to provide data but also the documents examined or the journals recorded or the researcher's own field notes, for example. In our study of nurses' values, the sample consisted of 121 nurses' poems and photographs numbering in excess of 700 individual entries.

Although there are no formulas to apply in determining sample size, a common rule of thumb is that data are collected until redundancy in the data occurs or the researcher finds that no new data are emerging. Experienced qualitative researchers, particularly ethnographers and grounded theorists, recommend that field research should be planned for a period ranging from several months to a year. Some methodologists (van Kaam, 1969, for example) specify large samples, but most are mute on the matter, leaving the number question open in deference to the more significant issue of adequacy of the database for the research question. Unlike quantitative research, in which statistical procedures determine the necessary sample size, qualitative research leaves the question open to judgment. This holds true even in the case study design; here, the case is the sample of one, but what the researcher identifies as sources of data about this one case is parallel to the concern with sample size in quantitative research.

In most qualitative designs, the sample is selected in accord with preestablished criteria or guidelines. These criteria should be described and, when possible, a plan to collect demographic data descriptive of research participants will enable the researcher to provide an account of this dimension of the context for the study.

Data-Collection Procedures, Ethics (How Will Data Be Solicited from These Sources?)

When the researcher has decided what form(s) of expression will constitute the data for the project, the next question concerns how, when, and where to solicit those expressions. Our study of nurses' values is illustrative of this aspect of the plan. In this study, the aim was "to enhance understanding about nursing perspective: the human values, value conflicts, and value questions expressed by nurses in their poems and photographs" (Munhall & Oiler, 1987). Multiple possibilities presented themselves for data generation concerning nursing perspective. From among them, we selected nurses' expressions in poetry and photography, in the recognition that these expressions might provide a more direct path to values than interview or questionnaire, for example. The idea of using nurses' esthetic expressions seemed particularly congruent with our phenomenological orientation as well as with our appreciation of the preverbal nature of nursing perspective for most nurses. Still, decisions needed to be made concerning how to solicit these esthetic expressions. A call for nurses' poems and photographs became the method for solicitation and was distributed as widely as our resources allowed. The call was published as a classified advertisement in The American Nurse, and fliers were distributed to 300 hospitals randomly selected from a national listing of hospitals accredited by the Joint Commission on Accreditation of Hospitals (JCAH), all Sigma Theta Tau chapters, and all newsletter editors of state nurses associations. Alternatively, nurses might have been asked to write poems or to take photographs for this research project, they might have been asked to respond to selected works of art, or they might have been interviewed about their nursing practices.

Questions and problems of gaining access to data include obtaining informed consent and plans for negotiating ground rules in an ongoing way. (Readers are referred to Chapter 19 for further detail concerning the ethics of qualitative studies and to the methods chapters for additional considerations for data-collection procedures.) For studies that are conducted over a period of time, a time frame for data-collection points should be tentatively planned.

Data Management (How Will Data Be Managed During the Data-Collection Process?)

A variety of strategies for managing qualitative data are described in this text as well as in the many references cited for expanded readings on qualitative methods. Typically, interview data are transcribed to facilitate the researcher's contemplation of the data during analysis. Field notes are often formatted to enable the researcher to record observations and to facilitate his or her reflections on the research process and the simultaneous data-analysis process.

Data Analysis (How Will Data Be Analyzed?)

Data-analysis procedures in qualitative research have drawn criticism because of their ambiguous nature. Despite the development of a variety of strategies to make the process of analysis explicit and reproducible, there remains a fundamental ambiguity that is inherent in the creativity of the process. Many methodologists have listed analytic steps that may be adopted to the satisfaction of all concerned. The use of expert judges to validate the researcher's analysis is commonplace, as is the practice of validating findings with research participants. Ironically, these strategies, which were developed largely to quell the concerns about bias in the research, sometimes have the effect of limiting the researcher's interpretations.

The importance of data analysis as a creative process cannot be overemphasized. It remains, regardless of the strategies employed to systematize it, a unique rendering of the meaning(s) of the phenomenon under study. The expression researcher-as-instrument in its widest sense refers not only to the researcher's influence (through his or her orientations) on what is studied and how it is studied, but also to the possibilities and limits of his or her sense making in data analysis. Like other creative acts, data analysis is a matter of composing an order and does claim to be the only possible order that could be brought to bear. Despite the difficulty of articulating in any precise way exactly how insights and orders are achieved, we offer the following guidelines for data analysis as having been useful for others. We suggest that strategies be planned that will help to:

1. Ponder the meaning of data in parts and as a whole and on repeated occasions.
2. Search for repeated instances that support each interpretation.
3. Reach for complex interpretations to account for variations in the data; contradictions in the data sometimes call attention to "real" contradictions in people's lives.
4. Use all the data available, including field notes, the literature, and any other sources of inspiration. Do not be limited to transcribed interview data merely because they seem more scientific.
5. Identify the technical aspects of data analysis. If data-analysis procedures from one of the qualitative methods is useful, adopt it in the design. Recognize that what you are doing is adopting a procedure rather than an entire design (unless, of course, you are).
6. Relate the findings to preexisting knowledge, keeping in mind that, although the project may be an end in itself in some ways, to qualify as science, it must be entered into a dialogue with one's colleagues. In the proposal phase, merely indicating a plan to do this may be sufficient. Some concepts, theories, and research may be identified in the proposal as a function of reviewing the literature for the purposes cited earlier; other relevant literature may be a part of the discovery *in* the research process, and this may need to be explained as part of the flexibility required in qualitative studies.

Reliability and Validity (How Will Reliability and Validity Be Ensured?)

Although questions of rigor may be adequately addressed in other sections of the proposal, they are sufficiently troublesome for many readers to warrant repetition in the method section. Here, the particular strategies that the researcher will use to ensure reliability and validity should be described in whatever language was used to explain the meaning of rigor in the selected design earlier. The strengths of the selected design and its application in the study should be emphasized, but limitations also should be acknowledged. Sample size and generalizability should not be listed as limitations, because they do not hold the same meaning for qualitative research and would serve to obfuscate the proposal by mixing paradigms (unless, of course, mixed paradigms are part of the study).

IMPLICATIONS AND THE FORM
OF THE RESEARCH REPORT

All qualitative studies produce description that is intended to be full and rich with detail. Standard forms for communicating research findings are generally concerned with efficiency, are thus in opposition to the primary purpose of qualitative research, and present troublesome challenges to qualitative researchers. There are, however, multiple options for the form of such descriptions, some of which aid the researcher in meeting the challenges; others call for new forms of communication in the discipline.

Expository writing is generally the form selected, with some variation based on the qualitative design selected; in a grounded-theory study, for example, figures and models often complement the presentation of the theory. Colaizzi's (1978) phenomenology produces what he referred to as an exhaustive description of essences, which encapsulates recurring themes in interview data. Presentation of qualitative themes in tabulated lists is a common format. Miles and Huberman (1984) described a variety of quantitatively inspired approaches to the presentation of findings that appeal to some. Other possibilities include vignettes and short stories or case study formats, even though case study design may not have been used. Selections from the data themselves may present options; for example, an exhibit of photographs might be arranged as the primary report format or as complementary to it.

The form of presentation will often be determined by the intended audience or the vehicle or both. Journal articles and dissertations, for example, will limit options dramatically. In many instances, findings may be presented in different ways for different audiences, serendipitously calling on the researcher to rewrite findings, which can be an occasion for continued refinement of the analysis. We now have a 15+-year accumulation of nursing literature on qualitative methodologies and on the debate about whether qualitative research is a legitimate tool of nursing science. In view of this accumulation, the attention given to the rationale for selection of a qualitative method and to elaborate explanations of the method itself may be attenuated in the interest of focusing more on the findings and their implications. In our view, the significance of findings for the discipline tend to be short-changed in many reports, a failing that is often attributed to the brevity required in journals and conference presentations. This practice can be changed now that there is greater sophistication in the discipline about qualitative approaches to knowledge development; the practice needs to change in order to apply qualitative research findings to nursing practices and subsequent nursing research.

In any case, the proposal should indicate tentative plans for discussion of the meaning of the findings and for disseminating findings. The discussion should bring the inquiry together as a whole, including scholarly reflection on the historical, scientific, and experiential contexts acknowledged in earlier sections of the proposal. In the course of data gathering, other aspects of these contexts and new contexts may have emerged, and they, too, should be related to the findings in order to enter them into the discipline's discourse about the phenomenon under study. One cannot predict the nature of the synthesis that is performed in the discussion, but the intention to perform a synthesis can be planned.

APPENDICES AND REFERENCES

As in any research proposal, communications relevant to the study, consent forms, and other supporting documents (such as an interview guide, if one is used) are appended to the proposal. References should reflect the researcher's mastery of relevant literature concerning the selected design as well as the phenomenon under study, particularly as it is understood and discussed in the nursing discipline.

Formats for the Research Proposal and Research Reports

In view of the interest in qualitative methodology and the discipline's relatively novice status in the use of qualitative designs, the final research report will be of interest not only for the research product but also for the research process. This observation does not distinguish qualitative research reports from those that spring from the dominant positivist paradigm, but it does suggest that the labor of explaining and defending the qualitative choice is meaningful.

Tables 24–1 and 24–2 provide outlines for a formal research proposal.[1] Overall, the first four sections of the proposal (Introduction: Aim of the study; Evolution of the study; Method of Inquiry: General; and Method of Inquiry: Applied) are usually consistent with dissertation requirements. Both sections on method require considerable expansion, first about the method itself to provide the background that is still necessary for readers to understand your qualitative approach. The applied-method section will be in accord with what actually happened in the research process. Specific illustrations of various features of the research process should be included to substantiate generalities. For example, in Haase's (1987) study of courage in hospitalized adolescents, the analytic steps of identifying significant statements in transcribed interview data, formulating restatements, and articulating formulated meanings are illustrated through the reporting of selected data. Alternatively, such illustrations might be introduced in the presentation and explanation of the design, an option that did not exist in the proposal phase.

Literature that was reviewed in data gathering should be cited in the Research Method section, and its use in the research process should be described. In those studies that postpone a formal review of scientific literature until the Discussion section, the literature review should be placed in that section. The Findings of the Inquiry and Reflections on the Findings sections are reported separately, with the material as indicated in the outline. The form of the Findings section is usually narrative, peppered with supportive "raw" data that might include quotations from participants, poems, or field note entries, for example. The aim of meaningful qualitative description should guide the researcher's choices among data-reporting forms and might include graphics as complementary to the narrative. In the Reflections section, the researcher delves deeply into the findings for meanings and understandings, as well as integrating the study's significance, substance, and importance to nursing. Appendices and references are modified as indicated by what actually transpired in the conduct of the research project.

---

[1] A full description with exemplars for these outlines can be found in Munhall (2000).

TABLE 24–1   Proposal for Qualitative Research Studies

1. Introduction: Aim of the Study
   (a) Phenomenon of interest
   (b) Perceived justification for studying the phenomenon
   (c) Phenomenon discussed within specific context (e.g., a lived experience, a culture, a human response)
   (d) Assumptions, biases, experiences, intuitions, perceptions related to belief that inquiry into phenomenon is important
   (e) Qualitative research method chosen with justification of its potential
   (f) Relevance to nursing
2. Evolution of the Study
   (a) Rationale
   (b) Historical context
   (c) Experiential context
3. Method of Inquiry: General
   (a) Introduction to specific method
   (b) Rationale for choosing method: philosophical and theoretical substantiation projected
   (c) Background of method
   (d) Outcome of method
   (e) Sources (individuals) whose methods will be followed
   (f) General steps or procedures of the method
   (g) Translation of concepts and terms
4. Method of Inquiry: Applied
   (a) Aim
   (b) Sample
   (c) Setting
   (d) Gaining access
   (e) General steps
   (f) Human subject considerations: informed consent, entry, departure, confidentiality, secrets, process consent—if and when situation should change
   (g) Strengths and limitations
   (h) Expected timetable
   (i) Actual feasibility of study—Is access cost possible?
5. Appendices
   (a) Supporting documents
   (b) Consent forms
   (c) Communication
6. References

TABLE 24–2 OUTLINE FOR REPORTING QUALITATIVE RESEARCH STUDIES

1. Aim of the Study
   (a) Same as the proposal but with more breadth.
   (b) Include new outline of remaining report.
2. Evolution of the Study
   (a) Same as proposal.
   (b) More breadth and depth.
3. Method of Inquiry: General
   (a) Same as proposal but more specific.
4. Method of Inquiry: Applied
   (a) As it happened.
5. Findings of the Inquiry
   (a) Findings are discussed according to the method. Example: In grounded-theory method, the aim is generation of theoretical constructs. In this section, then, the researcher would have findings from the process of
   • memoing
   • theoretical sampling
   • sorting
   • saturation
   • review of literature
   • the theory
   (b) With the ethnographic method, the findings may be reported in a smooth, flowing descriptive narrative. The aim of the narrative is to portray the full context, to the extent possible, that was discovered by exploring pieces of reality or experience or both. Review of other sources (literature, art, films) is a plus.
   (c) With phenomenology guiding the method, the findings will be reported differently. An example might include:
   • description of experiential themes
   • essences of experience
   • description of relations among essences
   • review of other sources (literature, art, films)
6. Reflections on the Findings:
   With preconceptions and ideas as discussed in the introduction;
   With existing literature and practice in the area of study;
   With the utilization of the method
   (a) Meanings and understandings
   (b) Implications of the study (for whom)
   (c) Relevance of the study (for whom)

TABLE 24–2   Continued

Integrate:
(d) Significance and substance
(e) Importance to nursing
(f) Suggestion for future inquiries
7. Appendices
   (a) Dissertation proposals and reports would include all necessary appendices (e.g., consent letters, tables, etc.).
8. References

THE ABSTRACT

Abstracts are commonly required for dissertations, by journals, and by research conference planners. Traditional formats are again troublesome for the qualitative researcher. Rather than sacrifice substance to form, we suggest that formats be modified to accommodate the nature of the qualitative paradigm. Table 24–3 presents an alternative that is consistent with the outlines for the proposals and reports and enables clear communication of the study for abstract form.

SUMMARY

In essence, a well-developed qualitative proposal provides:

1. A clear statement that specifies the phenomenon to be studied;
2. Documentation of a need for study, with specification of the significance of the study for nursing (or social science in general);
3. Acknowledgment of the researcher's *a priori* orientation(s) and perspective(s) with articulated questions about the attendant presuppositions;
4. Identification of the qualitative approach with a rationale for its selection; and
5. Specification of the design with attention to:
   a. what data are sought,
   b. how and when those data will be solicited,
   c. how relations with research participants will be initiated, maintained, and terminated,
   d. how data will be managed,

TABLE 24–3 OUTLINE FOR QUALITATIVE RESEARCH ABSTRACT

1. Aim of the Study
   (a) Phenomenon of interest
   (b) Relevance for nursing
2. Evolution of the Study
   (a) Rational, experiential, and historical contents
3. Method of Inquiry: General
   (a) Brief overview of purpose of method
   (b) Basic steps
   (c) Suggestion for future inquiries
4. Method of Inquiry: Applied
   (a) Brief overview of specific steps: sample, interviews, setting, procedures, consent, and data analysis
5. Findings of the Study
   (a) Brief synopsis of findings of study
6. Reflection on the Findings
   (a) Brief synopsis of the meaning, understandings, and possible implications of the study
   (b) Significance and substance briefly discussed

---

   e. how data will be analyzed and related to preexisting knowledge, and
   f. how findings will be reported.

Variation in the outline not only is possible (without transgressing the tenets of the qualitative paradigm), but also may be necessary or desired as determined by particular interpretations of the various qualitative designs or by the researcher's needs in a given situation or by both.

As long as qualitative research approaches have the status of being an oddity, qualitative methodology will require careful attention and explication. In our state of heightened consciousness about methods, however, it is helpful to recall Schutz's (1970) advice on the matter:

Methodology is not the preceptor or the tutor of the scientist. It is always his pupil, and there is no greater master in his scientific field who could not teach the methodologists how to proceed. But the really great teacher always has to learn from his pupils. . . . In this role, the methodologist has to ask intelligent questions about the technique of his teacher. And if those questions help others to think over what they really do, and perhaps to eliminate certain intrinsic difficulties hidden in the foundation of the scientific edifice where the scientists never set foot, methodology has performed its task. (p. 315)

With this advice in mind, every qualitative study stands to teach us something about methodology. To the extent that qualitative studies bring us closer to the lived realities of health care recipients and their nurses in common circumstances, qualitative methodology will also learn from the teacher of nursing practice.

REFERENCES

Colaizzi, P. (1978). Psychological research as the phenomenologist views it. In R. Valle and M. King (Eds.), *Existential phenomenological alternatives for psychology*. New York: Oxford University Press.

Glaser, B., & Strauss, A. (1967). *The discovery of grounded theory*. Chicago: Aldine.

Haase, J. (1987). Components of courage in chronically ill adolescents: A phenomenological study. *Advances in Nursing Science, 9*, 64–80.

Kirk, J., & Miller, M. (1986). *Reliability and validity in qualitative research*. Newbury Park, CA: Sage.

Knafl, K., & Howard, M. (1984). Interpreting, reporting, and evaluating qualitative research. *Research in Nursing and Health, 7*, 17–24.

Knafl, K., & Howard, M. (1986). Interpreting, reporting, and evaluating qualitative research. In P. Munhall & C. Oiler (Eds.), *Nursing research: A qualitative perspective*. Norwalk, CT: Appleton-Century-Crofts.

Lofland, J., & Lofland, L. (1984). *Analyzing social settings: A guide to qualitative observation and analysis*. Belmont, CA: Wadsworth.

Marshall, C., & Rossman, G. (1989). *Designing qualitative research*. Newbury Park, CA: Sage.

Miles, M., & Huberman, A. (1984). *Qualitative data analysis: A sourcebook of new methods*. Newbury Park, CA: Sage.

Munhall, P., & Oiler, C. (1987). Human values in nursing: Esthetic expressions. Poster presentation at the American Nurses Association, Council of Nurse Researchers International Nursing Research Conference, Washington, DC.

Munhall, P. (2000) *Qualitative Research Proposals and Reports: A Guide* (2nd ed.). Sudbury, MA: Jones and Bartlett.

Schutz, A. (1970). *On phenomenology and social relations*. Chicago: University of Chicago Press.

van Kaam, A. (1969). *Existential foundations of psychology*. New York: Doubleday.

Van Manen, M. (1990). *Researching lived experience: Human science for an action-sensitive pedagogy*. New York: SUNY Press.

25

Getting Qualitative Research Ideas and Help On-Line

Maureen Duffy

For graduate students contemplating their first piece of research, the idea of designing, implementing, and analyzing a research project can be daunting. Beginning researchers and students find it helpful to see what more experienced researchers are thinking and doing. For the more experienced researcher, it is fascinating to see what others are doing and to see the proliferation of serious qualitative studies in the social and health sciences. There is no better place to get a bird's-eye view of what is going on in the qualitative landscape than on the Internet.

It can take anywhere from 6 to 18 months for a refereed article to appear in print in an academic journal. The publication of a book can take the same amount of time or longer. Ideas, works-in-progress, and finished articles can be placed on the Internet in a matter of minutes, making the Internet what Marshall McLuhan would have called a "hot" medium. Although no serious student of research would ignore the world of scholarly journal articles or published books, few researchers would ignore the opportunity to keep up-to-date with the growing amount of information and inspiration about qualitative research that the Internet provides. There is an abundance of high-quality material related to qualitative research on the Internet.

Surfing the Net for qualitative research stuff can be fun and productive. It can seem a lot more like play than does sitting down and poring over a research text, however interestingly written the text may be. Many individual people and groups have spent an incredible amount of time pulling together some of the most helpful ideas about qualitative research and posting them on the Web, often on impressively organized Web sites. It would be a shame not to take advantage of the fruits of their work.

This chapter will provide directions to some of my favorite qualitative research Web sites. My hope is that you also will find these resources helpful as you begin your work. The chapter is not intended to be a comprehensive list of qualitative research sites, but rather a welcoming invitation to visit some Internet destinations that I enjoy. So, let us get started.

COMPREHENSIVE QUALITATIVE RESEARCH WEB SITES

A few Web sites provide a comprehensive array of all kinds of information about qualitative research. These Web sites are excellent jumping-off points for beginning and then narrowing your own search. They include a focus on multiple issues in qualitative research and have links to other quality resources.

Qualitative Research Resources on the Internet
http://www.nova.edu/ssss/QR/qualres.html

Ron Chenail at Nova Southeastern University in Fort Lauderdale, Florida, has been building a wonderful qualitative research Web site for more than a decade. Ron's Web site has an extensive list of links to qualitative research resources worldwide. He also has a collection of abstracts, posters, and full-text articles in qualitative research by a wide range of authors. Included in this collection of textual sources are articles about qualitative research in nursing, a review of qualitative research in psychotherapy, and many reports of specific research as well as contributions about methodological issues. Ron has also gathered a variety of qualitative research course syllabi from throughout the United States that teachers of qualitative research will undoubtedly find very helpful.

His Web site also houses *The Qualitative Report*, an on-line journal dedicated to qualitative research and critical inquiry. Although it is several years old now (1992), one contribution especially helpful to beginning qualitative researchers is Linda Wark's (http://www.nova.edu/ssss/QR/QR1-4/wark.html) list of journals in the health and social sciences, which are open to publishing qualitative research. Another useful article is Tony Heath's "The Proposal in Qualitative Research" (http://www.nova.edu/ssss/QR/QR3-1/heath.html). In this contribution, Tony Heath guides researchers through the proposal development process step by step. He makes concrete and specific suggestions for every part of the research proposal, from engaging the intended audience to describing data-analysis procedures. *The Qualitative Report* accepts submissions from students and professional researchers alike.

QualPage: Resources for Qualitative Research
http://www.ualberta.ca/~jrnorris/qual.html

Judy Norris's qualitative research Web site is an outgrowth of her passion for qualitative research and her generosity in making good ideas and resources available to others. She is always on the hunt for new ideas and warmly invites others to contribute new qualitative resources to her Web site. For beginning researchers, this Web site has an excellent research methods section. Here the Web visitor can learn about methods as diverse as action and participatory research, content analysis, ethnomethodology, grounded theory, historical research, narrative inquiry, and phenomenology by jumping to specific sites through the links that Judy provides.

This Web site also includes Judith Preissle's exhaustive lists of qualitative research discussions on the Web and e-mail resources. Judith hails from the University of Georgia and is a key player in the Annual Qualitative Research in Education Conference that is held in Athens, Georgia, every January, featuring acclaimed qualitative researchers. Students and professionals are encouraged to submit proposals for presentations at this conference. The conference also provides opportunities for beginning researchers to share their research projects with qualitative research faculty at the University of Georgia and to receive feedback and support.

Judy's site, *QualPage*, has an interesting selection of qualitative research presentations. One presentation that must be singled out is Joan Fleitas' "Band-Aids & Blackboards" (http://funrsc.fairfield.edu/~jfleitas/contents.html). This is a wondrous and colorful presentation of Joan's research about what happens when kids and teens live and go to school with chronic illness. She presents her research "findings" of the lived experience of chronically ill children in an interactive, story format. There is something at this Web site for kids, teens, parents, and teachers alike, as well as for qualitative researchers of all persuasions.

The Qualitative Research Page
http://www.oit.pdx.edu/~kerlinb/qualresearch/

Bobbi Kerlin's award-winning Web site includes an excellent qualitative research section. She provides an outstanding bibliography on qualitative research topics ranging from action research to photo-ethnography to journaling to oral history and narrative. She has bibliographies for validity and paradigms and case study and more. An endless source of lateral reading recommendations is available to the serious researcher here.

A somewhat unique feature of Bobbi's Web site is the section dealing with qualitative research software. Web-site visitors can learn about a whole array of software for voice transcription and for qualitative research data management. She also provides references and links to articles discussing the positives and negatives of using computer-based programs for data management and analysis and for articles comparing the widely used data-management systems. For those researchers interested in computer-assisted management of data and analysis, these resources are invaluable.

For those interested in theory, this Web site is a treasure trove. Post-modernism, critical theory, phenomenology, educational theory, sociological theory, and the theory of theory are all included, along with other theoretical perspectives and accompanying links, references, and resources. Bobbi's list of philosophers who have influenced educational, psychological, and postmodern thought is superb. She provides a biography of each thinker, an overview of his or her major ideas and work, fascinating miscellaneous information, references, and links to further information. Each time I visit Bobbi's Web site, I am filled with awe and gratitude for her amazing work and for her willingness to share so much.

Other invaluable tools for the qualitative researcher are available in Bobbi's section on "Planning & Preparing Research." Help in developing a research proposal and reflections on important issues in research ethics are included here. Ideas and sources for obtaining research grants also are provided. In qualitative research, obtaining grant money is often an overlooked aspect of the research process, and it is good to see the topic of funding included in this Web site. When you are all finished exploring this amazing Web site and come away with a lifetime's worth of reading about research and critical thought, click back to Bobbi's main homepage, called "Bobbi's Place." There, click on "The Grace of Great Things" and treat yourself to a retreat for your heart and soul that both quiets and inspires to action. This retreat can be found in the form of a 12-page essay by Parker Palmer titled "The Grace of Great Things: Recovering the Sacred in Knowing, Teaching, and Learning" (http://csf.colorado.edu/sine/transcripts/palmer.html).

The International Institute of Human Understanding

This institute, headed by Tricia Munhall, first started as The International Institute for Phenomenological Inquiry in 1994. In a twofold effort to become more inclusive, the name was changed to welcome all methods of inquiry that assist in human understanding and to become more interdisciplinary. All members of disciplines that focus on coming to understand being human are invited to join. The Institute sponsors an annual international conference, as well as workshops, and offers consultation and workshops on request. The philosophy, aims, and membership benefits can be found on its Web site, http://www.iihu.org. The annual conference is not to be missed!

SPECIALIZED QUALITATIVE RESEARCH WEB SITES

There are any number of specialized sites focusing on some aspect of qualitative research that a persistent Web surfer can find. The comprehensive sites described in the preceding section have links to hundreds of them. I am going to give you a preview of some of my personal favorites here.

ENQuIRE: East of Scotland Network for Qualitative Inquiry, Research and Education, University of Dundee

http://www.dundee.ac.uk/generalpractice/research/qualitat.htm

This site describes the work of a group of qualitative researchers in the area of health care research. The group offers advice and support, both formal and informal, to other researchers and is committed "To raising the profile of Qualitative Health Research by promoting excellence in design, process and reporting."

An interesting qualitative research course syllabus that contains simple, clear goals for the qualitative learning experience is posted on the Web site. Most interesting, though, are the abstracts and summaries of the research publications of group members. A grounded-theory study on medication-taking behavior in primary care is summarized. In another study, an action research design was used to find ways of incorporating adult and reflective learning methods into the general practice training year for physicians. The site also contains an advocacy statement for utilizing qualitative research methods in health care settings.

The ENQuIRE research group consists of six members. Aside from the interest in qualitative research that connects them, from their photographs, it looks as if you might also have to like hanging out in the snow and ice with spiked boots to belong.

Narrative Psychology Internet and Resource Guide

http://maple.lemoyne.edu/~hevern/narpsych.html

Father Vincent Hevern of Lemoyne College in Syracuse, New York, is the editor and manager of this sophisticated site about narrative theory and narrative psychology. Narrative perspectives in the humanities and social sciences focus attention on how people understand and make sense of the experiences of their lives. Exploring "meaning" is central to the process of narrative psychology, and qualitative methods are used to gather the meanings that people assign to events and situations. Narrative perspectives attend to the stories that people tell about themselves and others and to how human experience is embodied in story. Both personal and cultural stories are considered important and are regarded as interdependent.

Here, again, there are wonderful bibliographies that offer a lifetime of reading and learning. Resources about narrative in multiple disciplines including medicine, nursing, health care, and holocaust studies are provided. Resources for qualitative methods also are plentiful, in particular for interviewing techniques, case study, and oral history. The interested Web visitor can find information and resources about somewhat esoteric disciplines and techniques such as psychobiography or biographical psychology (these terms are used interchangeably).

There is a link to Father Hevern's fascinating related site titled "The Personal Documentary Center" (http://home.earthlink.net/~hevern/index.html) at which personal stories, journals, essays, and other kinds of personal documents can be found. Such documents are often used as data sources in qualitative research. Because there are so many resources and so much to read and think about at Father Hevern's Web sites, the Web visitor needs to guard against feeling overwhelmed.

Gary Shank: Privateer of the Semiotic Seas!
http://www.geocities.com/Athens/5260

I have not met Gary Shank, but I think I would probably like him a lot. When I see his e-mail address on the qualitative research discussion list, I approach his contributions with more interest and excitement than I do when some others contribute to a thread. In the midst of some really good ideas, some even brilliant, there is an honesty and vulnerability in Gary's writing that is very attractive. You can see this for yourself in Gary's own writings that are posted on his Web site. Among many other things, Gary is passionate about semiotics and the philosophy of Charles Sanders Peirce. You will find many resources for both at his Web site.

Gary's Web site is a little more randomly put together than the others on which I have commented here. But, remember, where there is no randomness, there is no creativity. At Gary's Web site, there is plenty of randomness and plenty of creativity. As well as articles and resources on qualitative research, semiotics, and C. S. Peirce, you can find Grateful Dead stuff and information about medievalists. Gary says that he's a closet one, whatever it is.

What you can also find at Gary's Web site is his essay on his 1996 trip to the Abbey of Gethsemani in Kentucky, where Thomas Merton, the Trappist monk, writer, social critic, and contemplative lived for about 27 years. Gary gives us a small glimpse into why he made this retreat as well as into the daily routine of life and prayer at the Abbey. I would like to end with one of Gary's reflections from this essay: "As a qualitative researcher, I see now that a large part of our vocation is to become, if you will, a secular contemplative. We are not just to record, to encode, to sort, and to list. We are called to interpret, to read into the depths of the world of experience." To continue the metaphor of the sacred, my hope is that, as you pursue this vocation of qualitative researcher, you will find at these Web sites tools for your calling, some fun, some new perspectives, and some inspiration for your work.